PHILIP L. HILLSMAN, M.D.

handbook of
OBSTETRICS & GYNECOLOGY

EIGHTH EDITION

handbook of

OBSTETRICS & GYNECOLOGY

RALPH C. BENSON, MD
Professor and Chairman Emeritus
Department of Obstetrics and Gynecology
Oregon Health Sciences University
Portland, Oregon

Illustrated by LAUREL V. SCHAUBERT

Lange Medical Publications
LOS ALTOS, CALIFORNIA 94022

1983

Published by APPLETON-CENTURY-CROFTS
For information, address Appleton-Century-Crofts,
25 Van Zant St., East Norwalk, CT 06856.

Lithographed in USA

Table of Contents

Preface

The eighth edition of *Handbook of Obstetrics & Gynecology* has been virtually rewritten, with the addition of much new material. All of this reflects the "information explosion" in this as in other medical specialties. The objective continues to be to provide a readily available source of practical current obstetric and gynecologic information for health care professionals.

This book is not intended to serve as a substitute for a primary textbook but does contain the essentials of diagnosis and treatment of obstetric and gynecologic disorders. Procedures and medications (with dosages and routes of administration, together with alternatives) are presented, but the choice is rarely inclusive or absolute.

This edition includes a new chapter on embryology of the female reproductive tract and new sections on physiologic changes during pregnancy, toxic shock syndrome, and hirsutism. The sections on fetal and neonatal organ function, infections during pregnancy, shoulder dystocia, sexually transmitted diseases, hemolytic disease of the newborn, shock and disseminated intravascular coagulation, urinary stress incontinence, and premenstrual tension have been extensively revised. Much new information has been incorporated into the sections on preeclampsia-eclampsia, high-risk pregnancy, fetal monitoring, and ultrasonography.

The popularity of this handbook overseas is suggested by the availability of translations in Spanish, Portuguese, Italian, and Polish. Serbo-Croatian and Japanese translations are in preparation. In addition, English editions for distribution in Asia are printed in Singapore, Taiwan, Korea, and the Philippines; and a Middle East edition, also in English, is published in Beirut.

I wish to thank my colleagues and readers here and abroad for their valued support and suggestions.

Ralph C. Benson, MD

Portland, Oregon
October, 1983

NOTICE

The author has been careful to recommend drug dosages that are in agreement with current official pharmacologic standards and the medical literature. Because all drugs may evoke idiosyncratic or toxic reactions, because drugs may interact with others in ways that modify therapeutic effectiveness and toxicity, and because some drugs are teratogenic, it is recommended that all clinicians review drug manufacturers' product information (eg, package inserts), especially in the case of new or infrequently prescribed medications. Furthermore, one must be thoroughly conversant with any drugs used in order to advise the patient about signs and symptoms of potential adverse reactions and incompatibilities.

The Author

Embryology of the Female Urogenital Tract | 1

FORMATION & EARLY DEVELOPMENT

As early as the first week following implantation of the fertilized ovum, an evagination of the hindgut forms the allantois, the tubular forerunner of the bladder. After the second week, the gut caudal to the origin of the allantois widens to form the cloaca, an incompletely developed urogenital ostium extending from the umbilical stalk to the rudimentary tail—virtually the extent of the inferior ventral aspect of the embryo—into which the gut, the allantois, and the mesonephric ducts open (Fig 1–1). In the fourth week, the cloaca begins to divide into a dorsal portion (the hindgut) and a ventral portion (the urogenital sinus). The tissue separating these 2 structures, the urorectal septum, inserts at the junction of the allantois and the gut. Separation is complete by the eighth week.

Initially, the cloaca does not open to the outside but ends abruptly in a thin partition, the cloacal membrane, which lies in a slight depression (the proctodeum, or anal pit) just anterior to the short tail segment. Normally, the membrane disintegrates by about the eighth week, opening the hindgut and the urogenital sinus to the exterior. The lower hindgut becomes the rectum; its exit is the anus. The external opening of the urogenital sinus is the urogenital ostium.

When the cloacal membrane fails to disintegrate, an imperforate anus results. In females, a rectovaginal fistula, the result of incomplete subdivision of the cloaca, will often be present as well.

DEVELOPMENT OF THE RENAL EXCRETORY APPARATUS

In the first stage of kidney development, the pronephros (primordial kidney) exists from the third to the fourth week of embryonic life. It may transport coelomic fluids. It consists of an incomplete duct with numerous lateral vestigial excretory tubules in the posterolateral mesoderm. The lateral tubules disappear, but the main duct persists and continues to develop longitudinally, becoming the mesonephric (wolffian) duct.

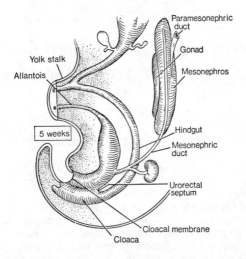

Figure 1–1. Diagrammatic left lateral view of urogenital system in relation to the hindgut at about 5 weeks. The paramesonephric duct does not appear until the sixth week but is shown here to indicate its position and downgrowth. (Reproduced, with permission, from Bacon RL: Chapter 1 in *Current Obstetric & Gynecologic Diagnosis & Treatment,* 4th ed. Benson RC [editor]. Lange, 1982.)

The mesonephros, the second stage in kidney development, extracts waste products from the coelomic fluid and blood. It is located in the lower thoracic, upper lumbar region of the embryo. The mesonephric duct extends caudally to join the cloaca, from which the bladder will later develop. Mesonephric tubules, together with neighboring blood vessels, soon form primitive glomeruli along the duct, the more cephalic of these degenerating as the more caudal ones develop. Degeneration of the mesonephric tubules is almost complete by the ninth week of embryonic life, but a few may persist in females as Gartner's duct or as the epoophoron or paroophoron. In males, the mesonephric duct becomes the epididymis and vas deferens. As the mesonephric tubules grow and degenerate, the metanephric diverticulum (ureteric bud) grows out from the mesonephric duct slightly cephalad to the cloaca to become the ureter and the metanephros, the true kidney.

The metanephros removes catabolic wastes from the blood and largely controls fluid and electrolyte balance. The metanephros and its ureter appear at about the fourth week on each side as a dorsolateral bud from the wolffian duct near the cloaca. These permanent kidneys develop rapidly. The ureter becomes independent of the wolffian ducts, and separate ureteral openings into the cloaca are formed promptly.

At about the fifth or sixth week, the ureter divides within the metanephric mass to form calices. Collecting and secretory tubules begin to radiate into the renal mesenchyme from the calices to connect with glomeruli, which appear in the renal cortex at about the same time. The metanephric excretory units develop as those of mesonephric origin atrophy, but the wolffian ducts remain, at least until sexual differentiation has occurred. The metanephros gradually migrates from the medial to the lateral aspect of both the wolffian and the müllerian ducts. As it migrates, it rotates about 90 degrees on its long axis. Meanwhile, the embryo elongates, mainly as a result of growth of the body segments, so that the kidney is ultimately situated in the dorsolumbar region and a long ureter develops.

The terminal wolffian ducts join the cloaca just below the juncture of the allantois and cloaca. Between the second and third months, the lower ends of the wolffian ducts progressively widen, the allantoic stoma opens appreciably, and the upper (urogenital) part of the cloaca becomes separated from the lower (rectal) portion. Thus, the bladder is formed from endodermal and mesodermal elements. Extreme maldevelopment results in exstrophy of the bladder.

The allantoic extension in the umbilical ligament and cord becomes the urachus, which may fail to obliterate late in fetal life. Urine may drain from an umbilical urachal fistula after delivery.

In males, the prostatic urethra develops from the terminal portion of the wolffian ducts, the membranous urethra from a subdivision of the urogenital sinus, and the penile urethra (in part ectodermal) from the closure of a groove beneath the phallus. In females, the origins are similar but there is, of course, no penile urethra and the prostate remains vestigial.

DEVELOPMENT OF THE ADRENAL (SUPRARENAL) GLANDS

The adrenal glands develop from cells that migrate into the region of the developing mesonephros as early as the fifth week. Each adrenal gland has a cortex composed of mesodermal cells that originate from the early urogenital ridge and a medulla composed of ectodermal cells that originate from the crest of neural folds in approximately the same somites as the cortical cells. Later, layering occurs, so that the medullary cells are covered by those of the cortex. Eventually, the adrenal glands occupy positions over the superior pole of the kidney on each side.

The fetal adrenal glands are relatively large. At term, they constitute about 0.2% of the body weight and are 20 times the size of those in the adult relative to body weight. This attests to their importance in fetal life. The large size is primarily due to the enlarged cortex. The fetal cortex comprises 80% of the cortex; it undergoes rapid degeneration at birth. The remaining 20%, the permanent cortex, does not become fully differentiated until almost 3 years after birth. Regression of the fetal cortex is not complete until adulthood.

Pelvic tumors that produce hormones associated with adrenal medullary cell types, eg, argentaffinomas, may involve the ovaries or retroperitoneal tissues. The tumor cells suggest primitive adrenal cells that may have been "lost" during their migration to the eventual site of the adrenal gland.

ORIGIN OF THE
FEMALE GENERATIVE DUCTS

An embryo 6 weeks of age reveals the beginnings of the müllerian ducts, which become the uterine tubes, uterus, cervix, and part of the vagina. On each side, these new channels develop parallel to the wolffian duct, just lateral to the mesonephric structures in the lumbodorsal mesenchyme. The müllerian system develops caudally and ventrally to converge and end near the cloaca (Fig 1–2). The cephalad portions of the müllerian ducts become the uterine tubes, which open to the peritoneal cavity. The upper end of the müllerian duct is often marked by a small persistent cyst (hydatid cyst of Morgagni) attached to one of the tubal fimbria. At the caudad end, the ducts fuse in the midline to form a central canal from which develop the uterus, cervix, and upper two-thirds of the vagina. Concomitantly, an invagination of the inferior part of the urogenital sinus is converted into the lower third of the vagina. Thus, endometrial and endocervical cells are of mesodermal (müllerian) origin, but exocervical and vaginal epithelium are derived from endodermal (urogenital sinus) cells.

The hymen is the vestige of the barrier between the descending müllerian core and the urogenital sinus. The uterus, cervix, and upper vagina are at first solid and then become septate. The cervix is the first part of the müllerian system to lose its longitudinal septum; then the vagina; and finally, at 4–5 months, the uterus. Partial or total failure of disappearance of these septa results in abnormal septa found in later life.

The wolffian ducts continue distally from below the ovary and pass just lateral to the uterus within the folds of the broad ligament; they traverse the peripheral tissues of the cervix and proceed down the anterolateral vaginal wall to the introitus. Normally, most of the unessential wolffian structures disappear, but mesonephric tubules may persist as the vestigial epoophoron and paroophoron within the mesovarium. Parovarian cysts and Gartner's cysts are benign neoplasms

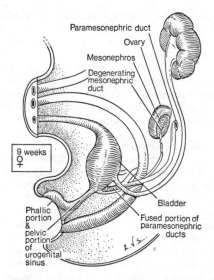

Figure 1–2. Diagram of female reproductive tract at an early stage of sexual differentiation (about 9 weeks). (Reproduced, with permission, from Bacon RL: Chapter 1 in *Current Obstetric & Gynecologic Diagnosis & Treatment,* 4th ed. Benson RC [editor]. Lange, 1982.)

of wolffian duct origin that may require excision. Carcinomas or cysts of wolffian origin are uncommonly discovered in females after birth.

ORIGIN OF THE GONADS

Primitive Stage

At about the fifth or sixth week of embryonic life, the genital ridges form in the right and left dorsolumbar regions within the coelomic cavity. These developments involve the medial aspect of the mesonephric mesenchyme on each side. The cephalad portions of the ridges become the gonads. Finally, the genital ridges separate from the mesonephros. A few mesonephric tubules may remain as vestiges in the epoophoron. Low cells of mesodermal origin line the coelomic cavity and cover the genital ridge. Concomitantly, primordial sex cells migrate from the yolk stalk across the gut mesentery into the cortex of the gonads. Meanwhile, broken columns of partially differentiated cells (Waldeyer's cords), which later become partially canalized (Pflüger's tubules), appear within the substance of the early gonad, apparently as a downgrowth of superficial cells.

Indifferent (Neuter) Stage

Before the sixth to seventh week after nidation, the gonads are sexually indistinct. Soon thereafter, the gonads differentiate into male or female structures according to the chromosomal inheritance of the fetus and hormonal influences. Sex hormones of endogenous or exogenous origin stimulate or retard full fetal genital development.

Stage of Ovarian Development

If the conceptus is destined to become a female, the sex cells seem to organize the mesenchymal elements of the gonad by the eighth week. Primordial clusters of ova develop as islands of cells containing one large primitive ovum surrounded by smaller, moderately differentiated cells that will become granulosa cells. Less well differentiated stromal cells become theca cells, and completely nondescript elements remain in the connective tissue series. Waldeyer's cords and the subsequent Pflüger's tubules, essential in testicular development but not required by the ovary, disappear in females. A few vestiges may remain, and these account for unusual cell patterns or even rare ovarian tumors such as Pick's adenoma.

ORIGIN OF THE EXTERNAL GENITALIA

The external genitalia of males and females are similarly derived from the cloacal ectoderm. The genital or cloacal tubercle and the coccygeal tubercle mark the anterior and posterior extensions of the proctodeum. The genital tubercle becomes the mons and clitoris in the female and the penis in the male. The anus forms just forward of the coccygeal tubercle. Labioscrotal folds develop on each side of the urogenital cleft. In females, these ridges become the labia. In males, scrotal pouches develop as fingerlike projections of the peritoneum, and the testes descend into these recesses through the inguinal canals after the 36th week.

In females, fatty tissue soon fills the labia majora. Although peritoneal downgrowths do form as in males, they are imperfect and are rapidly obliterated. In rare individuals, vestiges of the peritoneal extensions persist as cysts of the canal of Nuck. The distal end of the vagina is at first separated from the urogenital sinus by a membrane. If this barrier does not disintegrate properly, an imperforate or abnormally thick hymen results. The urogenital cleft remains patent, providing access to the vaginal introitus and the urethral meatus.

In males, the scrotal folds fuse in the midline, causing partial closure of the urogenital cleft and displacing forward the small remaining opening, the incompletely formed urethra. The genital tubercle rapidly becomes the penis. The remaining urogenital cleft defect closes completely when the edges of the ventral tract between the corpora cavernosa adhere to complete the terminal urethra. Because of these changes and the small size of the parts, the sex of the fetus cannot be determined clinically with confidence until after the 26th week.

2 | Anatomy & Physiology of the Female Reproductive System

The female reproductive system may be divided into the external and internal genitalia and their supporting structures.

The external genitalia (Fig 2–1), collectively termed the pudendum or vulva, comprise the following structures, all easily visible on external examination: mons veneris (mons pubis), labia majora, labia minora, clitoris, vestibule and external urethral meatus, Skene's glands (paraurethral glands), Bartholin's glands (vulvovaginal glands), hymen, fourchette, perineal body, and fossa navicularis. They present varying contours around the urogenital cleft, which lies anteroposteriorly between the vaginal and urethral openings. The contours of the external genitalia are determined by the bony configuration of the anteroinferior pelvic girdle as well as by the subcutaneous fat, muscle, and fascial arrangement.

The internal genitalia comprise the vagina, cervix, uterus, uterine (fallopian) tubes, and ovaries. They require special instruments for inspection; the intra-abdominal group can be examined visually only by laparotomy, laparoscopy, or culdoscopy (invasive methods) or by contrast ultrasonography or roentgenography (noninvasive methods).

The anatomy of the bony pelvis and the pelvic floor is discussed on pp 26–29.

EXTERNAL GENITALIA

MONS VENERIS
(Mons Pubis)

General Appearance

The mons veneris, a rounded pad of fatty tissue overlying the symphysis pubica, develops from the genital tubercle. It is not an organ but a region or a landmark. Coarse, dark hair normally appears over the mons early in puberty.

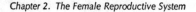

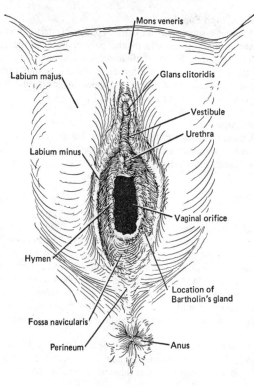

Figure 2-1. External female genitalia.

During reproductive life, the pubic hair is abundant, but after the menopause it becomes sparse. The normal female escutcheon is typically a "triangle with the base up," in contrast with the "triangle with the base down" male pattern.

Histology
The skin of the mons contains sudoriferous and sebaceous glands. The amount of subcutaneous fat is determined by nutritional and possibly by steroid hormonal factors.

Innervation
The sensory nerves of the mons are the ilioinguinal and genitofemoral nerves.

Blood & Lymph Supply

The mons is supplied by the external pudendal artery and vein. The lymphatics merge with those from other parts of the vulva and from the superficial abdomen. The crossed lymphatic circulation from the labia within the mons is of clinical importance, since it permits carcinoma metastases from one side of the vulva to appear in the inguinal glands of the opposite as well as the affected side.

Clinical Importance

Dermatitis is common in the pubic area. Edema may occur secondary to vulvar varicosities or to carcinomatous infiltration of the lymphatics. Cancer elsewhere in the vulva may also involve the mons.

LABIA MAJORA

General Appearance

In the adult female, these 2 raised, rounded, longitudinal folds of skin are the most prominent features of the external genitalia. They originate from the genital swellings extending down and backward from the genital tubercle; arising from the perineal body, they extend anteriorly around the labia minora to merge with the mons. The labia are normally closed in nulliparous women but then gape progressively with succeeding vaginal deliveries and become thin, with sparse hair in old age.

The skin of the lateral surfaces of the labia is thick and often pigmented; it is covered with coarse hair similar to that of the mons. The skin of the inner labia majora is thin and fine and contains no hairs.

Histology

The labia majora are made up of connective and areolar tissue, with many sebaceous glands. They are homologous to the scrotum. A thin fascial layer similar to the tunica dartos of the scrotum is found within the labia just below the surface. The round ligaments of the uterus pass through the canal of Nuck to end in a fibrous insertion in the anterior portion of the labia majora.

Innervation

Anteriorly, the labia majora are supplied by the ilioinguinal and pudendal nerves. Laterally and posteriorly, they are innervated by the posterior femoral cutaneous nerve.

Blood Supply

The labia majora are supplied by the internal pudendal artery, derived from the anterior parietal division of the internal iliac (hypogastric) artery; and by the external pudendal artery (from the femoral artery). Drainage is via the internal and external pudendal veins.

Clinical Importance

No special function is performed by the labia majora. A cyst of the canal of Nuck is often mistaken for an indirect inguinal hernia. Adherence of the labia in infants may indicate vulvitis. External force or the complications of labor may cause vulvar hematoma.

LABIA MINORA

General Appearance

The labia minora are small, narrow, elongated folds of skin between the labia majora and the vaginal introitus. They are derived from the skin folds beneath the developing clitoris. Normally, the labia minora are in apposition in nulliparas, concealing the introitus. Posteriorly, the labia minora merge at the fourchette. The labia are separate from the hymen, which is an individual structure marking the vaginal entrance or introitus. Anteriorly, each labium merges into a median ridge that fuses with its mate to form the frenulum of the clitoris and an anterior fold that becomes the prepuce of the clitoris.

The lateral and anterior surfaces of the labia minora are usually pigmented; their inner aspect is pink and moist, resembling the vaginal mucosa.

Histology

The labia minora have neither hair follicles nor sweat glands but are rich in sebaceous glands.

Innervation & Blood Supply

The innervation of the labia minora is via the ilioinguinal, pudendal, and hemorrhoidal nerves.

The labia minora are not truly erectile, but a rich vasculature permits marked turgescence with emotional or physical stimulation. They are supplied by the external and internal pudendal arteries.

Clinical Importance

The labia minora tend to close the introitus. They increase in size as the result of ovarian hormonal stimulation. After the menopause, they all but disappear unless estrogens are administered. Squamous cell carcinoma of the vulva often originates in the labia minora; sebaceous cysts also develop in these structures. The presence of adherent labia minora in the infant is usually due to inflammation. Fusion may indicate sexual maldifferentiation.

CLITORIS

General Appearance & Histology

This 2- to 3-cm-long homolog of the penis is found in the midline slightly anterior to the urethral meatus. It is composed of 2 small, erectile corpora, each attached to the periosteum of the symphysis, and a diminutive structure (glans clitoridis) that is generously supplied with sensory nerve endings. The glans is partially hooded by the labia minora.

Innervation & Blood Supply

The clitoris is supplied by the hypogastric and pudendal nerves and pelvic sympathetics and by the internal pudendal artery and vein.

Clinical Importance

Cancer of the clitoris is rare, but it is extremely serious because of early metastases. The inguinal and femoral nodes are usually involved first.

VESTIBULE & URETHRAL MEATUS

General Appearance & Histology

The triangular area between the labia minora anteriorly, onto which the urethra opens, is the vestibule. It is derived from the urogenital sinus and is covered by delicate stratified squamous epithelium.

The urinary meatus is visible as an anteroposterior slit or an inverted V. Like the urethra, it is lined by transitional epithelium. The vascular mucosa of the meatus often pouts or everts. This makes it appear more red than the neighboring vaginal mucosa.

Innervation & Blood Supply

The vestibule and terminal urethra are supplied by the pudendal nerve and by the internal pudendal artery and vein.

Clinical Importance

Caruncles, as well as squamous cell or transitional cell carcinoma, may develop in the urethrovestibular area.

PARAURETHRAL GLANDS
(Skene's Glands)

General Appearance & Histology

Immediately within the urethra on its posterolateral aspect are 2 small orifices leading to the shallow tubular ducts or glands of Skene, which are wolffian duct remnants. The ducts are lined by transitional cells and are the sparse equivalent of the numerous male prostatic glands.

Blood Supply

Like the vestibule and urethral meatus, Skene's glands are supplied by the internal pudendal artery and vein.

Clinical Importance

Skene's glands, which supply minor amounts of mucus, are especially susceptible to gonococcal infection, which may be first evident here. Following successful antigonorrheal therapy, nonspecific infection with other purulent organisms is common. With recurrent skenitis, destruction of the ducts with electrocautery may be necessary.

PARAVAGINAL OR VULVOVAGINAL GLANDS & DUCTS
(Bartholin's Glands & Ducts)

General Appearance & Histology

Just inside the lower vagina, on either side, are 2 tiny apertures. A narrow duct, 1–2 cm long, connects each of these apertures with a small, flattened, mucus-producing gland that lies between the labia minora and vaginal wall. These are paravaginal or vulvovaginal glands, or Bartholin's glands, the counterpart of Cowper's glands in the male. The ducts are lined with transitional epithelium.

Innervation & Blood Supply

The internal pudendal nerve, artery, and vein serve Bartholin's glands.

Clinical Importance

Bartholin's glands secrete mucus that acts as a lubricant during coitus. Gonorrhea frequently causes Bartholin's ducts to become abscessed and cystic, although the glands themselves are usually not affected. Nonvenereal bacterial infections occasionally result in this complication. Primary adenocarcinoma is a rare neoplasm in the external genitalia, but it may originate in Bartholin's glands. Transitional cell epidermoid carcinoma of Bartholin's duct may also occur.

HYMEN

General Appearance & Histology

The hymen, a circular or crescent-shaped membrane just inside but separate from the labia minora, marks the entrance to the vagina. The hymen is a thin, moderately elastic barrier that partially or, in rare instances, completely occludes the vaginal canal. It is a double-faced epithelial plate covering a matrix of fibrovascular tissue.

Innervation & Blood Supply

The hymen is supplied by the pudendal and inferior hemorrhoidal nerves, arteries, and veins.

Clinical Importance

A tight hymen may result in painful gynatresia, in which case hymenotomy or dilatation will be required. The remnants of the lacerated hymen following intercourse or delivery are called carunculae hymenales (myrtiformes). Hymenal or perineal scars may cause dyspareunia.

PERINEAL BODY, FOURCHETTE, & FOSSA NAVICULARIS

General Appearance

The perineal body includes the skin and underlying tissues between the anal orifice and the vaginal entrance. It is supported by the transverse perineal muscle and the lower portions of the bulbocavernosus muscle.

The labia minora and majora converge posteriorly to form a low ridge called the fourchette. Just beyond this fold, extending about 1 cm anteriorly to the hymen, is a shallow depression called the fossa navicularis.

Innervation & Blood Supply

These structures are supplied by the pudendal and inferior hemorrhoidal nerves, arteries, and veins.

Clinical Importance

These structures are often lacerated during childbirth and may require repair. Because of their vascularity, an early or deep episiotomy can result in the loss of several hundred milliliters of blood; faulty repair may be followed by dyspareunia or by reduced sexual satisfaction.

SKIN GLANDS

Small and large coiled subcutaneous sweat glands are situated all over the body except beneath mucocutaneous surfaces, eg, the labia minora or vermilion border of the lips.

Normally, the fluid secretion of small coiled (eccrine) sweat glands, which have no relationship to hairs, has no odor.

Large coiled (apocrine) sweat glands that open into hair follicles are found over the mons, the labia majora, and the perineum as well as in the axillas. These glands, which begin to secrete an odorous fluid at puberty, are more active during menstruation and pregnancy. The sweat glands are controlled by the sympathetic nervous system.

Hidradenomas are tumors that originate in sweat glands. Rarely, they are malignant.

Sebaceous glands are associated with and open into hair follicles. However, on the labia minora, where hairs are absent, sebaceous glands open on the surface. At puberty, an oily secretion with a slight odor is produced. The fluid lubricates and protects the skin from irritation by vaginal discharge. Gland secretion is mediated by hormonal and psychic stimuli. The activity of the sebaceous glands diminishes in old age.

Sebaceous cysts, almost invariably benign but often infected, develop from sebaceous glands.

INTERNAL GENITALIA

VAGINA

General Appearance

The vagina (Fig 2–2) is a thin, muscular, partially collapsed rugose canal 8–10 cm long and about 4 cm in diameter. It extends from the urogenital cleft to the cervix and curves upward and posteriorly from the vulva. The cervix protrudes several centimeters into the upper vagina to form recesses called the fornices. Since the posterior lip of the cervix is longer than its anterior lip, the posterior fornix is deeper than the anterior fornix. The vaginal dimensions are reduced during the climacteric, and all fornices, especially the lateral ones, become more shallow.

The vagina lies between the bladder and rectum and is supported principally by the transverse cervical ligaments (cardinal ligaments, Mackenrodt's ligaments) and the levator ani muscles.

The peritoneum of the posterior cul-de-sac (pouch of Douglas) and the posterior vaginal fornix are close together at the vaginal vault, a detail of surgical importance.

Histology

The vagina is lined by stratified squamous epithelium, which is thick and folded transversely in the nulliparous woman. Many of these rugae are lost with repeated vaginal delivery and after the menopause. Normally, no glands are found in the vagina.

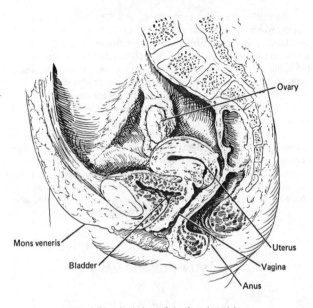

Figure 2–2. Midsagittal view of the female pelvic organs.

Innervation & Blood Supply (See Fig 2–4.)

The nerve supply to the vagina is via the pudendal and hemorrhoidal nerves and the pelvic sympathetic chain. The blood supply is from the vaginal artery, which is derived from a descending branch of the uterine artery, and from the middle hemorrhoidal and internal pudendal arteries. It is drained by the pudendal, external hemorrhoidal, and uterine veins.

The lymphatic drainage of the lower vagina is directed toward the superficial inguinal nodes; that of the upper vagina is to the presacral, external iliac, and hypogastric nodes. This is important in vulvovaginal infections and cancer spread.

Clinical Importance

Vaginal discharge (leukorrhea) is common and may be due to local or systemic disorders. Infections of the lower reproductive tract are the most common cause of leukorrhea; estrogen depletion (senile or atrophic vaginitis) and estrogen or psychic stimulation are other causes.

Primary cancer of the vagina is very rare, but secondary carcinoma of the vagina, most frequently from extension of cervical cancer, is not uncommon.

CERVIX

General Appearance

The cervix of the nonpregnant uterus (Fig 2–3) is a conical, moderately firm organ about 2–4 cm long and about 2.5 cm in outside diameter. A central spindle-shaped canal communicates with the uterus above and the vagina below. About half the length of the cervix is supravaginal and is close to the bladder anteriorly.

Childbirth lacerations account for most cervical distortions. The external os, which is initially round and only a fraction of a centimeter in diameter, may gape as a result of these tears. Even in the absence of distortions, however, it is customary to refer to the cervix as having anterior and posterior lips.

The cervix is supported by the uterosacral ligaments and transverse cervical ligaments (cardinal ligaments, Mackenrodt's ligaments).

Histology

The intravaginal portion of the cervix is covered by stratified squamous cells, which usually extend to just inside the external os. The

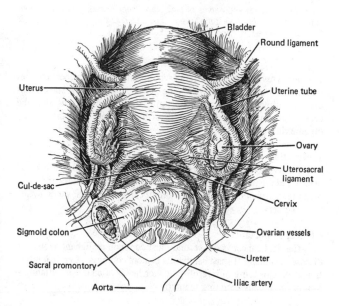

Figure 2–3. Pelvic organs (superior view).

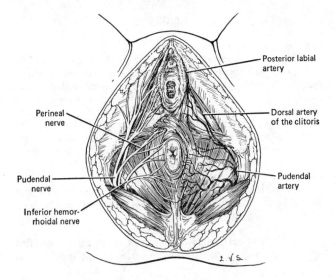

Figure 2–4. Arteries and nerves of perineum. (Reproduced, with permission, from Krantz KE: Chapter 2 in *Current Obstetric & Gynecologic Diagnosis & Treatment*, 4th ed. Benson RC [editor]. Lange, 1982.)

countless crevices that give the cervix a honeycombed appearance on transection were once believed to be glands, but it is now known that they are infoldings of a mucus-secreting membrane. Peripherally, the cervix contains circular muscle fibers that connect with the uterine myometrium above.

Innervation & Blood Supply (See Fig 2–4.)

Innervation of the cervix is via the second, third, and fourth sacral nerves and the pelvic sympathetic plexus. The cervical artery and vein, major branches of the uterine circulation, carry most of the blood to and from the cervix.

Clinical Importance

Cervical cancer is the second most common malignant neoplastic disease in women. (Breast carcinoma is more common.) Cervical infection is a major cause of infertility; leukorrhea is often due to inflammation of the mucus-secreting membrane.

BODY & FUNDUS OF THE UTERUS

General Appearance

The uterus (Figs 2–2 and 2–3) is a muscular organ with a narrow central cavity situated deep in the true pelvis between bladder and rectum. It is shaped like an inverted pear. The adult nonpregnant uterus is approximately 7–8 cm long and about 4 cm in its widest diameter. The uterine tubes join the uterus, one on either side, about two-thirds of the distance to the top of the uterus. That portion of the uterus above the tubal insertion is called the fundus; below the insertion is the body, or corpus, of the uterus, which is continuous with the supravaginal segment of the cervix. In the nulliparous woman, the uterus and cervix are usually directed forward at almost a right angle with the long axis of the vagina, but 25–35% of women will have a retroverted or retroflexed uterus.

Except for the anteroinferior portion of the corpus, which is covered by the bladder, the uterus is covered by peritoneum.

The uterus is supported by (1) the muscular round ligaments (ligamentum teres), each of which originates in the fundus laterally and ends in a labium majus; (2) the broad ligaments, wide peritoneal folds sweeping laterally from either side of the corpus to the lateral pelvic walls; (3) the uterosacral ligaments, fibrous strands that originate in the cervico-uterine junction and insert into the periosteum of the sacrum; (4) the transverse cervical ligaments (cardinal ligaments, Mackenrodt's ligaments); and (5) the levator ani muscles and accompanying fascia.

Histology

The uterine wall is composed mainly of interwoven smooth muscle fibers, which are especially thick in the fundal portion. This muscular meshwork is perforated by the vascular supply. The cavity is small and lined by endometrium, which thickens, bleeds, desquamates, and regenerates periodically during reproductive life.

Innervation (See Fig 2–5.)

Efferent impulses leave the uterus via S2–4. The afferent impulses reach the central nervous system via the posterior roots of T5–12, L1, and S2–4 and carry sympathetic stimuli.

Blood Supply

The uterine circulation is derived from the uterine and ovarian arteries and veins. During pregnancy especially, these channels anastomose freely within the uterus, and a much greater vasculature develops to supply not only the hyperplastic, hypertrophic uterus itself but also the growing placenta and fetus. Interlacing, contracting muscle fibers account for control of uterine bleeding after delivery.

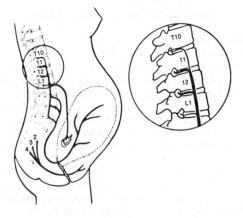

Figure 2–5. Parturition pain pathways. Afferent pain impulses from the cervix and uterus are carried by nerves that accompany sympathetic fibers and enter the neuraxis at T10, T11, T12, and L1. Pain pathways from the perineum travel to S2, S3, and S4 via the pudendal nerve. (Reproduced, with permission, from Bonica JJ: The nature of pain of parturition. *Clin Obstet Gynaecol* 1975;**2**:511.)

Lymphatics

Embryologically, the uterine lymphatic system is derived from venous channels. Lymph drainage from the uterus is directed to the iliac, aortic, sacral, and inguinal lymph glands. Nevertheless, the lymphatics of the uterus and neighboring organs intermingle, permitting progressive and retrogressive flow.

Clinical Importance

The uterus is capable of enormous expansion to accommodate the products of conception. During pregnancy, it increases in weight from about 90 g to about 1 kg, and its capacity increases more than 4000-fold. Normally, the fertilized ovum implants in the uterine endometrium, where it develops through the embryonal and fetal stages. Delivery prior to viability (24 weeks) constitutes abortion and, almost invariably, death of the fetus. After viability, the likelihood of survival of the newborn increases in direct proportion to the gestational age of the fetus.

Uterine tumors cause gynecologic problems such as abnormal uterine bleeding and pelvic pain. Developmental anomalies also result in obstetric complications, particularly dystocia.

Cancer of the uterine corpus is the second most common malignancy of the female genitalia, exceeded only by cervical carcinoma.

UTERINE TUBES
(Fallopian Tubes, Oviducts)

General Appearance

The uterine tubes are a pair of delicate peristaltic ducts 10–12 cm in length. Each extends posterolaterally from the cornu of the uterus and opens into the peritoneal cavity just below and medial to the ovary on the same side. The diameter of the canal varies from 1–2 mm at either end to more than twice that in the mid portion. The distal tube is connected with the ovary by a single elongated fimbria that retains the ovary and tubal extremity in close proximity.

Histology

The uterine tubes are composed of thin, superficial longitudinal and deep circular smooth muscle layers. They are lined by cuboidal epithelium (endosalpinx), which is similar to endometrium but has a sparse stroma. Many filmy longitudinal plicae, or folds, characterize the endosalpinx, especially in the distal half of the tube. The uterine tubes are encased in a peritoneal fold called the mesosalpinx, which is a portion of the broad ligament of the uterus.

Structurally, the uterine tubes vary in different segments. The distal end of the tube, which communicates with the peritoneal cavity through a minute opening (abdominal ostium), is fimbriated and almost erectile when turgid. The cavity of the distal 2–3 cm of the tube is termed the infundibulum, because of its cornucopialike shape. Continuous with this segment and about 6–8 cm long is the ampulla, which is somewhat dilated. The narrower isthmus, 1–2 cm long, extends from the ampulla to the uterine wall. The portion of the tube within the uterus proper (the interstitial segment) is about 1 cm long. The lumen of the tube is narrowest (1 mm) at this end.

Innervation & Blood Supply

The nerve supply to the uterine tubes is similar to that of the uterus. The blood supply to the proximal portions of the tubes is via the uterine artery; to the distal portions, blood supply is via both the uterine and ovarian arteries. Drainage is via the uterine and ovarian veins. The ampulla drains laterally through the mesosalpinx and broad ligaments to the hypogastric and iliac nodes. The isthmus and infundibulum drain toward lymph nodes supplying the uterus and ovaries.

Clinical Importance

The ovum is fertilized in the mid portion of the uterine tube and, after 3–4 days of movement down the tube, implants in the uterine endometrium. If both tubes are completely occluded, conception cannot occur. With partial occlusion, the fertilized ovum may be retained within the tube and result in tubal pregnancy. Infection of the tube (salpingitis) with resultant scarring, occlusion, and infertility is a common sequela of septic abortion or gonorrhea. Carcinoma of the tube is rare.

OVARIES

General Appearance

The ovaries (female gonads) (Figs 2–2 and 2–3) are a pair of whitish, ovoid, flattened, firm organs, about $1.5 \times 3 \times 3.5$ cm, found in the true pelvis. In the nullipara, each ovary usually rests almost vertically against the peritoneum of the lateral pelvic wall in a shallow depression, the ovarian fossa. This space is bounded medially by the obliterated umbilical artery, laterally by the ureter and uterine vessels, and inferiorly by the obturator nerve and its accompanying artery and vein. The fimbriated end of the uterine tube often curls up and over the superior medial aspect of the ovary.

The ovary is suspended between the lateral pelvic wall and the uterus by the mesovarium, which is part of the posterior segment of the broad ligament of the uterus. The mesovarium does not surround or cover the ovary but fuses with its superficial epithelial layer. It is also loosely attached to the uterus by a bandlike ovarian ligament that traverses the broad ligament.

Histology

The ovary is composed of a germ cell (ovum)-containing cortex and a vascular medulla. The cortex, the outer one-third to one-half of the ovary, is covered by a single layer of cuboidal cells, falsely called the germinal epithelium because ova are not derived from this tissue. The cortical stroma is composed of characteristic spindle-shaped or oat-shaped cells surrounding numerous small, variably placed vesicular spaces (graafian follicles). The inner one-half to two-thirds of the ovary, the medulla, is devoid of follicles but contains loose stroma and a rich vasculature.

In the newborn, the ovarian cortex contains thousands of ova (oocytes) in various stages of development. Before puberty, each ovum is surrounded by a single layer of epithelial cells and is termed a primordial follicle and ovum. These follicles, each measuring about 0.25 mm in diameter, contain a single eccentrically placed, large, well-developed sex cell with a granular hyperchromatic nucleus. The epithelial layer is composed of small, flattened, darkly-staining granulosa cells. Immediately surrounding the ovum is a cavity filled with clear serous fluid.

After puberty, the primordial follicles may become graafian follicles under gonadotropic hormone stimulation. Gonadotropic hormones stimulate certain follicles cyclically, so that crops of ova begin maturing approximately once a month. The original flattened cells become cuboidal and more numerous. As they multiply, they separate into 2 layers: the tunica interna, which is the inner vesicular layer; and the tunica externa, which is composed of flattened, smaller cells. Immediately surrounding the eccentrically placed ovum and lining the entire cavity are granulosa cells, or the granulosa membrane. The fluid within the cavity is called the liquor folliculi. It contains a high concentration of estrogens, which are produced by follicular cells.

About once a month a small number of follicles begin to develop, but only 1–2 graafian follicles reach full development and rupture to extrude the ova. The empty follicle, now termed a corpus luteum, produces both estrogens and progesterone. Partially matured follicles, still containing their ova, regress and finally disappear (atresia).

If pregnancy occurs, the corpus luteum becomes even larger and more productive of steroid sex hormones. If pregnancy fails to occur, the corpus luteum degenerates, menstruation occurs, and after a number of months the corpus luteum becomes a hyalinized remnant called a corpus albicans. An extensive circulation within the ovary is apparent during adult life, so that each maturing follicle is well vascularized. During the climacteric, the ovary becomes less vascular and more dense.

Innervation & Blood Supply

The nerves and blood vessels of the ovary traverse its suspensory ligament and enter and leave the hilum within the mesovarium. The ovarian arteries arise from the aorta just below the renal arteries and anastomose freely with branches from the uterine artery. A venous network within the mesovarium (pampiniform plexus) directs blood into the uterine and ovarian veins. The right ovarian vein empties into the inferior vena cava, and the left ovarian vein drains into the left renal vein.

Nerves from the dorsal roots of T10 and L1 and fibers from the pelvic and lumbar sympathetics accompany the arteries and veins.

The lymphatics of the ovary join those of the uterus to drain to the iliac and aortic nodes.

Clinical Importance

The ovary performs numerous functions:

(1) It is the repository for the female primordial sex cells (ova). In ovarian dysgenesis (ovarian agenesis of Turner), no primordial ova are present and the individual is sterile.

(2) It is the site for the production, "ripening," and monthly release of mature ova during reproductive life. Infertility results if ova fail to mature properly (eg, in phase defects of the menstrual cycle) or are not released (eg, "trapped ovum," retention of a fully developed ovum when the primary follicle fails to rupture because of either adhesions of

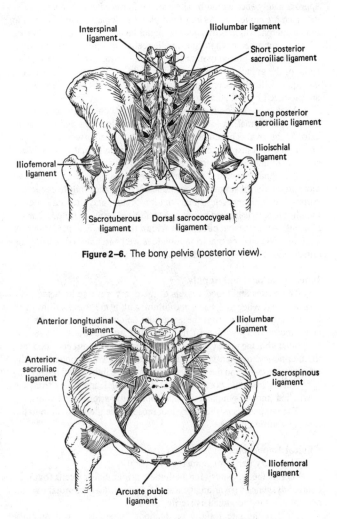

Figure 2–6. The bony pelvis (posterior view).

Figure 2–7. The bony pelvis (superior view).

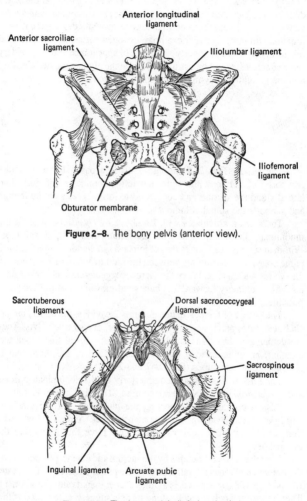

Figure 2–8. The bony pelvis (anterior view).

Figure 2–9. The bony pelvis (inferior view).

the ovary to a neighboring organ or a thickened ovarian tunica due to perioophoritis).

(3) It produces steroid sex hormones (luteal function). If the ovary does not produce these hormones (estrogens, progestogens, and androgens) in proper amounts, normal female growth, development, and function will not occur. For example, estrogen deficiency in childhood results in dwarfism; at puberty, in failure of appearance of the secondary sex characteristics and menstruation; and at the climacteric, in infertility and the involutional symptoms of the climacteric.

BONY PELVIS

The pelvis (Figs 2–6 through 2–9) is a basin-shaped structure composed of 4 bones: the right and left innominates anteriorly and laterally and the sacrum and coccyx posteriorly. It rests on the femurs and supports the spinal column.

The sacrum articulates with L5 above by an arthrodial joint; the innominate bones articulate with the femurs below by enarthroses. Within the pelvis itself are 2 types of joints: a synchondrosis uniting the 2 pubic bones, and diarthroses between the sacrum and ilium and between the sacrum and coccyx. When the sacrococcygeal joint is not ankylosed, a slight involuntary forward and backward movement of the coccyx is possible.

The design of the pelvic bones forms 2 cavities: the upper, larger, shallower false pelvis and the lower, smaller, deeper true pelvis. They are demarcated from one another by the iliopectineal line (linea terminalis), an oblique ridge on the inner surface of the ilium that is continued onto the pubes (Figs 2–7 and 2–9).

The false pelvis is bounded anteriorly by the abdominal muscles and posteriorly by the vertebral column. The flat, shallow, funnellike false pelvis aids in supporting the intestines, but the uterus is within the true pelvis when the woman is erect. Abdominal constriction, obesity, tumors, and pregnancy also force the uterus into the true pelvis.

The true pelvis is bounded by the sacrum and coccyx posteriorly, by the innominate bones laterally, and by the pubes anteriorly. The posterior portion of the true pelvis is 3 times deeper than its anterior segment. The shape of the pelvic cavity along its axis suggests a bent tube with a considerably shortened anterior curve.

The upper limit of the true pelvis is the slightly heart-shaped brim, superior strait, or inlet. The lower limit, which forms an anteroposterior ellipse, is the inferior strait or outlet (Figs 2–7 and 2–9).

No 2 pelves are identical; size and shape vary according to individual, familial, and racial characteristics. Disease may further modify the features of the bony pelvis.

THE PELVIC FLOOR

The pelvic floor (Figs 2–10 and 2–11) consists of muscle, ligaments, and fascia arranged in such a manner as to support the pelvic viscera; provide sphincterlike action for the urethra, vagina, and rectum; and permit the passage of a term infant. It is composed of the upper and lower pelvic diaphragms and the vesicovaginal and rectovaginal septa, which connect the 2 diaphragms, the perineal body, and the coccyx. Accessory structures include the transverse cervical (cardinal or Mackenrodt's) ligaments and the gluteus maximus muscles.

The upper pelvic diaphragm is a musculofascial structure made up of endopelvic fascia, the uterosacral ligaments, and the levator ani muscles (including the pubococcygeus portion). The lower musculofas-

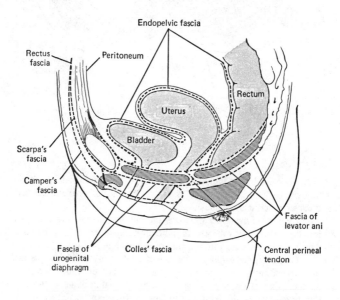

Figure 2–10. Fascial planes of the pelvis. (Modified after Netter.)

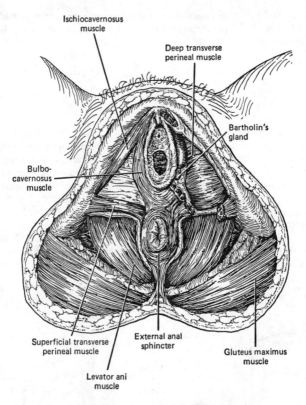

Figure 2–11. Pelvic musculature (inferior view).

cial pelvic diaphragm includes the urogenital diaphragm and the sphincter muscles at the vulvar outlet (ischiocavernosus, bulbocavernosus, and transverse perineal muscles).

All parts of the upper and lower musculofascial diaphragms anchor into the perineal body directly or indirectly, like spokes into the hub of a wheel or shroud lines into the ring of a parachute.

For reciprocal support, the layers of the pelvic diaphragms are interwoven and superimposed. They are not fixed but move upon one another. This makes it possible for the birth canal to dilate to capacity during passage of the fetus and to close postpartum.

The pelvic floor is perforated centrally by 3 tubular structures:

urethra, vagina, and rectum. Each traverses the pelvic floor at an angle, which enhances the sphincterlike action of the pelvic muscles.

The tissues of the musculofascial diaphragm play an important role in providing both support and resilience: The connective tissue provides support but no recoil; the fascia gives strength but no elasticity; the elastic tissue has resilience but little strength; and the voluntary and smooth muscle provide stretch and recoil with limited tolerance.

Weakness, laceration, or relaxation of the pelvic floor may be due to neurologic injury or injury during childbirth, or it may be of congenital or involutional origin.

PHYSIOLOGY

PUBERTY

At about age 9–11, puberty marks the end of childhood and the beginning of adolescence. Maturity follows 6–7 years later. Puberty includes the following sequence of events: thelarche (breast development), adrenarche (pubic and axillary hair growth), a growth spurt, and, finally, menarche (the onset of menstruation).

With puberty, the rather constant annual gain in height and weight that typifies childhood changes dramatically. A sudden increase in the rate of growth occurs, along with striking physiologic and psychologic changes. Finally, the growth rate peaks and then slows, and growth ultimately stops when adult size is achieved.

Puberty begins with maturation of the hypothalamus, which regulates release of the tropic hormones to the pituitary. Neuroreleasing hormones produced in the hypothalamus and stored in nerve endings are transmitted to the pituitary via a minute vascular network in response to central nervous system signals and steroid sex hormone levels.

During infancy and childhood, the gonadotropic releasing hormone, luteinizing hormone-releasing hormone (LHRH), and the hormones it controls, follicle-stimulating hormone (FSH) and luteinizing hormone (LH), are maintained at low levels by minimal secretion of estrogen by the immature ovary. During cumulative growth, the catecholamine content of the hypothalamus increases. Finally, a critical level of these neurostimulatory substances is reached, and hypothalamic inhibition of LHRH is diminished. An increase in production of FSH and LH results, and a new, higher negative feedback level is established. In this way, the ovaries are stimulated to produce more steroid sex hormones, which activate target areas and stimulate the development of secondary sex characteristics.

With continued maturation, production of other tropic hormones—corticotropin (ACTH), thyrotropin (TSH), and growth hormone (GH)—increases also. Thus, pituitary and ovarian hormones approach adult values in composition and concentration 3–4 years after the onset of puberty.

Thelarche

The first sign of puberty is the development, between ages 9 and 11, of a so-called bud or thickening of the duct system beneath each nipple, caused by increased estrogen production. Over the next 5–7 years, estrogen stimulates increased breast development and also gradually induces vaginal changes: thickening of the vaginal mucosa, an increase in vaginal cellular exfoliation, production of cervical mucus, and a decrease in vaginal fluid pH.

Adrenarche

The progress of maturation is marked at about age 11–12 by the appearance of pubic hair. Axillary hair usually appears after pubic hair growth is complete. However, some females develop only scant axillary hair. Adrenarche is an expression of ACTH-adrenocortical (adrenogenic) function.

Growth Spurt

The growth spurt, technically expressed as increased linear growth velocity in centimeters per year, occurs at about age 11–12 in girls and is complete by about age 13½. (In boys, the growth spurt begins about 1–1½ years later and terminates 1–2 years later.) Growth hormone and steroid sex hormones are responsible for about 9 cm of linear growth at the peak of the growth curve.

Skeletal changes are especially apparent during postpuberal growth, although all parts of the body participate in growth. Usually, the legs lengthen first, then shoulder breadth increases, and then the trunk lengthens. Concomitantly, the pelvis enlarges, and the internal dimensions increase. Girls approach maximal height by age 17–18. (Boys at that age will still grow 2–3 cm more.) Fusion of the epiphyses, a function of increased steroid sex hormones, terminates growth.

Menarche

Menarche occurs at about age 11–13, after the growth rate has slowed and breast development is well advanced. A popular theory holds that menstruation begins when a critical weight (about 45 kg [100 lb]) is attained following other adolescent changes. Early menstrual cycles usually are anovulatory and therefore may be unpredictable in time, amount, and duration. Regular, perhaps crampy ovulatory periods usually begin 1–2 years after menarche.

MENSTRUATION

General Considerations

Menstruation, or normal periodic uterine bleeding, is a physiologic function that occurs only in female primates. It is basically a catabolic process and is under the influence of pituitary and ovarian hormones. Its onset, the menarche, occurs usually between the ages of 11 and 14 years; its termination, the menopause, normally occurs between the ages of 45 and 55 years, although radiologic or surgical intervention may cause artificial menopause at an earlier age.

The interval between menstrual periods varies according to age, physical and emotional well-being, and environment. The normal menstrual cycle is commonly stated to be 28 days, but intervals of 24–32 days are still considered normal unless cycles are grossly irregular. At both the beginning and the end of reproductive life, the cycle is likely to be irregular and unpredictable owing to failure of ovulation. Most gynecologists therefore make a distinction between ovulatory and anovulatory menstruation. Upon reaching maturity, approximately two-thirds of women maintain a reasonably regular periodicity, barring pregnancy, stress, or illness.

The average duration of menstrual bleeding is 3–7 days, but this also may vary.

The amount of blood lost in menstruation averages about 70 mL, but many presumably normal women lose considerably more than this each month. Women under age 35 years tend to lose more blood than those over age 35.

Menstrual discharge contains principally blood, desquamated endometrial and vaginal epithelial cells, cervical mucus, and bacteria. Prostaglandins have been recovered from menstrual blood together with enzymes and fibrinolysins from the endometrium. The latter prevent clotting of menstrual blood unless bleeding is excessive. Nonetheless, small, fragile, fibrin-deficient vaginal clots may form because of the presence of mucoprotein and glucose in an alkaline environment.

The following factors are believed to influence menstrual bleeding: (1) fluctuations in ovarian hormone, pituitary hormone, prostaglandin, and enzyme levels; (2) characteristics of the endometrium (phase, receptivity to hormones); (3) activity of the autonomic nervous system; (4) vascular changes (stasis, spasm-dilatation); and (5) other factors, such as nutrition and psychologic states.

Endometrial Factors (See Fig 2–12 and p 37.)

The degree of maturation of the endometrium reflects estrogen and progesterone stimulation. For the first 10–14 days after the onset of menstrual bleeding, the endometrium proliferates as a result of a rising estrogen titer. For the next 2 weeks, progesterone "ripens" the lining,

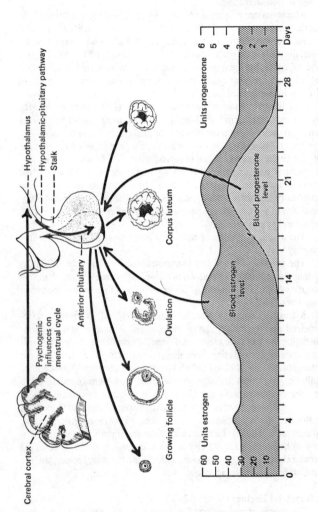

Figure 2–12. Menstrual cycle (hormones, histologic changes, basal body temperature).

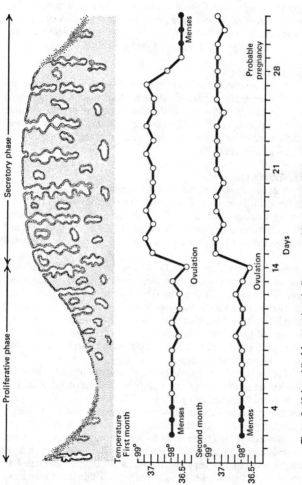

Figure 2–12 (cont'd). Menstrual cycle (hormones, histologic changes, basal body temperature).

and ovulatory type bleeding finally results from this secretory phase endometrium.

In cases of atrophic or hypertrophic endometrium, estrogen alone—in minimal amounts or in excessive or continued amounts, respectively—is found. Critical fluctuations in the titer of estrogens then result in anovulatory bleeding from a nonsecretory endometrium. The flow is usually heavier and lasts longer with hyperplastic endometrium, in contrast to that with atrophic endometrium.

Autonomic Factors

A few myelinated and nonmyelinated nerves are present in the endometrium and myometrium. These nerves terminate in simple end organs in the tunica adventitia of the blood vessels of the endometrium and in the inner layers of the myometrium itself. It would seem that both sensation and endometrial-myometrial vascular control are mediated by such an arrangement.

Vascular Factors

Vascular changes in the endometrium are obviously involved in menstruation. Five types of bleeding have been observed: (1) arterial bleeding with formation of a minute hematoma; (2) arterial bleeding without hematoma formation; (3) diapedesis; (4) venous bleeding; and (5) secondary bleeding from a previously ruptured, poorly thrombosed vessel.

Blood is supplied to the endometrium by 2 types of arterioles: a tortuous (spiral) type near to or surrounding the endometrial glands that supplies the functionalis layer, or outer two-thirds of the endometrium; and short straight vessels that supply only the basalis layer, or inner one-third of the endometrium. The basalis is not shed but remains as a reservoir of tissue for regeneration of the stroma and surface of the endometrial glands. Only the superficial coiled arteries are involved directly in menstrual bleeding.

For the first week after the onset of menstrual bleeding, the spiral arterioles are short and relatively straight. During the period of thickening of the endometrium, they lengthen. The vessels grow more rapidly than the endometrium, however, so that they become coiled, particularly in the mid portion of the functionalis.

In monkeys (and probably in humans also), just before menstrual bleeding begins, a rapid endometrial regression caused by marked estrogen-progesterone depletion results in buckling of the coiled arterioles in the functionalis, stasis of the blood within the arteriovenous channels, necrosis of the terminal arteriolar walls, constriction of these arterioles within the basalis, and periodic relaxation and hemorrhage from these peripheral branches.

Four to 24 hours before the onset of menstruation, periodic (every

60–90 seconds) vasoconstriction of the coiled arterioles apparently causes a type of "blanch and blush" phenomenon resulting from relaxation and contraction of the vessel musculature. At this time, there seems to be considerable dehydration of the endometrium. Bleeding soon follows from various areas in the endometrium.

Prostaglandins

The presence of noxious substances in menstrual blood has been suspected for centuries. Prostaglandins—largely of the PGF group—are present in considerable amounts in endometrium and menstrual blood. Prostaglandins cause intense arterial spasm and smooth muscle contraction, and this may explain dysmenorrhea of obscure origin. They are probably the cause of the vasoconstriction in the endometrium that precedes dilatation and menstrual bleeding.

Other Factors

Numerous other factors can profoundly affect the menstrual cycle and flow. Undernutrition and other metabolic disturbances, inadequate rest, and emotional tension may have an effect upon the cycle.

THE TYPICAL MENSTRUAL CYCLE

The menstrual cycle is mediated by complex neuroendocrine mechanisms. Releasing (RH) or inhibitory (IH) hormones produced in the hypothalamus are transmitted to the anterior pituitary via a minute vascular system. A single releasing hormone, luteinizing hormone-releasing hormone (LHRH), has been identified for the gonadotropins follicle-stimulating hormone (FSH) and luteinizing hormone (LH). Prolactin secretion is controlled by prolactin-releasing hormone (PRH) and prolactin-inhibiting hormone (PIH).

With the proper coordination of releasing and inhibiting substances, the anterior lobe of the pituitary secretes still other tropic hormones—thyrotropin (TSH), corticotropin (ACTH), growth hormone (GH), and melanocyte-stimulating hormone (MSH)—all of which are important to reproductive physiology.

In contrast with the anterior lobe of the pituitary, the posterior lobe is linked with the hypothalamus by nerves. The posterior pituitary hormones vasopressin and oxytocin are secreted in the hypothalamus and stored in the posterior pituitary. Vasopressin (antidiuretic hormone, ADH) controls plasma osmolality and is released by impulses from the supraoptic and paraventricular nuclei. Oxytocin, which causes uterine muscular and myoepithelial breast ductal cell contraction and thus stimulates both labor and lactation, is released by complex neuroendocrine mechanisms and probably by other mechanisms as well.

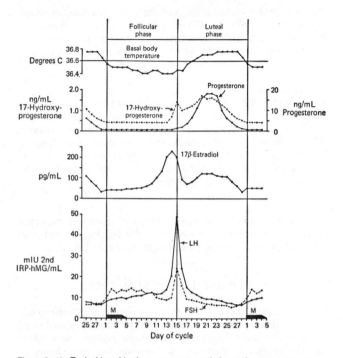

Figure 2–13. Typical basal body temperature and plasma hormone concentration during a normal 28-day human menstrual cycle. M, menstruation; IRP-hMG, international reference standard for gonadotropins. (Reproduced, with permission, from Midgley AR in: *Human Reproduction.* Hafez ESE, Evans TN [editors]. Harper & Row, 1973.)

Normal menstrual cycles are carefully regulated by gonadotropin secretion (Fig 2–13). With the onset of each cycle, follicles ready for maturation are stimulated to develop by FSH. One (rarely more) outstrips the others to form a prominent graafian follicle. Regression of the remaining follicles then ensues. Meanwhile, estrogen is produced by the theca lutein cells of the follicles. On the eighth or ninth day of the cycle, the estrogen level stops rising and LH and FSH levels begin to fluctuate. On about the 14th day, a sudden LH surge triggers rupture of the follicle and thus ovulation (extrusion of the ovum). Slight bleeding occurs, and the empty follicle soon becomes filled with clotted blood (hemorrhagic follicle). LH and prolactin stimulate luteinization of the granulosa cells, and a corpus luteum is thus formed. The granulosa lutein cells produce progesterone, which peaks on about the 23rd or 24th day. If fertilization and nidation of the ovum (pregnancy) have not occurred by this time, the corpus luteum regresses. The levels of progesterone and estrogen decline thereafter to reach a critical level on about the 28th day, when endometrial bleeding (menstruation) occurs.

Prolactin may not be as important in maintenance of the corpus luteum in humans as in laboratory animals. Only slight variations in the titer of this substance have been recorded during the menstrual period, but much higher levels are reached during pregnancy. Very high levels of prolactin are the rule during lactation.

Ovarian endocrine function is mediated by the gonadotropins FSH and LH. Both stimulate production of estrogen. After the LH surge, more estrogen and, now, progesterone are secreted. The follicle theca cells are the major site of estrogen elaboration, whereas the luteinized granulosa cells of the corpus luteum synthesize progesterone. The principal ovarian estrogens are estrone (E_1), estradiol (E_2), and small amounts of estriol (E_3). Ovarian stromal cells normally produce small amounts of androgen, largely androstenedione. If pregnancy does not occur, a rapid fall in estrogen and progesterone levels begins on about the 24th day of the cycle; low levels of these hormones are reached early in menstruation.

Endometrial Changes (See Figs 2–12 and 29–2.)

During reproductive life, the endometrium undergoes continuous cyclic change. For each cycle, it is generally considered to pass through 4 phases that correspond to ovarian hormone activity and can be identified by endometrial biopsy.

A. Proliferative Phase: The proliferative (estrogenic) phase may vary considerably in duration but is usually consistent with each individual. It is about 14 days in a 28-day cycle.

The early proliferative phase starts on about the fourth or fifth day of the cycle, just before the end of menstruation, and lasts 2–3 days. The end of this phase coincides with about the seventh day of the classic cycle. Surface epithelium is repaired but is thin or defective; its thickness depends upon the loss of tissue during menstrual bleeding. Glands are straight. Nuclei of epithelial cells are pseudostratified, and mitoses are frequent. Stromal cells show relatively large nuclei and little cytoplasm. There are few phagocytes.

The midproliferative phase coincides with about the tenth day of the cycle. It differs from the early proliferative phase only in degree. The surface is more regular, the glands more tortuous, and glandular cells pseudostratified. Thickness of the endometrium is increased.

The late proliferative phase occurs on about the 14th day of the average cycle. The surface is undulating; stromal cells are closely packed; and variable amounts of extracellular fluid are lost. Thickness is about as before, but with greater cellular concentration. The glands are increasingly tortuous and contain minimal secretion. There is no glycogen in the fluid.

B. Ovulatory Phase: Ovulation occurs on about the 14th day of a 28-day cycle. Because there is no appreciable change in the endometrium within the 24–36 hours following ovulation, one cannot distinguish between the 14th- and 15th-day endometrium. Distinctive changes appear in gland cells on the 16th day and thereafter, indicating corpus luteum activity and, presumably, ovulation.

C. Secretory (Progestational) Phase: (This phase technically begins with ovulation.) On the 16th day, tortuosity of the glands is increased, there are many mitotic figures, and the glycogen-laden basal vacuoles appear. On the 17th day, the most pronounced vacuolization of cells occurs. Almost two-thirds of the basal portion of such glands contains glycogen-laden fluid. Slight edema is noted. Mitoses are rare. On the 18th day, secretion of fluid within the glands is apparent. (This corresponds to the time when the ovum is free within the uterine cavity and must derive nourishment from uterine secretions.) On the 22nd day, the glands are more tortuous but there is less secretory activity. Considerable mucoid secretion is seen in their lumens. Stromal edema is now at the peak. (This may facilitate implantation of the ovum.) The high points of secretory activity and stromal edema coincide with the period of greatest corpus luteum activity. From the 24th to the 27th days, edema regresses and the stromal cells metamorphose into elements suggestive of decidua cells. The first change is noted in cells around the spiral arterioles, with the appearance of mitotic figures in the perivascular stroma. The glands become more and more tortuous, with serrations of their walls. Secretion of gland cells diminishes. There is infiltration by polymorphonuclear neutrophils and monocytes. Finally, necrosis and slough develop.

If pregnancy occurs, active secretion and edema persist. Glands become more feathery and serrated. The predecidua is not immediately accentuated except around the ovum. The presence of all 3 (secretion, edema, and predecidua) strongly suggests early pregnancy even though the patient has not yet missed a menstrual period.

D. Menstrual Phase: The endometrial edema and degenerative changes that occur at the end of the secretory phase cause tissue necrosis that is irregularly distributed throughout all endometrial layers except the basalis. The necrosis causes blood vessels to open, producing scattered small hemorrhages that enlarge and coalesce into propagating hematomas, which in turn cause endometrial shedding and further rupture of small vessels. Shedding of tissue fragments usually begins in a patchy fashion about 12 hours after bleeding starts in ovulatory cycles, although an entire cast of the endometrial cavity is separated in so-called membranous dysmenorrhea. This painful condition results from sudden separation of the entire secretory endometrial lining, presumably because the sequence of events described above is abnormally rapid and complete.

About two-thirds of the endometrium is presumed to be lost with each ovulatory menstruation. By the time brisk flow ceases, tissue shrinkage and separation have occurred over the greater portion of the surface of the uterine cavity.

After a menstrual period of 4–7 days, bleeding gradually diminishes. Regional ooze is reduced by constriction and thrombosis of the remaining undamaged coiled arterioles, so that spotting finally ceases.

The interval between ovulation and menstruation is normally almost exactly 14 days. In contrast, the preovulatory period, the interval from the first day of menstruation to the day of ovulation, may vary from 7–8 days to over a month. This variability of the preovulatory period accounts for the variability of the interval between menstrual periods.

Changes in Cervical Mucus & Vaginal Cytology

A. Cervical Mucus: The amount and consistency of cervical mucus varies during the menstrual cycle. If a smear of cervical mucus is allowed to dry in air without fixation and examined under a microscope, characteristic patterns of crystallization can be identified at various stages. At the time of ovulation, the mucus dries to a striking fernlike pattern (fern test). Before and after ovulation and during pregnancy, other characteristic granular patterns can be observed.

At about the time of ovulation, the cervical mucus becomes extremely clear and liquid in contrast to the yellowish, viscid mucus normally observed during the extreme pre- and postovulatory phases of the cycle. Just before ovulation, a drop of endocervical mucus can be stretched into a thin cobweblike strand 6 or more centimeters long. This quality (''spinnbarkeit'') is related to a high estrogen level and altered saline content.

B. Vaginal Cytology: Vaginal cytology reflects estrogen and progesterone variations and is distinctive during each of the 4 stages of the life span (Fig 2–14).

During reproductive life, the vaginal cytology is characteristic of pregnancy or of the phase of the menstrual cycle. During the late follicular (preovulatory, proliferative) phase (days 12–15 of the menstrual cycle), a cytologic smear of vaginal fluid normally appears estrogenic, with many pyknotic epithelial cells and few white blood cells. After ovulation, the smear appears progestational, containing curling and clustering epithelial cells and occasional white blood cells; this is evidence of the luteal phase. A smear during pregnancy is marked by smaller, clumped, navicular epithelial cells with a high glycogen content and relatively few white blood cells.

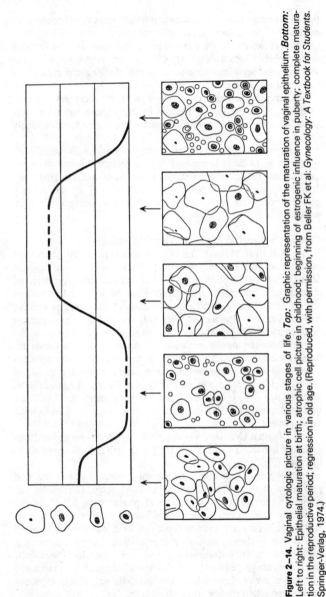

Figure 2–14. Vaginal cytologic picture in various stages of life. *Top:* Graphic representation of the maturation of vaginal epithelium. *Bottom: Left to right:* Epithelial maturation at birth; atrophic cell picture in childhood; beginning of estrogenic influence in puberty; complete maturation in the reproductive period; regression in old age. (Reproduced, with permission, from Beller FK et al: *Gynecology: A Textbook for Students.* Springer-Verlag, 1974.)

Systemic Changes

During the preovulatory phase of the menstrual cycle, resting temperatures taken each morning will usually be low (< 36.6 °C [98 °F]). Activity, infection, inadequate sleep, and alcoholic beverages before retiring can cause an elevated temperature the following morning. On the day of ovulation, the temperature dips, then rises sharply almost one degree Fahrenheit (0.5 °C) and remains elevated until just before the menstrual period, when it begins to fall toward the low preovulatory levels (Figs 2–12 and 2–13). This occurs only in ovulating women.

Other systemic changes associated with uterine bleeding after ovulation are as follows: (1) Extracellular edema, which is the cause of premenstrual weight gain. (2) Muscle sensitivity or hypertonicity, producing irritability and agitation. (3) Vascular alterations, including pelvic hyperemia and increased capillary fragility or a tendency toward bruising. (4) Mastalgia due to increased breast size and turgescence. (5) Headache, including menstrual migraine, which appears to be a hormonally mediated vascular headache.

ANOVULATORY CYCLES

In anovulatory cycles, the maturation and differentiation of the endometrium caused by progesterone does not occur, and the sequence of events is therefore greatly altered. The period is qualitatively similar to an ovulatory one, but minimal coiling of the spiral arterioles probably can cause only small fissures and no propagating hematomas. The peeling away of the functionalis layer thus takes place only imperfectly in the proliferative or hyperplastic endometrium. Bleeding from terminal arteriolar loops must occur, but tissue loss is minimal. The endometrium continues to proliferate from month to month, with the result that hemorrhage finally ensues in subsequent periods from this grossly thickened tissue.

THE MENOPAUSE & CLIMACTERIC
(See Chapter 28.)

PHYSIOLOGIC CHANGES DURING PREGNANCY

Physiologic adjustments during pregnancy often suggest borderline deficiencies or disease states, eg, reduced red blood cell count, increased sedimentation rate, breathlessness. Therefore, a proper understanding of such changes is important for correct management of the obstetric patient.

Certain physiologic variations are normal in pregnancy and usually require only recognition and reassurance. Pathologic disorders call for explanation to the patient and a plan of treatment that is best for mother and fetus.

Weight Gain & Energy Requirements

The recommended weight gain during the first half of pregnancy is approximately 1 lb per month; during the second half, when marked fetal growth occurs, the recommended gain is 1 lb per week. The weight gain at term is approximately 25 lb. The fetus and placenta contain about 500 g of protein and account for about half of the total weight increase during pregnancy.

The average daily energy requirement for a mature nonpregnant woman is about 2200 kcal. With pregnancy, an additional 300 kcal/d is needed beginning late in the first trimester.

Metabolic & Chemical Changes

A. Proteins:

1. Serum albumin and globulins–The serum albumin level drops slightly during pregnancy until term and rises to normal nonpregnant levels several months postpartum. Total serum globulin levels rise slightly during pregnancy and return to normal after the puerperium.

2. Serum fractions–The levels of some serum fractions (eg, β-lipoprotein, α_1-antitrypsin, transferrin) rise considerably until term but soon fall to normal values postpartum. Thyroxine-binding prealbumin remains at essentially the same level throughout gestation.

3. Immunoglobulins–In normal pregnancy, the IgA level drops slightly, that of IgG gradually declines, the IgD level increases markedly, and IgM remains essentially unchanged. However, in preeclampsia or the nephrotic syndrome, the IgA level remains unchanged, that of IgG falls, the IgD level falls considerably—for unknown reasons—and the IgM level increases.

4. Alpha-fetoprotein–Alpha-fetoprotein, an α-globulin, is synthesized in the fetal liver and intestine. Peak levels of this substance are reached at 13–14 weeks and decline gradually during the remainder of pregnancy. If the fetus has an open neural tube defect or upper gastrointestinal tract obstruction, α-fetoprotein levels are greatly increased in both amniotic fluid and maternal serum. Alpha-fetoprotein is also increased in chronic fetal distress, with fetal death, and in normal multiple pregnancy.

B. Carbohydrates: Pregnancy is considered to be diabetogenic because during pregnancy (1) women predisposed to diabetes become chemical diabetics but revert to normal carbohydrate metabolism postpartum; (2) glucose tolerance test curves are altered, making it difficult to compare even normal nonpregnant women with normal pregnant women; (3) insulin is released by the pancreas more rapidly and in greater amounts, while, on the other hand, cellular sensitivity to insulin is reduced; and (4) fasting is followed by a more rapid drop in plasma glucose, amino acids, and insulin than in the nonpregnant state, resulting in a greater rise in free fatty acids and ketone bodies—the so-called accelerated starvation of pregnancy.

Pregnant women have an increased need for carbohydrate. The fetal demand for glucose seems partly responsible for this, despite the fact that the insulin molecule is too large to cross the placental barrier. Several maternal and fetoplacental hormones mediate for this increased carbohydrate requirement.

During pregnancy, the maternal level of free cortisol is increased, and insulin is secreted more rapidly. Increased levels of estrogens blunt the action of insulin while they cause higher plasma levels of both insulin and free cortisol. Progesterone increases the output of insulin but decreases its cellular utilization. Glucagon, which remains unchanged during pregnancy, can be discounted as a cause of altered carbohydrate metabolism.

Human chorionic somatomammotropin (hCS), formerly called human placental lactogen (hPL), a protein hormone elaborated by the syncytiotrophoblast, increases peripheral utilization of glucose while it stimulates lipolysis. This increases plasma levels of glycerol and free fatty acids. Thus, hCS increases energy production from fat and makes glucose available to the fetus.

C. Lipids: Relative hyperlipidemia is a feature of pregnancy. Plasma levels of total lipids, serum triglycerides, and free fatty acids are all increased. Plasma levels of cholesterol and total phospholipids almost double during the second and third trimesters, reaching values of 250–300 mg/dL and approximately 400 mg/dL, respectively.

D. Water: A gross increase in body water amounts to an excess of 1–2 kg at term. This may be much greater in obese and edematous patients. Numerous factors late in pregnancy, including altered renal excretion, play a part in this increase. Almost half of all normotensive patients without proteinuria have some dependent edema. More importantly, women with preeclampsia usually have generalized edema.

E. Minerals:

1. Iron–A normal pregnancy requires approximately 1 g of elemental iron, or 4–5 mg/d. Of this, 300 mg is needed by the fetus and placenta, about 500 mg augments the maternal hemoglobin mass, and the remainder is lost in bleeding during delivery and the puerperium. Maternal iron stores are small, and absorption is limited; therefore, a daily supplement of 30–60 mg of elemental iron is recommended. If anemia is diagnosed or hemorrhage develops, more iron should be prescribed.

2. Calcium–In addition to maternal needs, the fetus requires about 30 g of calcium during pregnancy. Most of the calcium and phosphorus for fetal growth is acquired after the fourth month of pregnancy.

Maternal stores of calcium are inadequate to supply the amounts needed during pregnancy. Assimilation of calcium from the gastrointestinal tract is not especially good, even with normal gastrointestinal function and adequate vitamin D intake. The FDA recommends a daily allowance of 1200 mg of calcium and 400–500 IU of vitamin D. With osteomalacia or prolonged inactivity, increased supplements of both calcium and vitamin D are required.

3. Phosphorus–Maternal stores of phosphorus, like those of calcium, are inadequate during pregnancy. The daily recommended phosphorus intake for pregnant women is 1200 mg. Absorption of both phosphorus and calcium is best with an alkaline medium; therefore, these supplements should be given well before or between meals.

4. Sodium–Retention of sodium and water in the extracellular fluid is a physiologic response to pregnancy. Sodium and water levels return to normal soon after delivery.

5. Potassium–Changes in the plasma potassium level during pregnancy are less marked but generally parallel those of sodium until delivery, when a prompt return to normal prepregnancy values follows.

6. Chloride–The plasma level of chloride falls early in pregnancy but rises by the second trimester to pregestational levels, where it remains without significant variation to term.

7. Magnesium–Hemodilution produces a slight reduction in the plasma magnesium level during pregnancy. The change is apparently inconsequential.

8. Trace elements–Animal studies suggest that small supplements of zinc, copper, manganese, and chromium are necessary during pregnancy. However, specific definitive studies in humans are lacking.

F. Folic Acid: Folates are essential for the increased erythropoiesis that occurs in both mother and fetus. The recommended daily dose of folic acid is 0.8 mg, but more should be given to patients with multiple pregnancy, anemia, or alcoholism and to those taking anticonvulsant medication, eg, phenytoin.

G. Acid-Base Balance: Progesterone increase has a central effect on ventilation. The increase in the progesterone level during pregnancy causes an increase in pulmonary tidal volume that results in a decrease in P_{CO_2} of approximately 5 mm Hg. This occurs as early as the tenth week of pregnancy. This drop in P_{CO_2} is accompanied by a slight rise in plasma pH, the reduction in base being about 2 mEq/L. Hence, in pregnancy there is minimal respiratory alkalosis balanced by slight metabolic acidosis. During labor, these acid-base changes become more marked, but values return to normal at about 3 weeks postpartum.

Skin & Hair Changes

Pregnancy induces hyperpigmentation of the skin of the face ("mask of pregnancy"), areolas and nipples, lower abdominal midline (linea nigra), and axillas and pudendum in most women, especially those with dark complexions. These changes, which begin in mid pregnancy and recede during the puerperium, are caused by melanocyte-stimulating hormone (MSH), an anterior pituitary hormone that concentrates melanin granules in the cytoplasm of epidermal cells.

Striae gravidarum are pink to violet-colored streaks over the breasts, abdomen, thighs, and buttocks that appear during late pregnancy in many women. Striae are not "stretch marks" but result from alterations in dermal collagen caused by increased levels of adrenal corticoids. Although stretching of the skin may influence the distribution of striae, it is not the cause. After delivery, striae fade to become permanent superficial silvery scars.

Palmar erythema and spider angiomas—small telangiectasias over the neck, chest, and arms—are presumed to be due to increased estrogen levels during pregnancy. Palmar erythema disappears postpartum; the small red angiomas fade but remain.

Epulis is a sensitive, hypertrophic gingival lesion that bleeds easily. One or more of these may develop after the first trimester of pregnancy. Epulis suggests a pyogenic granuloma, but the disorder may be more comparable to spider angiomas. Epulis disappears spontaneously after delivery, and dental surgery is rarely required.

Some generalized hair growth may be noted during pregnancy. However, a moderate to severe hair loss, or telogen effluvium, occasionally occurs 3–4 months postpartum; this is the result of metabolic and endocrine changes. The hair loss is a reversal of the anagen (hair growth) pattern that prevailed during pregnancy. Hair loss may continue for up to 6 months, but if there are no significant health problems, regrowth will occur without therapy in a few months. The patient should be reassured that the hair will grow back.

Respiratory Changes

Nasal hyperemia due to increased estrogen levels during pregnancy may result in nosebleeds (epistaxis).

The diaphragm is elevated during pregnancy, but the ribs are flared so that there is little net change in thoracic capacity. There is a slight increase in the respiratory rate, but the vital capacity does not change significantly. Tidal volume is increased, so that the ventilation rate rises to about 10 L/min—an increase of more than 40%.

The lungs are somewhat compressed by the elevated diaphragm, and for this reason the functional residual capacity is decreased. This, together with the increased tidal volume, allows a much more effective mixing of gases, so that the alveolar ventilation increases by about 65%.

The marked increase in ventilation rate results in a lowered alveolar P_{CO_2} and a decrease in blood bicarbonate. There is no change in blood pH. Oxygen consumption increases by almost 20% during pregnancy.

Cardiovascular Changes

A. Hemodynamic Changes: The heart rate gradually accelerates 15–20 beats per minute by term. The cardiac stroke volume varies greatly but is normally 65–70 mL. With this, the cardiac output increases by approximately 1.5 L/min by the tenth week, remaining at about 6–7 L/min to term.

There is no significant change in systolic blood pressure in normal pregnancy, but a slight decrease in diastolic blood pressure does occur as a consequence of decreased peripheral resistance. The pulse pressure is increased.

There is no change in venous pressure in the upper body, but there is a marked increase in venous pressure in the lower extremities in the supine, sitting, or standing position. Venous pressure rises from about 10 to about 30 cm of water. In some women, lying down for long periods causes decreased return of blood to the heart, decreased cardiac output, a fall in blood pressure, and edema.

B. Arteriovenous Oxygen Difference: The arteriovenous oxygen difference (A-V O_2 difference) rises from approximately 3.3 mL of oxygen per deciliter of blood in the late first trimester to about 4.5 mL/dL at term. This is the result of a disproportionate increase in circulating hemoglobin and cardiac output as contrasted with the basal oxygen consumption.

C. Changes in Heart Sounds: The intensity of the 2 components of the first heart sound increases during pregnancy. Because of a slightly earlier closure of the mitral valve, a split first sound may be heard. There are no significant changes in the second heart sound during pregnancy. A third and even a fourth heart sound may be identified in an occasional normal pregnant woman after the 20th week of pregnancy.

A slight to moderate systolic murmur to the left of the sternal margin is commonly heard in patients during late pregnancy. This is an indication of increased blood flow. Near term, a precordial systolic murmur from the mammary artery, or even a venous hum over engorged breast veins, may be noted. Any diastolic murmur requires investigation.

D. Changes Visible on X-Ray: In late pregnancy, the heart is displaced upward and to the left because of elevation of the diaphragm. The cardiac silhouette may be little changed from that observed before pregnancy. However, a slight enlargement of the heart with prominence of the pulmonary conus may be noted, and straightening of the upper left cardiac shadow is not uncommon. In the right anterior oblique view, the anterior wall of the esophagus is seen to be indented by the heart.

E. Electrocardiographic Changes: Normal variations in the ECG during pregnancy include a slight left axis deviation, flattening or even inversion of the T wave in lead III, low-voltage QRS complexes, and Q waves in lead III. Ectopic beats and supraventricular tachycardia are neither unusual nor serious.

F. Hematologic Changes:

1. Blood volume–In the first half of pregnancy, the increase in total blood volume is greater than that in red cell volume; in the second half, the reverse is true. The total blood volume increases 1–2 L during pregnancy; it returns to normal prepregnant levels about 2 weeks after delivery.

2. Red blood cells–Pregnancy-induced erythropoiesis begins at about the 16th week, and the total red cell mass expands about 25% during pregnancy if iron stores are adequate. A slight decline in hematocrit occurs during pregnancy; this is because the increase in blood volume exceeds the increase in red cell volume. The red cell volume returns to normal by the second week postpartum.

3. White blood cells and platelets–Beginning in mid pregnancy, the white blood cell count increases gradually, most of the increase being polymorphonuclear leukocytes. It reaches a maximum of about 14,000/μL at term and returns to normal by the end of the first week following parturition. The lymphocyte count normally remains unchanged. A slight decrease in platelet count occurs during pregnancy.

4. Coagulation factors–All plasma clotting factors except XI and XIII increase during pregnancy. Fibrinolytic activity is depressed. Thus, pregnancy is, at least in vitro, a state of hypercoagulability. Clotting factors are rapidly consumed during and after delivery, but thromboembolic phenomena due to stasis, trauma, or infection are 3 times more common postpartum, when most of the coagulation factors have returned to near prepregnancy values, than antepartum.

Gastrointestinal Changes

Changes in appetite, nausea and vomiting, and indigestion or constipation are common during pregnancy. Pancreatic and hepatic function is altered, enteric secretion is reduced, and absorption of fluid is increased.

The cause of nausea and vomiting is unknown, although emotional tension and increased hCG levels may play a role. Profuse salivation (ptyalism) may occur for unknown reasons. A blunted sense of taste may explain the desire of some pregnant patients for salty foods or flavorful condiments. Pica may also occur during pregnancy.

Slowing of peristalsis and relaxation of the musculature of the gastrointestinal tract in pregnancy, due mainly to estrogen-progestin effects, may cause heartburn (pyrosis). Heartburn is due to regurgitation of gastric contents into the lower esophagus secondary to relaxation of the cardiac sphincter and reverse peristalsis. Temporary hiatus hernia is common during pregnancy and may be part of the heartburn syndrome. The symptom is most likely to occur when the patient is lying down or bending over.

Gastric emptying time and acid and pepsin secretion are reduced during pregnancy. The small intestine is less motile, but absorption of nutrients, including iron, is adequate. The hypotonicity of the colon during pregnancy permits increased water absorption—perhaps secondary to higher levels of circulating angiotensin and aldosterone—which results in reduced bulk. Thus, constipation is more common and more troublesome during pregnancy.

The gallbladder and liver become somewhat hypotonic, with consequent bile stasis. Cholestatic jaundice and the formation of gallstones are therefore more common during pregnancy. Most liver function tests are unchanged—serum bilirubin, lactic dehydrogenase (LDH), serum glutamic-oxaloacetic transaminase (SGOT), and serum glutamic-pyruvic transaminase (SGPT) levels are normal—but serum alkaline phosphatase is elevated and serum cholinesterase reduced. Excretion of sulfobromophthalein by the liver is decreased during pregnancy.

Renal Changes

Dilatation of the renal hila, calices, and ureters is notable after the first trimester of pregnancy but usually regresses to normal by the end of the puerperium. The right collecting system exhibits greater dilatation because of compression by the enlarged, dextrorotated uterus. Bilateral vesicoureteral reflux often occurs during pregnancy. Thus, pregnant women are most susceptible to urinary tract infection.

Functional changes in the kidney include increased renal plasma flow (RPF) in the first and second trimester and an increase of about 50% in the glomerular filtration rate (GFR) during early pregnancy because of increased blood volume and renal blood flow, lowered oncotic pressure, and endocrine changes. The RPF and GFR fall in the final month of pregnancy.

Urea, creatinine, and uric acid are all excreted more effectively during pregnancy, so that the blood concentrations of these substances normally are lower than in the nonpregnant state. More glucose and lactose are excreted during pregnancy. Most amino acids are eliminated more rapidly and in larger amounts during pregnancy. Ascorbic acid and folate are also more readily excreted during pregnancy.

Fluid volume and composition are regulated by renal control of the excretion of sodium and water. Estrogen and cortisol and the renin-angiotensin-aldosterone system contribute to the changes in sodium and water homeostasis during pregnancy. The greatly increased GFR during pregnancy causes a considerable increase in sodium filtration, but tubular reabsorption of sodium is increased, resulting in the positive sodium balance needed to allow for fetal requirements and the increased maternal blood volume. Proportionately more water than sodium is retained during the third trimester. This contributes to the commonly observed dependent edema of late pregnancy.

Reproductive System Changes

The uterus undergoes obvious major changes during pregnancy. It increases markedly in size, so that the capacity is increased about 500-fold. The contractility of the uterus increases, and after the first trimester, irregular contractions may be felt by the patient and the examiner. These contractions become stronger and more frequent as term approaches.

The coiled uterine arteries gradually straighten to permit better circulation to the enlarged uterus. Uterine blood flow gradually increases during pregnancy, so that at term it is approximately 500 mL/min. This flow is greatly diminished during uterine contractions.

The cervix becomes much softer and more congested as gestation progresses. These changes are apparent even in early pregnancy. There is marked hypertrophy of the endocervical glands, with a resultant increase in the amount of cervical mucus. The cervix becomes shorter (effaced) and slightly dilated as term approaches. This is particularly notable in multiparous individuals.

The vagina also becomes much softer and more congested. There is considerable loosening of the connective tissue to permit greater distensibility. An increased amount of glycogen in the epithelial cells normally occurs. Exfoliation of the hypertrophic mucosa is increased, producing an increase in the volume of vaginal secretion. An increased lactic acid content that causes a lowering of the pH to 4.0–6.0 is usual.

The ovaries enlarge only slightly during gestation. The prominent corpus luteum of pregnancy maintains gestation until about the sixth week, when it shrinks in size while the trophoblast assumes the major production of progesterone and other hormones required by pregnancy. Slightly raised pink decidual patches are often seen over the ovaries, peritoneum, and oviducts. There are no other significant changes in the oviducts during pregnancy.

An enormous increase in the size of the uterine and ovarian veins is characteristic of pregnancy.

The breasts enlarge, and congestion is so great that breast tenderness is common in early pregnancy. Superficial veins become apparent. The breasts become more firm as a result of an increase in the alveoli. The nipples become larger, darker, and more erectile. Hypertrophy of sebaceous glands in the areolas produces small protrusions known as

Montgomery's tubercles. Colostrum may be expressed after the second trimester, but this is more likely as full term approaches. Lactation is the result of interaction of estrogen, progesterone, hCS, prolactin, and oxytocin.

Musculoskeletal Changes

Pregnant women develop significant changes in stance, posture, and gait. A considerable increase in lumbar lordosis and increased flexion of the neck are both necessary compensations for balance. Moreover, relaxation of the periarticular supports, which may be due to relaxin, results in increased motility of the pelvic joints. These changes and increased weight-bearing are responsible for the fatigue and the back pain, muscle pain, and even nerve root pain that occur in pregnancy.

Endocrine Changes

A. Anterior Pituitary Hormones: The pituitary gland enlarges slightly during pregnancy, and characteristic "pregnancy cells" develop in the anterior lobe. The production of most pituitary hormones remains unchanged during gestation, but FSH and GH levels decrease. Prolactin is the only pituitary hormone to increase. There is a steady rise in the prolactin level to term, when it increases 10-fold over nonpregnant values. Prolactin does not cross the placental barrier.

Despite high prolactin levels, lactation does not occur during pregnancy because of the inhibitory effect of estrogen. With normal pituitary, thyroid, and adrenal function, delivery triggers a fall in serum estrogen levels, and milk production begins. Suckling stimulates periodic prolactin secretion, but the levels needed to maintain lactation are lower than during pregnancy. The highest prolactin level occurs immediately postdelivery. Prolactin levels return to normal 3–4 weeks postpartum if the mother does not nurse her infant. Lactation can be suppressed by inhibition of prolactin secretion; synthetic ergots such as bromocriptine are safe and highly effective for this purpose.

The fetal pituitary also secretes prolactin, and by term, the fetal serum and amniotic fluid prolactin levels exceed maternal levels. It is postulated that prolactin is important to fetal osmotic regulation.

B. Posterior Pituitary Hormones: The levels of posterior pituitary hormones remain unchanged during pregnancy. During labor, a small amount of oxytocin is released by both the mother and the fetus, although labor does not seem to depend upon such stimulation. Women who have undergone removal of the posterior pituitary can experience normal labor. Nonetheless, during the second stage of labor, a burst of oxytocin occurs in normal women. This aids in evacuation of the uterus and helps to control bleeding.

Nursing causes oxytocin release via a breast-to-pituitary neural reflex. Oxytocin makes the myoepithelial cells of the breast contract, causing ejection of milk. Oxytocin is essential for milk ejection in humans.

Vasopressin production and function are unchanged during pregnancy, labor, and the puerperium.

C. Thyroid Hormones: The thyroid increases in size during pregnancy, and although the basal metabolic rate rises, this is not due to thyroid activity, ie, the normal pregnant woman remains euthyroid. The increased gland size is due to hyperplasia of the glandular tissue and increased vascularity. Much of the increase in basal metabolic rate is due to increased growth and oxygen consumption by the pregnant uterus, the fetus, and the placenta.

Iodine uptake by the thyroid is increased during pregnancy, as is urinary excretion of iodine. *Caution:* Radioactive iodine should not be administered during pregnancy, since it can damage the fetal thyroid gland. Estrogen stimulates an increase in the level of thyroxine-binding globulin (TBG) early in pregnancy. This results in increased levels of circulating thyroxine (T_4) and triiodothyronine (T_3), but the levels of free T_4 and T_3 remain unchanged, and their peripheral utilization does not change.

The fetal thyroid does not synthesize thyroid hormones during the first trimester, but iodine uptake by the fetal thyroid can be demonstrated after the 13th week. Thyrotropin (TSH) and T_4 do not cross the placental barrier to the fetus readily. Estrogens and TBG do cross the placenta to stimulate the fetal thyroid.

D. Parathyroid Hormone (PTH): The major function of the parathyroid glands is to regulate calcium and phosphorus metabolism. Hypoparathyroidism is marked by hypocalcemia, and hyperparathyroidism causes demineralization of bone, hypercalcemia, and hypercalciuria. Pregnancy normally induces a slight rise in maternal production of PTH during the first trimester. The calcium required for fetal growth is transported from mother to fetus via the placenta. Severe, chronic hyperparathyroidism causing osteitis fibrosa cystica is rare during pregnancy except in patients with long-standing renal disease.

E. Adrenal Hormones: The increased estrogen levels during pregnancy cause a rise in plasma transcortin that results in a large increase in bound cortisol and corticosterone in the circulation. A smaller increase in free cortisol and corticosterone is caused by altered hepatic function and elevated progesterone levels. The concentration of testosterone rises in response to the increased levels of testosterone-binding globulin caused by estrogen; however, this is not of clinical importance.

The estrogens estriol, estradiol, and estrone are secreted in greater amounts during pregnancy. Dehydroepiandrosterone (DHEA) from both mother and fetus is a necessary precursor for estradiol and estrone synthesis, and estriol is formed from 16-hydroxydehydroepiandrosterone sulfate from the fetus. Estriol is conjugated in the maternal liver and excreted by the kidney; thus, maternal plasma and urine estriol levels can be used as indicators of fetal well-being.

The considerable increase in aldosterone production after the first trimester of pregnancy may be mediated by progesterone. Increased activity of the renin-angiotensin system during pregnancy also stimulates increased adrenal production of aldosterone. Renin is produced in the kidney and angiotensin from α_2-globulin produced in the liver.

F. Ovarian Hormones: Ovarian production of progesterone and the estrogens increases rapidly in early pregnancy in response to a sudden rise in hCG production by the trophoblast. After the sixth to eighth weeks, ovarian production of these hormones declines, but the placenta takes over this function, ensuring adequate progesterone and estradiol to maintain gestation. The serum progesterone concentration reaches a plateau at about the 36th week and remains at this level until delivery. Thereafter, significant amounts of progesterone are not produced again until ovulation resumes.

The maternal serum level of 17-hydroxyprogesterone falls with declining function of the corpus luteum in early pregnancy but rises again about 1 month before term. The rise is probably due to production of the hormone by the fetal adrenal gland.

G. Prostaglandins: During pregnancy, the prostaglandins have numerous vital but as yet poorly understood functions. These include roles in the regulation of uterine blood flow and resistance to the pressor effects of angiotensin II. Prostaglandins are important to the compliance of the cervix and, because they enhance the effects of oxytocin, to the initiation and quality of labor. Prostaglandins have also been implicated in dysmenorrhea and in the development of preeclampsia-eclampsia.

Diagnosis of Pregnancy & the Duration of Pregnancy | 3

DIAGNOSIS OF PREGNANCY

Although most women appear for prenatal care convinced they are pregnant, in about one-third of cases it is difficult to make a definite clinical diagnosis before the second missed period. This is due to the variability of the physical changes, obesity, poor patient relaxation, and the possibility of tumors. A record of the time and frequency of coitus may be of help in the diagnosis of pregnancy. The grave emotional and perhaps legal consequences of misdiagnosis suggest caution; if there is doubt, reexamination should be scheduled 3–4 weeks later. If earlier confirmation is requested, a pregnancy test may be performed, but even the most sensitive—radioimmunoassay for the β subunit of hCG—may not be 100% accurate.

Pregnancy causes both obvious and subtle changes that involve many organ systems but are most pronounced in the reproductive system (see p 41). Because these subjective and objective alterations vary widely, the diagnostic criteria of pregnancy are classified as (1) presumptive, (2) probable, and (3) positive.

Presumptive Manifestations of Pregnancy

The following signs and symptoms are presumptive evidence of pregnancy, but even 2 or more are not diagnostic.

A. Symptoms:

1. Amenorrhea–Conception is usually followed by cessation of menses due to the rising titer of hCG. For unknown reasons, about 25% of pregnant women experience slight painless bleeding at some time during the first few months, either at the time of implantation or near the time of the expected period. The cause is not known.

2. Nausea and vomiting, distaste for food, and queasiness– These symptoms are reported by almost half of pregnant women during the first 3 months. Because it is most often noted upon arising, this reaction is called morning sickness; in some patients, however, it may occur only in the evening. Pungent smells or cooking odors frequently will precipitate gastric upset.

3. Breast tenderness and tingling–Engorgement of the breasts after the first weeks of pregnancy is caused by estrogen stimulation of the mammary duct system and progesterone stimulation of the alveolar components.

4. Urinary frequency and urgency–Estrogens and progesterone increase the turgescence of the bladder and urethra. Bladder irritability, urinary frequency, and nocturia are common in the first trimester.

5. Constipation–Constipation often develops early in pregnancy as a result of changing food habits or hormone-mediated hypoactive peristalsis; later, it may be caused by uterine enlargement, which displaces and compresses the intestines.

6. Fatigue–Lassitude and easy fatigability are noted by many pregnant women even a few weeks after the missed period. The cause is not known.

7. Quickening–Many primiparas perceive fetal movements at about the 16th week; multiparas, as early as the 14th week.

8. Weight gain–During pregnancy, a steady weight gain occurs from about the 10th to the 36th week, when it levels off. A sense of well-being in some, anxiety and compensatory overeating in others, or the mistaken impression that a pregnant woman should "eat for 2" is usually responsible for excessive gain.

9. Metabolic effects–These may be noted as early as the sixth week. Some pregnant women complain of a thinning and softening of the nails and joint relaxation.

10. Temperature–Elevation of the basal body temperature for longer than 3 weeks is presumptive evidence of pregnancy.

B. Signs:

1. Skin pigmentation–Facial melasma (chloasma) and darkening of the skin over the forehead, the bridge of the nose, and the malar prominences ("mask of pregnancy") occur to a variable degree in most pregnant women after the 16th week. Pigmentation of the nipples and areolas appears at about the same time. The linea nigra (pigmented linea alba) is noted after the third month and is particularly marked in brunets. In primigravidas, it follows the uterine fundus to the umbilicus; in multigravidas, the linea nigra reappears in its entirety early in the second trimester. Pigmentation is caused by pituitary melanotropin, which stimulates the melanophores in these areas particularly.

2. Epulis–Hypertrophic gingival papillae are often seen after the first trimester of pregnancy.

3. Leukorrhea–Increased cervical mucus and pronounced exfoliation of vaginal epithelial cells are caused by augmented estrogen-progesterone levels during pregnancy.

4. Breast changes–

a. Enlargement and vascular engorgement of the breasts begin at about the sixth or eighth week after conception.

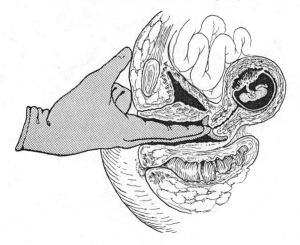

Figure 3–1. Softening of the cervix.

b. Secondary areola (a pink periareolar flush) and enlargement of the circumlacteal sebaceous glands (Montgomery's tubercles) may be noted at approximately 6–8 weeks and are due to steroid sex hormone stimulation.

c. Colostrum (''pre-milk'' secretion) is produced mainly by the actions of prolactin and progesterone and may be expressed after the 16th week.

5. Abdominal enlargement–Protuberance of the lower abdomen is usually evident after the 14th week.

6. Pelvic organ changes–See Figs 3–1 to 3–5.

a. Cyanosis of the vagina (Chadwick's sign, Jacquemier's sign) is present by about the sixth week.

b. Softening of the tip of the cervix is occasionally noted as early as the fourth or fifth week of pregnancy; however, fibrosis, infection, or scarring may prevent softening until late in pregnancy.

c. Softening of the cervico-uterine junction often occurs as early as the fifth or sixth week. A soft spot is first noted anteriorly in the midline of the uterus near the junction of the body and the cervix (Ladin's sign). A wider zone of softness and compressibility at the lower uterine segment (Hegar's sign) is the most valuable sign of early pregnancy and can usually be noted by the sixth week. Ease in flexing the fundus on the cervix (McDonald's sign) generally appears by the seventh or eighth week.

d. Irregular softening and slight enlargement of the fundus at the

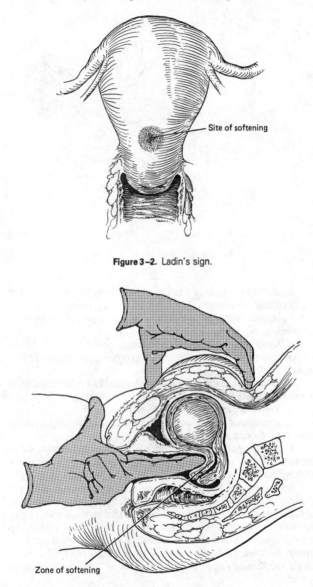

Figure 3–2. Ladin's sign.

Figure 3–3. Hegar's sign.

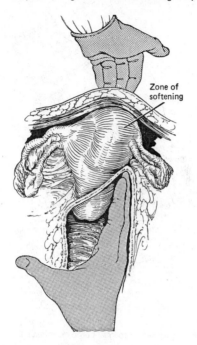

Figure 3–4. Piskacek's sign.

site of or on the side of implantation (Von Fernwald's sign) occurs by about the fifth week. When implantation is in the region of a uterine cornu, a more pronounced softening and almost tumorlike enlargement may occur (Piskacek's sign).

e. Generalized enlargement and diffuse softening of the corpus of the uterus are usually present after the eighth week of pregnancy.

f. The bony and ligamentous structures of the pelvis are also involved in the changes due to the reproductive process. The joints will develop a slight but definite relaxation. This is most noticeable in the symphysis, which may separate to an astonishing degree during pregnancy.

Probable Manifestations of Pregnancy

   A. **Symptoms:** Same as presumptive symptoms, above.
   B. **Signs:**
   1. **Uterine enlargement**–Correlation of uterine size with the dura-

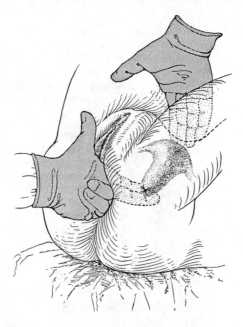

Figure 3–5. Bimanual pelvic examination.

tion of amenorrhea or the date of conception is significant from the sixth
to the 28th week. After 28 weeks, changes in the shape of the fundus, the
varying position of the fetus, and increased amniotic fluid may make
such a relation invalid.

2. Uterine souffle (bruit)–After the 16th week, a rushing sound
synchronous with the mother's pulse can often be heard bilaterally just
above the symphysis. It is due to increased blood flow to the uterus
through arteries of increased diameter and usually indicates pregnancy.

3. Uterine contractions (Braxton Hicks sign, Hicks's sign)–
Upon bimanual examination (Fig 3–5), irregular uterine contractions
may be felt after the 28th week, especially in asthenic women. These are
usually not painful, in contrast with the contractions of premature or
actual labor.

4. Positive pregnancy test–See Tables 3–1 and 3–2.

Positive Manifestations of Pregnancy

A. Symptoms: No subjective evidence of pregnancy can be accepted as diagnostic.

B. Signs: Any one of the following signs is medical and legal proof of pregnancy. They are usually not present until after the fourth month.

1. Auscultation of fetal heartbeat–One must be able to hear distinctly *and count* the fetal heartbeat. It is faster than the mother's and resembles the tick of a watch under a pillow. Auscultation is generally possible in slender women after the 17th–18th weeks. Electronic identification of the fetal heart pulse using Doppler ultrasound is possible after the 12th week.

2. Palpation of fetal outline–After the 24th week, the fetal outline may be identified in many pregnant women.

3. Recognition of fetal movements–

a. Active movements are usually palpable after the 18th week.

b. By the 16th–18th weeks, passive movements of the fetus can often be elicited by abdominal and vaginal palpation. A firm tap on the uterine wall or vaginal fornix displaces the fetus as a "floating body," which can then be felt as a thrust as it moves back to its accustomed position (ballottement). Ascites and tumors must be excluded.

4. X-ray demonstration of fetal skeleton–An oblique view of the abdomen may reveal fetal bones as early as the 12th week. An anteroposterior film may not disclose a definite skeleton until the 16th week because of the interference of bowel shadows and the variable density of the sacrum. *Caution:* X-ray films should be avoided whenever possible during pregnancy to protect against gonadal damage and the possibility of genetic abnormalities.

5. Ultrasonography–Ultrasonography records high-frequency sound waves as they are reflected from anatomic structures. Repeated bursts of sound waves from a transducer are transmitted through tissues. Between transmissions, the transducer is switched to act as an echo receiver. Since the tissues have different densities, each returns a different echo depending upon the energy reflected. This echo signal is electronically measured and converted into a 2-dimensional picture (sonogram) of the area under examination.

The following are examples of types of ultrasonography and their clinical uses:

a. The A mode allows mainly linear measurement and may suffice for determining intrapelvic diameters or fetal dimensions such as the fetal biparietal distance.

b. The B mode provides spatial reconstruction imaging of the reflected ultrasound waves. An advanced type of B mode ultrasonography is real-time ultrasonography, which gives rapid, sequential spatial reconstruction of reflected ultrasound waves to show motion. B mode gray scale imaging uses a television display and reconstruction of images to reveal broad amplitude differences and give better resolution. This is the equivalent of fluoroscopy because cinema type imaging is possible; thus, fetal movements such as respiratory or cardiac activity can be accurately observed. This dynamic system is most useful in obstetrics.

Ultrasonography uses no ionizing radiation when employed for diagnosis. It is noninvasive but may be used in conjunction with invasive procedures, eg, to guide or control needle insertion, as in amniocentesis or to obtain a needle biopsy. Ultrasonography has no demonstrable biologic side-effects and causes no somatic or genetic damage. There is an extremely high safety factor for both mother and fetus; innumerable repeat examinations are possible. Transverse and longitudinal spatial reproductions with this method give data in 3 dimensions. Moreover, ultrasonographic equipment is relatively inexpensive, and examinations can be performed at much less cost than arteriography or computerized tomography (CT scan). Some disadvantages of ultrasonography are that contrast media have not been developed to extend the applicability of the method and that most of the equipment is not automated, so that considerable skill and experience are required to use it effectively.

Ultrasonography may have its greatest application in obstetrics. Pregnancy can be diagnosed as early as the fourth week, and twins have been identified during the sixth week. Hydatidiform mole can be diagnosed and abortion predicted. With frequent (often weekly) ultrasonographic measurements, determination of fetal growth as an index of fetal health becomes extremely accurate. Fetal respiratory movements, swallowing, and voiding can be studied. The site and extent of the placenta can be mapped.

Diagnostic ultrasonography is also an accurate means of identifying and localizing pelvic masses and estimating their size. The overall accuracy is excellent, although occasional errors may occur because of overinterpretation of bowel loops or misinterpretation of small lesions at the lower limit of resolution. Whatever the problem, the physician and the ultrasonographer should collaborate in arriving at an interpretation of the recording.

6. Fetal electrocardiography–A fetal ECG can first be recorded at about the 84th day of pregnancy (12 weeks).

DIFFERENTIAL DIAGNOSIS OF PREGNANCY

All of the presumptive and probable symptoms and signs of pregnancy, as well as positive clinical and laboratory test results indicative of pregnancy, can be caused by other conditions.

Differential Diagnosis of Symptoms

A. Amenorrhea: *Caution:* Progestogens, eg, hydroxyprogesterone or oral contraceptive tablets, which are capable of causing abnormal fetal development, must not be administered to promote withdrawal bleeding in the differential diagnosis of nonpregnancy amenorrhea and early pregnancy.

1. Psychic factors–Hypothalamic (psychogenic) amenorrhea, emotional shock, fear of pregnancy or sexually transmitted disease, intense desire for pregnancy (pseudocyesis).

2. Endocrine factors–Exercise-associated amenorrhea; early menopause; lactation; pituitary, thyroid, adrenal, or ovarian dysfunction.

3. Metabolic factors–Anemia, malnutrition, climatic changes, diabetes mellitus, degenerative disorders.

4. Obliteration of the endometrial cavity by infection, curettage (Asherman's syndrome).

5. Systemic disease (acute or chronic)–Infections such as tuberculosis or brucellosis; cancer.

B. Nausea and Vomiting:

1. Emotional disorders–Pseudocyesis, anorexia nervosa.

2. Gastrointestinal disorders–Enteritis, peptic ulcer, hiatus hernia, appendicitis, intestinal obstruction, "food poisoning" (bacterial contamination of foods, toxins, allergens).

3. Acute infections–Influenza, encephalitis.

C. Breast Tenderness: Premenstrual tension, hyperestrinism (due to hormone therapy or anovulatory cycles), chronic cystic mastitis, pseudocyesis.

D. Urinary Frequency: Urinary tract infection, cystocele, pelvic tumors, emotional tension.

E. Quickening: Increased peristalsis, "gas" (especially in women preoccupied with thoughts of pregnancy), abdominal muscle contractions, shifting abdominal contents.

Differential Diagnosis of Signs

A. Epulis: Local infection, dental calculus, vitamin C deficiency.

B. Lactiferous Secretion: Persistent manual breast stimulation, residual fluid from a previous pregnancy, galactorrhea.

C. Abdominal Enlargement: Obesity of rapid onset, relaxation of abdominal muscles (as often occurs in pseudocyesis), pelvoabdominal tumors, tympanites, ascites, ventral hernia.

D. Leukorrhea: Infections and tumors of the vagina and cervix, psychically induced excessive cervical mucus.

E. Vaginal and Cervical Color Changes: Premenstrual turgescence, "pelvic congestion syndrome," venous obstruction due to pelvic tumor or infection.

F. Changes in Consistency, Size, and Shape of Cervix and Uterus: Premenstrual engorgement, notable in multiparas with uterine hypertrophy; uterine tumors, usually myomas; tubo-ovarian cysts closely adherent to the uterus; cervical stenosis and hemato-, muco-, or pyometra.

Table 3–1. Immunologic tests for pregnancy.

Method	Materials	Results
Direct coagulation	Latex particles coated with anti-hCG + serum or urine	Coagulation if hCG is present (pregnant).
Inhibition of coagulation	Anti-hCG + serum or urine **plus** Sensitized red cells **or** Latex particles coated with hCG	Coagulation if hCG is absent (not pregnant); inhibition if hCG is present (pregnant).

Diagnosis of Pregnancy

A. Elevation of Basal Body Temperature (BBT) for Longer Than 2 Weeks: This may be due to pregnancy, but it is necessary to rule out corpus luteum cyst, hCG or progesterone therapy, and faulty thermometer or incorrect methods of taking or recording the temperature.

B. Pregnancy Tests: (Tables 3–1 and 3–2.) The term pregnancy test is a misnomer because the current tests do not detect pregnancy per se but only one of the compounds associated with pregnancy: hCG. Moreover, these tests are also used to screen for complications of pregnancy (eg, hydatidiform mole) and even disorders unrelated to pregnancy (eg, germ cell testicular tumors).

A radioimmunoassay (RIA) for the β subunit of hCG is the most sensitive (earliest) pregnancy test. This test can be completed within 24 hours. It may be positive as early as the second day following implantation of the ovum or the 23rd day of the menstrual cycle in which a pregnancy occurs. This is about 5 days before the first menstrual period is missed.

Diagnosis of Previous Pregnancy

This diagnosis can never be made with certainty, but a reasonably accurate opinion can often be obtained. Examination of the breasts, including areolar pigmentation; palpation of the abdominal wall; and examination of the abdomen for striae and the vulva for episiotomy scars may give useful clues. The vaginal canal may be more relaxed in a parous woman, and the external cervical os usually appears as a transverse slit or stellate gap rather than a small circular opening as in the nulliparous patient.

Diagnosis of Fetal Death

Fetal death is as important a diagnosis as pregnancy. Failure of uterine growth and 2 negative pregnancy tests represent presumptive evidence of fetal death. However, pregnancy tests measure the hormones of the trophoblast, some of which may remain viable for some time after the fetus has died.

Table 3–2. Some representative pregnancy tests currently available.*†

Trade Name	Manufacturer	Principle‡	Method Sensitivity (mIU/mL)	Reaction Time
Pregnosis (slide)	Roche	AI	1500–2500	2 min
Sensi-Tex (tube)	Roche	AI	250	1½ h
Gest State (slide)	Fisher	AI	2000–4000	2 min
hCG Test	Hyland	AI	2000–8000	2 min
Pregnosticon (tube)	Organon	AI	750	2 h
Pregnosticon (Accu-spheres)	Organon	AI	750–1000	2 h
Pregnosticon (slide)	Organon	AI	1000–2000	2 min
Pregnosticon Dri-Dot	Organon	AI	1000–2000	2 min
Gravindex	Ortho	AI	3500	2 min
DAP Urine	Wampole	DA	2000	2 min
DAP Serum	Wampole	DA	2000	2 min
UCG (tube)	Wampole	AI	1500	2 h
UCG (slide)	Wampole	AI	2000	2 min
Biocept-G	Wampole	RRA	200	1 h
hCG (β-subunit, qualitative)	Radioassay Systems Laboratories, Inc.*	RIA	40	2 h
Preg/Stat β-hCG (qualitative)	Serono	RIA	15	1 h
β-hCG (quantitative)	Serono	RIA	3.12	3 h
β-hCG (quantitative)	Serono	RIA	1.56	18 h

*Reproduced, with permission, from Danforth D (editor): *Obstetrics and Gynecology,* 4th ed. Harper & Row, 1982.

†Data from published reports or manufacturers' information.

‡AI, agglutination inhibition; DA, direct agglutination; RRA, radioreceptor assay; RIA, radioimmunoassay.

In later pregnancy, cessation of fetal movement may be the first abnormal sign noted by the mother. The uterus may cease to enlarge over a period of 2–3 weeks. Fetal heart tones may now be absent. Certain signs and symptoms of pregnancy may disappear, eg, breast enlargement or skin pigmentation, or weight may be lost. Ultrasonography or x-ray of the fetus often shows evidence of fetal death: overlapping of the skull bones (Spalding's sign); gas in the fetus, especially in the great vessels (Robert's sign), spinal canal, or skull; and an abnormality of fetal position as evidenced by exaggeration of the spinal curvature. Some of these signs depend upon changes in fetal tissue due to maceration. Hence, if questionable ultrasonographic or x-ray findings are noted, a repeat examination should be performed. Amniocentesis may reveal concentrated dark brown fluid, which is diagnostic of fetal death.

DURATION OF PREGNANCY & EXPECTED
DATE OF CONFINEMENT (EDC)

Pregnancy in women lasts about 10 lunar months (9 calendar months). The average length of pregnancy is 266 days. The median duration of pregnancy initiated by a known single sexual exposure is 269 days. An authenticated case of a pregnancy of 360 days' duration with the delivery of a normal newborn that survived is on record.

In the absence of medical or obstetric complications, the physician's prediction regarding the duration of pregnancy is influenced by the patient's obstetric history: Some women tend to have long or short gestations, and primiparas tend to have slightly longer gestations than multiparas.

Nägele's Rule (See also Inside Back Cover.)

The expected date of confinement (EDC) or estimated date of delivery cannot be precisely calculated.

It has become traditional to calculate the EDC from Nägele's rule: Add 7 days to the first day of the last menstrual period (LMP), subtract 3 months, and add 1 year (EDC = [LMP + 7 days] − 3 months + 1 year). For example, if the first day of the LMP was June 4, the EDC will be March 11 of the following year.

Nägele's rule is based on a 28-day menstrual cycle with ovulation occurring on the 14th day; in calculating the EDC, an adjustment should be made if the patient's cycle is shorter or longer than 28 days.

The discrepancies caused by 31-day months and the 29-day variation in February of leap year are not correctable by Nägele's rule. Nevertheless, it provides an acceptable estimate of the EDC.

Only 4% of patients will deliver on the EDC after spontaneous labor. Most (60%) will deliver within 2 weeks of the EDC. One should regard "term" as a season or period of maturity, therefore, and not as a particular day.

Height of Fundus on Abdominal Wall

Until about the sixth month, the height of the fundus on the abdominal wall provides a rough estimate of the duration of pregnancy. The anteverted fundus is palpable just above the symphysis at 8–10 weeks; halfway between the symphysis and the umbilicus at 16 weeks; and at the umbilicus at 20–22 weeks (Fig 3–6).

TERM PREGNANCY

The diagnosis of term pregnancy is generally based on the estimated period of gestation and fetal measurements. Term is reached when the

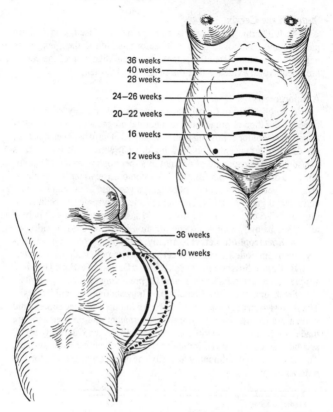

Figure 3–6. Height of fundus at various times during pregnancy.

pregnancy has persisted for at least 37 weeks. Under the best circumstances, such an infant has a 95% chance of surviving the first 28 days of life (neonatal period). Full term (ideal maturity) is reached at 40 weeks of gestation. The chance for survival at full term is raised to 99%.

When there are discrepancies in the dates, other observations (see below) will be required to diagnose term or full-term states.

Engagement

In nulliparas, a zero or plus station (Fig 6–6) suggests a term pregnancy. In multiparas, it is strong evidence that term has been reached.

Status of the Cervix

At full term, the cervix is soft, partially effaced, and slightly patulous and has moved from a posterior situation to the apex of the vaginal vault. Complete effacement and partial dilatation of the cervix are unequivocal evidence that the pregnancy is at term.

Amniocentesis

Amniotic fluid or its cellular inclusions can be analyzed to determine the duration of pregnancy. In a normal pregnancy, accurate determination of 3 of the following values denotes that term has been reached: (1) Creatinine concentration > 2 mg/dL; (2) absence of bilirubin as measured at a wavelength of 450 nm in a spectrophotometer; (3) amniotic fluid osmolality < 250 mosm/L; (4) amniotic (fetal) fat-laden cells = 10% or over 20 orange cells per high-power field after staining with commercial grade Nile blue sulfate; (5) a lecithin/sphingomyelin (L/S) ratio of 2–2.5 or a strongly positive rapid surfactant test (RST, ''bubble test''; see below), a clinical determination based on the L/S ratio.

A. Spectrophotometry: Normally, bilirubin becomes unmeasurably low in amniotic fluid at 37 weeks unless hemolytic disease exists.

B. Rapid Surfactant Test (RST, "Bubble Test"): This is a simple, rapid, and reliable technique for predicting fetal lung maturity.

Fresh amniotic fluid is obtained by transabdominal amniocentesis. The fluid is centrifuged at 2000 rpm for 15 minutes, and the supernatant is then drawn off. Two dilutions of supernatant and 95% ethanol are made—1:1 and 1:2. The tubes are capped and shaken vigorously for 30 seconds and then observed for the appearance of bubbles at the surface. The predicted fetal pulmonary maturity has been correlated with the L/S ratio as follows:

Predicted Fetal Pulmonary Maturity	L/S Ratio	RST
Mature	>2	Complete ring of bubbles persists 15 minutes at the 1:1 and 1:2 dilutions.
Intermediate	1.5–2	Complete ring of bubbles persists 15 minutes at 1:1 dilution only.
Immature	<1.5	No complete ring of bubbles at either dilution.

C. Phosphatidylglycerol Test: Phosphatidylglycerol constitutes about 10% of surfactant phospholipids, and its presence appears to improve the functioning of lung surfactant. Spot tests for phosphatidylglycerol are available, but the results must be interpreted with care.

X-Ray Visualization of Fetal Ossification Centers

To avoid genetic and developmental alterations, x-ray exposure of the mother and her fetus is contraindicated except in urgent situations. Ultrasonographic measurements of the fetus to determine gestational age are more accurate and far safer than x-ray films.

Ultrasonography

In early or mid pregnancy, the crown-rump length (CRL) as determined by ultrasonography can be translated into a reasonably accurate estimate of fetal age (Table 3–3). In late pregnancy, the dimensions of the fetal skull can be measured within 2 mm of the actual size as determined at delivery. A biparietal diameter of 9.8 cm or more is usually found with fetal maturity. The length of long bones and chest and abdominal girth have also been used as guides to fetal maturity. Ul-

Table 3–3. Crown-rump length (CRL) measurement as a determinant of fetal age.[*]

Menstrual Maturity (Weeks + Days)	CRL (mm)		Menstrual Maturity (Weeks + Days)	CRL (mm)	
	Mean	2 SD		Mean	2 SD
6 + 2	7.0	3.3	10 + 0	33.0	7.2
6 + 3	6.5	1.4	10 + 1	33.8	7.6
6 + 4	7.0	4.6	10 + 2	35.2	7.3
6 + 5	6.5	4.2	10 + 3	36.0	7.9
6 + 6	10.0	2.6	10 + 4	37.3	9.7
7 + 0	9.3	2.3	10 + 5	43.4	7.7
7 + 1	10.3	8.0	10 + 6	40.1	7.1
7 + 2	11.8	5.7	11 + 0	46.7	6.1
7 + 3	12.8	4.8	11 + 1	43.6	7.2
7 + 4	13.4	6.7	11 + 2	47.5	6.2
7 + 5	15.4	3.6	11 + 3	48.8	5.9
7 + 6	15.4	4.4	11 + 4	49.0	9.5
8 + 0	17.0	4.9	11 + 5	54.0	9.8
8 + 1	19.5	5.7	11 + 6	56.2	9.5
8 + 2	19.4	6.2	12 + 0	58.3	9.4
8 + 3	20.4	5.0	12 + 1	56.8	7.2
8 + 4	21.3	3.8	12 + 2	59.4	6.6
8 + 5	20.9	2.4	12 + 3	62.6	8.6
8 + 6	23.2	3.6	12 + 4	63.5	9.5
9 + 0	25.8	6.0	12 + 5	67.7	6.4
9 + 1	25.4	4.6	12 + 6	66.5	8.2
9 + 2	26.7	4.4	13 + 0	72.5	4.2
9 + 3	27.0	2.8	13 + 1	69.7	8.5
9 + 4	32.5	4.2	13 + 2	73.0	15.1
9 + 5	30.0	10.0	13 + 3	77.0	8.5
9 + 6	31.3	5.5	13 + 4	...	...
			13 + 5	...	...
			13 + 6	76.0	5.7
			14 + 0	79.6	7.8

[*]Reproduced, with permission, from Robinson HP, Fleming JEE: A critical evaluation of sonar "crown-rump length" measurements. *Br J Obstet Gynaecol* 1975;82:702.

trasonography can also be used to assess fetal growth and development and can be employed as early as the 13th week of gestation.

PROLONGED PREGNANCY
(Postdate or Extended Pregnancy)

Although human pregnancy has extended to 360 days with delivery of a normal infant, prolonged pregnancy, by definition, is pregnancy that extends 2 or more weeks beyond the EDC as calculated from the LMP (280 + 14 = 294 days or 42 weeks). Living anencephalic monsters have been retained for as long as 389 days before spontaneous labor and delivery.

Although some women consistently carry normal pregnancies beyond the EDC, serious concern may be raised because (1) an accurate determination of the end point of pregnancy is not yet available, and (2) the perinatal mortality rate for offspring delivered after prolonged pregnancy is 2–3 times that reported at term. Nevertheless, the hazards of postmaturity largely relate either to primiparas, especially those over 35 years of age, or to obstetric patients with complications such as malposition, isoimmunization, or hypertension.

Clinical Possibilities

(1) The pregnancy is *not* prolonged, and thus there is no threat to the fetus because of postmaturity.

(2) The pregnancy *is* prolonged.

a. Good placental function indicates no fetal jeopardy.

b. Acute placental insufficiency indicates new fetal jeopardy.

c. Chronic placental insufficiency indicates continued fetal jeopardy.

An accurate menstrual history is most helpful, with the LMP dated or even described in a diary or on a calendar. In estimating the EDC, some patients' long menstrual cycles or their use of hormone therapy must be considered.

Correlation of the History & Physical Examination

(1) If good correlation of the duration of pregnancy from the LMP is established after the first 2 prenatal visits, the EDC calculated from the initial LMP is verified.

(2) If poor correlation exists, 2 separate records in the chart should be made: the EDC from menstrual history and the EDC from initial examination.

(3) Ultrasonography should be performed at 12 weeks to clarify the gestational age. When one examination between 12 and 20 weeks is compatible with physical examination, accept the EDC calculated from

ultrasonography. If the patient is more than 20 weeks pregnant, obtain 2 serial ultrasonograms to confirm the EDC based on the initial examination.

Note: The EDC cannot be calculated when the fetal biparietal diameter is greater than 9.5 cm.

Diagnosis of Prolonged Pregnancy

The diagnosis of prolonged pregnancy can be based on ultrasonography (see above) or can be made without further corroboration at 42 weeks if the pregnancy continues with good correlation between the LMP and the physical examination. If initial observations are started at less than 20 weeks of gestational age as calculated from the physical examination, 3 of the following 4 criteria must be met before the diagnosis is considered established: (1) 36 weeks have elapsed since a positive pregnancy test. (2) 32 weeks have elapsed since Doppler recording of fetal heart tones. (3) 24 weeks have elapsed since recorded fetal movements. (4) 22 weeks have elapsed since fetal heart tones were noted by auscultation.

Other studies can be done to support the diagnosis but are not required (eg, amniotic fluid analysis to determine the L/S ratio, the creatinine concentration, or both).

Management

(1) When the diagnosis is confirmed, induce labor, monitor continuously, and observe for meconium when the membranes rupture.

(2) When diagnosis is uncertain, manage expectantly and obtain further confirmation; await additional indications for delivery.

Expectant Management (Observation Versus Delivery)

(1) Obtain weekly fetal activity determination (FAD).

(2) Assess cervical effacement and dilatation weekly.

(3) Utilize amnioscopy to detect meconium in amniotic fluid.

(4) Obtain serial plasma estriol determinations.

If induction is not indicated, consider the past obstetric history, the age of the mother, and other risk factors. Reevaluate the diagnosis of prolonged pregnancy. If the diagnosis is firm, induce labor. If there are doubts regarding the diagnosis, observe the patient further.

4 | The Placenta, Fetus, & High-Risk Neonate

THE PLACENTA & ITS STRUCTURES

Fertilization

Beginning on about the 14th day of the average ovulatory menstrual cycle, the uterine glands develop the feathery contour characteristic of pregnancy endometrium, and the stromal cells assume the polygonal shape of decidua cells. This preparation for implantation of the fertilized ovum is influenced by progesterone (elaborated by the corpus luteum) and, to a lesser extent, by estrogens.

Following capacitation (preparation of the ovum for entry of spermatozoa) and fertilization, which usually occurs in the outer portion of the uterine tube, the ovum develops into the embryonic blastocyst. About 3–4 days are required for the blastocyst to reach the uterus, and implantation ensues 5–6 days later. During the entire period prior to implantation, the embryo depends upon adherent granulosa cells and perhaps nutrient fluids within the tube and uterus for sustenance (histotrophic phase of embryo).

Implantation

The chorion, the outermost layer of the fertilized ovum, serves for nutrition and protection of the embryo and consists of an inner mesodermal layer and an outer ectodermal layer, the trophoblast. Initially the trophoblast is a poorly defined syncytium, but it soon develops into 2 tissue types: an inner, distinctly cellular cytotrophoblast (Langhans' stria) and an outer, confluent but differentiated plasmotrophoblast (syntrophoblast).

The trophoblast produces proteolytic enzymes capable of rapid destruction of endometrium and even myometrium. They enable the embryo to erode deeply and without delay into the functionalis layer of the endometrium (but usually not beyond the compacta). Deeper invasion (placenta accreta) is prevented by formation of Nitabuch's stria, a layer of hyalinized fibrin just beyond the advancing trophoblast.

Normally, the blastocyst implants on the fifth or sixth day after entry into the uterus, most commonly in the decidua lining the anterior or

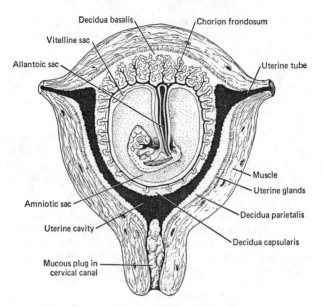

Figure 4–1. Relationships of structures in the uterus at the end of the seventh week of pregnancy.

posterior wall of the fundus. The site of nidation heals immediately. Three decidual areas can now be recognized: (1) decidua capsularis (reflexa), that portion of the uterine mucosa immediately overlying the embryo; (2) decidua basalis, beneath the embryo; and (3) decidua parietalis, the remainder of the uterine lining (Fig 4–1). The decidua capsularis disappears as the embryo grows to fill the uterine cavity. The decidua basalis is the site of future development of the placenta.

By 10–11 weeks, the amnion, chorion, and attenuated decidua capsularis, which compose the membranes of the amniotic cavity, contain sufficient fluid to come into apposition with the decidua parietalis to obliterate the uterine cavity for the duration of pregnancy.

PLACENTATION

Fetoplacental Circulation

Following implantation, small lacunae develop in the plasmotrophoblast. These later become confluent. The lacunae (future intervillous spaces) fill with maternal blood by reflux from previously tapped veins. An occasional maternal artery then opens, and a sluggish circulation is established (hematotrophic phase of embryo).

The lacunar system is separated by trabeculae, many of which develop buds or extensions. Within these branching projections, the cytotrophoblast forms a mesenchymal core. The core is later canalized, and connections are established with other potential blood vessels. The vascularized tufts, each within a maternal blood space, are now referred to as villi.

The most extensive ramification of the villous tree occurs on the part of the chorion closest to the maternal blood supply (chorion frondosum). This is the site of the future placenta. Scattered villi also form over the remainder of the chorion (chorion reflexa) but soon atrophy, leaving a smooth surface (chorion laeve).

The villous system is more like an inverted tree than an inverted chandelier. The branches pass obliquely downward and outward within the intervillous spaces. This arrangement probably permits preferential currents or gradients of blood, as in the liver. Nevertheless, such an arrangement undoubtedly encourages intervillous fibrin deposition, which is commonly seen in the mature placenta.

Cotyledons (subdivisions of the placenta) can be identified early in placentation. They are separated by columns of thin fibrous tissue, the placental septa. The septa contain no vessels. Communication within each cotyledon is provided by fenestrations. In contrast, intercotyledonous septa contain few openings. Some communication betwe.n cotyledons does exist, however, via the subchorionic lake in the roof of the intervillous spaces.

Fetal blood flow between villi probably does not occur. Hence, the concept of the placenta as a sponge is not anatomically accurate.

Uteroplacental Circulation

A. Veins: Many randomly placed venous orifices can be identified over the entire decidua basalis (basal plate of the placenta). They remain numerous throughout gestation. These veins have no sphincters, and there is no arteriolization of the veins to suggest comparison of the placenta to an arteriovenous fistula.

The human placenta has no peripheral venous collecting system. Collection of venous outflow is a function frequently ascribed to a marginal sinus. Less than one-third of the blood drains from the placenta at its margin. A marginal sinus is not seen even in the early placenta, and subchorionic marginal lakes are not commonly found in the mature placenta. Occasionally, dilated maternal vessels are found beneath the periphery of the placenta; these have been described as wreath veins, or venous lakes. They may or may not communicate with the intervillous spaces, and their significance is still debated. Nonetheless, one of these

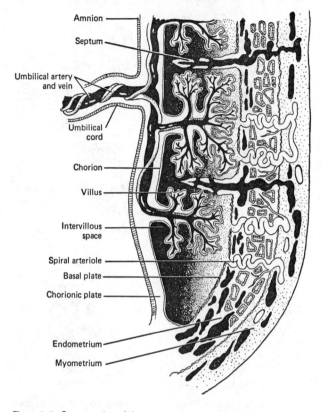

Figure 4–2. Cross section of the mature placenta. (Modified after Netter.)

thin-walled veins may be torn during premature marginal separation of the placenta, resulting in the bleeding problem erroneously called marginal sinus rupture. Actually, the problem is marginal separation of the placenta.

B. Arteries: In contrast to the veins, the arteries are grouped closer to the decidual attachments of the intercotyledinous septa. As the placenta matures, thrombosis decreases the number of arterial openings into the basal plate. At term, the ratio of veins to arteries is 2:1, approximately that found in other mature organs.

Even in an area beneath a well-formed placenta, some spiral arterioles empty into the intervillous spaces, but many remain coiled and

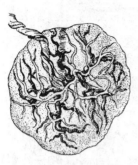

Figure 4–3. Normal placenta.

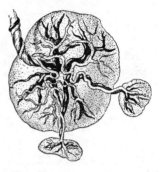

Figure 4–4. Succenturiate placenta.

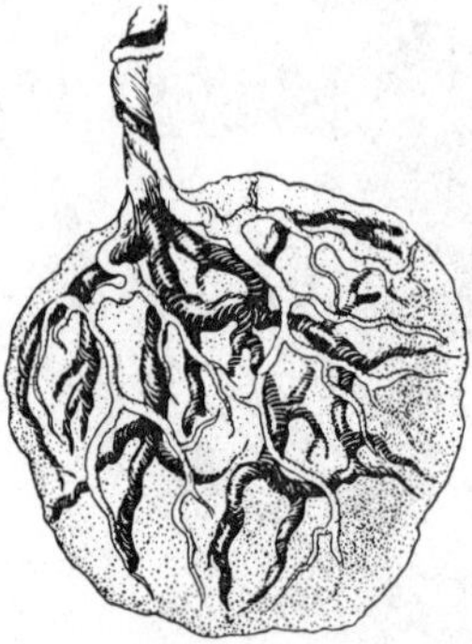

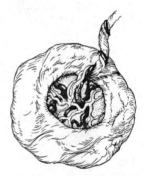

Figure 4–5. Marginal insertion, or battledore, placenta.

Figure 4–6. Marked circumvallate, or extrachorial, placenta.

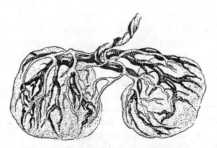

Figure 4–7. Bipartite placenta.

compressed. Arterioles supplying the intervillous spaces appear circuitous and angulated because of fixation of the vessels and growth of the placenta. The tortuosity creates baffles, or points of deflection, that tend to slow the afferent bloodstream.

Near their entry into the intervillous spaces, the terminal maternal arterioles lose their elastic reticulum. Since the distal portions of these vessels are lost with the placenta, bleeding from this source can be controlled only by uterine contraction.

THE MATURE PLACENTA*

The mature placenta (Fig 4–2) is a blue-red, rounded, flattened, meaty organ about 15–20 cm in diameter and 3 cm thick. It weighs 400–600 g, or about one-sixth the normal weight of the newborn. The umbilical cord (funis) extends from the fetal surface of the placenta to the umbilicus of the fetus; the fetal membranes arise from the placenta at its margin. In multiple pregnancy, one or more placentas may be present depending upon the number of ova implanted and the type of segmentation that occurs. The placenta is derived from both maternal and fetal tissue. At term, about four-fifths of the placenta is of fetal origin.

The maternal portion of the placenta is composed of compressed sheets of decidua basalis, remnants of blood vessels, and, at the margin, spongy decidua. Irregular grooves or clefts divide the placenta into cotyledons. The maternal surface is torn from the uterine wall at birth and as a result is rough, red, and spongy.

The fetal portion of the placenta is composed of numerous villi, branched terminals of the fetal circulation that provide for transfer of metabolic products. The villous surface, which is exposed to maternal blood, may be as much as 50 m^2 (165 sq ft). The fetal capillary system within the villi is almost 50 km (27 miles) long. Most villi are free within the intervillous spaces, but an occasional anchor villus attaches the placenta to the decidua basalis. The fetal surface of the placenta is covered by amniotic membrane and is smooth and shiny. The umbilical cord vessels course over the fetal surface before entering the placenta.

Platental Types

The normal placenta is shown in Fig 4–3. Occasionally, the placenta may have one or more succenturiate (satellite) lobes (Fig 4–4). These are attached to the main body of the placenta by a bridging major fetal artery and vein covered by intervening membranes.

In the common marginal insertion placenta, or battledore placenta

*Placenta previa is discussed in Chapter 11.

(Fig 4–5), the cord inserts at the periphery of the placenta. The battle-dore placenta poses no special problems.

In about 5% of deliveries, a yellowish opaque band of fibrous tissue will be seen to cover the fetal surface of the placenta at the periphery. Such placentas are circumvallate or circummarginate (extrachorial) placentas (Fig 4–6).

A bipartite placenta (Fig 4–7) is uncommon. The placenta is divided into 2 separate lobes but united by primary vessels and membranes.

In velamentous insertion of the cord, which is rare, the cord ends at the membranes where primary branching of the cord vessels occurs.

Umbilical Cord (Funis)

The umbilical cord is a gray, soft, coiled, easily compressible structure that connects the fetus with its placenta. It averages 50 cm in length and 2 cm in diameter and is covered by a thin layer of stratified squamous epithelium comparable to fetal skin. The cord contains a framework of loose fibrous connective tissue and is filled with a mucoid material (Wharton's jelly). Normally, the cord contains 2 arteries that carry deoxygenated blood from the fetus and one vein that supplies the fetus with oxygenated blood. The cord usually has an eccentric insertion into the placenta. One umbilical artery is absent in about 1% of single-tons and 6% of twins, and about 50% of these infants have other structural anomalies.

Fetal Membranes

The chorion and amnion arise from the placenta at its margin to envelop the fetus. They strip easily from the fetal surface of the placenta and can be separated from one another by careful dissection.

The amnion is a double-layered translucent membrane; its outer layer is mesodermal connective tissue, and its inner layer is ectoderm. The amnion may be considered an extension of the skin of the fetus. Although it consists generally of a few layers of stratified squamous cells, patches of low cuboidal cells are also seen. Thickened squamous areas are occasionally observed, especially near the umbilical cord.

The placental membranes contain the amniotic fluid and provide a barrier against infection for the fetus. They provide a 2-way exchange system for fluids, electrolytes, and hormones between the mother and fetus.

(Note: A check for completeness of the membranes at delivery is essential to avoid infection or bleeding associated with retained products of conception.)

Amniotic Fluid

At term, the fetus is submerged in about 1 L of clear watery fluid (though up to 2 L may be normally present) of low specific gravity (about 1.008) and mild alkalinity (pH about 7.2). The amniotic fluid protects the fetus from direct injury, aids in maintaining its temperature, allows free movement of the fetus, minimizes the likelihood of adherence of the fetus to the amniotic membrane, and allows for hormonal, fluid, and electrolyte exchange. It acts as a repository for fetal secretions and excretions. It contains fetal squamous debris, flecks of vernix, a few leukocytes, and small quantities of albumin, urates, and other organic and inorganic salts. The calcium content of amniotic fluid is low (5.5 mg/dL), but the electrolyte concentration is otherwise equivalent to that of maternal plasma. Hormones (eg, estriol) are found in the amniotic fluid in small amounts.

Amniotic fluid is variously considered to be a secretion of the amnion, a vascular transudate, or fetal urine. It is probably all 3, but the first is most important. Approximately 350–375 mL of amniotic fluid is replaced each hour. Retention of only a few milliliters per hour will soon result in polyhydramnios (> 2 L of amniotic fluid), while excessive clearance will cause oligohydramnios (< 300 mL of amniotic fluid at term).

PHYSIOLOGY OF THE PLACENTA

The placenta has 2 principal functions: It acts as a transfer organ for metabolic products, and it produces or metabolizes the hormones and enzymes necessary for the maintenance of pregnancy. It thus acts as a lung, a gastrointestinal tract, a kidney, and a complex of ductless glands for the conceptus.

Like any other organ, the placenta lives and "breathes." It derives most if not all of its nourishment from maternal blood. The metabolic activity of the placenta may be measured by its oxygen consumption. The placenta is a poorly compensated organ, however. Continued growth of the placenta is feasible only to a point, and its functional capacity and oxygen consumption decline in late pregnancy.

Hemodynamics

Prior to labor, placental filling occurs whenever the uterus contracts (Braxton Hicks contractions). At these times, the maternal venous exits are closed but the thicker-walled arteries are only slightly narrowed. When the uterus relaxes, blood drains out via the maternal veins. Blood is thus not squeezed out of the placenta with each contraction, nor does it enter in appreciably greater amounts during relaxation.

There is little short-circuiting of blood from an arterial opening to an adjacent venous outlet, because the arterial pressure of the maternal blood (60–70 mm Hg) actually causes it to be squirted into the low-pressure (20 mm Hg) intervillous space. Maternal arterial blood is directed toward the chorionic plate, whereas venous blood in the placenta tends to flow along the basal plate and out. This establishes circulation currents.

Maternal blood flow through the placenta at term is about 500 mL/min, whereas only about 400 mL of fetal blood circulates through the placenta each minute.

The slow rate of circulation within the placenta is offset by the capacity of the placenta, which exceeds that of the vessels supplying and draining it, as well as by the excess of maternal over fetal blood. Changes in maternal blood pressure therefore have only a gradual effect on the intervillous blood pressure in the placenta. Mechanisms to improve placental transfer are few, however. An increased rate of rhythmic uterine contractions is helpful; but strong, prolonged labor contractions are detrimental to the placental and fetal circulation. An increased fetal heart rate tends to expand the villi during systole, and this is a minor aid in circulatory transfer.

The pressure gradient within the fetal circulation changes slowly with the mother's posture, fetal movements, and physical stress. The pressure within the placental intervillous space is about 10 mm Hg when the pregnant woman is lying down. After she stands for a few minutes, this pressure exceeds 30 mm Hg. In comparison, the fetal capillary pressure remains at about 20 mm Hg.

The Placental Barrier

The human placental barrier is represented initially by 2 layers of trophoblastic cells that separate the maternal and fetal bloodstreams. The outer layer is the syntrophoblast, or plasmotrophoblast; the inner layer is the cytotrophoblast, or Langhans' stria. After the third month, the cytotrophoblast normally loses its continuity, and the cells become less numerous. Therefore, in late pregnancy, the only separation between maternal blood and the fetal vascular endothelium is the syntrophoblast, a single cell layer that is, in essence, a transfer membrane. However, this is a poor barrier, only a limited number of high molecular weight substances (eg, insulin, hCG) are completely blocked. Thus, the term "barrier" is something of a misnomer. Nonetheless, the placenta serves as a time barrier rather than a concentration barrier in most instances. If a drug can be absorbed through the maternal gastrointestinal tract, it can cross the placenta; but passage takes time, and the presence of a drug in the cord blood does not necessarily mean that the drug has reached effective levels in the fetal brain. It takes almost 40 minutes for thiopental to achieve an anesthetic level in the fetal brain but only 5 minutes for the mother to be anesthetized.

Placental Transfer

Transfer across the placental barrier is accomplished by at least 5 different processes: simple diffusion, facilitated diffusion, active transport, pinocytosis (engulfment of particles by cells), and leakage through defects.

A. Simple Diffusion: Substances required for the maintenance of fetal life and the elimination of its waste products are handled largely by diffusion across the placental barrier. Included in this group are oxygen, CO_2, water, electrolytes, and urea. Fetal and maternal blood have similar diffusion constants, so that passage of these substances is rapid in either direction. Large quantities of certain substances are involved; near term, almost 4 L of water clears the placenta each hour.

Fortunately, the fetal oxygen requirements are less than those of the newborn. Oxygen tension in the intervillous space is only about half that in the maternal pulmonary veins. The fetus is compensated to a degree, at least, because fetal hemoglobin carries slightly more oxygen than adult hemoglobin. Moreover, fetal blood also eliminates CO_2 better than the blood of the newborn.

Substances of low molecular weight (< 1000) diffuse across the placenta with ease. Thyroxine, thiamine, and many drugs, including alcohol and morphine, are in this group. Large molecules (MW > 1000) such as blood proteins and chorionic gonadotropin do not pass the placental barrier by diffusion.

B. Facilitated Diffusion: Certain substances important to the fetus (eg, glucose) are transported across the placenta more rapidly than is possible by simple diffusion. In these instances, a carrier system functions with the chemical gradient, but the system may become saturated at high concentrations. (This mechanism differs from active transport, which operates against the gradient.)

C. Active Transport: The placenta concentrates certain substances (eg, amino acids) during their transit from mother to fetus. Enzymatic mechanisms probably are responsible for the selective transport of essential nutrients. This cannot be explained by differential protein building or by other identified processes.

D. Pinocytosis: Ultramicroscopy has shown moving pseudopodial projections of the plasmotrophoblastic layer that reach out, as it were, to surround minute amounts of maternal plasma. These particles are carried across the cell virtually intact and released on the other side, whereupon they promptly gain access to the fetal circulation. This process may work both to and from the fetus, but how selective it is has not been determined. Complex proteins, small amounts of fat, and perhaps immune bodies may traverse the placenta in this way.

E. Leakage Through Defects: Trophoblastic endothelial junctions may "leak" small amounts of plasma and blood cells. Maternal and fetal blood may mix as a result of any of the following processes:

1. Degenerative changes, eg, subchorionic fibrin accumulation ("fibrinoid" degeneration), which may cause necrosis within the area;

Table 4–1. Embryonic and fetal growth and development.

Fertilization Age (weeks)	Crown-Rump Length*	Crown-Heel Length*	Weight*	Gross Appearance	Internal Development
Embryonic Stage					
1	0.5 mm	0.5 mm	?	Minute clone free in uterus.	Early morula. No organ differentiation.
2	2 mm	2 mm	?	Ovoid vesicle superficially buried in endometrium.	External trophoblast. Flat embryonic disk forming 2 inner vesicles (amnioectomesodermal and endodermal).
3	3 mm	3 mm	?	Early dorsal concavity changes to convexity; head, tail folds form; neural grooves close partially.	Optic vesicles appear. Double heart recognized. Fourteen mesodermal somites present.
4	4 mm	4 mm	0.4 g	Head is at right angle to body; limb rudiments obvious, tail prominent.	Vitelline duct only communication between umbilical vesicle and intestines. Initial stage of most organs has begun.
8	1.7 cm	3.5 cm	2 g	Eyes, ears, nose, mouth recognizable; digits formed, tail almost gone.	Sensory organ development well along. Ossification beginning in occiput, mandible, humerus (diaphysis), and clavicles. Small intestines coil within umbilical cord. Pleural, pericardial cavities forming. Gonadal development advanced without differentiation.
Fetal Stage					
12	5.8 cm	11.5 cm	19 g	Skin pink, delicate; resembles a human being, but head is disproportionately large.	Brain configuration roughly complete. Internal sex organs now specific. Uterus no longer bicornuate. Blood forming in marrow. Upper cervical to lower sacral arches and bodies ossify.

16	13.5 cm	19 cm	100 g	Scalp hair appears. Fetus active. Arm-leg ratio now proportionate. Sex determination possible.	Sex organs grossly formed. Myelinization. Heart muscle well developed. Lobulated kidneys in final situation. Meconium in bowel. Vagina and anus open. Ischium ossified.
20	18.5 cm	22 cm	300 g	Legs lengthen appreciably. Distance from umbilicus to pubis increases.	Sternum ossifies.
24	23 cm	32 cm	600 g	Skin reddish and wrinkled. Slight subcuticular fat. Vernix. Primitive respiratorylike movements.	Os pubis (horizontal ramus) ossifies. Viability possible.
28	27 cm	36 cm	1100 g	Skin less wrinkled; more fat. Nails appear. If delivered, may survive with optimal care.	Testes at internal inguinal ring or below. Astragalus ossifies. Less than 10% survive with the best of care.
32	31 cm	41 cm	1800 g	Fetal weight increased proportionately more than length.	Middle fourth phalanges ossify. About 60% survive with specialty care.
36	35 cm	46 cm	2500 g (for Caucasian)	Skin pale, body rounded. Lanugo disappearing. Hair fuzzy or wooly. Earlobes soft with little cartilage. Umbilicus in center of body. Testes in inguinal canals; scrotum small with few rugae. Few sole creases.	Distal femoral ossification centers present. About 70–80% survive with individual care.
40	40 cm	52 cm	3200+ g	Skin smooth and pink. Copious vernix. Moderate to profuse silky hair. Lanugo hair on shoulders and upper back. Earlobes stiffened by thick cartilage. Nasal and alar cartilages. Nails extend over tips of digits. Testes in full, pendulous, rugous scrotum (or labia majora) well developed. Creases cover sole.	Proximal tibial ossification centers present. Cuboid, tibia (proximal epiphysis) ossify. Over 95% survive with good care.

*Approximate.

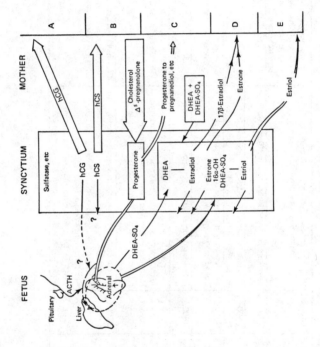

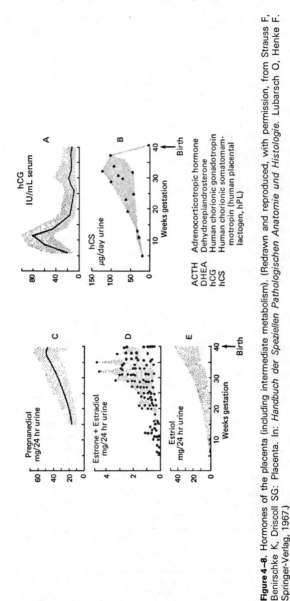

Figure 4-8. Hormones of the placenta (including intermediate metabolism). (Redrawn and reproduced, with permission, from Strauss F, Benirschke K, Driscoll SG: Placenta. In: *Handbuch der Speziellen Pathologischen Anatomie und Histologie.* Lubarsch O, Henke F. Springer-Verlag, 1967.)

ACTH   Adrenocorticotropic hormone
DHEA   Dehydroepiandrosterone
hCG   Human chorionic gonadotropin
hCS   Human chorionic somatomam-
       motropin (human placental
       lactogen, hPL)

intervillous fibrin deposition with ischemic necrosis of the villi; infarction of a small portion of the placenta or even of entire cotyledons following the occlusion of a branch of the umbilical artery; and syncytial degeneration or incomplete loss of investment of villi (partially "naked" villi).

2. Functional stresses, eg, stretching of the villous tree during increased fetal intracapillary pressure or relaxation of the villous tree after fetal capillary contraction.

3. Infection, eg, tuberculous placentitis, granulomatous lesions of coccidioidomycosis, or pyogenic abscess of the placenta.

4. Trauma, eg, premature separation of the placenta (especially abruptio placentae) or manipulation of the uterus.

5. Abnormal development of the placenta, eg, hydatidiform mole or choriocarcinoma with local necrosis.

Hormone Changes During Pregnancy
(See Figs 4–8 and 4–9.)

With the onset of pregnancy, the pattern of circulating hormones changes abruptly from that of the normal menstrual cycle.

A. Estrogens: Estrogens are produced in ever-increasing amounts by the syncytiotrophoblast. The placenta cannot produce the required estrogen precursors but synthesizes estrogens from precursors supplied by the mother and the fetus. The most potent estrogen, 17β-estradiol, is derived from dehydroepiandrosterone from both mother and fetus and from testosterone of maternal ovarian origin. This estrogen, like the weakest estrogen, estriol, increases approximately 1000-fold from the onset of pregnancy to term. Estrone, metabolized principally from androstenedione synthesized from maternal cholesterol and fetal and maternal dehydroepiandrosterone, increases only 100-fold over the nonpregnant level; and, although it seems therefore to be of minor importance, estrone together with estradiol is vital for fetal growth and development. Estriol, the largest fraction of the total estrogens during pregnancy, is largely produced from fetal 16-hydroxydehydroepiandrosterone. Since the fetal precursors are such an important source of estriol, estriol determinations in maternal plasma or urine are used as measures of fetal well-being (eg, in diabetes mellitus or preeclampsia).

B. Progestogens: 17α-Hydroxyprogesterone declines to very low levels after an initial slight elevation about 2 weeks after the beginning of pregnancy. It is probably produced by the corpus luteum, whose function is almost totally taken over by the placenta after pregnancy is well established. In contrast, progesterone, which is produced by the placenta, increases daily after the beginning of pregnancy to more than double the prepregnancy value. Progesterone is metabolized about equally by the maternal liver and by the fetal liver and adrenal cortex. The final metabolites are 20α-dihydroprogesterone and pregnanediol.

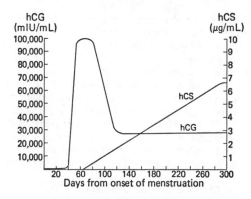

Figure 4–9. hCG and hCS levels in peripheral circulation during pregnancy. (Reproduced, with permission, from Dignam WJ: Chapter 3 in *Current Obstetric & Gynecologic Diagnosis & Treatment,* 4th ed. Benson RC [editor]. Lange, 1982.)

Progesterone is a precursor principally of the glucocorticoids and mineralocorticoids of the fetus. Progesterone can also be synthesized in the placenta from acetates or cholesterol; the estrogens cannot. The concentration of progesterone and its metabolite pregnanediol may be an index of placental function, independent of the fetus. Certainly, a failing placenta cannot support the fetus. Hence, falling pregnanediol (or estriol) values indicate that the pregnancy is in serious jeopardy.

C. hCG: Chorionic gonadotropin (hCG) is produced by the cytotrophoblast. Its concentration rises sharply after implantation of the fertilized ovum and reaches a peak value of about 60,000 mIU/mL around the eighth week, then falls sharply to a lower level by about the 120th day and remains at this level to term. It disappears from the circulation within 2 weeks after delivery. hCG is secreted directly into the maternal plasma, virtually none reaching the fetal blood. hCG is luteotropic and, like LH, stimulates the production of progesterone, 17-hydroxyprogesterone, and estrogens. The physiologic role of hCG, particularly in later pregnancy, is not known. It is apparently important for maintenance of the corpus luteum in very early pregnancy, but after the first few weeks of gestation the corpus luteum itself is no longer essential to the maintenance of pregnancy. Recent studies suggest an immunologic role for hCG (may inhibit lymphocyte response to "foreign placenta").

Because of its rapid rise early in pregnancy and continued high output throughout gestation, tests for hCG in the urine have formed the basis for virtually all pregnancy tests. Immunologic tests for hCG have supplanted animal assays. The α subunit of hCG is nearly identical with that of LH, but their β subunits differ. Thus, radioimmunoassays for the β subunit of hCG in serum have become the most sensitive tests, allowing very early accurate diagnosis of pregnancy.

hCG is not absolutely specific for pregnancy. Small amounts are secreted by a variety of gastrointestinal and other tumors, and it is measured in individuals with suspected tumors as a "tumor marker."

D. FSH: Plasma follicle-stimulating hormone (FSH) rapidly falls to scarcely detectable levels about 10 days after ovulation, never rising again until ovulation occurs several months or more after delivery. The activity of the anterior pituitary is probably suppressed by hCG and later by prolactin.

E. hCS: Chorionic somatomammotropin (hCS), formerly called human placental lactogen (hPL), is chemically and biologically related to growth hormone (GH). It is produced by the syncytiotrophoblast and secreted directly into the maternal circulation. The titer rises in almost linear fashion from the second month to delivery. hCS is lactogenic and has most of the actions of GH. It appears to function as a "maternal growth hormone of pregnancy," increasing nitrogen, potassium, and calcium retention and decreasing glucose utilization. hCS is largely responsible for the diabetogenic effect (resistance to insulin) seen during pregnancy. Since serum hCS levels are proportionate to placental weight, the hCS level has been used to screen for multiple pregnancy. Low hCS levels are a sign of placental insufficiency.

F. Other Protein Hormones: The placenta also produces chorionic thyrotropin (CT) but not corticotropin.

Complete sex steroid hormone (estrogen and progesterone) production by the placenta alone is impossible because the necessary enzymes are lacking. However, the fetal and maternal adrenal cortices produce the precursors needed for placental synthesis of the hormones. This is the basis for the concept and term "maternal-fetal-placental unit."

Estrogens are bound to serum albumin in the maternal circulation and are therefore metabolized slowly. Progesterone, on the other hand, is unbound and is metabolized rapidly. Thyroxine (T_4) is bound to α-globulin and prealbumin. Corticosteroids are held in relatively inactive form in plasma by transcortin. Thus, the titer of hydroxycorticosteroids is high during pregnancy, although frank Cushing's syndrome is uncommon.

PLACENTAL DISORDERS

Placental Insufficiency (Dysmaturity)

Placental insufficiency is an obstetric concept used to explain fetal growth retardation, dysmaturity, or otherwise unaccounted for fetal death. Small placentas and fetuses are associated with glomerulonephritis and long-standing hypertension, cyanotic heart disease, and systemic lupus erythematosus. Small placental size or early placental aging can result in progressive reduction of the placenta as an effective anabolic-catabolic fetal organ.

A persistently failing placenta may cause chronic or prolonged fetal distress manifested by subnormal fetal growth, apparent in severe diabetes mellitus or preeclampsia. Acute placental insufficiency, as with premature separation of the placenta, may cause sudden, acute fetal distress.

Clinical signs of placental insufficiency are failure of the uterus to enlarge at the normal rate, oligohydramnios (common), a small or malnourished infant, and frequently, a placenta that is smaller than average for gestational age. Pathologic examination of placental tissue shows microinfarcts, diffuse perivillous fibrin deposition, and occlusion of vessels of the villous system, all of which imply reduced function.

Serial plasma or 24-hour urinary estriol levels may be used to assess maternal-fetal-placental function. Plasma and urinary levels of estriol rise progressively to term during the second half of pregnancy; at term, the range of plasma estriol is 4–25 ng/dL and that of urinary estriol is 8–37 mg/24 h. Estriol levels are higher in multiple gestation, but they fail to rise normally with molar pregnancy, anencephaly, or placental sulfatase deficiency. Moreover, considerable variability in estriol levels is common in late pregnancy; hence, single determinations are neither reliable nor adequate. Be this as it may, a sudden sustained fall in serial estriol levels occurs in fetal death, and a slow (or rapid) drop usually is observed when serious fetal jeopardy develops, eg, dysmaturity, preeclampsia-eclampsia, diabetes mellitus.

Placental Infection (Placentitis)

Placentitis is a bacterial or viral infection usually involving the fetal surface of the placenta, particularly the chorion and amnion near the insertion of the umbilical cord. Placentitis generally is a sequela to chorioamnionitis. A "steamy" or milky appearance of the membranes due to the presence of inflammatory cells and exudative products is characteristic of chorioamnionitis and placentitis. Perivascular leukocytic infiltration of the cord and placental fetal vessels is typical of omphalitis or placentitis. Focal infection involving the villi and even the decidual plate may occur. Puerperal sepsis, a major cause of maternal death and disability, commonly begins with placentitis. Fetal pneumonia, omphalitis, and septicemia also are serious complications associated with chorioamnionitis and placentitis.

Placental Infarcts

Infarcts of the placenta, which appear as red to pale, firm areas containing degenerating villi and fibrin, are quite common. They result from interference with the maternal blood supply to the intervillous space. The trophoblast is dependent upon the maternal rather than the fetal blood supply, so that occlusion of a maternal artery supplying a major cotyledon will result in the ischemic necrosis of a large portion of that vascular unit. This occurs more often with preeclampsia-eclampsia than during normal pregnancy.

Intervillous thrombosis with extensive fibrin deposition is common also. When intervillous thrombosis is extensive, placental insufficiency and fetal growth retardation or fetal death may develop.

Tumors of the Placenta or Membranes

Except for hydatidiform mole and choriocarcinoma (see below), tumors of the placenta are rare. The only common benign tumor is chorioangioma, which is probably a chorionic mesenchymal hamartoma. This abnormality has been associated with fetal maldevelopment of one of twins, perhaps because of shunting of blood.

Amnion nodosum is an uncommon abnormality of the amnion that may represent evidence of disease of this membrane or of incorporation of fetal extradermal derivatives. It is characterized grossly by small pearly irregularities on the fetal surface of the amnion that can be shown microscopically to be plaques of benign squamous cells. Amnion nodosum is associated in most cases with oligohydramnios and major abnormalities of the fetal urinary tract or, more rarely, the gastrointestinal tract.

Placental Vascular Anomalies

A 2-vessel cord (absence of one umbilical artery) occurs about once in 500 deliveries. The cause may be aplasia or atrophy of the missing vessel. For unknown reasons, the anomaly is more common in blacks than whites but is equally frequent in primiparas and multiparas. Other congenital malformations will be diagnosed in about half of newborns with 2-vessel cords, but no particular organ system is likely to be involved. Abnormally early delivery is not an associated problem, but undergrowth of the offspring is common.

True knots, generally in abnormally long cords, are noted in about 1% of deliveries. Loose knots are unimportant, but tight knots cause cord compression and fetal distress and may cause death of the fetus.

FETAL NUTRITION

There are 3 stages of fetal nutrition: (1) Absorption: Minimal quantities of tubal and uterine fluid are taken in by the fertilized ovum during the 3–4 days before nidation. (2) Histotrophic transfer: Strategic and waste materials are passed between the early embryo and decidua for at least 2 months before the establishment of an effective fetal circulation. (3) Hematotrophic transfer: Anabolic and catabolic products cross the placental barrier by both active and passive processes.

FETAL-NEONATAL PHYSIOLOGY

CARDIOVASCULAR FUNCTION

Unmistakable hematopoiesis begins in the liver, spleen, and mesonephros at about the second month of gestation, although clumps or islands of blood cells may be seen in the yolk sac during the first 1–2 months of fetal life. The fetus shows a relative leukocytosis, the white cell count being 15–20 thousand/μL at term. Very early in human development, all the circulating red cells are nucleated; by the third month, only about 10% of the red cells still retain their nuclei; and at term, only 5–8% are nucleated. Premature as well as mature infants are polycythemic by adult standards, having red cell counts of 4–6 million/μL. Macrocytic erythrocytes are typical of the entire fetal period. Fetal and adult red cells have the same life span, approximately 120 days.

A gradual relative increase in hemoglobin occurs as the fetus develops. Normally, the hemoglobin totals about 20 g and the hematocrit 40–60% at term. Fetal hemoglobin (hemoglobin F) is the type present from the 13th week until about the 24th week, when adult hemoglobin (hemoglobin A) appears. At term, 15–45% of the hemoglobin is type A. After delivery, the proportion of hemoglobin A in the infant's blood increases rapidly; in most instances, less than 2% of the hemoglobin detected at age 1 year is hemoglobin F.

Ferritin, the iron storage protein essential to the production of hemoglobin, is present in the placenta as early as the first month and increases in amount through the sixth month. Ferritin appears in the fetal liver during the second and third months and may be recovered from the spleen after the fourth month. In contrast with the newborn and the adult, it is absent from the intestines. The relative amount of ferritin in the fetus does not vary significantly during gestation.

Fetal blood is slightly more saturated with oxygen than maternal blood. This heightened affinity for oxygen is due more to increased permeability of the fetal erythrocytic membrane than to the type of hemoglobin contained, but hemoglobin F augments the oxygen-carrying capacity of fetal blood.

Environmental changes occurring in the abrupt transition from intrauterine life to an independent existence necessitate certain circulatory adaptations in the newborn. These include diversion of blood flow through the lungs, closure of the ductus arteriosus and foramen ovale, and obliteration of the ductus venosus and umbilical vessels (see p 93).

Infant circulation has 3 phases (Figs 4–10 to 4–12): (1) the predelivery phase, in which the fetus depends upon the placenta; (2) the intermediate phase, which begins immediately after delivery with the infant's first breath; and (3) the adult phase, which is normally completed during the first few months of life.

Predelivery Phase

The umbilical vein carries oxygenated blood from the placenta to the fetus. At the umbilicus, the vein branches and enters the liver; a small branch, the ductus venosus, bypasses the liver to enter the inferior vena cava directly.

Blood from the inferior vena cava enters the right heart, and most of it is immediately shunted through the widely patent foramen ovale into the left atrium. A smaller quantity enters the pulmonary artery. From the left atrium, the oxygenated blood passes into the left ventricle and thence into the ascending aorta. The head, coronary arteries, and upper extremities are thus well supplied with oxygenated blood. Only a small amount of blood from the left ventricle flows into the descending aorta.

Blood returning from the head enters the right atrium via the superior vena cava. From the right atrium, it flows into the right ventricle and thence into the pulmonary artery. A small amount of the pulmonary arterial blood goes to the lungs; most flows directly into the descending aorta via the ductus arteriosus.

Most of the blood in the descending aorta returns to the placenta via the hypogastric (internal iliac) arteries, from which the umbilical arteries branch. The remainder circulates through the lower extremities and abdominal pelvic viscera and then into the inferior vena cava, whence it is returned, along with the large volume of oxygenated blood from the placenta, to the right heart. The cycle is then repeated.

Blood reaches the inferior vena cava by 3 routes: (1) around the liver via the ductus venosus (oxygenated blood); (2) from the liver via the hepatic and portal veins (oxygenated and deoxygenated blood); and (3) from the lower extremities via the iliac veins (deoxygenated blood). The largest volume of blood in the inferior vena cava, however, is oxygenated blood from the placenta.

The right atrium receives oxygenated blood from the inferior vena

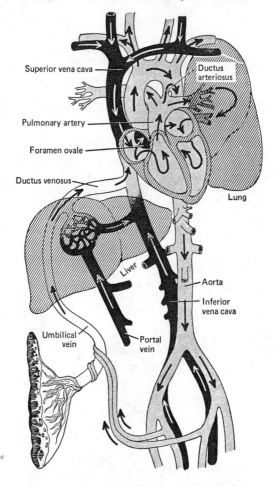

Figure 4–10. Fetal circulation.

cava and deoxygenated blood from the superior vena cava. The structure and position of the foramen ovale between the right and left atria are such, however, that the stream of blood is split; most of the blood from the inferior vena cava passes through the foramen ovale into the left atrium; the blood from the superior vena cava is directed into the right ventricle.

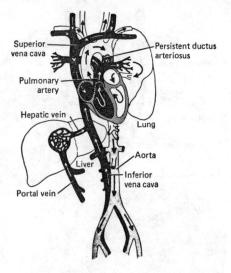

Figure 4–11. Circulation immediately after delivery.

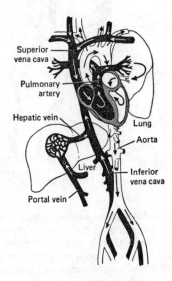

Figure 4–12. Normal circulation.

Fifty to 60% of the cardiac output goes to the placenta, which offers a low resistance; about 35% perfuses body tissue; and only 10–15% passes through the more resistant pulmonary bed.

The oxygen tension of blood (P_{O_2}) in the umbilical vein is considerably lower than that of arterial or even venous blood after birth. In the fetal circulation itself, blood oxygen saturation varies widely (umbilical vein, 80%; left ventricle, 60%). This is only about 30% of the normal adult P_{O_2}.

Intermediate Phase

At birth, 2 events alter fetal hemodynamics: (1) ligation of the umbilical cord causes an abrupt though transient rise in arterial pressure; and (2) a rise in plasma CO_2 and fall in blood P_{O_2} help to initiate regular breathing.

With the first few breaths, the intrathoracic pressure of the newborn remains low (−40 to −50 mm Hg); after distention of the airways, however, the pressure rises to the normal adult level (−7 to −8 mm Hg). The initially high vascular resistance of the pulmonary bed is probably reduced by 75–80%. Pressure in the pulmonary artery falls by at least 60%, whereas pressure in the left atrium doubles.

In the fetus, the high resistance of the pulmonary bed causes most of the deoxygenated blood in the pulmonary artery to enter the descending aorta via the ductus arteriosus. With expansion of the lungs and the drop in resistance of the pulmonary bed in the newborn, most of the blood from the right ventricle enters the lungs via the pulmonary artery. Further, the increased arterial pressure reverses the flow of blood through the ductus arteriosus: blood flows from the high-pressure aorta to the low-pressure pulmonary artery.

If the foramen ovale remained patent, the increased pressure in the left atrium would result in backflow into the right heart. However, the anatomic configuration of the foramen is such that the increased pressure causes closure of the foramen by a valvelike fold situated in the wall of the left atrium.

The neonatal circulation is complete with closure of the ductus arteriosus and foramen ovale, but adjustments continue for 1–2 months, when the adult phase begins.

Adult Phase

The ductus arteriosus usually is obliterated in the early postnatal period, probably by reflex action secondary to an elevated oxygen tension and the action of epinephrinelike metabolites. If cortisol was administered to the mother, closure of the infant's ductus arteriosus may be delayed. If the ductus remains open, a systolic crescendo murmur that diminishes during diastole (''machinery murmur'') is often heard over the second left interspace.

Obliteration of the foramen ovale is usually complete in 6–8 weeks, with fusion of its valve to the left interatrial septum. The foramen may remain patent in some individuals, however, with few or no symptoms. The obliterated ductus venosus from the liver to the vena cava becomes the ligamentum venosum. The occluded umbilical vein becomes the ligamentum teres of the liver.

The hemodynamics of the normal adult differ from those of the fetus in the following respects: (1) venous and arterial blood no longer mix in the atria; (2) the vena cava carries only deoxygenated blood into the right atrium, whence it is pumped into the pulmonary arteries and thence to the pulmonary capillary bed; and (3) the aorta carries only oxygenated blood from the left heart via the pulmonary veins for distribution to the rest of the body.

RESPIRATORY FUNCTION

Gas Exchange

Gas exchange in the fetus occurs in the placenta. The gases are transferred by diffusion across a membrane, and the rate of exchange is proportionate to the difference in partial pressure of each gas. Gas exchange is measured by Fick's law of diffusion.

$$\frac{\text{Amount of gas}}{\text{transferred}} = \frac{\text{Surface area}}{\text{Thickness of membrane}} \times \text{Time} \times \frac{\text{Partial pressure}}{\text{difference}} \times \text{D (Diffusion)}$$

Until about the 12th week, placental permeability is low because of the small surface area of the placental "lake" and the early relative thickness of the trophoblastic membrane. However, from 12 to 32 weeks, the membrane thins and the surface area steadily increases. Obviously, active metabolism of the placenta itself requires considerable oxygen, but this makes quantitation of oxygen transfer difficult.

In any event, the partial oxygen pressure (P_{O_2}) of fetal blood is less than that of maternal blood. Although this is not compatible with extrauterine life, it is adequate for the fetus because the fetus can adjust to lower oxygen tensions and can even survive brief periods of anaerobic metabolism. Fetal blood is polycythemic (ie, it contains a relatively greater proportion of red blood cells) and contains mostly hemoglobin F, which has a higher affinity for oxygen than does hemoglobin A.

Both the P_{CO_2} and the CO_2 content of fetal blood are slightly greater than these values in the mother's blood, and as a result, CO_2 tends to diffuse from fetus to mother for elimination.

Breathing

The normal fetus makes respirationlike movements that can be detected by ultrasonography or cineroentgenography during the last half of pregnancy. The activity normally increases to term. Dysmaturity or other fetal jeopardy, heavy sedation, or narcotic analgesic administration to the mother reduces respirationlike movements.

The first breath of the newborn normally occurs within the first 10 seconds after delivery. It is really a gasp, the result of central nervous system reaction to sudden changes in pressure and temperature and other stimulation. With the first breath, a slight increase in P_{O_2} may activate chemoreceptors to send impulses to the central nervous system respiratory center and then to the respiratory musculature. A rhythmic but rapid breathing sequence, similar to that of the infant, usually follows. Meanwhile, amniotic fluid drains from the respiratory tree or is absorbed. If the lungs are mature, good expansion and gas exchange should follow. However, if inadequate phospholipid surfactant is present (L/S ratio < 2), as in the immature newborn, the surface tension at the air-fluid (membrane) interface in the alveoli will remain high, the alveoli will not expand, and respiratory distress secondary to atelectasis will promptly ensue.

With the onset of breathing, the circulatory changes described above occur.

GASTROINTESTINAL FUNCTION

The gastrointestinal tract is not truly functional until after birth because the fetus is nourished via the placenta. Nonetheless, the fetus swallows and absorbs considerable amniotic fluid beginning early in the second trimester. Therefore, it is presumed that the gastrointestinal tract plays some role in fetal fluid balance.

Meconium is produced during late pregnancy, but the amount is small. Passage of meconium in utero occurs only with asphyxia, which increases intestinal peristalsis and relaxation of the anal sphincter.

Secretory and absorptive functions of the gastrointestinal tract are accelerated after delivery. At birth, most digestive enzymes are present, but the gastric contents are neutral. Nonetheless, acidity soon develops. The initial neutrality may briefly delay the growth of vitamin K-producing bacteria in the bowel.

The newborn can assimilate simple solutions immediately after birth but cannot digest food (milk) until after the second or third day following elimination of excessive gastric mucus. During the early neonatal period, milk normally progresses slowly through the stomach and upper intestine. Large bowel peristalsis increases promptly after delivery, and the newborn normally produces 1–6 small stools per day. Absence of stool within 48 hours after birth indicates intestinal obstruction.

HEPATIC FUNCTION

Intrahepatic erythropoiesis in the fetus begins during the eighth week. Histologically, the liver is well-developed by mid pregnancy. During fetal life, the liver acts as a storage depot for glycogen and iron, but metabolic liver functions are carried out by the placenta and maternal liver. Hence, hepatic function—particularly catabolic functions involving enzymatic processes—really begins at delivery. All things considered, the younger the newborn in gestational age, the poorer its liver function. Liver function gradually improves during the neonatal period and infancy, assuming proper food, freedom from infection, and a favorable environment. Actually, reasonably complete liver function is not achieved until several months after birth.

At birth, there are many liver deficiencies. Hepatic production of fibrinogen and coagulation factors II, VII, IX, XI, and XII is low. Liver stores of vitamin K are deficient because vitamin K must be formed by bacteria in the intestine. These deficiencies predispose the infant to hemorrhage during the first few days of life.

Hepatic gluconeogenesis (formation of glucose from amino acids) and storage of glucose are not well established in the newborn. Moreover, carbohydrate-regulating hormones such as cortisol, epinephrine, and glucagon may be insufficient initially. As a consequence, neonatal hypoglycemia is common after stressful stimuli such as exposure to cold or malnutrition.

Glucuronidation is limited during the early neonatal period, so that bilirubin is not readily conjugated for excretion as bile. After physiologic hemolysis of excess red blood cells in the first week after birth, or with pathologic hemolysis in hemolytic disease of the newborn, jaundice occurs. If marked hyperbilirubinemia develops, kernicterus may ensue.

In the newborn period, many drugs (eg, sulfonamides, chloramphenicol) are poorly metabolized by the liver. Moreover, numerous inborn errors of metabolism (eg, galactosemia) may be diagnosed soon after birth.

RENAL FUNCTION

The kidneys are unnecessary for fetal growth and development, as demonstrated by a rare infant born with renal agenesis. The placenta and maternal lungs and kidneys normally maintain fetal fluid and electrolyte balance.

The kidney is not fully developed even at term. Renal immaturity is reflected in limited kidney function. The glomerular filtration of the newborn is only about 50% of that of an adult. Urine concentration and tubular resorption of sodium and phosphate are also reduced. Even so, considerable fluid and electrolyte variability can be managed successfully by the newborn. With renal agenesis or congenital obstructive uropathy, oligohydramnios is present.

ENDOCRINE FUNCTION

After delivery, the newborn must assume the endocrine functions provided earlier by the mother. The transition is not always smooth, however. For example, the regulation of blood glucose concentration and its effect on fat and protein synthesis are functions of insulin. During the first 12 hours of life, there may be a serious drop in blood glucose followed by a period of instability that is usually corrected by adjustment of insulin production and insulin stimulation of hepatic glycogen storage and release.

The anterior pituitary is active in utero, and its function continues uninterrupted after birth. The functions of the fetal posterior pituitary are unknown.

The fetal thyroid is active. At term, T_4 (thyroxine) and T_3 (triiodothyronine) levels are similar to those of the mother. Immediately following delivery, there is a temporary increase in T_4.

The newborn is slightly hypoparathyroid for a short time; thus, parathyroid regulation of intestinal absorption, transport, and balance of calcium and phosphorus initially may be less than optimal. A slightly high serum phosphorus level and low serum calcium level are usual for a while. Hypocalcemia increases the susceptibility to tetany, but calcium and vitamin D may be given orally or parenterally to correct this.

The relative importance and activity of the fetal adrenal is suggested by its size—larger than the kidney during much of fetal development. The adrenal cortex is stimulated by fetal ACTH; maternal ACTH does not cross the placental barrier. Cortisol is produced by the outer (adult) zone of the cortex, and increasing amounts of this hormone may play a part in the initiation of labor. This is supported by the observation that anencephalic monsters do not produce ACTH; their adrenal cortices are hypoplastic and inactive, and such pregnancies are unusually prolonged. The principal hormone of the inner (fetal) zone of the adrenal cortex is dehydroepiandrosterone, an essential precursor of the estrogens needed to maintain pregnancy.

The adrenal medulla produces small amounts of catecholamines, which are important in vascular regulation.

Fetal ovarian or testicular function is obscured by maternal production of large amounts of estrogen and progesterone during pregnancy. Brief vaginal discharge or bleeding by female newborns and temporary enlargement of the breasts of newborns of both sexes reflect the effects of increased maternal estrogens, progesterone, and prolactin.

Other fetal or neonatal changes may result from maternal dysfunction, eg, infants born of diabetic mothers may have pancreatic B cell hyperplasia and produce large quantities of insulin.

CENTRAL NERVOUS SYSTEM FUNCTION

The functional development of the central nervous system is too complex even to be summarized here. Nonetheless, it is apparent that the brain is only partially developed and functional at term. However, the brain doubles its weight by the end of the first year of life and triples it by the end of the fifth year. The rate of growth then slows, but adult development is achieved at about the time of puberty.

The fetus and a "spinal animal" are comparable neurologically because both have only basic reflexes. Between 10 and 20 weeks of gestational age, the human fetus displays several basic motor patterns that are later integrated into specific actions. The first jerky patterns of the second trimester become the functional movement patterns that allow the fetus to move about in utero. After mid pregnancy, these motor patterns mature in a manner similar to the mature repertoire of the newborn. Clues to future central nervous system development may be found in the study of these various fetal motor patterns, and failure to progress at various stages seems to indicate subsequent cerebral dysfunction. Disease, trauma, or poor postnatal care may irreparably damage or retard central nervous system development.

The body temperature of a newborn must be maintained within a very narrow range. This is most important because the fetal temperature is about 0.5 °C above that of the mother prior to and even during labor, and immediately after delivery, a fall of at least 2–3 °C occurs as a result of loss of protection provided by the uterus and amniotic fluid, evaporative heat loss, and the relatively large surface area of the newborn. If moderate chilling occurs, the mature newborn can produce compensatory body heat by nonshivering thermogenesis, catabolism of so-called brown fat to effect a short-term increase in body heat. If this warming is inadequate, shivering (which is more stressful) normally follows. Preterm infants or those who are narcotized, asphyxiated, or traumatized may be incapable of maintaining a reasonable body temperature by any means and may die.

Maternal hypoxia during labor or delivery or hypoxia of the infant during the early postnatal period may be especially hazardous for the newborn. Such asphyxiated infants often have Apgar scores of 1–4. Some die in the neonatal period; and some who survive, particularly immature newborns, will develop cerebral palsy, neurologic defects, or mental retardation. Moreover, infection, trauma, or congenital anomaly may further compound the effects of asphyxia. Although many jeopardized newborns apparently recover from asphxia, whether they will achieve their full genetic potential is uncertain. Consequently, prevention and proper treatment of fetal-neonatal asphyxia are imperative.

HIGH-RISK PREGNANCY

A high-risk pregnancy is one that imposes a definite or probable increased hazard to the life or health of the mother or offspring. The risk may be due to maternal or fetal problems or to treatment of these problems. Any pregnancy considered to be at risk must be evaluated with reference to the prognosis for the mother and offspring.

Disorders that involve an added risk for the mother or fetus include prepregnancy problems, obstetric disorders such as complications of labor and delivery, and maternal medical or surgical disorders. The fetus or newborn alone may be at risk due to genetic abnormalities, placental dysfunction, untimely delivery, or umbilical cord complications.

Socioeconomic and cultural factors strongly influence perinatal mortality and morbidity rates. Education, family support, nutrition, access to the health delivery system, and other related details determine the success or failure of pregnancy. This explains in part why women of the more prosperous class in any given culture are generally more successful than women in less fortunate circumstances in giving birth to healthy infants and have lower maternal and neonatal morbidity and mortality rates. Good emotional health, living conditions, and personal health habits also improve the likelihood of successful pregnancy.

The incidence of high-risk pregnancy depends upon the definitions used, which are somewhat arbitrary, and the community under consideration. In the USA, at least 20% of all pregnancies are at increased risk, and these patients account for most instances of maternal and perinatal mortality and morbidity.

Pathogenesis

At least 60% of fetal and over 50% of neonatal deaths are associated with only 5 of a long list of obstetric complications: breech presentation, premature separation of the placenta, preeclampsia-eclampsia, multiple pregnancy, and urinary tract infection. Certain less common complications (eg, eclampsia, cord prolapse) also cause an inordinately high proportion of perinatal losses. Unwanted pregnancy, ignorance, exposure to toxic products, and unwillingness or inability to obtain good early obstetric care also relate to high-risk pregnancy. Whatever the problem, prevention, early diagnosis, and proper treatment will greatly reduce the perinatal mortality and morbidity rates.

Table 4–2. Teratogenic and fetotoxic drugs.*

Maternal Medication	Fetal or Neonatal Effect
Established teratogenic agents	
Antineoplastic agents	Multiple anomalies, abortion.
Antimetabolites (amethopterin, flu-orouracil, DON, 6-azauridine, etc)	
Alkylating agents (cyclophosphamide, etc)	
Antibiotics (amphotericin B, mito-mycin, etc)	
Estrogens, diethylstilbestrol	May cause clear cell carcinoma of cervix or vagina, genital anomalies, or infertility in offspring of patient.
Other sex hormones (androgens, proges-togens)	Masculinization, advanced bone age.
Thalidomide	Fetal death or phocomelia; deafness; cardiovascular, gastrointestinal, or genitourinary anomalies.
Organic mercury	Cerebral palsy
Polychlorinated biphenyls (PCBs) (con-taminants in manufacture of rice, cooking oil)	"Cola"-colored neonates with other developmental defects.
Possible teratogens	
Insulin (shock or hypoglycemia)	Anomalies.
LSD	"Fractured chromosomes," anomalies.
Sulfonylurea derivatives	Anomalies.
Vitamin D	Cardiopathies.
Fetotoxic drugs	
Analgesics, narcotics	
Heroin, morphine	Neonatal death or convulsions, tremors.
Salicylates (excessive)	Neonatal bleeding.
Cardiovascular drugs	
Ammonium chloride	Acidosis.
Hexamethonium	Neonatal ileus.
Reserpine	Nasal congestion, drowsiness.
Coumarin anticoagulants	Fetal death or hemorrhage.
Ethanol	Fetal alcohol syndrome.
Poliomyelitis immunization (Sabin)	Death or neurologic damage.
Sedatives, hypnotics, tranquilizers	
Meprobamate	Retarded development.
Phenobarbital (excessive)	Neonatal bleeding.
Phenothiazines	Hyperbilirubinemia.
Smallpox vaccination	Death or fetal vaccinia.
Tetracyclines	Dental discoloration and abnormalities.
Thiazides	Thrombocytopenia.
Tobacco smoking	Undersized babies.
Vitamin K (excessive)	Hyperbilirubinemia.

*Modified from Benson RC: Chapter 12 in *Current Medical Diagnosis & Treatment 1983*. Krupp MA, Chatton MJ (editors). Lange, 1983.

Table 4–3. Teratogenicity drug labeling now required by FDA.*

Category A: Well-controlled studies have not disclosed any fetal risk.

Category B: Animal studies have not disclosed any fetal risk or have suggested some risk not confirmed in controlled studies in women, or there are no adequate studies in women.

Category C: Animal studies have revealed adverse fetal effects; there are no adequate controlled studies in women.

Category D: Some fetal risk, but benefits may outweigh risk (eg, life-threatening illness, safer effective drug). Patient should be warned.

Category X: Fetal abnormalities in animal or human studies; risk not outweighed by benefit. **Contraindicated in pregnancy.**

*These 5 categories established by the FDA are based on the potential for causing birth defects in infants born to women who use the drugs during pregnancy. By law, the label must set forth all available information on teratogenicity.

Disorders contributing to an increased risk during pregnancy may be maternal problems (eg, thyroid dysfunction or hypertensive cardiovascular disease), placental abnormalities (eg, placenta previa), cord complications (eg, cord compression or vasa previa), or fetal problems (eg, genetic abnormalities or twin-to-twin transfusion).

Abnormal development or disordered function depends upon the individual disorder, compensatory mechanisms, and mode of treatment. Medication given to the mother may benefit her but be deleterious to the fetus; for example, all uracil drugs cross the placenta promptly and are goitrogenic for the fetus.

Diagnostic Evaluation

A. Initial Screening: Initial screening of the gravida must include the following:

1. Complete general physical examination–This should include height, weight, development, etc, and diagnosis of systemic disease, dysfunction, or abnormality.

2. Pelvic evaluation with special reference to the following–

a. Uterus–Configuration, size, fundal height, patient girth, fetal size (estimate), fetal presentation, position, engagement, amount of amniotic fluid.

b. Cervix–Position, epithelialization, effacement, dilatation.

c. Spine, pelvis, and extremities–Abnormalities, measurement of pelvic diameters.

3. Laboratory tests–Hematocrit, urinalysis, urine culture, nontreponemal serologic test for syphilis, rubella and other antibody screening, blood type, Rh determination, vaginal cytologic smear for infection, hormonal status, and malignant elements. Special studies may be required for particular problems (eg, glucose tolerance test in diabetes mellitus).

Table 4—4. High-risk obstetric categories. (After Wigglesworth.)

History of Any of the Following:

Hereditary abnormality (osteogenesis imperfecta, Down's syndrome, etc).

Premature or small-for-dates neonate (most recent delivery).

Stillbirth or birth-damaged neonate.

Congenital anomaly, anemia, blood dyscrasia, preeclampsia-eclampsia, etc.

Severe social problem (teenage pregnancy, drug abuse, chronic alcoholism, etc).

Long-delayed or absent prenatal care.

Age < 18 or > 35 years.

Teratogenic viral illness or dangerous drug administration in the first trimester.

A fifth or subsequent pregnancy, especially when the mother is > 35 years of age.

Prolonged infertility or essential drug or hormone treatment.

Significant stressful or dangerous events in the present pregnancy (critical accident, excessive exposure to irradiation, etc).

Heavy cigarette smoking.

Diagnosis of Any of the Following:

Height < 60 inches or a prepregnant weight of 20% less than or over the standard for height and age.

Minimal or no weight gain.

Obstetric complications (preeclampsia-eclampsia, multiple pregnancy, hydramnios).

Abnormal presentation (breech, presenting part unengaged at term, etc).

A fetus that fails to grow normally or is disparate in size from that expected.

A fetus > 42 weeks' gestation.

B. Antenatal Visits: Antenatal visits should be more frequent for high-risk than for normal obstetric patients. This allows for more accurate appraisal of the course of the pregnancy and identification and correction of problems (eg, anemia, urinary tract infection). Obstetric disorders that may require special treatment or decisions (eg, preeclampsia-eclampsia, uterine bleeding) must be identified early. Antenatal visits also provide the opportunity for education about hygiene, nutrition, use of drugs, and care of the newborn; for assessment of emotional well-being; and for counseling if this is needed.

C. Assessment of Fetal Growth, Maturity, and Well-Being:

1. Indirect (noninvasive) methods–

a. Calculation of gestational age of the fetus (last menstrual period, basal body temperature, date of quickening, first fetal heart tones).

b. Growth of uterus (fundal height, patient's girth).

c. Engagement.

d. Roentgenography (anomalies). (*Caution:* Except in urgent situations, x-ray exposure of the mother and fetus is contraindicated.)

e. Ultrasonography (fetal biparietal diameter, anomalies).

f. Determination of maternal plasma or urinary estriol.

2. Direct (invasive) methods–

a. Amniocentesis–Enzyme studies, osmolality, creatinine content, bilirubin concentration, L/S ratio, percentage of fat-laden cells (see p 66); culture, cytochemistry, and chromosome studies on amniotic fluid cells.

b. Amniography (anomalies, placental situation). With increasing availability of ultrasonography, the number of indications for amniography is decreasing.

c. Amnioscopy.

Differential Diagnosis

A ''large for dates'' uterus may indicate multiple pregnancy, hydramnios, or uterine tumors. A uterus that is smaller than expected from the last menstrual period (LMP) may signify dysmaturity of the fetus (placental insufficiency), oligohydramnios, overestimation of the duration of pregnancy, or fetal disease (eg, rubella, cytomegalovirus disease) or anomaly.

Treatment

Maternal disease must be treated cautiously and properly to avoid harm to the fetus. Fetal perinatal mortality and morbidity rates can sometimes be reduced by extension of gestation—eg, in the case of premature labor, multiple pregnancy, placenta previa, cervical incompetence, slight premature separation of the placenta, or thyroid dysfunction. Judicious early delivery may be necessary to rescue the fetus if the membranes rupture before 34 weeks or in preeclampsia-eclampsia, severe isoimmunization, clinical diabetes mellitus, persistent urinary tract infection, considerable hydramnios, or placental insufficiency.

Prognosis

Improved obstetric care has reduced the maternal mortality rate in the USA from 66 per 100,000 births in 1930 to 9.9 per 100,000 in 1978. Nonetheless, some obstetrics patients still die of preventable disorders. Moreover, the present perinatal mortality rate in the USA is about 30 per 100,000 births, and at least one-third to one-half of these losses could have been avoided. It is likely that less rigid dietary restrictions for weight control during pregnancy could further reduce infant mortality rates. Socioeconomic factors undoubtedly play a role. The vast majority of maternal and perinatal deaths occur in high-risk pregnancies.

ASSESSMENT OF THE FETUS IN HIGH-RISK PREGNANCY

Assessment of the Fetus During Pregnancy

A. Duration of Pregnancy: Determination of the duration of pregnancy must be accurate. One must consider the LMP, the height of the fundus, the date of quickening, and the fetal biparietal diameter as measured by ultrasonography. X-ray identification of ossification centers may be used to determine the age of the fetus, but because x-ray exposure of the fetus is contraindicated, this method should only be used in urgent situations.

B. Amniocentesis: Developmental or heritable disorders, including sickle cell or Tay-Sachs disease, should be sought by amniocentesis (prenatal genetic diagnosis).

C. Alpha-Fetoprotein Determination: High levels of α-fetoprotein, a fetal central nervous system metabolite associated with congenital neural tube defects in the offspring, can be detected in maternal serum and in amniotic fluid. Anencephaly and spina bifida are the most common anomalies associated with high α-fetoprotein values. Utilizing this biochemical "marker," prenatal screening of women 12–20 weeks pregnant can identify a seriously malformed fetus early enough to permit abortion, if this is acceptable.

The incidence of congenital neural tube defects in the general population is 0.5%. However, if the family history reveals this problem in a young member, the risk of the fetus having a major anomaly is greatly increased.

Patients whose serum α-fetoprotein values are +2 standard deviations above the mean almost always have infants without neural tube defects. False-negative tests are rare, but occasional false-positive tests do occur when the values exceed this level. Therefore, gravidas with abnormal or equivocal serum α-fetoprotein values should be evaluated by amniocentesis and gray scale ultrasonography to detect fetal abnormality. False-positive diagnoses may be further reduced by adding a quantitative acetylcholinesterase assay; acetylcholinesterase levels are significantly elevated in open neural tube defects.

D. Maturity of Fetus: The physiologic maturity of the fetus can be determined by testing color of the amniotic fluid, L/S ratio, creatinine content, bilirubin concentration, or fluid osmolality or by the oxytocin challenge test (see below).

E. Estriol Determinations: For fetuses in potential jeopardy, one of the best indices of fetal distress is a series of determinations of the maternal serum or urinary estriol concentration. An abnormal estriol level may or may not indicate a fetal problem. A rapid fall of serial estriol values usually indicates serious deterioration of the fetus; a rising or normal estriol level definitely indicates a healthy fetus.

The most reliable test is the serum unconjugated estriol assay. Maternal urine estriol values measure conjugated estriol and are acceptable if a 24-hour specimen can be guaranteed.

1. Clinical indications–

a. Diabetes mellitus–

(1) Class A–If fetal blood glucose levels are normal, do estriol

assays only after 40 weeks. If there is a history of stillbirth or preeclampsia-eclampsia, manage as for classes B–H.

(2) Classes B to H–Obtain estriol determinations twice a week at 28 weeks, 3 times a week at 32 weeks, and daily at 34 weeks. With poor control of diabetes or the development of complications, begin assessments earlier than 28 weeks.

b. Preeclampsia-eclampsia and other disorders–Obtain estriol values 2–3 times a week for outpatients but daily for hospitalized patients. In all cases, evaluate the situation clinically with nonstress and stress tests.

c. Estriol values are of no value to detect hemolytic disease in the fetus. Moreover, maternal steroids, ampicillin, renal disease, placental sulfatase deficiency, or oxytocin induction of labor may greatly alter estriol values.

2. Interpretation–A significant fall in urinary or serum estriol is defined as $\geq 40\%$ of the average of the 3 *highest and consecutive* previous values.

Date	Estriol Value	
3/4/83	23.5	
3/5/83	19.0	
3/6/83	23.9	
3/7/83	24.4	
3/8/83	25.4	3 highest
3/9/83	25.0	consecutive
3/10/83	27.0	values
3/11/83	19.8	
3/12/83	11.5	

$$\frac{11.5}{25.6} \times 100 = 44.9\%$$

If the urine collection is adequate, the percentage drop in both urinary estriol and estriol/creatinine (E/C) ratio will be comparable. A 24-hour specimen is usually required. The E/C ratio can sometimes be used as a substitute for 24-hour collection, but at least a 12-hour urinary output must be obtained to ensure an accurate result.

A significant rapid fall of estriol indicates serious, perhaps critical fetal jeopardy. Lack of rise indicates uteroplacental insufficiency that may require termination of pregnancy. In contrast, other problems, eg, antibiotic effect, congenital malformation, do not require early delivery.

Assessment of Fetal Health in Labor

(1) Consider pertinent details in the history, the general physical and obstetric examination, pelvimetry, and fetal heart tones (monitored externally or internally).

(2) Appraise the character and progress of labor, eg, Friedman's curve (see Fig 6–3) and the passage of blood or meconium-stained amniotic fluid.

(3) Identify fetal distress, ie, abnormal fetal heart rate (FHR) patterns (direct or indirect), with special attention to bradycardia or late severe variable deceleration, and acidosis in samples of fetal scalp blood.

FETAL MONITORING

The traditional stethoscopic monitoring of fetal heart tones to assess fetal well-being is inadequate because periodic auscultation of the fetal heart rate (FHR) often fails to detect fetal compromise until irreversible damage has occurred. Patients who are known to be at high risk are candidates for fetal monitoring, but its use may soon be extended to most obstetric patients who deliver in hospitals because of the obvious benefits. Unfortunately, fetal monitoring equipment is expensive.

The most important indices to fetal health are the FHR patterns associated with uterine contractions. Significant changes during contractions may be subtle and within the normal range. Hence, beat-to-beat recording becomes most important. For these reasons, monitoring equipment has been developed to display uterine activity and the FHR synchronously.

Changes in the degree of FHR irregularity between uterine contractions may also be significant in the appraisal of fetal well-being. A loss of this irregularity may indicate fetal compromise. Hence, rate circuitry that computes a rate for each beat-to-beat interval is now incorporated in better fetal monitoring equipment.

Fetal monitors currently available provide either external or internal sensing of the FHR and the associated contraction sequence and a permanent record of the data.

External Fetal Monitoring

Most external fetal monitors utilize an ultrasound transducer applied to the mother's abdominal wall. This detects fetal heart activity and triggers the rate-computing circuit of the unit. A disadvantage of ultrasonic detection of the FHR is the inherent irregularity of the rate recording because of the relatively indistinct signal from the transducer. This contrasts with the sharp signal input of the R wave of the ECG used in direct or internal monitoring. Moreover, external monitoring prevents interpretation of changes in baseline irregularity. Another criticism of external fetal heart monitoring is that what may appear to be normal or increased variability may be artifact because of the ultrasound pickup. If the baseline appears smooth when an ultrasound transducer is used, the

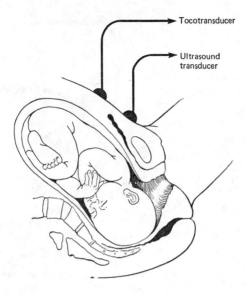

Tocotransducer

Ultrasound
transducer

Figure 4–13. External fetal heart rate monitoring. (Redrawn, with permission, from Hon EHG: *Hosp Pract* [Sept] 1970;5:91.)

variability of the true FHR may be decreased. Thus, variability of the FHR cannot be accurately determined with ultrasound.

A tocotransducer that responds to changes in pressure transmitted from the uterus to the abdominal wall is used to monitor uterine activity. Unfortunately, the external monitor does not provide quantitative data regarding the intensity of uterine contractions—only their frequency and duration are recorded for clinical interpretation. Moreover, the patient may be quite uncomfortable because of the constricting belt that holds the transducer. In addition, the input signals often are distorted when the patient moves or if the belt is loosened. Obesity may further reduce the quality of the external FHR recording.

One technical problem is that the abdominal transducer often must be readjusted or reapplied to ensure good recording. Moreover, if the tocotransducer becomes wet, it may not function.

On the other hand, because external fetal monitoring is noninvasive, it is almost devoid of clinical complications.

Internal Fetal Monitoring

A. General Considerations: Internal fetal heart monitoring during

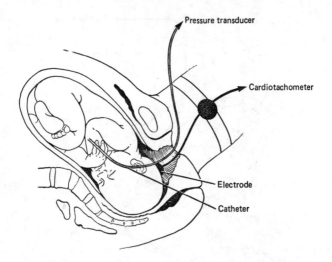

Figure 4–14. Internal fetal heart rate monitoring. (Redrawn, with permission, from Hon EHG: *Hosp Pract* [Sept] 1970;5:91.)

labor yields data that are relatively free of artifacts caused by patient movement, but it cannot be used before the cervix is dilated about 2 cm and rupture of the membranes has occurred to permit placement of the scalp electrode. Nevertheless, when the cervix is ''open'' and a pressure transducer attached to an intrauterine catheter can be inserted, an accurate record of intrauterine pressure usually can be obtained. Thus, the intensity of contractions can be determined and an abnormal elevation of uterine tone between contractions recognized. This information is useful clinically, especially when oxytocin induction or augmentation of labor is considered or when premature separation of the placenta occurs.

Internal FHR monitoring has become more practical with the advent of the spiral fetal scalp electrode. The fetal R wave is used by the rate-computing circuit of the internal fetal monitor to develop a beat-to-beat recording that accurately depicts baseline irregularity and the widest ranges of the FHR.

Clinical problems attributable to internal FHR monitoring are few. Serious fetal scalp infection is rare. Perforation of the uterus has been reported; slight placental bleeding, also due to the intrauterine catheter transducer, has occurred, but amnionitis can rarely be ascribed to the instrumentation.

Internal fetal monitoring may be complicated by damage or malfunction of the pressure transducer. Occasionally, the transducer, which must lie within the uterine cavity, may slip down into the vagina; it must then be reinserted into the uterus. Air bubbles, pressure leaks or kinks in the catheter system, loose valves, a defective stopcock, or a damaged cable or coupling may cause a recording failure. The pressure transducer must be properly calibrated to atmospheric pressure.

Technical internal monitoring problems are few. However, if the internal electrode is applied to the cervix accidentally, the mother's heart rate will be recorded instead of the fetal heart rate.

Most obstetric services require physician management of internal fetal monitoring systems, but nurses share in the observation of patients. Nurses often initiate and maintain external monitoring. Unfortunately, the quality of these data may deteriorate in late labor, and internal monitoring may be required.

Representative portions of the FHR record, including abnormal strip recordings, usually are retained as part of the patient's chart. Some hospitals microfilm selected segments for the record.

Although the procedure is formidable and worrisome to some, most obstetric patients accept fetal monitoring as a part of better perinatal care and insurance against fetal damage or death.

B. Indications: Intrapartum fetal monitoring should be used if one or more of the following high-risk factors are present:

1. History–Maternal age under 16 or over 35 years, previous cesarean section, diabetes mellitus, significant cardiac or hypertensive disease, moderate or severe isoimmunization, other serious disorders.

2. Prenatal factors–Multiple pregnancy, preeclampsia-eclampsia, moderate or severe anemia, pyelonephritis, uterine bleeding, polyhydramnios, fetal growth retardation or compromise (abnormal clinical or laboratory tests), premature labor, meconium-stained amniotic fluid, postdatism (42 weeks or more), abnormal fetal heart tones, other serious disorders.

3. Intrapartum factors–Augmentation of labor, dysfunctional labor, uterine bleeding, prolonged first or second stage of labor, abnormal fetal heart tones—including tachycardia ($> 160/min$) or bradycardia ($< 120/min$)—conduction anesthesia (including paracervical block), other serious disorders.

C. Evaluation: To evaluate the state of the fetus during FHR monitoring, first determine the baseline FHR (normal: $120–160/min$) and establish the baseline variability (normal: ± 5 beats/min). Then observate for the following:

1. Tachycardia–(FHR $> 160/min$.) This is indicated by an elevated baseline lasting for over 30 minutes. Tachycardia may be the result of maternal or fetal infection (fever) and may represent fetal distress. Hence, the problem should be investigated.

2. Bradycardia–(FHR $< 120/min$.) Fetal distress is present when

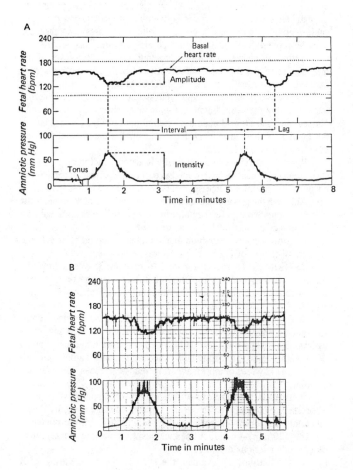

Figure 4–15. Fetal heart rate tracings. *A:* Schematic tracing. *B:* Early deceleration. (Reproduced, with permission, from Babson SG et al: *Management of High-Risk Pregnancy and Intensive Care of the Neonate,* 3rd ed. Mosby, 1975.)

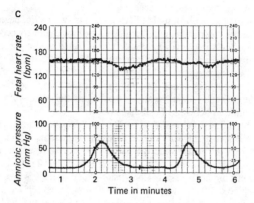

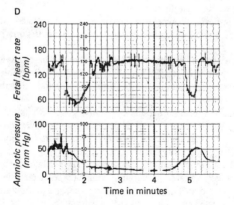

Figure 4–15 (cont'd). Fetal heart rate tracings. *C:* Late deceleration. *D:* Variable deceleration. (Reproduced, with permission, from Babson SG et al: *Management of High-Risk Pregnancy and Intensive Care of the Neonate,* 3rd ed. Mosby, 1975.

the FHR is less than 100/min. This may be due to hypoxia or cord compression.

3. Abnormal FHR patterns–

a. Early deceleration–The FHR pattern is symmetric, beginning with a uterine contraction and returning to the baseline in concert with the uterine pressure curve. **Probable cause:** Fetal head compression mediated via the vagus nerve. **Conclusion:** No fetal distress.

b. Late deceleration–The FHR pattern is similar to that of early deceleration but with onset *after* the peak of the uterine contraction. **Probable cause:** Hypoxia that affects the fetal central nervous system or myocardium. **Conclusion:** Fetal distress.

c. Variable deceleration–The slope of this pattern is more angular than the symmetric early or late deceleration patterns. The onset is irregular and inconstant, and the pattern has no consistent temporal relationship to the uterine contraction. **Probable cause:** Transient compression of umbilical vessels. **Conclusion:** Fetal distress is present if, over a period of 30 minutes or more, the pattern occurs repeatedly and the FHR falls below 70, these changes lasting over 30 seconds with each contraction.

d. Periodic accelerations–These are associated with uterine contractions. **Probable cause:** Brief, partial umbilical cord compression. **Conclusion:** No fetal distress.

e. Nonperiodic accelerations–These are associated with fetal movement. **Probable cause:** Fetal activity. **Conclusion:** No fetal distress.

f. Decreased baseline variability–Decreased baseline variability indicates nonfunctioning FHR control mechanism. **Probable cause:** Fetal acidosis or maternal medication. **Conclusion:** Possible fetal distress.

In interpreting abnormal FHR patterns, judge each pathologic pattern as slight, moderate, or marked depending on the level and duration of bradycardia. The greater the severity of late or variable deceleration, the greater the fetal acidosis.

Fetal scalp blood sampling is indicated (1) when late deceleration or persistent severe variable deceleration occurs, (2) when meconium staining of the amniotic fluid is associated with unusual or abnormal FHR patterns, or (3) when confusion exists regarding the cause of decreased baseline variability, eg, fetal acidosis (pH ≤ 7.20) or maternal medication.

Treatment of Fetal Distress

The objectives of the treatment of fetal distress are to maintain or restore utero-placental-fetal blood flow and acid-base balance.

A. Medical Measures:

1. Change the gravida's position, eg, from supine to lateral recum-

bent, to relieve aorta–vena cava compression or umbilical cord compression.

2. If induction or augmentation of labor is in progress, discontinue oxytocin administration to reduce the frequency, intensity, and duration of uterine contractions.

3. Administer oxygen by face mask at 6 L/min to reduce fetal hypoxia.

4. Obtain a fetal scalp blood sample to determine the level of compromise. (If scalp blood pH is ≤ 7.20, delivery without delay is indicated.)

5. Type and cross-match the mother's blood for possible transfusion.

6. Prepare for operation; summon the anesthesiologist and pediatrician on call.

B. Surgical Measures: Deliver the fetus in the safest, most expeditious manner.

Prognosis

The prognosis for the infant is good if prompt, safe rescue is possible. The prognosis for the mother is also good if skillful, uncomplicated forceps delivery or cesarean section can be accomplished.

DAILY FETAL MOVEMENT COUNTS

Frequent movements of the fetus as perceived by the mother have been a reassuring sign for centuries, and investigators have reported a marked decrease in fetal movements during fetal distress or just prior to fetal death.

Comparisons of daily fetal movement counts (DFMC) with movements recorded electronically for a 12-hour period have revealed that almost 90% of all fetal movements can be identified by the mother. This simple, cost-free ''test'' should be utilized, especially in complicated pregnancies.

Normally, the number of fetal movements decreases late in pregnancy. However, in uteroplacental insufficiency (fetal distress), fetal movement decreases markedly, ceasing at fetal death. Although the test has not yet been standardized, fewer than 10 fetal movements in a 12-hour period probably warrants a nonstress and perhaps a stress test.

NONSTRESS TESTING

The nonstress test is an appraisal of fetal well-being based upon the observation that the normal fetus will produce characteristic FHR patterns but the unhealthy fetus will not. Average baseline variability and acceleration of the FHR in response to fetal movement indicate that the fetus is not in jeopardy and has a good reserve. This is assessed by external fetal monitoring without stimuli (stress) to the fetus. Nonstress testing of this type also has been termed fetal activity acceleration determination.

If the fetal central nervous system is depressed because of hypoxia, acidosis, or drug overdosage, often the baseline variability is reduced and FHR acceleration with fetal movement is absent. These patterns may also be noted during fetal sleep. Thus, monitoring should continue for 20–30 minutes longer until the fetus becomes active, or the fetus should be stimulated by abdominal palpation.

Major indications for nonstress testing are a history of stillbirth or serious anomaly, drug abuse or alcoholism, possible asphyxia or other circulatory problem (eg, meconium-stained amniotic fluid prior to labor, hemoglobinopathy, Rh isoimmunization), suspected intrauterine growth retardation, medical complications of pregnancy (eg, diabetes mellitus of classes B–H, chronic renal disease, systemic lupus erythematosus), hypertensive disorders complicating pregnancy, and prolonged pregnancy.

The first nonstress test is rarely required before the 28th week of pregnancy. The maternal history or status generally indicates the time for the first test—eg, about the 32nd week in severe diabetics or if there is a history of stillbirth or onset of severe preeclampsia.

Procedure

(1) The patient should be placed in bed in the semi-Fowler position at about 30 degrees of elevation.

(2) The maternal blood pressure should be recorded on the FHR record every 10 minutes.

(3) The time must be recorded on the FHR record every 10 minutes.

(4) Record for 20 minutes. If the test is reactive (see below), end the test; if nonreactive, continue for another 20 minutes; if the test remains nonreactive, proceed to the oxytocin challenge test (contraction stress test)—do not manipulate the fetus.

Interpretation

The test is reactive if there are 4 or more accelerations of FHR that reach > 15 beats/min above the baseline and are at least ≥ 15 seconds in duration in a 20-minute period. A nonreactive test does not meet the criteria for the reactive test.

Management

If the test is nonreactive, perform oxytocin challenge test (contraction stress test). If the test is reactive, repeat in 7 days.

THE OXYTOCIN CHALLENGE TEST (OCT)
(Contraction Stress Test)

The oxytocin challenge test (OCT), a useful but still incompletely quantified method of determining fetal well-being, is a stress test based upon the fact that uterine contractions decrease uteroplacental blood flow. Before onset of labor, mothers with obstetric problems associated with uteroplacental compromise (eg, small-for-dates fetus) are candidates for the OCT method of fetal evaluation. Contraindications include previous cesarean section, placenta previa, and women at high risk for premature labor, eg, those with incompetent cervix, multiple pregnancy, or ruptured membranes with a premature offspring. The test must be done after viability is well established, generally after the 34th week.

Although prognostication is difficult, the incidence of neonatal death and morbidity is much higher in patients with a positive OCT than in high-risk patients with a negative OCT.

Procedure

The gravida is placed in the semi-Fowler position and slightly on one side. An external FHR monitor (ultrasound, phonocardiograph, or skin electrocardiographic leads from the mother's abdomen) and a uterine activity monitor are placed on the mother's abdomen. FHR and uterine activity are observed for 10–30 minutes (baseline). Oxytocin is then administered by controlled intravenous infusion (IVAC, Harvard Pump, or comparable device) controlled at 0.5 mU/min. Oxytocin dosage is slowly increased until at least 3 contractions develop in a 10-minute period. Slow (every 20 minutes) step-up may be required, but hyperstimulation—contractions at intervals of 2 minutes or less or contractions over 90 seconds in duration—must be avoided or fetal distress and emergency cesarean section may be necessary.

Interpretation

The OCT requires 1½–2 hours to perform, and interpretation depends upon strict adherence to the protocol. Twenty to 40% of positive OCTs are falsely positive.

(1) A positive OCT is one in which persistent late deceleration occurs—a drop in FHR with onset at or beyond the peak of uterine contraction. The minimal degree of deceleration in FHR (beats per minute) has not been acceptably defined. Some authorities have agreed on 5, and others regard any perceptible deceleration as significant. Nonetheless, decelerations must occur with most contractions and persist.

When the OCT is positive, about 10% of fetuses will die within 1 week if undelivered. When the state of the cervix is favorable, a closely monitored labor may be chosen, but in most cases a convincingly positive OCT is an indication for cesarean section, because almost 75% of these patients who are allowed to go into labor have late decelerations.

A patient with a positive OCT should not be delivered preterm solely on the basis of the positive OCT; the fetus must have a mature L/S ratio. Before vaginal delivery of any high-risk patient is attempted, an internal electrode should be placed and the patient monitored by direct means during labor.

(2) A suspicious or equivocal OCT, hyperstimulation, or unsatisfactory test cannot be interpreted and must be repeated in 24 hours.

(3) A negative OCT is temporarily reassuring, but the outcome of any high-risk pregnancy must be guarded. Intrauterine death is unlikely to occur within 7 days with a negative OCT. The OCT should be repeated in 1 week, with estriol monitoring in the meanwhile. If labor, unfavorable symptomatology, or serious laboratory indices (eg, falling estriol levels) develop, the need for cesarean section must be assessed.

Prenatal Care | 5

HISTORY & PHYSICAL EXAMINATION

A thorough medical history and physical examination early in pregnancy provide the groundwork for the diagnosis and treatment of disorders that may compromise pregnancy. Knowing the patient's general health problems permits the obstetrician to interpret developing symptoms correctly and treat complications promptly. Good antenatal care is preventive medicine of a high order because it provides an opportunity for screening gravidas to identify high- versus low-risk patients.

Vital Statistics

The following information should be recorded by the physician for each patient:

(1) Date of first examination, and unit or hospital number.

(2) Patient's full name, address, telephone number, husband's given names.

(3) Patient's occupation. This may be helpful in interpreting symptoms caused by fatigue, exposure to industrial hazards, or occupational tensions.

(4) The date of marriage, especially of a primigravida, may alert the physician to possible problems regarding the patient's attitude toward the pregnancy. The question of abortion, adoption, or keeping the child is often best raised at this time.

(5) Husband's age, height, weight, race, national origin, and occupation. The physical inheritance of the father is of significance in anticipating hereditary disorders.

History of Present Pregnancy

The patient is more concerned with the present pregnancy than with those that have occurred in the past. A sincere interest in her current status will help the physician to establish good rapport.

A. Symptoms, Signs, Infections, Injuries: The patient's complaints may include breast tenderness, nausea, headache, constipation, or other minor problems. Ask specifically about drug ingestion and about infections and injuries in early pregnancy.

B. Menstrual History: The patient's menstrual history should include age at menarche, average interval between periods, duration and amount of flow, pain and its relation to flow, presence or absence of intermenstrual bleeding (note day of cycle), existence of significant leukorrhea or other abnormalities, date of onset and character of the last menstrual period (LMP), date of the previous menstrual period (PMP), and date of quickening, if present, in relation to the LMP. The expected date of confinement (EDC) can then be calculated. Pregnant women occasionally experience painless, quasiperiodic bleeding. In such instances, ultrasonography or knowing the date of the PMP may be necessary to determine the EDC.

History of Previous Pregnancies

For each previous pregnancy, whether completed successfully or not, the following information should be recorded:

A. Termination: Date (month and year); name of hospital and name of physician.

B. Complications: Describe complications and note whether they were antepartal, intrapartal, or postpartal. The occurrence of preclampsia-eclampsia, infection, or hemorrhage should be described fully. Suspect serious complications if the patient was hospitalized before the onset of labor or for more than 5 days after delivery.

C. Labor:

1. Record whether labor was spontaneous or induced and the reason for induction.

2. Note the duration of each pregnancy in comparison with its EDC. A consistent pattern of early or late delivery may be apparent.

3. Length of labor–The length of previous labors is helpful in anticipating and preparing for problems of dystocia or precipitate delivery. One should attempt to determine the duration of "strong labor" rather than the interval between onset of contractions or admission to the hospital and delivery. Long labors may indicate dystocia (due to fetal disproportion) or inadequate, uncoordinated contractions. Dystocia may recur if similar problems develop again. If previous labors have been brief or precipitate at term (3 hours or less), induction may be indicated.

D. Delivery:

1. Method of delivery (vaginal, cesarean), presentation (vertex, breech), and whether assisted or not (forceps, version, extraction).

2. Anesthesia–Type used, whether it was satisfactory, and any problems.

3. Complications of previous deliveries can often be inferred from the patient's statements regarding the perineum. "A few stitches"

usually indicates a routine episiotomy or minor lacerations, and "no stitches" indicates a relaxed perineum. "Many stitches" may indicate tears that required extensive repair.

E. Previous Children at Birth:

1. Birth weight–The birth weights of each of the patient's children help to determine the weight pattern, maturity, and maternal disease (eg, diabetes). If the infant was delivered at home, the reported birth weight may be inaccurate.

2. Condition–A damaged ("marked") child usually implies a difficult delivery. Developmental abnormalities (eg, cardiopulmonary anomalies) should be suspected if the infant's color was unusual ("blue baby").

3. Sex–If sex-linked disorders exist in previous children, the same possibility exists for the expected infant if it is the same sex.

F. Breast Feeding: Note whether the patient nursed any of her previous infants and for how long. Reevaluation of previous failures may indicate whether the mother will want to nurse the expected infant.

G. Present Health of Children: Record if the children are living and well. A stillbirth or death of a child under 1 year of age is obstetrically significant.

Medical History

Record all important illnesses and *all* medications, allergies, drug sensitivities, and blood transfusions. Fertility studies and contraceptive methods should be included also.

Surgical History

List and give dates of all operations and serious injuries. Of particular importance are surgery or trauma to the pelvic floor, pelvis and its contents, urinary tract, bowel, or abdominal wall.

If the patient has had one or more cesarean deliveries, note the type, indications, whether there was a trial of labor, and special surgical problems or postoperative complications. Such information is necessary in determining how the fetus may have to be delivered.

Family History

List medical, genetic, and psychiatric disorders that may affect the patient or her offspring, eg, diabetes mellitus, cancer, or mental disease.

History by Systems

A careful system review often provides clues to the existence of significant diseases omitted from the history. Symptoms or signs should be recorded for all organ systems.

Patient's Attitudes

   A. Anesthesia and Analgesia: Note any fear the patient may have of anesthesia. Assess her pain threshold, ie, how soon in labor she may require analgesics.

   B. Emotional Balance: Estimate the patient's general emotional stability. Is she uncertain or confident? Does she want the infant? Observe alterations of mood at subsequent visits.

Antepartal Notes

   From the initial office visit until delivery, a continuing record of the progress of the pregnancy must be maintained. Include symptoms, signs, habits, contacts or exposures to illnesses, medications, pulse, temperature, weight, blood pressure, cervical and fundal changes, fetal progress, and laboratory tests. Return visits and periodic examinations provide successive assessments of fetal growth, maturity, and well-being.

Physical Examination

   Conduct the general examination much as any other routine physical examination. Serious diseases are often first noted during an obstetric physical examination (eg, anemia, tuberculosis, breast tumors). Pay particular attention to the following:

   A. General Examination: Record systolic and diastolic blood pressure at each antenatal visit. A significantly elevated blood pressure together with generalized edema and proteinuria indicate the onset of preeclampsia-eclampsia. Note body build and state of nutrition. Palpate the breasts, examine the nipples, and auscultate the heart and lungs.

   1. Skin and hair–Metabolic disorders (eg, hypothyroidism) are often first manifested by dermatologic changes.

   2. Mouth–Evaluate oral hygiene and check for epulis. If necessary, encourage the patient to see her dentist.

   3. Thyroid–Slight physiologic enlargement of the thyroid gland occurs in about 60% of pregnant patients.

   4. Abdomen–Consider especially the following:

   a. Uterine size, shape, and consistency. The height of the fundus above the symphysis should be measured and recorded.

   b. Hernias–Umbilical, inguinal, femoral, and lumbar hernias often become larger during pregnancy.

   c. Masses–Organs and tumors must be identified.

   5. Extremities–Note development, deformity, and restriction of movement of legs, arms, and back. Varicosities and edema must be explained and treated.

   6. Posture and body mechanics–These should be noted.

   B. Pelvic Examination: A thorough, stepwise pelvic examination can be performed at any time before term and is most important for each new obstetric patient. Gloves and instruments must be clean but need not be sterile unless gross infection is present or likely to occur during the examination or operative procedure. Pay particular attention to the following:

1. Vulvar and vaginal varicosities–These may bleed at delivery.

2. Cervix and uterus–Examine as described in Chapter 6. Near term, it is essential to note the degree of effacement and dilatation of the cervix. Record the site and extent of previous lacerations of the cervix; tears may recur at these sites at delivery.

3. Pelvic masses–Distinguish between ovarian and other pelvic tumors and retroperitoneal tumors. Suspected cancer, severe pain, or dystocia at previous deliveries may be indications for removal of certain pelvic tumors before term.

4. Pelvic measurements–In most cases, clinical appraisal of the pelvis by an experienced physician is adequate. If a pelvis is thought to be inadequate and precise pelvic measurements are needed, x-ray pelvimetry or ultrasonography (or both) should be used (see below). Those clinical measurements likely to afford a reasonably good estimate of the pelvic outlet and inlet diameters are as follows:

a. Biischial diameter (BI)–(Normal: ≥8 cm) This is also known as the transverse diameter of the outlet or the bituberous, intertuberous (IT), or tuberischial (TI) diameter. It is the distance between the inner margins of the ischial tuberosities, which can be measured above the

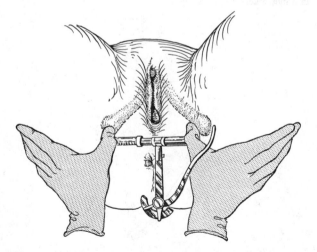

Figure 5–1. Measurement of biischial diameter (BI) with Thoms's pelvimeter.

anus. It constitutes the hypotenuse of the anterior pudendal triangle. The actual distance between the bony margins is 11 cm or more, but when measured through the soft tissues, the value is 8 cm or more for a normal pelvis. During delivery, the fetal head (average biparietal diameter: 8 cm) impinges on the pubic rami or, in the case of an occiput anterior presentation, at the points where the BI is measured. Thoms's and Williams' outlet pelvimeters are useful for accurate measurement of the BI (Fig 5–1).

b. Posterior sagittal diameter of the outlet (PS)–(Normal: 8–9.5 cm) This measurement is taken directly with the rectal finger touching the sacrococcygeal joint. The PS is the distance from the midpoint of the line between the ischial tuberosities to the external surface of the tip of the sacrum (the tip of the rectal finger). Thoms's pelvimeter measures this indirectly (Fig 5–2). The PS is measured indirectly from the point corresponding to the midpoint of the BI to the base of the coccyx (sacrococcygeal joint) on its external (skin) surface. This measurement is usually 10.5–11 cm. Subtract 1–1.5 cm for bone and soft tissue.

Thoms's or Klein's rule: When the sum of the BI and the PS is more than 15 cm, an infant of normal size will usually pass without difficulty.

c. Anteroposterior diameter of the outlet (AP)–(Normal: ≥11.9 cm) This is the distance from the inferior border of the symphysis to the posterior aspect of the tip of the sacrum. A Martin or Breisky pelvimeter is generally used. This is virtually as accurate as x-ray measurement even in a moderately obese patient.

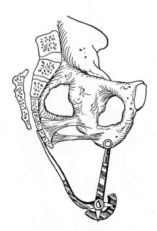

Figure 5–2. Posterior sagittal (PS) measurements with Thoms's pelvimeter.

A metal bar or ring 8.5 cm in diameter (equivalent to the biparietal diameter of the average term infant's head) can also be fitted beneath the pelvic arch between the pelvic rami as an estimate of the available space at the pelvic outlet.

d. Interspinous diameter of the mid pelvis – (Normal: ≥10.5 cm) This important measurement is usually obtained by x-ray, although with experience, the distance between the ischial spines can be directly measured with a Hanson's pelvimeter. Direct measurement causes

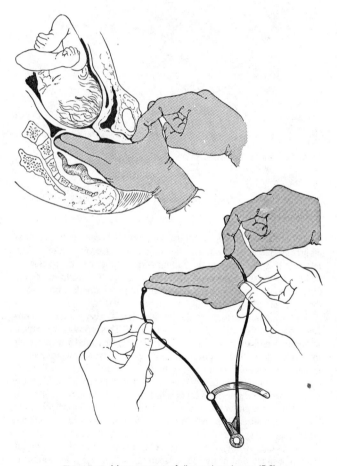

Figure 5–3 Measurement of diagonal conjugate (DC).

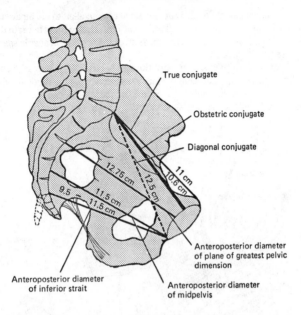

True conjugate

Obstetric conjugate

Diagonal conjugate

12.75 cm   12.5 cm   11 cm (10.6 cm)

9.5   11.5 cm   11.5 cm

Anteroposterior diameter
of plane of greatest pelvic
dimension

Anteroposterior diameter
of inferior strait

Anteroposterior diameter
of midpelvis

Figure 5–4. Pelvic measurements.

minor discomfort. When the vagina is relaxed, both ends of the pelvimeter are inserted into the vagina; when the vagina is narrow, one end of the instrument is inserted into the rectum and the other into the vagina. A DeLee or Breisky pelvimeter may be used, but these instruments are difficult to use transvaginally, especially in primigravidas, because of the pain caused by the rigidity of the narrow vault.

e. **Diagonal conjugate of the inlet (DC—also called the conjugata diagonalis, CD)**–(Normal: >11.5 cm) This is probably the most important single measurement of the pelvis. It is measured from the inner inferior border of the symphysis to the midpoint of the sacral promontory (or false promontory, whichever is shorter) (Figs 5–3 and 5–4). The true conjugate (conjugata vera, CV) is estimated from the DC. The CV is the distance from the anterior midpoint of the sacral or false promontory to the superior margin of the symphysis in the midline and is calculated to be 1.5 cm shorter than the DC; this represents the actual available anteroposterior space at the inlet (Fig 5–3). A DC of 11.5 cm or less or a CV of less than 10 cm indicates contracture of the pelvic inlet or superior strait; the likelihood of dystocia, assuming an average-sized infant, is inversely proportionate to this measurement.

5. Palpation–

a. Pubic arch–Trace the pubic arch with the examining fingers. The angle formed by the pubic arch (the angle of the rami at the pubis) is usually 110–120 degrees. If the angle is narrow (< 90 degrees), the BI may be considerably shortened. This is typical of an android pelvis.

b. Spines of the ischium–Consider the degree of prominence, sharpness, and extent of encroachment of the spines into the birth canal.

c. Sacrum–The contour, depth, and irregularities (eg, bosses of rickets, false promontory) are important. Record the curvature as "hollow" (deep), "average" (normally capacious), and "flat" (shallow).

d. Coccyx–By grasping the coccyx between the fingers of the examining hand with the other hand placed in the cleft between the buttocks, the direction of the coccyx, its degree of movement at the sacrococcygeal articulation, and local tenderness may be determined.

e. Sacrosciatic notch–(Normal: > 3 cm) The width of this space should be estimated in centimeters, not "fingerbreadths."

C. X-Ray Pelvimetry: X-ray pelvimetry (see p 381) is contraindicated except at term when cephalopelvic disproportion is anticipated. Record the measurements obtained, as well as average dimensions (see p 379) for comparison. Evaluate the inlet, mid pelvis, and outlet and determine the type of pelvis and the skull size, presentation, position, and relative size of the fetus.

D. Ultrasonography: Ultrasonography can be used to measure important pelvic or fetal skull diameters. However, considerable experience and skill are required for accurate mensuration.

Ultrasound may also be used for cephalometry (which is correlated with fetal weight), placental localization, volumetric appraisal of the growth of the placenta, diagnosis of molar or multiple pregnancy, determination of fetal placement, and detection of fetal abnormalities (anencephaly, hydrocephaly) and fetal death. Other uses include early identification of intrauterine or extrauterine pregnancy, mensuration of the uterine volume, demonstration of hydramnios or oligohydramnios, identification of uterine or ovarian tumors, and detection of foreign bodies.

E. Rectal Examination: Identify hemorrhoids and fissures.

Laboratory Tests

The following routine tests should usually be performed on the first antenatal visit or soon thereafter:

A. Urinalysis: A first morning specimen of voided urine and a 2-hour postprandial specimen should be tested at the second visit and a first voided specimen at every visit thereafter for protein and glucose. Instruct the patient to cleanse the urethral meatus with damp cotton and tell her how to obtain a "clean-catch" ("midstream") specimen while the urine is being passed. A clean-catch specimen is not contaminated with vaginal mucus and blood and gives almost the equivalent of a catheterized specimen.

If the specimen contains more than faint traces of protein or glucose, special tests for urinary tract disease and diabetes mellitus may be required.

B. Urine Culture: A screening culture should be done to detect asymptomatic urinary tract infection.

C. Hematocrit: Determine the hematocrit or hemoglobin level. If the hematocrit is less than 35% or the hemoglobin level is below 10 g/dL, the patient is anemic and further tests should be done to determine the cause of anemia. Iron and folic acid deficiencies are common causes of anemia in pregnancy and can be detected by determining serum levels of iron, ferritin, and folate. If these tests give normal results, less common causes of anemia (eg, β-thalassemia, vitamin B_{12} deficiency) should be investigated.

D. White Blood Cell Count and Differential Count: These tests should be done when infection or blood dyscrasia is suspected.

E. Serologic Studies:

1. ABO typing–Determine the blood type. If the patient has type O blood, the husband's blood type should be determined to check for possible ABO incompatibility. If incompatibility exists, the infant may develop hyperbilirubinemia.

2. Rh typing–If an Rh-negative woman carrying an Rh-positive fetus becomes sensitized to the fetal blood, hemolytic disease of the newborn (erythroblastosis fetalis) can occur. If the Rh antibody titer rises during pregnancy, the rise in titer should be verified; if it has risen significantly, amniocentesis is probably indicated.

All Rh-negative women carrying Rh-positive fetuses should be immunized with Rh$_0$ (D) immune globulin within 72 hours after abortion, amniocentesis, or delivery.

3. Typing for other red cell agglutinins–Certain familial agglutinins stimulate production of antibody in a person whose blood does not contain these antigens. The Kell, Duffy, Lutheran, Lewis, and Kidd factors are the most common of these, although they occur in only 2% of obstetric patients. The indirect Coombs test is used to demonstrate the presence of antibodies against these factors. If the test is positive, the particular antibody should be identified and the gravida monitored for a rising antibody titer, which indicates that isoimmunization is developing.

4. Serologic test for syphilis–All pregnant women should have a nontreponemal serologic test for syphilis at the time of the first prenatal visit. The VDRL (Venereal Disease Research Laboratory) test is most commonly used, but occasional false-positive results occur. Seroreactive patients should be evaluated promptly by a quantitative nontreponemal test and a fluorescent treponemal antibody absorption

(FTA-ABS) test. They should also be tested for gonorrhea (see below). If the FTA-ABS test is nonreactive and there is no clinical evidence of syphilis, treatment is not necessary. If the diagnosis of syphilis is positive or uncertain, treatment should be instituted and the patient monitored by periodic VDRL tests. A falling titer indicates that treatment is adequate; a rising titer indicates inadequate treatment or reinfection.

5. Rubella screening–All pregnant women who are not known with certainty to have had rubella (German measles) or who have not been immunized against this disease should be tested for rubella antibodies by the rubella hemagglutination inhibition (RHI) test. An RHI titer of up to 1:10 indicates immunity; a higher titer indicates relatively recent infection; and a lower titer indicates lack of immunity. Patients who are not immune to rubella should avoid contact with anyone who has or is suspected of having this disease. If exposure occurs, the RHI test should be repeated 3–4 weeks later; seroconversion indicates prenatal infection, and the risk to the fetus must be investigated. Therapeutic abortion may be warranted.

Nonimmune women should be vaccinated against rubella, but because the vaccine virus can infect the fetus, *vaccination should never be done during pregnancy*. Vaccinate immediately postpartum or later. Pregnancy should be avoided for at least 2 months after vaccination.

F. Cervical Cytologic Smears (Papanicolaou Smears): Antenatal screening for cervical intraepithelial neoplasia (CIN) is now routine. A Papanicolaou smear (see p 575) is also useful in the diagnosis of acute herpesvirus infection, although a negative report will not exclude this possibility; if herpesvirus infection is strongly suspected or cervical cytology suggests it, an attempt should be made to isolate and identify the virus.

G. Other Tests:

1. Tuberculosis–Women who have had tuberculosis or have had close contact with a tuberculous individual should be tested for this disease. Those known to react positively to tuberculin (eg, tine test) should have a chest x-ray; others should have a tuberculin skin test. If the test or x-ray is positive, request medical consultation for further evaluation and possible chemotherapy.

2. Gonorrhea–All patients with a positive serologic test for syphilis, a history of gonorrhea, or multiple sexual contacts should have cervical and anal specimens taken for culture for *Neisseria gonorrhoeae*. Patients found to have gonorrhea must be treated immediately (see p 523).

3. Hemoglobinopathy screening–All black patients who have not been tested previously should be screened by hemoglobin electrophoresis for hemoglobinopathies (eg, sickle cell disease) associated with increased maternal and fetal morbidity and mortality. Hemoglobins

SS, SC, and S-thai are the most common. Black husbands of patients with hemoglobin SS or SC should also be screened if this has not already been done. Genetic counseling may be advisable.

H. Special Studies: Other laboratory tests may be required for particular problems. If there is a history of significant renal or hypertensive disease, creatinine, creatinine clearance, and blood urea nitrogen tests and a 24-hour urine collection for determination of total protein should be done. Cardiac evaluation, including an ECG and chest x-ray, must be done if there is a history of chronic hypertension. A glucose tolerance test is required for frank or gestational diabetes. Antenatal screening of both parents for inherited metabolic disorders can sometimes substitute for genetic screening by amniocentesis. For example, Tay-Sachs disease, a congenital absence of the enzyme hexosaminidase A, is an autosomal recessive disorder; thus, if the enzyme is present in both parents and they are not carriers of the recessive gene, the infant will not have Tay-Sachs disease.

Diagnosis

Record whether the pregnancy is normal or abnormal and its duration.

Prognosis

Record an initial prediction of the outcome of the pregnancy (vaginal or cesarean delivery) and the likelihood of medical or surgical complications (eg, diabetes mellitus, inguinal hernia). The prognosis may be altered if obstetric problems develop later.

Anticipate disproportion, preeclampsia-eclampsia, and other likely problems.

THE NEW OBSTETRIC PATIENT

Communication, understanding, and rapport between the patient and the physician are vital to good prenatal care. The physician, the nurse practitioner, or the physician's assistant must explain what is required of the patient during pregnancy and why her full cooperation is necessary.

Explanatory books or short reviews of obstetrics for the layman are available through most bookstores.

PROCEDURE AT THE FIRST OBSTETRIC VISIT

After the history has been taken, the physical examination performed, and blood specimens obtained, the following should be done:

(1) Ask the patient to bring a first voided urine specimen at each subsequent visit.

(2) Arrange an appointment for the first return visit.

(3) Supply written prenatal care instructions and a booklet or library reference. Ask that the patient and her husband read them carefully before the next visit.

(4) Prescribe necessary medications.

(5) Answer questions and explain the costs of care.

(6) Order laboratory tests (see p 125).

MANAGEMENT OF NORMAL PREGNANCY

Visits & Examinations

Plan to see the patient in the office or clinic once a month until the 32nd week, every 2 weeks until the 36th week, and weekly thereafter until delivery—or more often if complications arise. Essential procedures at each visit are as follows:

(1) Ask the patient about her general health and any complaints.

(2) Weigh the patient and record her weight on the prenatal chart. Evaluate weight changes in comparison with the average curve and the plan for her total gain or loss during the pregnancy.

(3) Examine a urine sample for protein and glucose.

(4) Record the patient's blood pressure.

(5) Palpate the abdomen; measure and record the height of the rounded uterus above the symphysis; record any abnormal observations. Auscultate the fetal heartbeat. After the 28th week, estimate the presentation of the fetus. From the 32nd week on, in addition to the above, record the position of the fetus, the engagement of the presenting part, and an estimate of the weight of the fetus.

(6) Rectal or vaginal examinations may be done at virtually any time (in the absence of bleeding) to confirm the identity of the presenting part, establish its station, and determine the status of the cervix. These data are most important if labor is imminent or if induction is contemplated.

(7) The hematocrit or hemoglobin determination should be repeated at about the 32nd week of pregnancy; treat anemia vigorously before term. Repeat Rh testing (see p 214) at 32–36 weeks if isoimmunization seems likely.

MINOR DISCOMFORTS OF NORMAL PREGNANCY

Breathlessness

Breathlessness, not actual dyspnea, is common during pregnancy. In nonsmokers and others free of cough or allergic problems, breathlessness occurs as early as the 12th week of pregnancy; most women have this symptom by the 30th week.

Backache

Virtually all women suffer from at least minor degrees of lumbar backache during pregnancy. Fatigue, muscle spasm, and postural and other types of back strain, especially during the last trimester, are most often responsible. Relaxation of the pelvic joints from the action of steroid sex hormones and perhaps relaxin is also responsible. Backache can often be relieved by the following measures:

(1) Improved posture. The abdomen should be flattened, the pelvis tilted forward, and the buttocks "tucked under" to straighten the back.

(2) Moderately vigorous daily exercises to tone the muscles and maintain their strength.

(3) Wearing shoes with 2-inch heels tends to keep the shoulders forward and straighten the back, particularly when flat footwear has been worn extensively.

(4) A firm mattress. A sagging mattress may cause painful, prolonged flexion of the back (after exaggerated extension while erect). Bedboards between the springs and mattress are often helpful.

(5) Local heat and light massage relax tense, taut back muscles.

(6) A maternity girdle for back support may be indicated for patients with backache due to extreme lordosis or kyphoscoliosis or associated with obesity or multiple pregnancy.

(7) Aspirin, 0.3–0.6 g orally, may be adequate for mild distress.

(8) Orthopedic evaluation is necessary when disability results from backache. Note neurologic signs and symptoms indicative of intervertebral disk syndrome or radiculitis.

Syncope & Faintness

Syncope and faintness are common in early pregnancy. Vasomotor instability, often associated with postural hypotension, results in transient cerebral ischemia and pooling of blood in the legs and splanchnic and pelvic areas, especially after prolonged standing or sitting in a warm room. Hypoglycemia before or between meals, more common during pregnancy, may result in "lightheadedness" or even fainting. These attacks can be prevented by avoiding inactivity and by slow change of motion. Encourage the patient to eat 6 small meals a day rather than 3 large ones. Stimulants (spirits of ammonia, coffee, tea) are indicated for attacks due to hypotension; food will correct hypoglycemia.

Nausea & Vomiting (Morning Sickness)

About half of all pregnant women complain of nausea and sometimes vomiting, often upon arising, at some time during pregnancy. This is most common during the first 10 weeks. The cause of the nausea and vomiting is not known, but endocrine mechanisms undoubtedly play a part. Emotional factors are also involved, but the symptoms may be experienced even by women who do not know they are pregnant. There is undoubtedly a physiologic basis for the symptoms in many cases. A few women with "morning sickness" develop intractable vomiting (hyperemesis gravidarum; pernicious vomiting of pregnancy); in such cases, hospitalization is usually necessary to correct fluid and electrolyte imbalance.

Explanation, reassurance, and symptomatic relief are usually sufficient. If the patient can be convinced that little harm is likely to result from the complaint, she will usually feel better. Dietary changes are often helpful. Eating dry toast and jelly immediately upon arising and before the nausea begins helps some patients. Six small "dry" meals daily may be a good plan. Avoidance of disagreeable odors and rich, spicy, or greasy foods is important. Urge the patient to drink water or other fluids between meals to avoid dehydration and acidosis, which predispose to nausea.

If nausea is prolonged and severe and constitutes a serious threat to the health of the patient, meclizine, 25 mg 3 times daily before meals, may be effective. Phenobarbital, 15 mg orally 1–3 times a day, may be beneficial, but avoid continued use. **Note:** Many drugs that are harmless for a nonpregnant woman may have unforeseen or undesirable effects on the fetus. Therefore, during pregnancy, even well-known drugs should be administered only when absolutely indicated. (See also Table 4–2.)

Excessive Salivation (Sialorrhea or Ptyalism)

Ptyalism may be troublesome (especially during early pregnancy) because of associated nausea, interference with sleep, and loss of fluids, electrolytes, and enzymes. Up to 1500 mL of saliva a day may be produced. Drug stimulation (eg, mercury, bismuth), oral lesions, seventh nerve paralysis, and hysteria should be ruled out as causes. The problem subsides in late pregnancy or after delivery.

Treatment involves reassurance and insistence that the patient not spit or collect the saliva. Anticholinergic drugs such as belladonna extract, 8–15 mg, or methscopolamine bromide, 2.5 mg orally 4 times daily, are most helpful. *Caution:* These and similar drugs should be avoided in patients with glaucoma, marked gastric retention, or intestinal stasis.

Leukorrhea

A gradual increase in the amount of vaginal discharge must be expected throughout pregnancy. Augmented estrogen production increases the secretion of cervical mucus. Vaginal fluid is milk colored, thin, and nonirritating unless infection occurs. Persistent external moisture due to mucus may cause mild pruritus, but itching is rarely severe unless infection is present. Reassurance is usually all that is needed. Some patients may find protective pads helpful. Excessive leukorrhea accompanied by pruritus, or discoloration of the secretion, may indicate infection, which requires specific treatment (see p 517).

Urinary Symptoms

Urinary frequency, urgency, and stress incontinence are quite common, especially in advanced pregnancy. They are due to altered renal and bladder function caused by hormonal changes and to increased intra-abdominal pressure, reduced bladder capacity, and pressure of the presenting part upon the bladder.

In some cases, urinary frequency is due to urinary tract infection. Suspect urinary tract disease if dysuria or hematuria is reported.

When urgency is particularly troublesome, limit caffeine, spices, and alcoholic beverages. Prescribe a bladder sedative mixture:

R Tincture hyoscyamus	30
Potassium citrate	60
Water, qs ad	180

Give 4 mL in water orally every 4 hours as necessary. Comparable preparations that may be given are Urised, 1–2 tablets orally every 4 hours as necessary, and Levamine, 1 capsule every 2 hours as necessary.

Heartburn

Heartburn (pyrosis, "acid indigestion") results from gastroesophageal regurgitation. In late pregnancy, this may be aggravated by displacement of the stomach and duodenum by the uterine fundus. Heartburn is most likely to occur when the patient is lying down or bending over.

Almost 10% of all pregnant patients experience severe pyrosis during late pregnancy because of diaphragmatic hiatus hernia. This hernia is reduced spontaneously by parturition. Symptomatic relief, not surgery, is recommended.

Chewing gum, hot tea, and change of posture are helpful. In late pregnancy, antacid gels containing aluminum hydroxide and magnesium hydroxide to reduce gastric irritation are beneficial. Avoid antacids during early pregnancy because gastric acidity is already low.

Constipation

Constipation due to sluggish bowel function in pregnancy may be prevented by emphasizing fluids and laxative foods (whole fruit) and by using a stool softener such as dioctyl sodium sulfosuccinate. Moderate exercise and good bowel habits are also helpful. Mild laxatives (eg, milk of magnesia) are helpful, but purgatives (eg, castor oil) should be avoided because of the possibility of inducing labor. Mineral oil is contraindicated; it absorbs fat-soluble vitamins from the gastrointestinal tract, and lack of vitamin K is a cause of hemorrhagic disease of the newborn.

Hemorrhoids (See also Chapter 26.)

Hemorrhoids are frequent in pregnancy and may cause considerable discomfort. Straining at stool often causes hemorrhoids, especially in women prone to varicosities. Treat constipation early. At delivery, use elective low forceps with episiotomy when feasible.

An attempt should be made to replace the hemorrhoids gently, though this is rarely possible. Useful medical measures include warm (or cool) sitz baths and the local application of witch hazel compresses. Soothing, astringent anal suppositories, topical anesthetics, and laxatives may be of great help.

Surgical treatment is usually not indicated during pregnancy. Recently thrombosed, painful hemorrhoids can be incised under local anesthesia and the clot evacuated. Do not suture. Sitz baths, rectal ointments, suppositories, and mild laxatives are indicated postoperatively. Injection treatments to obliterate hemorrhoids during pregnancy are contraindicated; they may cause infection and extensive thrombosis of the pelvic veins and are rarely successful because of the great dilatation of many vessels.

Breast Tenderness

Physiologic breast engorgement may cause discomfort, especially during early and late pregnancy. A well-fitted brassiere worn 24 hours a day affords relief. Ice packs or cold compresses are temporarily effective. Hormone therapy is of no value.

Headache

Headache in pregnancy is a common, usually benign symptom. Headache is most disturbing during the first and third trimesters. Emotional tension is the most common cause. Refractive errors and ocular imbalance are not caused by normal pregnancy. The pregnant woman is usually more sedentary; she may read, sew, or watch television more despite eyestrain. Hormonal stimulation causes vascular engorgement of the nasal turbinates, and the resultant congestion contributes to sinusitis and headache, frequently accompanied by nosebleeds.

Severe, persistent headache in the last trimester must be regarded as symptomatic of preeclampsia-eclampsia.

The belief that pituitary swelling during normal pregnancy causes headache is without foundation.

Headaches usually require only reassurance, adequate rest, and mild analgesics (eg, aspirin). Mild sedatives such as diazepam (Valium), 5–10 mg orally, may be beneficial. Give nasal decongestants for acute nasal congestion. Ophthalmologic studies may reveal a need for corrective lenses. Emotional support may help to relieve anxiety and reduce emotional tension.

Ankle Swelling

Edema of the lower extremities not associated with preeclampsia-eclampsia develops in at least two-thirds of women in late pregnancy. Edema is due to sodium and water retention, increased venous pressure in the legs, varicose veins with venous congestion, prolonged sitting or standing, and elastic garters or knee-high stockings.

Treatment is largely preventive and symptomatic. The patient should elevate her legs frequently and sleep in a slight Trendelenburg position. Round garters or knee-high stockings, which interfere with venous return, should not be worn. Restrict excessive salt intake and provide elastic support for varicose veins (see below). Diuretics, particularly thiazide compounds, may reduce edema temporarily, but they may be harmful to the mother or fetus.

Varicose Veins

Varicosities may develop in the legs or in the vulva. The pregnant woman is usually a multipara, and a family history of varicosities is often present. Varices are due to weakness of the vascular walls and valves, increased venous stasis in the legs due to the hemodynamics of pregnancy, inactivity and poor muscle tone, and obesity. Pressure by the enlarging uterus on the venous return from the legs is a major factor in the development of varicosities. Although most varicose veins are asymptomatic, all are unsightly. Large or numerous varicosities cause muscle aching, edema, skin ulcers, and emboli. Venous stasis, trauma, and dermatitis contribute to phlebothrombosis and thrombophlebitis.

Early in pregnancy, the patient should be instructed to exercise, rest in the recumbent position, elevate her legs above the level of her body, wear loose clothing, and control weight gain. She should avoid vigorous massage and point-pressure over the legs.

Patients with significant varices in the lower legs should be fitted with elastic "stretch" stockings. Complete elastic leg hose are impractical. Cotton stockings are cooler and more absorptive than nylon hose.

Have the patient lie flat with one leg raised for a few minutes to empty the veins, then roll the elastic stocking on from the toe with the leg still elevated. Stockings should be worn at all times while the patient is up. In severe cases, elastic hose may even be worn during sleep.

Large vulvar varices cause pudendal discomfort. A vulvar pad wrapped in plastic film and snugly held by a menstrual belt or Jobst leotards gives relief.

Specific therapy (injection or surgical correction) of even small varicose veins usually is contraindicated during pregnancy.

Leg Cramps

Cramping or "knotting" of the muscles of the calf, thigh, or buttocks occurs suddenly after sleep or recumbency in many women after the first trimester of pregnancy. For unknown reasons, it is less common during the month before term. Sudden shortening of the leg muscles by stretching with the toes pointed precipitates the cramp. Leg cramps may be due to a reduced level of diffusible serum calcium or an increased serum phosphorus level. This follows excessive dietary intake of phosphorus in milk, cheese, meat, or dicalcium phosphate or diminished intake or impaired absorption of calcium. Fatigue in the extremities is a contributing factor.

Treatment should include curtailment of phosphate intake (less milk and nutritional supplements containing calcium phosphate) and increase of calcium intake (without phosphorus) in the form of calcium carbonate or calcium lactate tablets. Aluminum hydroxide gel, 8 mL orally 3 times a day before meals, adsorbs phosphate and may increase calcium absorption. Symptomatic treatment consists of leg massage, gentle flexing of the feet, and local heat. Tell the patient to avoid pointing her toes when she stretches her legs (eg, on awakening); this triggers a gastrocnemius cramp. She should practice "leading with the heel" in walking.

Abdominal Pain

Intra-abdominal alterations causing pain during the course of pregnancy include the following:

A. Pressure: Pelvic heaviness, a sense of sagging or dragging, is caused by the weight of the uterus on the pelvic supports and the abdominal wall. The patient should rest frequently in the supine or lateral recumbent position. A maternity girdle may provide relief.

B. Round Ligament Tension: Tenderness along the course of the round ligament (usually the left) during late pregnancy is due to traction on this structure by the uterus with rotation of the uterus and change of the patient's position. Local heat and measures as for pressure pain (see above) are effective.

C. Flatulence, Distention, Bowel Cramping: Large meals, fats, gas-forming foods, and chilled beverages are poorly tolerated by pregnant women. Mechanical displacement and compression of the bowel by the enlarged uterus, hypotonia of the intestines, and constipation predispose to gastrointestinal distress. Dietary modifications give effective relief. Regular bowel function should be maintained, using mild laxatives when indicated. Exercise and frequent change of position are also of value.

D. Uterine Contractions: So-called Braxton Hicks contractions of the uterus may be strong, sharp, and startling for some patients. The onset of premature labor must always be considered when forceful contractions develop. If they remain infrequent and brief in duration, the danger of early delivery is not significant. Phenobarbital, 30–60 mg orally 2–4 times daily; sedatives such as diazepam (Valium), 5–10 mg 3 times daily; or aspirin, 0.3–0.6 g 2–3 times daily, may be of value.

E. Intra-abdominal Disorders: Pain may be due to obstruction, inflammation, and other disorders of the gastrointestinal, urinary, neurologic, or vascular system or to pathologic pregnancy or tubal or ovarian disease. These disorders must be diagnosed and treated appropriately.

Fatigue

The pregnant patient is more subject to fatigue during the last trimester of pregnancy because of altered posture and extra weight. Anemia and other systemic diseases must be ruled out. Frequent rest periods are recommended.

NUTRITION IN PREGNANCY

Weight Gain

Until recently, many authorities encouraged restriction of weight gain during pregnancy, even to the point of recommending stringent weight reduction programs for overweight patients. A weight reduction program during pregnancy, even for the obese patient, is no longer recommended.

There has recently been a renewal of interest in the notion that increased maternal weight gain during pregnancy increases mean birth weight in the infant. The mother's prepregnancy weight and her weight gain during pregnancy are major determinants in the birth weight of the infant. Women who are in a low weight category (eg, < 55 kg) before pregnancy and gain a limited amount of weight (< 4500 g) during pregnancy have a notably higher incidence of low-birth-weight infants than heavier mothers who gain more weight during pregnancy.

Good maternal nutrition is a major determinant of normal fetal growth and development. Any gross deficiency of maternal circulation may interfere with both maternal and fetal nutrition. Obstetric patients with severe heart disease bear small babies probably as a result of poor circulation. Placental transport mechanisms may be adversely affected by nutritional deficiencies in the mother. The clinician should evaluate all relevant factors, including socioeconomic status and cultural habits, when considering the nutritional aspects of fetal growth and development.

The physician will be more successful as a nutrition counselor if emphasis is placed on what should be eaten rather than what should be avoided. However, one should discuss what to avoid during pregnancy when substitutes for necessary foods are the rule, eg, in the case of the teenager who subsists on soft drinks, potato chips, and hamburgers.

How much weight should a pregnant woman be allowed, or encouraged, to gain? The normal mean weight gain of pregnant women eating "to appetite" is difficult to determine for many reasons—not the least of which is the fact that, in the past, few pregnant patients who were studied had been permitted to eat as much as they wanted. The average weight gain of a healthy patient, excluding gain due to fat, is about 13 kg (28 lb). It should be remembered, however, that many patients will weigh more or less than the mean without apparent ill effects.

There is no convincing evidence that excessive weight gain, whether in the form of fat or water, causes preeclampsia-eclampsia. Nevertheless, the incidence of preeclampsia-eclampsia in the USA has declined markedly, and it seems likely that better nutrition may account for at least part of this improvement.

The rate of weight gain plays an important role in the diagnosis of preeclampsia-eclampsia. An increase of more than 1814 g (4 lb) per month in any 2 consecutive months in the last trimester will often presage preeclampsia-eclampsia.

Moderate weight gain is associated with the lowest incidence of low-birth-weight infants and neonatal death. The underweight woman with a small gain in weight during pregnancy should be considered a high-risk patient. The woman who gains excessive weight will have the usual problems of obesity. Individualization of diet seems the best course of action. Emphasis should be placed on good nutrition rather than on precise weight control.

Since up to 10% of body weight may be gained in the form of retained fluids before peripheral edema is apparent, the patient's weight and blood pressure should be checked carefully and repeatedly during pregnancy.

Dietary Requirements

The daily dietary allowances recommended by the Food and Nutrition Board of the National Academy of Sciences-National Research Council are listed in Table 5–1. These should be considered approximations, because adult patients who are ill or underweight and young girls who have not completed their growth will require larger allowances. In any event, a pregnancy diet should include the following daily components: milk, 1 L (or quart); one average serving of citrus fruit or tomato, a

Table 5-1. Recommended daily dietary allowance for women 18–50 years old, 64 inches tall, and weighing 120 pounds when not pregnant. (Food and Nutrition Board, National Academy of Sciences–National Research Council. Revised 1980.)

Nutrient	Nonpregnant	Increase Pregnant	Increase Lactating
Calories (kcal)	2000	+300	+500
Protein (g)	44	+30	+20
Vitamin A (RE)[1]	800	+200	+400
Vitamin D (IU)	200	+200	+200
Vitamin E (mg α-TE)[2]	8	+2	+3
Vitamin C (mg)	60	+20	+40
Folacin[3] (μg)	400	+400	+100
Niacin (mg NE)[4]	14	+2	+5
Thiamine (mg)	1.1	+0.4	+0.5
Riboflavin (mg)	1.3	+0.3	+0.5
Vitamin B_6 (mg)	2	+0.6	+0.5
Vitamin B_{12} (μg)	3	+1	+1
Calcium (mg)	800	+400	+400
Phosphorus (mg)	800	+400	+400
Iodine (μg)	150	+25	+50
Iron (mg)	18	+30–60	+30–60
Magnesium (mg)	300	+150	+150
Zinc (mg)	15	+5	+10

[1] Retinol equivalents. 1 RE = 1 μg retinol or 6 μg β-carotene.

[2] α-Tocopherol equivalents. 1 α-TE = 1 mg α-tocopherol.

[3] Refers to dietary sources as determined by *Lactobacillus casei* assay after treatment with enzymes to make polyglutamyl forms of the vitamin available to the test organism.

[4] Niacin equivalents. 1 NE = 1 mg niacin or 60 mg dietary tryptophan.

leafy green vegetable, and a yellow vegetable; and 2 average servings of lean meat, fish, poultry, eggs, beans, or cheese.

Supplemental Minerals & Vitamins

Milk is relatively inexpensive, and 1 L (or 1 quart) of cow's milk contains 1 g of calcium—approximately the daily intake recommended during pregnancy (1.2 g)—and 33 g of protein. Therefore, 1 quart of milk plus other food usually will provide adequate calcium intake. The milk need not always be in the form of a beverage but can be used in the preparation of food such as custard, junket, and soup. If the patient will not or cannot drink milk, substitute sources of calcium (eg, cheese, yogurt, ice milk, spinach) should be offered or a supplement such as calcium carbonate prescribed. Some patients—especially American Indians, foreign-born blacks, and Orientals—may have a disaccharidase deficiency that causes intolerance to lactose in milk. For these persons, protein, calcium, and vitamins must be supplied in other forms (eg, cheese, fish, fruits).

Supplemental iron is needed to prevent depletion of the maternal iron stores, especially during the latter part of pregnancy. About 30 mg of iron daily, in the form of a simple iron compound (ferrous gluconate or ferrous fumarate), provides sufficient iron to meet the requirements of pregnancy and protect iron stores.

Folic acid (folacin), 0.8 mg/d orally, should be given as a dietary supplement during pregnancy. Routine folate treatment will not harm a pregnant woman with unrecognized pernicious anemia.

A pregnant woman who consumes adequate quantities of properly prepared fresh foods needs no other vitamin or mineral supplements, but many women do not eat enough vitamin-containing foods. To make certain that the vitamin intake is adequate, half the daily recommended dietary allowances listed in Table 5–1 should be given in the form of a supplement. The common practice of recommending prenatal vitamin supplements is not harmful in the doses usually prescribed. Excessive ingestion of vitamins D and A may be harmful.

Although ample calcium and phosphorus are required by the mother for fetal anabolism, a relative excess of phosphorus may cause leg cramps (see p 135). Large quantities of milk, meat, cheese, and dicalcium phosphate (taken as a supplement) provide too much phosphorus.

Salt Restriction

Moderate amounts of salt- or sodium-containing foods are not harmful during normal pregnancy. The widespread practice of restricting sodium intake and prescribing diuretics at the same time is potentially dangerous. The requirement for sodium during pregnancy is increased slightly, and overemphasis on sodium restriction is not justified unless sudden weight gain or preeclampsia-eclampsia occurs.

Fluids

At least 2–3 quarts of fluid should be taken daily during pregnancy to accommodate metabolic processes and aid in elimination. This should normally include 1 quart of milk. Limitation of fluids will neither prevent nor correct fluid retention. Liquids containing no sodium will not contribute to edema in the absence of renal failure. Actually, increased intake of water aids slightly in the excretion of sodium.

OTHER CONCERNS IN PREGNANCY

Medications

It is wise to discourage the administration of drugs to pregnant women as much as possible because of reports of teratogenesis after drug administration in early pregnancy. In general, give drugs only when urgently required; avoid new and experimental drugs and all drugs that have been suggested as possible teratogens; and give drugs, when needed, in the lowest dosage consistent with clinical efficacy.

Record *all* drugs taken by the patient during pregnancy, and caution her about taking any drug without first discussing it with the physician.

Most drugs taken regularly before pregnancy (thyroid, aspirin, laxatives) may be continued during pregnancy on approval of the obstetrician (but see above). It may be necessary, however, to vary the medication or dosage appropriately as pregnancy progresses.

Steroid sex hormones, especially diethylstilbestrol, must not be administered to pregnant women because of the possible development of carcinoma of the cervix or vagina in the offspring.

Drugs with proved ill effects upon the fetus are listed in Table 4–2.

Alcoholic Beverages

Complete avoidance of alcohol is best, but an occasional alcoholic beverage may be permitted most pregnant patients. Excessive alcohol intake may cause fetal anomalies (fetal alcohol syndrome). If weight reduction is a problem, it must be remembered that alcohol stimulates appetite and is itself a significant source of calories: there are 160–175 kcal in a cocktail, 140 kcal in a highball with ginger ale; 96 kcal per 12-oz bottle of ''light'' beer; about 7–8 kcal per ounce of fortified or sweet dessert wine; and 80 kcal per 1-oz jigger of whiskey.

Smoking

Smoking even in moderation may be harmful to the pregnancy. Pregnant women should be encouraged not to smoke. Insist upon severe limitation or complete avoidance of smoking when chronic respiratory irritation, asthma, or persistent indigestion are related to smoking. The incidence of low birth weight is higher than normal in infants born to women who are moderate to heavy smokers (20 or more cigarettes a day) during pregnancy. Although smaller, these infants are not necessarily preterm. A slightly higher perinatal mortality rate must be expected in these infants. Lactation is not affected by smoking, nor is the nursing infant apparently harmed by limited smoking by the mother.

Immunizations

Live virus vaccines, especially those for measles, mumps, rubella, and typhoid fever, should be avoided during pregnancy because of risk to the fetus. Immunization against influenza, poliomyelitis, or yellow fever may be permitted if the pregnant woman is at increased risk of contracting one of these diseases.

Dental Care

If the patient neglects oral hygiene during early pregnancy, when nausea may be troublesome, hormonal hypertrophy and turgescence of the gums (epulis) will permit irritation and infection of the gingivae. Variations in salivary pH may contribute to dental caries. However, even with gross dietary calcium deficiency, decalcification of the mother's teeth does not occur as a result of pregnancy.

Necessary dental fillings or extractions may be performed during pregnancy, preferably under local anesthesia. Abortion or premature labor and delivery are not caused even by extensive dental surgery. Septicemia as a sequela to dental abscesses may complicate maternal cardiovascular or renal disease; antibiotics should be administered prophylactically in such cases.

Intercourse & Vaginal Hygiene

Coitus and douches very rarely contribute to spontaneous abortion and premature labor. Contraindications include premature labor, rupture of the membranes, bleeding, and genital herpesvirus infection. Intercourse should be avoided during the first month by women who are habitual aborters. Douching is seldom necessary and may be harmful. Forceful douches, especially with a hand bulb syringe, may produce air or fluid embolism.

Bathing

Bath water does not enter the vagina. Tub baths and swimming are not contraindicated in normal pregnancy. However, diving should be avoided because of possible trauma. Women in the last trimester of pregnancy are clumsy and have poor balance. For this reason, they should be cautioned about slipping and falling in the tub or shower.

Preparation for Breast Feeding

Most women who breast-feed successfully do so naturally without preparation. The advantages of nursing should be explained to the obstetric patient, and the final decision on whether to breast-feed should be reserved until the last trimester of pregnancy. Aversion and objections to breast feeding may be dispelled if encouragement and adequate information are provided. If the patient decides to nurse, institute predelivery breast and nipple care (see p 247).

The Figure

Pregnancy need not "ruin" the figure. Excessive weight gain, change in body habitus, altered posture, and breast enlargement are temporary. Attention should be given to personal appearance; and avoidance of excessive weight gain, continued daily exercise, and a well-fitted brassiere worn much of the time will help to preserve the figure. Some loss of abdominal tone is inevitable during pregnancy, and the healthiest attitude is simply to minimize and accept it temporarily; abdominal tone can be regained postpartum (see Chapter 9).

Exercise

Moderate exercise in work or sports is beneficial during pregnancy, but excessive exercise may be harmful to both mother and fetus. Strenuous sports like scuba diving or long-distance running require substantial physical effort that increases maternal oxygen consumption (which increases the risk of hypoxia) and the demand on cardiac reserve (which may result in decreased blood flow to the fetus). Women who have had early gestational losses or 2 previous preterm infants or who have uterine anomalies are at risk of early labor with overexertion.

Employment

Many women can continue to work full- or part-time during pregnancy. How long the pregnant woman can safely remain on the job depends upon the type of work, industrial hazards, the policy of the employer, and pregnancy complications. Women with sedentary jobs often work without difficulty beyond the 28th week of pregnancy, but others whose employment requires more physical exertion may find it advisable to take maternity leave earlier. Rest periods during the day may help to avoid undue fatigue.

Travel

The pregnant woman should avoid long and arduous travel. If a long journey is essential, air travel is best, but pregnant women should not fly in unpressurized aircraft unless oxygen is available. All commercial aircraft are now pressurized to 1525–2130 m (5000–7000 ft). Most airlines, to avoid possible delivery en route, will not permit women to fly during the last month of pregnancy.

Pregnant women who are traveling—especially those with pre-eclampsia, anemia, or isoimmunization—should get up to stretch and walk every 30–45 minutes to prevent venous stasis and reduced oxygen to the fetus. Travel will not cause abortion or premature labor, but the pregnant woman is jeopardized indirectly by travel because she may be far from her obstetrician in case of obstetric emergency, she is more likely to overexert herself and become fatigued, and dietary control and regular personal habits are not as easily maintained.

Danger Signals

Any vaginal bleeding, abdominal or pelvic pain, fever, generalized swelling, blurred vision, dysuria, markedly reduced urine output, escape of considerable fluid from the vagina, or other disturbing problems should be reported promptly to the physician.

Symptoms of Onset of Labor

Nulliparas in particular are anxious about how to recognize the onset of labor. Explain the usual symptoms of oncoming labor.

Course & Conduct of Normal Labor & Delivery | 6

Labor is the process by which the products of conception are normally delivered. It requires a coordinated, effective sequence of involuntary uterine contractions, which are usually augmented by voluntary contractions of the abdominal muscles. Labor may begin at any time during pregnancy, but the likelihood increases as full term approaches. Endocrine alterations are responsible for its onset and maintenance. True labor, under normal conditions, implies dilatation of the cervix and proceeds in a definite sequence to recovery of the placenta. False labor, very common in late pregnancy, is characterized by irregular, brief contractions accompanied by a mild aching sensation confined to the lower abdomen. No change in the character of the cervix occurs, and the presenting part does not descend. False labor has no significance except as a frequent cause of anxiety and premature admission to the hospital.

The beginning of true labor is marked by regular uterine contractions ("pains") that become increasingly more frequent, forceful, and prolonged.

The patient is usually aware of the contractions during the first stage. The severity of pain depends upon the fetopelvic relationships, the quality and strength of uterine contractions, and the emotional and physical status of the patient. Very few women experience no discomfort during the first stage of labor. With the beginning of true normal labor, some women describe slight low back pain that radiates around to the lower abdomen. Each contraction starts with a gradual buildup of intensity, and rather prompt dissipation follows the climax. Normally, the contraction will be at its height before discomfort is reported. Dilatation of the lower birth canal and distention of the perineum during the second stage of labor will almost always cause pain.

The fetal membranes, a protective barrier against infection, rupture before the onset of labor in about 10% of cases (premature rupture of the membranes). At full term, 9 pregnant women out of 10 will be in labor within 24 hours after rupture of the membranes. If labor does not begin within 24 hours after rupture, the case must be considered to be complicated by premature prolonged rupture of the membranes.

Just before the beginning of labor, a small amount of red-tinged mucus may be passed ("bloody show"). This is a plug of cervical mucus

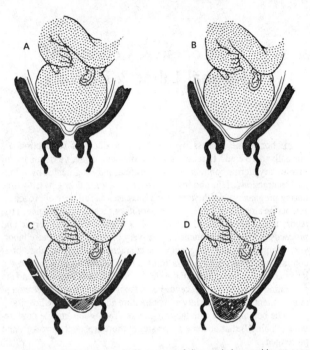

Figure 6–1. Dilatation and effacement of the cervix in a multipara.

mixed with blood and is evidence of cervical dilatation and effacement and, frequently, descent of the presenting part.

Premature labor can often be quelled by tocolytic drugs, eg, ritodrine.

THE COURSE OF NORMAL LABOR

There are 3 stages of labor: (1) the period from the onset of labor to full dilatation of the cervix, (2) the period from full dilatation of the cervix to delivery of the infant, and (3) the period from delivery of the infant to recovery of the placenta. The hour immediately after delivery of the placenta, during which time the danger of postpartal hemorrhage is great, is often referred to as the fourth stage of labor; it will be considered here as part of the third stage.

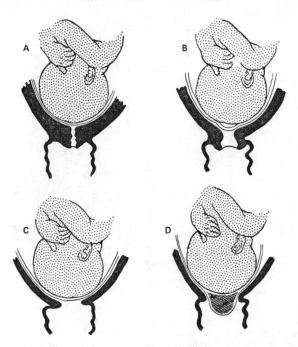

Figure 6–2. Dilatation and effacement of the cervix in a primipara.

The onset of the first stage begins with demonstrable, progressive dilatation and effacement of the cervix (Figs 6–1 and 6–2). It is often difficult to determine the exact time of onset, since the cervix may change very slowly or rapidly.

The first stage of labor ends with complete (10 cm) dilatation of the cervix. This stage is by far the longest, the average duration being about 13 hours for a primigravida and about 8 hours for a multipara. However, the first stage of labor may be less than 1 hour or more than 24 hours depending upon the parity of the patient; the frequency, intensity, and duration of uterine contractions; the ability of the cervix to dilate and efface; fetopelvic diameters; and the presentation, position, and size of the fetus.

The second stage of labor begins when the cervix becomes fully dilated and ends with the complete birth of the infant. The second stage lasts a few minutes to several hours, depending upon fetal presentation and position; fetopelvic relationships; resistance of maternal pelvic soft

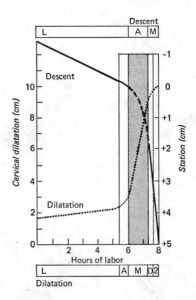

Figure 6–3. Composite mean curves for descent (solid line) and dilatation (broken line) for 389 unselected multiparas. Intervals: L, latent; A, acceleration; M, maximum slope; D, deceleration; 2, second stage. Relationship is shown between acceleration period of descent and maximum slope of dilatation (shaded area), between latent period of descent and latent plus acceleration phases of dilatation, and between maximum slope of descent and deceleration phase plus second stage. (Redrawn and reproduced, with permission, from Friedman and Sachtleben: *Am J Obstet Gynecol* 1965;**93**:526.)

parts; the frequency, intensity, duration, and regularity of uterine contractions; and the efficiency of maternal voluntary expulsive efforts.

The third, or placental, stage of labor is the period from birth of the infant to 1 hour after delivery of the placenta. The rapidity of separation and means of recovery of the placenta determine the duration of the third stage.

There is no unanimity of opinion about what constitutes prolonged labor. Some obstetricians use 24 hours or more as a criterion; others use 18–20 hours. Prodromal labor sometimes may be included erroneously.

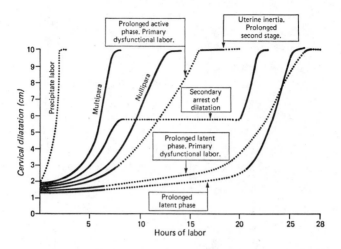

Figure 6–4. Major types of deviation from normal progress of labor may be detected by noting dilatation of cervix at various intervals after labor begins. (Reproduced, with permission, from Russell KP: Chapter 31 in *Current Obstetric & Gynecologic Diagnosis & Treatment,* 4th ed. Benson RC [editor]. Lange, 1982.)

MANAGEMENT OF THE FIRST STAGE OF LABOR

Initial Examination & Procedures

(1) Admit the patient if she has been registered in a hospital, or visit her at home if delivery there is anticipated.

(2) Obtain history of relevant medical details since the last examination.

(3) Take the patient's temperature, pulse, and blood pressure. Examine a clean-catch urine specimen for protein and glucose.

(4) Do a brief general physical examination.

(5) Palpate the uterus to determine the fetal presentation, position, and engagement (Fig 6–5). Auscultate the fetal heartbeat and mark the skin where the heartbeat is heard most clearly to facilitate subsequent examination and to note the shift and descent of the point of maximal intensity, which serves as evidence of internal rotation and descent of the fetus during labor.

(6) Note the frequency, regularity, intensity, and duration of uterine contractions and the tone of the myometrium between contractions. Observe the patient's reactions and her tolerance of labor. Restlessness and discomfort often develop as labor progresses.

(7) Check for vaginal bleeding or leakage of amniotic fluid. Nitra-

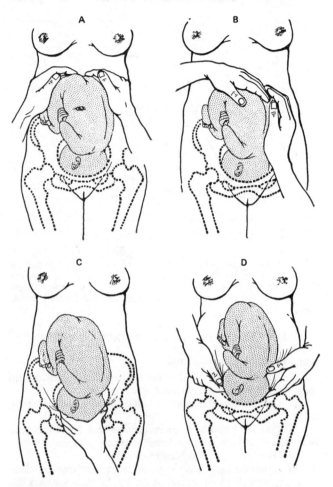

Figure 6–5. Determining fetal presentation *(A* and *B)*, position *(C)*, and engagement *(D)*. (The 4 maneuvers of Leopold.)

zine indicator paper will turn from green to yellow when moistened with
amniotic fluid (pH 7.0).

(8) Examine the patient rectally or vaginally with a surgically clean
glove. It is essential that the examiner wear a mask. This evaluation
should identify the presenting fetal part and the station of the presenting
part in relation to the level of the ischial spines. If the presenting part is at

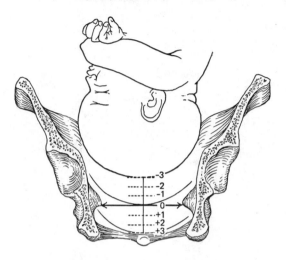

Figure 6–6. Stations of the fetal head.

the spines, it is said to be at "zero station"; if above the spines, the distances are stated in minus figures (−1 cm, −2 cm, −3 cm, and "floating"); if below the spines, the distances are stated in plus figures (+1 cm, +2 cm, +3 cm, and "on the perineum") (Fig 6–6).

(a) Dilatation of the cervical os is expressed as the diameter of the cervical opening in centimeters. A diameter of 10 cm constitutes full dilatation. A diameter of 6 cm or less can be measured directly; when the distance is more than 6 cm, however, it is often easier to subtract twice the width of the remaining "rim" from 10 cm. For example, if a 1-cm rim is felt anteriorly, posteriorly, and laterally, dilatation is 8 cm.

(b) Effacement of the cervix (Figs 6–1 and 6–2) is a process of thinning out that occurs before and, especially, during the first stage of labor. The cervix thins by retraction. In this manner, it "gets out of the way" of the presenting part, allowing more room for the birth process. Expression of mucus and compression aid in thinning of the cervix.

Effacement is expressed in percent. An uneffaced cervix is 0%, and a cervix less than about 0.25 cm thick is 100% effaced.

(c) The position of the presenting part can usually be confirmed by internal examination:

(i) Vertex presentations (Fig 6–7)–The fontanelles and the sagittal suture are palpated. The position is determined by the relation of the fetal occiput to the mother's right or left side. This is expressed as OA (occiput precisely anterior), LOA (left occiput anterior), LOP, etc.

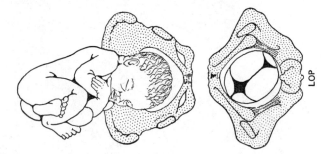

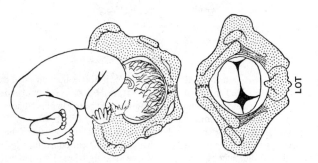

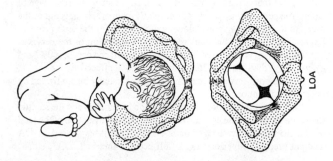

Figure 6–7. Vertex presentations.

(ii) Breech presentations are determined by the position of the infant's sacrum in respect to the mother's right or left side. This is expressed as SA (sacrum directly anterior), LSA (left sacrum anterior), LSP, etc.

(iii) Face presentations–Extension of the fetal head on the neck causes the face to be the presenting part. The chin, a prominent and identifiable facial landmark, is used as a point of reference. As with vertex presentations, the position of the fetal chin is related to the anterior or posterior portion of the left or right side of the mother's pelvis. This is expressed as RMP (right mentum posterior), etc.

(iv) Brow, bregma, or sinciput presentation is a presentation mid-way betweeen flexion and extension. It usually is a temporary presentation that converts during labor to face or occiput presentation.

(v) Transverse presentations–The long axis of the body of the fetus is perpendicular to that of the mother. One shoulder (acromion) will occupy the superior strait, but it will be considerably to the right or left of the midline. Transverse presentations are designated by relating the infant's inferior shoulder and back to the mother's back or abdominal wall. Thus, LADP (left acromio-dorso-posterior) indicates that the infant's lower shoulder is to the mother's left and the back is toward her back.

(vi) Compound presentations–Prolapse of a hand, an arm, or a foot or leg is a complication of one of the above presentations. These special or unusual presentations are generally recorded without abbreviations.

Preparation of the Patient for Labor

The following should be done after the internal examination at admission or at the onset of labor to be conducted in the home:

(1) Prepare and cleanse the pudendum. It is best to clip the hair short over the entire perineum and the labia and thoroughly wash with water and soap or surgical detergent.

(2) If delivery is not imminent, administer a warm tap-water or soapsuds enema to evacuate the lower bowel.

(3) A barbiturate, eg, pentobarbital sodium, 0.1–0.2 g, or diazepam (Valium), 10 mg, may be given to allay anxiety and enhance relaxation. Sedatives should not be administered before actual analgesia is required in most cases.

(4) Keep the patient in bed after the membranes have ruptured or labor has definitely begun.

(5) Allow only clear liquids by mouth during labor. Solid food is poorly assimilated, causes indigestion, and may be aspirated if vomiting occurs during general anesthesia or with eclamptic or epileptic convulsions. Offer tap water, tea, or fruit juices frequently to avoid dehydration.

(6) Analgesia should not be given until labor is definitely estab-

lished. The cervix should be dilated at least 3 cm. Analgesics must be ordered on an individual basis, considering each patient's anticipated obstetric problems, the quality of labor, and her desire to be alert or subdued.

Further Examinations & Procedures

(1) Electronic fetal monitoring (EFM) is but one means of fetal assessment, and although the internal type carries only slight risk, it is rarely a substitute for adequate clinical judgment.

Current retrospective and prospective data support the use of continuous internal EFM for high-risk obstetric patients (see p 109). Internal EFM is preferable to external EFM because it is more precise and comprehensive in appraising fetal status.

The physician may choose and the patient may accept continuous EFM even in low-risk cases, and a normal record is most reassuring to all concerned. Nonetheless, electronic monitoring of all obstetric patients is impractical and probably unnecessary considering the cost/benefit ratio.

(2) If continuous EFM is not used, auscultate the fetal heart tones (FHT) for 30 seconds following a uterine contraction at least every 30 minutes during the first stage, at least every 15 minutes during the second stage, when the membranes rupture and again within 30 minutes after the membranes rupture, and also if brisk bleeding occurs or if meconium passes (in other than vertex presentations). During the second stage (or with serious complications), record the FHT every 10–15 minutes or more often as indicated.

(3) Perform external and internal examinations as often as necessary to determine the progress of labor. However, too frequent vaginal or rectal examinations cause the patient discomfort and increase the incidence of intrauterine infection, particularly after rupture of the membranes. Descent and internal rotation of the fetus can often be determined by external palpation alone.

(4) Encourage the patient to void frequently. Palpate the abdomen occasionally for signs of bladder fullness. Catheterize if distention occurs or if voiding is obviously inadequate.

(5) Cleanse the vulvar region before and after internal examination, after defecation and voiding, or when soiling by vaginal secretions occurs.

MANAGEMENT OF THE SECOND STAGE OF LABOR
(Vertex Delivery)

Spontaneous delivery of the infant presenting by the vertex is divided into 3 phases: (1) delivery of the head, (2) delivery of the shoulders, and (3) delivery of the body and legs.

Final preparations for delivery should be completed by the time the presenting part reaches the pelvic floor (or sooner, if labor is progressing very rapidly).

Preparation for Delivery

Strict asepsis is required.

(1) Place the patient in a modified lithotomy position for delivery. The left lateral decubitus (Sims) position may be used if a spontaneous uncomplicated birth is anticipated.

(2) The physician and assistants must carefully scrub their hands and wear masks and sterile gowns and gloves as for a major surgical procedure. Any delivery may become surgically complicated. (See Chapter 15.)

(3) Administer anesthesia (eg, pudendal block). Gown and gloves must be changed if any contamination has occurred.

(4) Cleanse the pudendum with water and surgical detergent.

(5) Drape the patient with sterile towels and sheets so that the abdomen and legs are covered.

(6) Sterile instruments and necessary supplies previously designated should be arranged conveniently on a table or stand.

Delivery of the Head (See Figs 6–8 through 6–12.)

During the late second stage, the head distends the perineum and vulva with each uterine contraction, aided by voluntary efforts of the mother. A part of the scalp may even be visible. The presenting part recedes slightly during the intervals of relaxation but is said to "crown" when its widest portion (biparietal diameter) distends the vulva just before emerging.

Do not hasten delivery, or serious damage to the mother and child may occur. Steady and slow the speed of delivery as necessary to avoid pudendal laceration or unexpected extrusion of the infant's head. Sudden marked variations in intracranial pressure can cause cerebral hemorrhage. As the head advances, control its progress by pressure applied laterally beneath the symphysis, and maintain flexion of the head, when necessary, by pressure over the perineum.

Draw the perineum downward to allow the head to clear the perineal body. Pressure applied from the coccygeal region upward (modified Ritgen maneuver) will extend the head at the proper time and thereby protect the perineal musculature.

Episiotomy should be done when the infant's head begins to distend the introitus.

In vertex presentations, the forehead appears first (after the vertex), then the face and chin, and then the neck. The cord encircles the neck in about 20% of deliveries. In such cases, gently attempt to slip the cord over the head. If this cannot be done easily, doubly clamp the cord with

Table 6—1. Mechanisms of labor: vertex presentation.

Engagement	Flexion	Descent	Internal Rotation	Extension	External Rotation or Restitution
Generally occurs in late pregnancy or at onset of labor. Mode of entry into superior strait depends on pelvic configuration; occiput posterior is most common position.	Good flexion is noted in most cases. Flexion aids engagement and descent. (Extension occurs in brow and face presentations.)	Depends on pelvic architecture and cephalopelvic relationships. Descent is usually slowly progressive.	Takes place during descent. After engagement, vertex usually rotates to the transverse. It must next rotate to the anterior or posterior to pass the ischial spines, whereupon, when the vertex reaches the perineum, rotation from a posterior to an anterior position generally follows.	Follows distention of the perineum by the vertex. Head concomitantly stems beneath the symphysis. Extension is complete with delivery of head.	Following delivery, head normally rotates to the position it originally occupied at engagement. Next, the shoulders descend in a path similar to that traced by the head. They rotate anteroposteriorly for delivery. Then the head swings back to its position at birth. The body of the infant is delivered next.

Table 6–2. Mechanisms of labor: frank breech presentation.

Flexion	Descent	Internal Rotation	Lateral Flexion	External Rotation or Restitution
Hips: Engagement usually occurs in one of oblique diameters of pelvic inlet.				
	Anterior hip generally descends more rapidly than posterior, at both inlet and outlet.	Ordinarily takes place when breech reaches levator musculature. Fetal bitrochanteric rotates to AP diameter.	Occurs when anterior hip stems beneath symphysis; posterior hip is born first.	After birth of breech and legs, infant's body turns toward mother's side to which its back was directed at engagement of the shoulders.
Shoulders: Bisacromial diameter engages in same diameter as breech.				
	Gradual descent is the rule.	Anterior shoulder rotates so as to bring shoulders into AP diameter of outlet.	Anterior shoulder at symphysis, and posterior shoulder is delivered first (when body is supported).	
Head: Engages in the same diameter as shoulders. Flexes on entry into superior strait. Biparietal occupies oblique used by shoulders. At outlet, neck or chin arrests beneath symphysis, and head is born by gradual flexion.	Follows the shoulders.	Occiput (if a posterior) or face (if an occiput anterior) rotates to hollow of sacrum. This brings presenting part to AP diameter of outlet.		

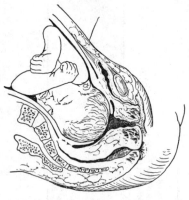

Figure 6–8. Engagement of LOA.

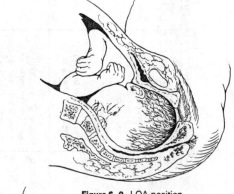

Figure 6–9. LOA position.

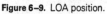

Figure 6–10. Anterior rotation of head.

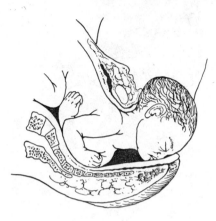

Figure 6–11. Extension of head.

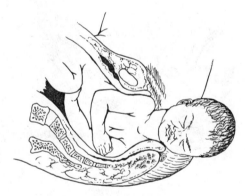

Figure 6–12. External rotation of head.

forceps, cut between the forceps, and proceed with the delivery. Wipe fluid from the nose and mouth, and then aspirate the oral passages with a soft rubber suction bulb or with a small catheter attached to a DeLee suction trap.

Before external rotation (restitution), which occurs next, the head is usually drawn back toward the perineum. This movement precedes engagement of the shoulders, which are now entering the pelvic inlet. From this time on, support the infant manually and facilitate the mechanism of labor.

Do not hurry! If the strength of the contractions seems to wane, be

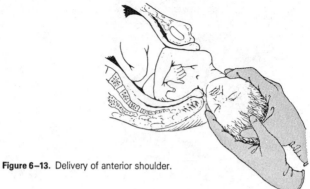

Figure 6–13. Delivery of anterior shoulder.

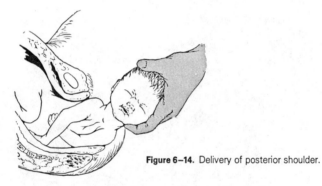

Figure 6–14. Delivery of posterior shoulder.

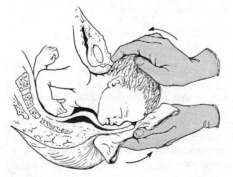

Figure 6–15. Modified Ritgen maneuver.

patient—labor will resume. Once the airway is clear, the infant can breathe and is not in immediate jeopardy.

Delivery of the Shoulders

Delivery of the shoulders should be slow and deliberate. The shoulders must rotate (or be rotated) to the anteroposterior diameter of the outlet for delivery.

Gently depress the head toward the mother's coccyx until the anterior shoulder impinges against the symphysis. Then lift the head upward. This will aid in delivery of the posterior shoulder. One may slip several fingers into the vagina at this point to assist in delivering the posterior arm. The anterior shoulder is next delivered from behind the symphysis. (At times it may be easier to deliver the anterior shoulder first.)

In vertex presentations, a hand may present after the head. This need not obstruct delivery of the shoulders. Merely sweep the infant's hand and arm over its face, draw the arm out, and deliver the other shoulder as outlined above.

Caution: Never exert pressure or strong anterior or posterior traction on the head, neck, or shoulders. Do not hook a finger into the child's axilla to deliver a shoulder; a brachial plexus injury (Erb or Duchenne), a hematoma of the neck, or shoulder injury may result.

Delivery of the Body & Extremities

The infant's body and legs should be delivered gradually by easy traction after the shoulders have been freed.

Immediate Care of the Infant

As soon as the infant is delivered, it should be held with the head lowered (no more than 15 degrees) to drain fluid and mucus from the oropharynx. A DeLee mucus trap catheter or comparable suction device is useful in clearing the air passages. Place the infant on a wheeled stand or tray the height of the delivery table or slightly lower. If it is below the level of the placental insertion, blood will drain readily from the placenta and cord to the newborn. This will amount to 30–90 mL before the cord is clamped or the placenta separates.

Resuscitate if necessary (see Chapter 7).

Some physicians place the child on the mother's abdomen. This contaminates the sterile field, however, and the infant is not secure there. Furthermore, with the infant on the mother's abdomen, blood may drain from the child into the cord and placenta.

Clamp and cut the cord as soon as it ceases to pulsate (or sooner if the infant is premature or distressed or if isoimmunization is probable). Examine the umbilical cord for 2 arteries and one vein. Apply a sterile cord clamp, cord tie of umbilical tape, or rubber band just distal to the skin edge at the cord insertion at the umbilicus. Cover the cord stump with a dry gauze dressing.

Wipe the eyelids with moist cotton. Instill 1 drop of 1% aqueous silver nitrate solution into each eye. The silver nitrate must be freshly prepared or expressed from commercial wax "pearls" that maintain the safe concentration. Penicillin is more effective and less harmful than silver nitrate, but the law in most states requires the use of silver nitrate.

Apply means of identification (necklace, bracelet, etc.).

Thoroughly examine the infant and record weight, total length, crown-rump length, shoulder circumference, circumference of the head, and cranial diameters. Note facial, peripheral, genital, or other abnormalities. The newborn should be received into warm sterile towels or blankets and must not be allowed to become chilled. When feasible, the mother should be allowed to hold the infant. The infant is then transferred to the nursery for further observation and care.

Immediate Care of the Mother Postpartum

Carefully inspect the perineum, vagina, and cervix for lacerations, hematomas, or extension of episiotomy incisions.

The extent of laceration of the birth canal may be designated roughly in degrees: (1) In first-degree lacerations, only the mucosa or skin (or both) is damaged. Bleeding is usually minimal. (2) Second-degree lacerations include tears of the mucosa or skin (or both) plus disruption of the superficial fascia and the transverse perineal muscle. (The anal sphincter is spared.) Bleeding is often brisk. (3) Third-degree lacerations involve the above structures plus the anal sphincter. Moderate blood loss is to be expected. (4) Fourth-degree lacerations include the above structures and entry into the rectal lumen. Bleeding may be profuse, and fecal soiling is inevitable.

Sulcus lacerations, urethral and cervical damage, etc, are designated specifically.

MANAGEMENT OF THE THIRD STAGE OF LABOR

Traction on the cord before placental separation and "kneading" the fundus to separate the placenta (Credé maneuver) must be avoided because this can lead to hemorrhage, uterine inversion, shock, and infection.

Maternal morbidity and mortality rates increase in proportion to the degree of blood loss and the duration of the third stage of labor. A uterus that contracts and remains contracted rarely bleeds excessively. Immediate manual separation and extraction of the placenta from the fundus of the uterus is an effective direct technique, but strict asepsis and, often, effective anesthesia are required. Less dangerous and generally satisfactory indirect methods are discussed below.

Delivery of the Placenta

Normal placental separation is manifested first by a firmly contracting, rising fundus. The uterus becomes smaller and changes in shape from discoid to globular. The umbilical cord becomes longer as the placenta descends. There is a palpable and visible prominence above the symphysis (if the bladder is empty) and a slight gush of blood from the vagina. These signs normally appear within about 3–4 minutes after delivery of the infant. The placenta should present at the internal os after 4–5 firm postpartum (uterine) contractions, when it is expressed into the vagina for delivery.

These signs are not often confused with other conditions. However, it is well to remember that uterine anomaly, a second undelivered infant, feces, a tumor, and lacerations of the birth canal can mimic many of the signs of normal placental separation.

The placenta is attached to the uterine wall only by anchor villi and thin-walled blood vessels, all of which eventually tear. In some instances, the placental margin separates first; in others, when the central portion of the placenta is freed initially, bleeding from the retroplacental sinuses may assist placental separation. Incomplete separation, usually due to ineffectual uterine contractions, may allow the retroplacental blood sinuses to remain open, so that severe blood loss may result.

As the placenta passes from the uterus into the vagina, it may present by either its shiny fetal surface or its roughened maternal surface. These have been termed the Schultze and Duncan mechanisms, respectively, but such designations are archaic and without significance. However, an understanding of the sequence of events of placental separation and blood loss is essential to correct management.

Complications of the Third Stage of Labor

The complications that may occur during the third stage of labor are hemorrhage, shock, and infection. These may be due to any of the following causes:

A. Uterine Inertia and Uterine Atony: Uterine inertia may be followed by uterine atony after birth of the infant. This occurs in prolonged labor, polyhydramnios, multiple pregnancy, myomas of the uterus, traumatic delivery, hemorrhage and excessive analgesia, and cessation of stimulation after anesthesia and delivery.

B. Entrapment or Incomplete Removal of the Placenta:

1. Uterine abnormalities–(a) Anomalies of the uterus or cervix may cause restriction and retention of the placenta. (b) Weak, ineffectual uterine contractions do not constrict the placental site sufficiently to force separation. (c) Tetanic uterine contractions, formation of a uterine constriction ring, or closure of the cervix may trap the placenta.

2. Placental abnormalities–Increased uteroplacental cohesion or partial or complete placenta accreta may create an unusually firm utero-

A

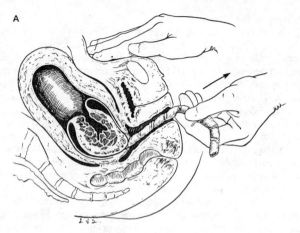

B

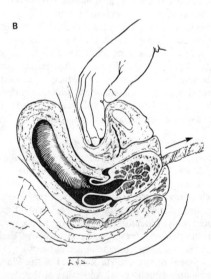

Figure 6–16. Brandt-Andrews maneuver. *A:* Traction is extended on the cord as the uterus is gently elevated. *B:* Pressure is exerted between the symphysis and the uterine fundus, forcing the uterus upward and the placenta outward, as traction on the cord is continued. (Reproduced, with permission, from Benson RC [editor]: *Current Obstetric & Gynecologic Diagnosis & Treatment,* 4th ed. Lange, 1982.)

placental union. Abnormalities of placentation at term include the following: (a) low-lying placenta (placenta previa); (b) cornual implantation of the placenta, or nidation in a separate portion of a subseptate or arcuate uterus; (c) succenturiate lobe; and (d) placenta accreta, complete (about one per 8000 deliveries) or partial (about one per 4000 deliveries).

3. Mismanagement of the third stage of labor–(a) Manipulation of the fundus before separation of the placenta stimulates tetanic, not rhythmic, fundal contractions. (b) Parenteral administration of ergot preparations too early or too late causes sustained uterine or cervical contractions that may trap the placenta. (c) Improper anesthetic management (especially deep anesthesia) may depress uterine motility and prevent contractions.

C. Uterine Inversion: Inversion may be partial or complete.

D. Failures of Aseptic Technique: Contamination may occur, eg, bacterial contamination of the cervix may occur at the introitus when the fundus is used as a piston to expel the placenta.

Techniques of Recovery of the Placenta

When the uterus is firmly contracted, the mother, if she has not been anesthetized, may be able to bear down during a contraction to expel the separated placenta. If spontaneous delivery does not occur, the following techniques may be used.

A. Pastore Technique:

1. Stand to the patient's left and elevate the fundus with the fingers of the right hand.

2. If the placenta separates, massage the fundus gently; otherwise, leave it alone until contractions occur.

3. Place the left hand flat over the abdomen with the fingers above the symphysis.

4. When contractions occur and the placenta separates, squeeze the fundus gently and push it downward slightly with the right hand.

5. Prevent the fundus from entering the pelvis by holding the left hand above and behind the symphysis. The placenta can be felt to slide beneath the hand through the lower uterine segment into the cervix or vagina.

6. Lift the fundus upward to leave the placenta free in the vagina.

7. Extract the placenta from the vagina by gentle cord traction.

B. Brandt-Andrews Technique (Modified) (Fig 6–16):

1. Immediately after delivery of the infant, clamp the umbilical cord close to the vulva. Palpate the uterus gently without massage to determine whether firm contractions are occurring.

2. After several uterine contractions and a change in size and shape indicate separation of the placenta, hold the clamp at the vulva firmly with one hand, place the fingertips of the other hand on the abdomen, and

press between the fundus and symphysis to elevate the fundus. If the placenta has separated, the cord will extrude into the vagina.

3. Further elevate the fundus, apply gentle traction on the cord, and deliver the placenta from the vagina.

C. Manual Separation and Removal of the Placenta:

1. Prepare the perineum and vulva again with detergent and antiseptic solution. Change gloves and redrape the operating field.

2. Making the hand as narrow as possible, insert it gently into the vagina and palpate for defects in the vagina and cervix. Slowly probe through the cervix with the fingers, taking care not to lacerate or forcefully dilate the canal. (Moderately deep anesthesia may be required if considerable delay has occurred.)

3. Locate the placenta and separate it if this can be done easily. Do not attempt to force separation against unusual resistance (placenta accreta).

4. Palpate the fundus for defects or tumors.

5. Remove the hand, grasping the completely separated placenta, or leave the placenta in the uterus if it is firmly adherent (placenta accreta). Hysterectomy will probably be required in the latter case.

Procedures That Minimize Complications During the Third Stage

The following program will usually prevent entrapment of the placenta and conserve blood:

(1) Give oxytocin (Pitocin), 0.5 mL intramuscularly, immediately after delivery of the infant.

(2) Recover the placenta by the Pastore or Brandt-Andrews technique.

(3) After delivery of the placenta, give ergonovine (Ergotrate), 0.2 mg intramuscularly.

(4) Elevate and compress the uterus manually to express all clots. (Clots may form when brisk bleeding occurs, especially from vaginal and cervical lacerations. Slight bleeding from the uterus ordinarily clots and liquefies to pass finally as fluid blood.)

(5) If bleeding continues and intravenous fluids have not been started, insert a No. 16 or No. 18 needle into a large vein and administer 5 units (0.5 mL) of oxytocin in 1 L of 5% glucose in water. Have cross-matched blood available.

(a) Examine the lower genital tract for lacerations.

(b) Explore the uterus *without anesthesia,* if possible, for retained products of conception and rupture of the uterus.

(6) Give a second dose of ergonovine intravenously.

(7) Repair lacerations quickly.

Emergency Treatment

Sudden, massive hemorrhage, especially following instrumental vaginal delivery, requires immediate sterile exploration of the birth canal and uterus to control bleeding. Abruptio placentae, rupture of the uterus, and gross cervical or vaginal lacerations require immediate definitive treatment.

(1) Extract the separated placenta or manually separate and withdraw the afterbirth.

(2) Palpate the uterine cavity for tumors, defects, or anomalies.

(3) Administer oxytocin (Pitocin), 0.5 mL intramuscularly immediately and 0.5 mL rapidly thereafter by intravenous drip.

(4) Examine the cervix and suture significant bleeding lacerations; inspect the vaginal canal and repair defects.

If rupture of the uterus is discovered, prepare for immediate laparotomy.

Treatment of Complications

When hemorrhage is due to disseminated intravascular coagulation, replace blood loss with fresh whole blood and administer heparin or cryoprecipitate to restore the clotting mechanism (see p 272). *Caution:* Never operate until the coagulation mechanism is restored to normal. If the patient continues to bleed excessively, prepare for hysterectomy even in a primipara—preferably under cyclopropane or other light anesthesia. Do not give spinal or—unless in combination with another agent—thiopental anesthesia, since these types of anesthesia tend to be associated with hypotension and prolonged depression of vital functions. In most instances, packing the uterus is only a temporary expedient: One cannot make certain that the uterus will not relax; and also, the pack may hold the sinuses open rather than closed.

Blood replacement is almost invariably inadequate. Estimates are often only half or less than half of the actual loss. Using skin color, pulse, respiration, blood pressure, central venous pressure, and patient response as guides, replace blood loss and treat shock.

Consider uterine (and often vaginal) packing in the following cases: (1) gross cervical laceration when assistance for repair is not immediately available, (2) rupture of the uterus while waiting for an operating room in which to do a laparotomy, (3) cases of placenta previa after placental extraction when bleeding continues from uncollapsed blood vessels in the lower uterine segment even when the fundus is well contracted, (4) when it is necessary to retain a uterus replaced after inversion, (5) when it is necessary to temporarily control paravaginal and vulvar hematomas, and (6) after evacuation of a large hydatidiform mole.

In general, packing can be avoided by the proper use of intravenous oxytocics, elevation and gentle massage of the uterus, and proper management of the third stage of labor.

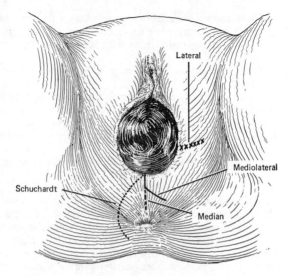

Figure 6–17. Types of episiotomy.

AIDS TO NORMAL DELIVERY

EPISIOTOMY (PERINEOTOMY); REPAIR OF EPISIOTOMY & LACERATIONS

An episiotomy is a pudendal incision to widen the vulvar orifice to permit easier passage of the infant. It should be used in most primiparas and many multiparas.

The advantages of episiotomy are that it prevents perineal lacerations, relieves compression of the fetal head, shortens the second stage of labor by removing the resistance of the pudendal musculature, and can be repaired more successfully than a jagged tear.

Episiotomy is indicated (1) when a tear is imminent, (2) in most operative deliveries, and (3) to facilitate delivery of a premature infant.

Types of Episiotomy (See Fig 6–17.)

The tissues incised by an episiotomy are (1) skin and subcutaneous tissues, (2) vaginal mucosa, (3) the urogenital septum (mostly fascia, but also the transverse perineal muscles), (4) intercolumnar fascia or superior fascia of the pelvic diaphragm, and (5) the lowermost fibers of the puborectalis portions of the levator ani muscles (if the episiotomy is mediolateral and deep).

A. Median: This is the easiest episiotomy to accomplish and to repair and is certainly the most bloodless. Following repair, it is more comfortable for the mother. It consists of incising the median raphe of the perineum almost to the anal sphincter. The disadvantage of this procedure is that it is occasionally accidentally extended to a third- or fourth-degree laceration (see p 160).

B. Mediolateral: The mediolateral incision is widely used in operative obstetrics because of its safety. The incision is made downward and outward in the direction of the lateral margin of the anal sphincter. The choice of a right or left incision depends upon the position of the presenting part and the expertise of the operator in repairing an oblique defect. A right mediolateral episiotomy widens the introitus slightly more (on the right) than a left mediolateral episiotomy does if the infant presents in an LOA, LOP, LSA, LMA, or any position in which the small parts are to the right. This is particularly important in forceps delivery and when the infant is large because it relieves stretch where the tension is greatest, thereby preventing lacerations. It also avoids the extension of an episiotomy when placed on the opposite side.

C. Schuchardt: This is a maximally-extended mediolateral episiotomy carried deep into one vaginal sulcus and curved downward and laterally part way around the rectum. Although rarely required, it is of great help in the difficult delivery of a large head or a restricted decomposition of a breech and in the correction of shoulder dystocia. It is also used in vaginal surgery requiring wide exposure.

D. Lateral: Lateral episiotomy affords very little relaxation of the introitus, is associated with profuse bleeding, and is difficult to repair. This incision has no merit and should be abandoned.

Timing of the Episiotomy

Episiotomy should be done when the head begins to distend the perineum, immediately preceding application of forceps, and just prior to breech extraction or internal podalic version. The slight reduction in blood loss achieved by delaying episiotomy until after forceps insertion and articulation is less important than a satisfactory application of the blades and a good episiotomy repair.

Repair of Episiotomy & Lacerations (See Figs 6–18 and 6–19.)

Episiotomy repair is actually a fascial repair and not merely the suture of muscle.

Interrupted or continuous suture or a combination of both may be used if catgut is chosen. Chromic catgut, No. 000, is usually selected. Carefully reapproximate the edges of the divided muscles and fascia.

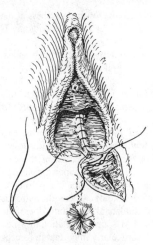

1. Continuous suture of mucosa with inverted suture of perineal body

2. Mucosal suture continued in skin and tied with inverted suture

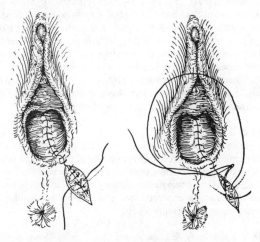

3. Closure of levator ani and perineal musculature

4. Skin closed subcutaneously

Figure 6–18. Episiotomy repair.

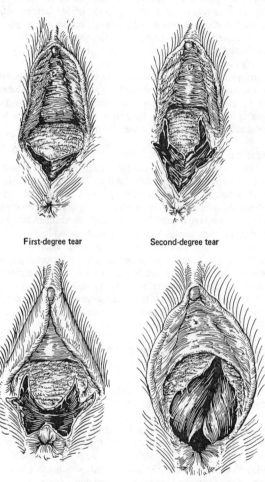

First-degree tear

Second-degree tear

Third-degree tear

Complete
(fourth-degree) tear

Figure 6–19. Perineal tears.

Avoid mass ligatures and tension on sutures; do not tie the sutures too tightly, or pain will occur later. In general, buried sutures cause less discomfort than sutures that protrude through and are tied over the skin.

Interrupted, removable nonabsorbable sutures such as No. 00 nylon are occasionally used when a rapid closure is desired or a grossly infected wound is to be repaired.

In repair of fourth-degree lacerations, close the rectal wall with fine interrupted catgut sutures tied within the lumen of the bowel. Reapproximate the ends of the rectal sphincter with interrupted catgut sutures, preferably in the perimuscular fascia rather than the friable muscle itself. Then suture lacerations in the more superficial structures.

Postpartum Observation

The mother should remain in the delivery or recovery room for at least 1 hour after delivery of the placenta. Observe her vital signs and note her reactions. Record the blood pressure and the pulse rate and regularity every 15 minutes, or oftener if necessary. Support the uterine fundus, and massage it gently and frequently to maintain firm contraction. Express clots occasionally and estimate blood loss.

Be alert to complaints of severe perineal pain suggestive of hematoma formation. A rapid pulse and increasing hypotension indicate impending shock, usually due to continued or excessive blood loss. Severe headache and hyperreflexia may precede eclampsia.

Do not release any patient to ward or room care until her condition is sufficiently improved and stable to permit convalescent status.

USE OF OXYTOCICS

Oxytocics are employed after delivery to reduce blood loss to prevent subinvolution of the uterus and endometritis. Two principal products are used: ergot preparations and oxytocin (natural or synthetic).

A. Oxytocin: Oxytocin (Pitocin or Syntocinon—nearly pure oxytocin), 0.5 mL (5 IU of extract), is administered at or immediately after delivery of the infant and repeated in the same dose following recovery of the placenta. *Caution:* Never use posterior pituitary extract (Pituitrin), because it contains vasopressin, which can cause sudden hypertension, coronary occlusion, and asthmatic crises.

B. Ergot Preparations: Ergonovine maleate (Ergotrate) or methylergonovine maleate (Methergine), 0.2 mg intramuscularly, may be given immediately after the placenta is delivered. *Caution:* These drugs have pressor effects and should not be administered to patients with hypertension. To minimize the possibility of hypertensive reactions and cardiovascular accidents, do not administer ergot preparations intravenously unless they are diluted in 50 mL or more of fluid.

OUTLET FORCEPS
(Elective Outlet Forceps)

Outlet forceps are used to extend the head and to guide the infant beneath the symphysis and over the perineum. Outlet forceps are used only when the vertex is on the perineum and extension is beginning.

Outlet forceps are used in the following circumstances: (1) When spontaneous expulsion is inhibited by analgesic or anesthetic drugs. Caudal or spinal anesthesia diminishes the patient's voluntary expulsive efforts, and outlet forceps are used in most of these cases. (2) When uterine inertia delays or prevents delivery of an infant whose vertex is distending the perineum. (3) When fetal distress is discovered during the late second stage. (4) When laceration of the introitus is likely. In such cases, a prophylactic episiotomy is also performed.

Caution: Use of outlet forceps, like other surgical procedures, is safe only with a skilled operator. The availability of outlet forceps delivery does not justify shortening the second stage by means of low or mid forceps extraction.

OBSTETRIC ANALGESIA, AMNESIA, & ANESTHESIA

Pain in childbirth is due to traction upon the adnexal, uterine, and cervical supports; pressure upon the ureters, bladder, urethra, and bowel; dilatation of the cervix and lower birth canal; hypoxia and the accumulation of catabolites in the myometrium; and fear, severe tension, and anxiety. The type of pain reported may be an ache in the back or loins (referred pain, perhaps from the cervix), a cramp in the uterus (due to fundal contraction), or a "bursting" or "splitting" sensation in the distal genital canal or pudendum (due to dilatation of the birth canal).

Dystocia, usually quite painful, may be due to cephalopelvic disproportion; tetanic, prolonged, or dysrhythmic uterine contractions; intrapartal infection, and many other causes.

The following types of pain relief are in use today: (1) positive conditioning of the patient (hypnosis); (2) hypnotics; (3) analgesics, which increase the patient's pain threshold; (4) amnesics, which obscure the memory of pain and associated disagreeable experiences; (5) regional anesthesia, which interrupts afferent pain pathways; and (6) general anesthesia, which prevents central perception of discomfort. Some of these are useful in home as well as in hospital delivery. Others can be used only in hospitals where equipment and specially trained professional personnel are available.

Types of Analgesics, Amnesics, & Anesthetics
A. Positive Conditioning: Positive conditioning of the receptive

patient, including hypnosis, during late pregnancy or early labor may reduce tensions and limit the need for pain relief medication.

B. Narcotic Analgesics: The commonly employed analgesics are narcotic drugs.

Injectable narcotics in the usual doses elevate the pain threshold by 50% or more; establish a state of relaxation, indifference, and euphoria or apathy; and induce lethargy and sleep. Most drugs in this group have a peak action in less than 90 minutes and a duration of effect of at least 2–3 hours. Nausea, vomiting, cough suppression, intestinal stasis, and diminution in the frequency, intensity, and duration of uterine contractions in the early first stage of labor are common undesirable side-effects. Minimal or no amnesia is achieved. Morphine or comparable opiates will not prevent or stop premature labor. Narcotics adversely affect the infant by depressing all of its central nervous system functions, especially activity of the respiratory center. Gestational age, weight, trauma, and long labor enhance the susceptibility of the infant to narcosis.

C. Inhalant Analgesics: Inhalant analgesics include trichloroethylene (Trilene) and nitrous oxide. Both of these gases are nontoxic if given with adequate air or oxygen. Inhalators for self-administration of these gas mixtures for brief periods during labor contractions are most useful and popular.

D. Sedatives (Hypnotics): The sedatives slow mentation, reduce perception of sensory stimuli, and increase receptivity to suggestion. They are poor analgesics and do not raise the pain threshold appreciably in conscious subjects. Amnesia does not occur. Labor may be slowed by large doses of sedatives, especially when they are given too early in the first stage.

Barbiturates are frequently given with or before a narcotic or other analgesic. Secobarbital, 0.1 g, may be administered orally in early labor; and meperidine or morphine may be administered later, when progress is more advanced. However, because serious fetal depression occurs, the barbiturates and narcotics should rarely be administered together.

Barbiturates should not be used alone for obstetric analgesia because the required dosage is dangerous to the fetus, which is extremely sensitive to central nervous system depression by these drugs. Periodic apnea and even abolition of all movements outlast the effects of the barbiturates on the mother.

E. Amnesics: The prototype of this group of drugs is scopolamine, which blots out memory astonishingly well. Unfortunately, this drug has no analgesic action and sometimes seems to lower the pain threshold. Furthermore, its effects are unpredictable: some patients become somnolent or stuporous; others restless, hallucinating, and delirious. (**Note:** Although amnesia during labor and delivery may have technical advantages, there is evidence that a woman "spared" recollection of her delivery experience may reject her offspring.)

Hydroxyzine (Vistaril) and diazepam (Valium) are examples of popular tranquilizers. Diazepam is useful in the first stage of labor because it has an effective tranquilizing action and also reduces the amount of analgesic drug required. It has a long half-life. Reports reveal that its use in the first stage of labor in dosages of 5–15 mg every 4 hours does not have a deleterious effect upon the newborn.

F. Potentiating Drugs: Phenothiazine drugs potentiate certain of the desirable (as well as a few of the undesirable) effects of the analgesics, amnesics, and general anesthetics.

G. Inhalation Anesthetics: This group includes a number of potent agents that can often be used for major operative procedures.

The inhalants discussed with analgesic drugs are not used as general anesthetics because they are too dangerous to be used alone to induce deep surgical anesthesia. For a more complete consideration of anesthetic procedures useful in obstetrics and gynecology, the reader is referred to standard textbooks on anesthesiology.

H. Thiobarbiturates: Intravenous anesthetics such as thiopental (Pentothal) and thiamylal (Surital) are widely used in general surgery. However, in less than 7 minutes after injection into the mother's vein, the concentrations of the drug in fetal and maternal blood will be equal. Even when rapid delivery is accomplished under thiopental anesthesia, for example, the infant may be so severely narcotized that resuscitation is difficult. Intravenous anesthesia should rarely be used in obstetric delivery.

I. Regional Blocks: A needle guide such as the Iowa trumpet (Fig 6–20) is useful in pudendal and paracervical anesthetic blocks. The thumb ring and the trumpet-shaped opening of the guide facilitate the entry and direction of the needle. The standard Iowa trumpet is 5½ inches long; a 6½-inch 22-gauge spinal needle will protrude slightly beyond the guide.

1. Paracervical anesthesia–Paracervical anesthesia (Fig 6–21) is administered when the cervix is dilated 4 cm or more. It relieves pain until the presenting part reaches the lower vagina, whereupon a pudendal and perineal block or other anesthetic procedure will be required. It is simple and effective and rarely disturbs the mother, but labor may be retarded briefly. Exceptional instances of sensitivity to the medication (tachycardia, syncope, convulsions) require supportive measures. Fetal bradycardia due to rapid or excessive (> 5 mL of anesthetic) drug absorption may be a serious side-effect.

Paracervical block may cause fetal bradycardia associated with decreased placental blood flow and, perhaps, a reflex mechanism. Therefore, this type of anesthesia should be used only in normal term deliveries.

A 5- or 6-inch needle with a guide or a lead shot affixed to it is used so that the point can be inserted 0.1–0.2 cm into the tissues. Inject 5 mL

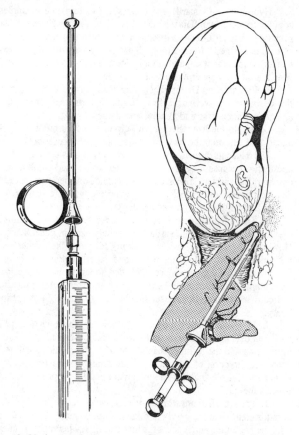

Figure 6–20. Iowa trumpet assembled.

Figure 6–21. Paracervical submucous block.

of procaine, 1% aqueous solution (procaine is preferred because of its safety), or a long-acting local anesthetic about 2 cm lateral to the cervix on both sides. If the presenting part is so far down that the lateral fornix cannot be reached easily, 5 mL injected as high as possible into each lateral vaginal wall will give considerable relief of discomfort during the second stage of labor.

    2. Pudendal and perineal block–(Fig 6–22.) This permits spontaneous, breech, low forceps, or even mid forceps delivery with little or

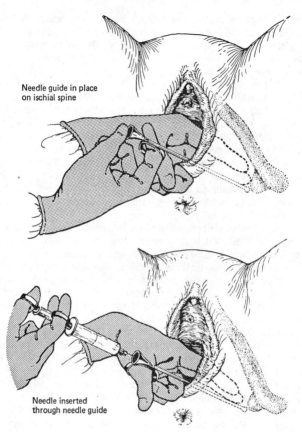

Needle guide in place
on ischial spine

Needle inserted
through needle guide

Figure 6–22. Use of needle guide (Iowa trumpet) in transvaginal anesthetic block.

no pain. It is extremely safe and simple, and the patient maintains her ability to cooperate during labor. The infant is not depressed, and blood loss is minimal. Disadvantages include regional discomfort during the injection and the 5-minute wait for the anesthetic to take effect.

Knowledge of the innervation of the lower birth canal is required for successful administration of pudendal and perineal local anesthesia. The 2 important nerves to be blocked on each side of the vagina are the pudendal and the posterior femoral cutaneous nerves. The pudendal nerve lies near the inner aspect of the ischial spine and should be blocked there. The posterior femoral cutaneous nerve may be injected beneath the inferior medial border of the tuberosity of the ischium. The descending branches of the ilioinguinal nerve supply the clitoral region. The pudendum and the perirectal zone are innervated by the hemorrhoidal nerve. The procedure is as follows:

a. Develop a wheal of 0.5–1% procaine (or equivalent) at the base of each labium majus. Perform all injections through this site.

b. Palpate the ischial spines vaginally or rectally. Slowly guide a 4- or 5-inch, 20- or 21-gauge spinal needle toward each spine while injecting a small amount of procaine ahead of the advancing point. Aspirate, and if the needle is not in a vessel, deposit 5 mL of anesthetic below each spine. This blocks the right and left pudendal nerves. Refill the syringe when necessary, leaving the needle in place, and proceed in a similar manner to anesthetize the other areas specified. Keep the needle moving while injecting, and avoid the vaginal mucosa and periosteum, which are sensitive.

c. Withdraw the needle about 3 cm and redirect it toward an ischial tuberosity. Inject 3 mL near the center of each tuberosity to anesthetize the inferior hemorrhoidal and lateral femoral cutaneous nerves.

d. Withdraw the needle almost entirely and then slowly advance it toward the symphysis pubica almost to the clitoris, keeping it about 2 cm lateral to the labial fold and about 1–2 cm beneath the skin. Injection of 5 mL of procaine on each side beneath the symphysis will block the ilioinguinal and genitocrural nerves.

If the above procedure is unhurried and skillfully done, there will be only slight discomfort during injections. Prompt flaccid relaxation and good anesthesia for 30–60 minutes can be expected.

J. Epidural Caudal Anesthesia: Caudal anesthesia may be given continuously, ie, during the latter portion of the first and all of the second stage of labor; or terminally, as a single injection just before delivery. Special training is required to administer caudal anesthesia. The advantages of caudal anesthesia are that it causes no fetal asphyxia, the mother remains conscious to witness the birth, blood loss is minimal, vaginal and perineal structures remain relaxed, and headache does not occur. The technique must be exact, however, and inadvertent massive (high) spinal anesthesia occasionally occurs. Undesirable reactions include rapid absorption syndrome (hypotension, bradycardia, hallucinations, convulsions) and postpartal backache and paresthesia. The incidence of persistent occiput posterior positions is increased because the infant's head is not normally rotated on the relaxed pelvic floor; forceps rotation and delivery is therefore more often necessary. A considerable quantity of anesthetic agent must be injected: 35 mL of 1.5% piperocaine (Metycaine) or equivalent.

K. Spinal Anesthesia: Spinal anesthesia is widely used not only to alleviate the pain of delivery but also to relieve pain during the late first and entire second stages of labor. Short-acting agents are employed for the former; more potent and long-acting drugs are necessary for the latter. Brief or minimal spinal anesthesia is far safer than prolonged spinal anesthesia, which is not recommended for obstetric use. The advantages of spinal anesthesia are that no fetal hypoxia occurs, blood loss is minimal, the mother remains conscious during delivery, no inhalation anesthetics or analgesic drugs are required, the technique is not difficult, and good relaxation of the pelvic floor and lower birth canal is achieved. Anesthesia is achieved within 5–10 minutes, and there are fewer failures than with caudal anesthesia. The dosage of spinal anesthetic is small, and hypotension is rare with these doses. Complications are fewer and easier to treat. For cesarean section, tilting the patient about 15–20 degrees to the left by elevating her right hip should avoid vena caval compression by the uterus and possible fetal distress. Spinal headache occurs in 5–10% of patients, however, and operative delivery is more often required because voluntary expulsive efforts are eliminated. Hypotension may occur. Respiratory failure may develop if the anesthetic ascends as a result of rapid injection or straining by the patient.

The procedure is as follows:

1. With the patient lying on her side or sitting up, inject 40 mg of procaine (0.8 mL of 5% solution) or comparable drug slowly into the third or fourth lumbar interspace between contractions. Elevate the patient's head on a pillow immediately after the injection. Tilt the table up or down to achieve a level of anesthesia at or near the umbilicus. Anesthesia will be maximal in 10–15 minutes and will last 1 hour or longer.

2. Record blood pressure and respirations every 5–10 minutes.

3. Give oxygen for respiratory depression and mild hypotension. If the blood pressure falls markedly, also administer vasopressors such as ephedrine, 25 mg intravenously.

L. General Anesthesia: For cesarean section, many physicians prefer general anesthesia induced by intravenous thiopental followed by nitrous oxide inhalation and succinylcholine chloride by intravenous drip. Considerable experience is required. Another "balanced anesthetic," light barbiturate-nitrous oxide-halothane, may be used similarly. In either case, ventilation of the intubated patient must be manually controlled.

General Comments & Precautions

(1) A patient who is psychologically prepared for her experience will require far less medication. Anticipate and dispel the mother's fears during the antenatal period and in early labor. Never promise a painless labor.

(2) Nurse anesthetists, trained by and working under the close

supervision of physician anesthesiologists, generally function very well in obstetrics. They are usually permitted to administer inhalation or parenteral analgesia and anesthesia.

(3) Individualize treatment, because each patient reacts differently. Unfavorable reactions occur to all drugs.

(4) Always think in terms of normal maternal-fetal physiology rather than the requests of the patient and her family. An overly demanding patient and a yielding physician are a perfect combination for tragedy.

(5) Be familiar with the drug you intend to administer. Know its limitations, dangers, and contraindications as well as its advantages.

(6) Do not render the patient unconscious in the first stage of labor. Some pain relief may be necessary, and relaxation may speed labor; but total amnesia and analgesia may be detrimental to the mother and her infant. Mild degrees of fetal asphyxia are not easily discernible but are often harmful.

(7) Avoid injections in an area of skin infection.

(8) Spinal, caudal, and other anesthetic blocks are surgical procedures requiring scrupulous preparation and aseptic technique.

Treatment of Complications

A. Early Delivery: If labor terminates earlier than planned, a narcotic antagonist may reverse the depressive effect of an opiate but will intensify the barbiturate effect.

B. Resuscitation of the Mother*: If a potentially lethal dose of anesthetic is given, proceed as follows:

1. Establish a patent airway (hyperextend the head; if necessary, insert a tracheal tube).

2. Aspirate mucus, blood, vomitus, etc, with a tracheal suction apparatus. Use a laryngoscope for direct visualization of air passages.

3. Administer oxygen by artificial respiration if respirations are absent or weak. If high spinal anesthesia has occurred, continue to "breathe" for the patient until paralysis of the diaphragm has dissipated.

4. Give antihistamines intravenously (eg, diphenhydramine, 15–25 mg) and oxygen by mask for drug sensitivity (rarely indicated).

5. Give vasopressors intravenously (ephedrine, 10–20 mg). Place the patient in the flat positive position with the feet elevated, and give plasma, plasma expanders, and blood transfusion for traumatic or hemorrhagic shock.

6. Specifically treat cardiac arrhythmias, arrest, failure, etc, if a heart disorder is the basic problem.

C. Spinal and Caudal Complications: Reactions to or complications of spinal or caudal anesthesia are best prevented by using the

---

*Resuscitation of the newborn is discussed in Chapter 7.

minimal effective dosage and the lowest possible concentration of anesthetic drug. The anesthetic should be injected slowly, with frequent aspiration. Unless contraindicated, vasoconstrictor drugs may be used to reduce systemic absorption of the anesthetic.

Untoward effects may be due to sensitivity, rapid absorption, overdosage, or inadvertent intravascular injection. The type of reaction is unpredictable and is related to the dosage and rate of absorption of the drug and the medical status of the patient. Two types of reaction may follow systemic absorption: (1) Slow onset: Stimulation, leading to agitation, vertigo, blurred vision, nausea, tremors, convulsions, hypotension, and cardiovascular depression or respiratory arrest. (2) Rapid onset: Depression, leading to respiratory arrest, cardiovascular collapse, or cardiac arrest.

Prompt recognition and treatment are imperative: (1) Intubate the patient; maintain a patent airway; administer oxygen. (2) Give small doses of a short-acting barbiturate, diazepam, or muscle relaxant to control convulsions. (3) Support the circulation with vasopressor drugs as indicated. (4) Utilize external cardiac massage for cardiac arrest.

Prognosis

The prognosis is excellent for mother and infant when physician anesthesiologists and obstetricians work as a team and a 24-hour anesthesiology service is available.

INDUCTION OF LABOR

Induction of labor by medical or surgical means should be performed only upon specific indications. Elective induction or induction for minor or controversial reasons (''meddlesome midwifery'') often increases maternal and fetal morbidity and mortality.

Indications

Indicated induction of labor, especially in the treatment of abnormal pregnancy (preeclampsia-eclampsia, pyelonephritis), usually reduces maternal and fetal morbidity and mortality. The following indications for induction of labor are valid in 5–8% of pregnancies:

(1) Maternal infections (pyelonephritis, diverticulitis) that often fail to resolve and are likely to become more severe unless pregnancy is interrupted.

(2) Uterine bleeding with partial placental separation or partial placenta previa.

(3) Preeclampsia-eclampsia unresponsive or only temporarily responsive to therapy.

(4) Diabetes mellitus.

Table 6–3. Bishop score.*

Cervical Criteria	Score			
	0	1	2	3
Effacement (%)	0–30	40–50	60–70	80
Dilatation (cm)	0	1–2	3–4	5–6
Station of vertex (−3 to +3 scale)	−3	−2	− 1, 0	+1, +2
Consistency	Firm	Medium	Soft	. . .
Position	Posterior	Midposition	Anterior	. . .

*Reproduced, with permission, from Bishop EH: A pelvic scoring for elective induction. *Obstet Gynecol* 1974;24:266.

(5) Renal insufficiency.

(6) Premature rupture of the membranes after the 36th week.

(7) Previous precipitate delivery in a woman who cannot be transported quickly to a hospital.

(8) Marked polyhydramnios.

(9) Placental insufficiency (dysmaturity).

(10) Isoimmunization (erythroblastosis).

(11) Elective or indicated second-trimester abortion.

Contraindications

(1) Cephalopelvic disproportion.

(2) Floating or deflected vertex or unfavorable presentation (including breech and multiple pregnancy).

(3) Firm, closed, uneffaced posterior cervix. (A vaginal examination must be performed before induction so that "ripeness" of the cervix can be confirmed.)

(4) Previous cesarean section or extensive myomectomy.

(5) Maternal cardiac disease (functional class III or IV).

(6) Grand multiparity (more than 5 pregnancies). With oxytocin, the uterus may rupture.

Dangers of Induction

A. For the Mother: In many cases, induction of labor exposes the mother to more distress and discomfort than judicious delay and subsequent vaginal or cesarean delivery. The following hazards must be borne in mind: (1) emotional crisis (fear and anxiety); (2) failure of induction and subsequent attempts to institute labor or to deliver the fetus; (3) uterine inertia and prolonged labor; (4) tumultuous labor and tetanic contractions of the uterus, causing premature separation of the placenta, rupture of the uterus, and laceration of the cervix; (5) intrauterine infection; (6) postpartal hemorrhage; (7) hypofibrinogenemia; and (8) amniotic fluid embolization.

B. For the Fetus: An induced delivery exposes the infant to the risks of prematurity if the EDC has been inaccurately calculated. Prolapse of the cord and infection may follow amniotomy. Violent labor or trauma in delivery may result in damage due to hypoxia or physical injury.

Bishop Score

Bishop has devised a scoring system (Table 6–3) to predict the outcome of induction when no contraindications, eg, placenta previa, exist. A Bishop score of 9 or more indicates that labor may be induced with only a small chance of failure.

Methods of Induction

A. Medical Methods:

1. Oxytocin–Parenteral administration of a very dilute solution of oxytocin is the most effective medical means of inducing labor. (**Note:** Fetal monitoring is always required during medical induction or stimulation of labor. Ergot preparations cause sustained contractions and must not be used before delivery for any reason. Posterior pituitary extract [Pituitrin] should never be used because of the vasoconstricting and antidiuretic effect of the vasopressin it contains.) Oxytocin exaggerates the inherent rhythmic pattern of uterine motility, which often becomes clinically evident during the last trimester and increases as term is approached.

The dosage of oxytocin must be individualized. The administration of oxytocin is really a biologic assay: the smallest possible effective dose must be determined for each patient and then utilized to initiate labor.

Note: Constant observation by qualified attendants (preferably the physician) is required if this method is used. It is the physician's responsibility (not the nurse's) to determine that the correct amount of oxytocin has been added to the infusion bottle and that a given number of drops per minute will deliver a specific oxytocin dose in milliunits (mU) per minute.

In most cases, it is sufficient to add 0.1 mL of oxytocin (1 unit, Pitocin or Syntocinon) to 1 L of 5% dextrose in water. Thus, each milliliter of solution will contain 1 mU of oxytocin.

Begin induction or augmentation at 1 mU/min. Increase oxytocin arithmetically by 2-mU increments—eg, 1, 3, 5, etc, mU/min—at 15-minute intervals.

When contractions of 50–60 mm Hg (internal monitor pressure) or 40–60 seconds (on the external monitor) occur at intervals of 2½ to 4 minutes, the oxytocin dose should not be increased further. If contractions cease or become weak and ineffectual after a satisfactory start, the infusion may be resumed.

2. Prostaglandins–Prostaglandin E_2 (PGE_2), 0.5 mg orally initially and then 1 mg/h orally for up to 24 hours, is almost as effective as intravenous oxytocin for induction of labor. Nausea or diarrhea may be a side-effect.

PGE$_2$, 5 mg in a gel applied to the cervix the night before induction at term, "ripens" the cervix, enhancing the likelihood of initiation of labor.

3. Enemas and purges–Enemas and purges for the induction of labor by reflex uterine hyperactivity may be harmful, are often unsuccessful, and are not recommended.

B. Surgical Methods:

1. Amniotomy is the easiest and surest way to induce labor. Release of amniotic fluid shortens the muscle bundles of the myometrium; the strength and duration of the contractions are thereby increased, so that a more rapid contraction sequence follows. Amniotomy causes few complications and is not painful.

The membranes should be ruptured at the internal os with a hook or other sharp instrument. Do not displace the infant's head upward to drain off amniotic fluid. Keep the patient in bed in Fowler's position after amniotomy so that slow drainage of fluid can occur. Anticipate labor within 6 hours if the patient is at term.

2. Stripping of the membranes (alone) is not recommended, since the result is unpredictable. Rupture increases maternal morbidity, may lead to bleeding from a low-lying placenta, may cause rupture of the membranes and prolapse of the cord with a high presenting part, and is painful.

If delivery within 12–24 hours is vital for the well-being of mother or infant and induction is unsatisfactory, cesarean section without delay must be considered.

• • •

"NATURAL CHILDBIRTH"

In modern obstetrics, numerous procedures and drugs are used to reduce discomfort and shorten labor. The techniques range from elective induction of labor to continuous conduction analgesia-anesthesia and prophylactic forceps delivery. Admittedly, overenthusiastic or ill-advised use of such methods may complicate parturition and, perhaps, "cheat" the mother of the satisfaction to be gained from a significant natural experience. For these reasons, Grantly Dick Read postulated that fear results in tension, which in turn causes pain, and that this can retard and intensify the discomforts of labor and delivery. Adequate knowledge about the mechanics of childbirth, emotional and physical preparation, and the confidence thus gained will often reduce pain and tension. Read urged the abandonment of "meddlesome midwifery"—ie, interference, manipulation, or "management"—and a return to supportive therapy based upon good physician-patient rapport and positive psychologic and physical conditioning of the patient. Good antenatal care is implied, and suitable pain relief is given when necessary even though the patient is encouraged to rely largely upon her own resources. Read's precepts are sound and should continue to receive the respectful attention of the profession. However, so many individual variations and interpretations of these concepts have evolved that the patient or physician using the term "natural childbirth" must always carefully define exactly what is meant. Nothing could be more "natural" than childbirth.

PSYCHOPROPHYLAXIS: LAMAZE TECHNIQUE FOR PREPARED CHILDBIRTH

The psychoprophylaxis program of preparation for childbirth emphasizes body-building exercises, relaxation, breathing techniques, and comfort aids. It has been most successful in alleviating tension and pain during labor. A trained teacher (often a nurse or midwife) assists the patient in physical education and relaxation procedures. Exercises such as sitting in "tailor" fashion, squatting, and abdominal and pelvic floor. muscle contractions are employed. Relaxation concentrates on muscle groups and includes command contraction-relaxation. Breathing techniques involve chest (not abdominal) breathing. The intercostal muscles are used, but the diaphragm is relaxed. (In abdominal breathing, the diaphragm tenses with a contraction, so that it may actually press down on the uterus and interfere with relaxation.)

During the first stage of labor, slow, deep chest breathing is used. Rapid, shallow breathing and panting are recommended just before full dilatation of the cervix, immediately prior to the phase of voluntary expulsive efforts.

During the second stage of labor, pushing alternates with panting. The patient sits in the tailor position, holding her flexed knees from the outside. This allows her to brace during bearing-down efforts. Panting between contractions helps relaxation.

Light massage of the back, pressure on the sacrum, and lying "on the side of the occiput" are aids to comfort.

This preparation for childbirth generally requires 6–8 weeks of practice sessions. Self-confidence and ability to cope with the labor process are improved by such a program, which is especially popular in France and Russia.

LE BOYER TECHNIQUE

"Gentle birth," the clinical application of Le Boyer's concepts ("birth without violence"), attempts to recreate features of the intrauterine environment in the delivery room. Spontaneous delivery is desirable for the program. A quiet, darkened room free of bright lights, gentle handling, and immersion of the newborn in a water bath (37 °C for 10–15 minutes) immediately after severance of the cord seem to calm the infant after what may have been a frightening, traumatic experience. After the bath, the newborn is given to the mother to suckle and cuddle.

Little definite pediatric information exists regarding the good or bad effects of gentle birth. However, infant bonding should be enhanced with this method; little extra time is required; no expensive equipment is necessary; and no increase in maternal or infant sepsis has been reported.

THE FATHER

The father is the man who "shares pregnancy" with the mother in the psychologic sense. Much has been said of the mother, her needs, and her relationship to the child, but the expectant or new father has been a somewhat neglected factor in the process. The complexity and urgency of his needs are many. Preparation for parenthood actually begins well before courtship and marriage, but the mother's pregnancy is the beginning of the transition leading to fatherhood. Recognition of the father's concerns leads to discussion and solution of many human problems that surround the expectation of a new infant.

Fathers-to-be experience at least 5 time periods that often overlap: (1) realization or confirmation of pregnancy, (2) awareness of changes in the mother's body and the presence of fetal movements, (3) anticipation of approaching labor, (4) involvement in the delivery process, and (5) new parenthood.

Fears that the father's presence in the delivery room would create a nuisance, add to confusion, or cause infection or legal conflicts have not been justified by events. Men who have participated with their wives in preparation for childbirth have been helpful, comforting, and reassuring. The delivery room experience is almost always an ego-building one for the father. With the father in the delivery room, it has proved easier for the physician and the parents to welcome a normal newborn as well as to cope with the birth of a defective offspring.

The father may act as a coach in addition to the nurse-physician team by assisting with comfort measures (eg, bringing cool drinks, giving back rubs). He may be an almost constant companion to the patient to offset the loneliness and anxieties of labor. He can be a messenger, to report problems or call for help and interpret his wife's needs and wishes to the nurse and doctor.

Whether or not the father has participated in parent education classes, he can receive "on-the-job training" and play his role. The nurse or physician should (1) familiarize the father with the maternity unit, the labor room, the Father's Room, and the medical personnel; (2) allow the father to participate actively in the delivery room or permit him to wait for progress information; (3) indicate to the father when his presence and assistance may be most helpful; and (4) teach him comfort measures without requiring that he assume responsibility for the observation or management of labor.

Supportive measures the father can offer include many aspects of physical care of his wife as well as encouragement and comfort. He deserves to be kept informed of the patient's progress and needs and to be allowed to help where he can. A well-informed participating father can contribute greatly to the health and well-being of the mother and child, to the benefit of the family relationship and his own self-esteem. All of these factors may prevent or greatly minimize many postpartum psychologic problems.

7 | The Infant

IMMEDIATE CARE OF THE NEWBORN

General Measures

In most instances, the cord should not be clamped until it ceases to pulsate, so that fetal blood in the placenta and cord will flow into the newborn circulation by gravity. However, the cord should be clamped immediately if the infant is premature or immature, if the infant is behaving abnormally though apparently not asphyxiated (distressed infant), or if erythroblastosis fetalis is a possibility. Transfer the newborn to a warmed incubator, bassinet, or crib. Determine the Apgar score (Table 7–1) at 1 and 5 minutes after birth. Examine the infant (see p 193).

Tie and dress the cord, instill silver nitrate or an antibiotic solution into the eyes, and apply an identification bracelet only when the infant is out of danger. Observe every infant closely for at least 1 hour for signs of cardiorespiratory distress.

Apgar Score

Immediate evaluation of the newborn by the Apgar method is a valuable routine procedure. The objective signs listed in Table 7–1 are

Table 7–1. Apgar score of newborn infant.

	Score		
	0	1	2
A Appearance (color)	Blue or pale	Body pink, extremities blue	Completely pink
P Pulse (heart rate)	Absent	<100	>100
G Grimace (reflex irritability in response to stimulation of sole of foot)	No response	Grimace	Cry
A Activity (muscle tone)	Limp	Some flexion of extremities	Active motion
R Respiration (respiratory effort)	Absent	Slow, irregular	Good, crying

evaluated 1 minute and 5 minutes after complete delivery of the infant, and the degree of response in each category is recorded as 0, 1, or 2; the total is the Apgar score. Infants who are severely depressed at birth should be observed constantly.

An Apgar score of 10 is a "perfect" infant score. This rating is uncommon even for mature, spontaneously delivered infants. An Apgar score of 7–9 indicates a normal or slightly depressed infant; a score of 4–6, one who is moderately depressed; and a score of 0–3, a severely depressed infant. About 9 out of 10 normal infants will score 7 or above at birth. Newborns with Apgar scores of 6 or above usually do not require special treatment.

The Apgar rating at birth must be made a part of the permanent health record.

ASPHYXIA NEONATORUM & RESUSCITATION

Most newborns breathe in less than 1 minute after birth. Those who do not begin to breathe within 1–2 minutes, for whatever cause, are developing asphyxia. Prolonged hypoxia during or after delivery is almost always associated with central nervous system damage, eg, cerebral palsy, mental retardation, epilepsy, or death.

Etiology

Asphyxia of the newborn may be due to the following:

A. Maternal Disorders: Marked anemia, eclampsia, uterine tetany, severe hypotension or shock, hemorrhage.

B. Fetal or Neonatal Disorders: Trauma, central nervous system disorders (cysts or tumors), pulmonary hypoplasia, congenital pulmonary or cardiovascular anomalies, depression of the respiratory center during labor and delivery due to maternal analgesics or anesthetics, fetomaternal transfusion, obstructed airway (mucus, meconium, blood), isoimmunization, syphilis.

C. Placental and Umbilical Disorders: Hydatidiform mole, intervillous fibrin deposition, infarction, hemorrhage due to premature separation of the placenta or placenta previa, cord occlusion (compression or prolapse and obstruction).

Many causes of respiratory distress of the newborn can be diagnosed by physical examination promptly after delivery. Nonetheless, supportive care is vital.

Prevention

Avoid giving large, frequent doses of analgesics to the woman in labor, especially within 1 hour of delivery. Curtail sharply all medications for relief of pain in premature labor or when operative delivery is likely. Use conduction anesthesia, especially pudendal block, whenever possible.

Avoid high-pressure insufflation of air or oxygen and inept instrumentation, since they may cause emphysema, pneumothorax, or pneumomediastinum.

Resuscitation

A person skilled in resuscitation should be present if operative delivery, premature birth, or a serious obstetric problem is anticipated.

A. Emergency Measures:

1. Severely depressed infant (Apgar score 0–3)–Support the infant in the head-down position to drain amniotic fluid, blood, and mucus from the nasopharynx. Gently aspirate the infant's throat and nose with a small, soft rubber catheter attached to a DeLee mucus trap. Avoid rough handling, and keep the infant warm. If meconium has been passed in utero or if thick viscid mucus is difficult to aspirate, perform direct laryngoscopy.

If the heartbeat cannot be heard, begin external cardiac massage by applying moderate finger pressure over the mid sternum (depress the sternum about 2 cm) 30–40 times a minute. Follow with laryngoscopy (see below) and oxygen therapy. Consider intracardiac injection of epinephrine (see p 190).

2. Moderately depressed infant (Apgar score 4–6)–Support the infant, aspirate the nose and throat, handle gently, and keep warm. Extend the infant's neck and insert a pharyngeal airway (see below).

B. Special Methods of Treatment:

1. Laryngeal intubation and aspiration–Intubate the larynx and aspirate if meconium was passed in utero or if thick viscid mucus is difficult to aspirate; if depression (asphyxia) is severe; if pulmonary expansion is incomplete or unequal; or if persistent, repeated retraction of the thorax occurs in the immediate postdelivery period.

2. Transfusion–Prepare for transfusion or blood replacement in infants with serious isoimmunization.

3. Laryngoscopy–

a. Extend the neck by elevating the infant's shoulders with a folded towel or by allowing the head to extend over the edge of the table. (*Caution:* Do not overextend the neck.)

b. Open the infant's mouth by applying pressure on the chin.

c. Hold the laryngoscope in the left hand (if right-handed) in order to leave the right hand free for manipulation of the suction tube.

d. Insert the laryngoscope blade into the angle of the infant's mouth; center the blade when the glottis is visible.

e. Tilt the tip of the instrument upward to raise the epiglottis out of the line of vision. This will expose the trachea.

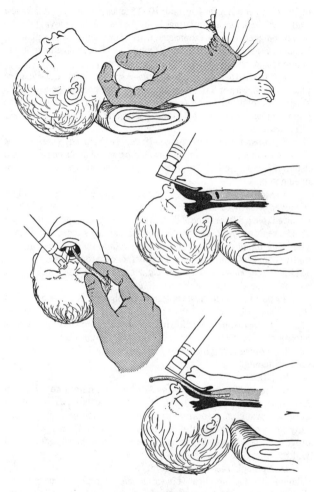

Figure 7–1. Resuscitation of the newborn.

f. Slip an endotracheal tube into the laryngoscope slot; under direct vision, pass the tube into the trachea as far as the flange.

g. Remove the laryngoscope carefully so that the endotracheal tube is left in place.

h. Gently aspirate any free fluid or mucus.

i. Direct short puffs of hydrated oxygen into the tube (at a pressure of 15–20 cm of water for 1 second, 10–15 times per minute). If the chest wall rises, the lungs are inflating. If the thorax does not move, the tube may be plugged or in the esophagus. Check heart action by auscultation. Continue regular, brief insufflations until spontaneous breathing occurs and the heart rate is over 110 beats per minute.

4. Mouth-to-mouth breathing–Aspirate fluid and insert a pharyngeal airway or Safar mouthpiece. By cheek action, gently blow a small quantity of *mouth* air (never air exhaled from the lungs) into the infant's mouth and nose 10–15 times per minute. Allow time for release of air between puffs.

5. Consultation and x-rays–If depression persists despite the above measures, secure further consultation and obtain a chest x-ray to determine expansion of the lungs and seek congenital anomalies or pneumothorax.

6. Stomach aspiration–Aspirate the stomach (*after* resuscitation) if delivery was by cesarean section, if placental insufficiency may have occurred (see p 87), or if the abdomen is markedly distended or the infant chokes repeatedly. (*Caution:* Do not aspirate the stomach of a small premature infant under any circumstances; little fluid will be present, and the danger of trauma is great.) Apply suction through a No. 10 or No. 12 Rausch or other soft rubber catheter with a DeLee mucus trap attached. Use slight epigastric pressure.

Suspect intestinal atresia or tracheoesophageal fistula (see p 199) if the catheter meets obstruction or if there is 30 mL or more of aspirate.

7. Transfusion–For pallid infants who have probably lost blood as a result of placental laceration or cord injury, promptly transfuse whole type O, Rh-negative blood into the umbilical vein. Do not wait for cross-matching.

8. Drugs–

a. Narcotic antagonists–Administer naloxone (Narcan Neonatal), 0.01 mg/kg intravenously, intramuscularly, or subcutaneously; or levallorphan (Lorfan), 0.05 mg intravenously or intramuscularly, to combat the effect of narcotics. (*Caution:* Do not give these drugs to the newborn if the mother has received barbiturates or the infant will become more depressed.)

b. Epinephrine–Inject 0.15 mL of epinephrine, 1:1000 aqueous solution, into the umbilical vein in moderately asphyxiated infants or directly into the heart through the fourth interspace to the left of the sternum in severely asphyxiated infants.

c. Glucose–Inject 10 mL of 10% glucose solution in water into the umbilical vein if the infant is severely anoxic.

d. Stimulants–Respiratory stimulants are of no value in initiating breathing. Caffeine and sodium benzoate, 6–10 mg/kg into the umbilical vein or intramuscularly, may stimulate the infant once breathing begins.

e. Antibiotics–Administer broad-spectrum antibiotics when severe intrapartal infection occurs or when resuscitation is prolonged and difficult. Treatment may have to be continued for 3–4 days.

Prognosis

The prognosis depends upon the mother's health, complications of labor and delivery, the maturity and condition of the newborn, and the success of resuscitation.

NEONATAL RESPIRATORY PROBLEMS
(Severely or Moderately Depressed Newborns)

Atelectasis

Atelectasis, the normal state of the lung prior to delivery, may persist as patchy atelectasis for several days after initiation of breathing. Then, if all goes well, full expansion of the lung is the rule. However, persistent extensive atelectasis occurs in congenital bronchial obstruction or after aspiration-retention of inspissated mucus, blood, or meconium. Disordered central nervous system function secondary to hemorrhage may be responsible for atelectasis also. Expect incomplete expansion of the lungs with pneumothorax or diaphragmatic hernia.

The newborn with atelectasis often is slightly cyanotic, but this may decrease with crying or oxygen therapy. Shallow, rapid, irregular respirations are typical, and suprasternal or intercostal retractions may be observed. Fine rales may be heard. X-ray films should reveal areas of increased density, usually in both lungs.

The cause of congenital atelectasis will determine the treatment. Change the position of the infant frequently, stimulate crying, and humidify the air to 80% in the crib. Antibiotic therapy may be indicated if complications such as pneumonitis develop.

The prognosis of congenital atelectasis is generally good unless serious basic problems such as diaphragmatic hernia are responsible.

Air Block

Air block is acute respiratory distress resulting from sudden pneumothorax, pneumomediastinum, or pneumopericardium. It is usually a complication of resuscitation, particularly in immature infants, and occurs in 1–2% of newborns.

Unforeseen dyspnea, hyperpnea, and cyanosis follow air block. Marked suprasternal and infrasternal retractions are notable, but there is little accompanying movement of the chest. With unilateral air block, the normal side will be larger. Hypertympany on the affected side, evidence of a mediastinal shift, and reduced intensity of the heart sounds are to be expected.

Treatment includes oxygen therapy and aspiration of air from the site of accumulation in severe cases. Absorption of more than a small amount of air is unlikely.

The prognosis is good with proper treatment except in premature newborns or infants with other serious complications.

Spontaneous Respiratory Distress Syndrome (RDS); Hyaline Membrane Disease of the Lungs

Spontaneous respiratory distress syndrome is progressive or persistent respiratory difficulty, with the development—within hours of delivery—of a so-called hyaline membrane within the proximal bronchioles of newborns who die of this disorder. The actual cause is still a matter of debate, but immaturity of surfactant synthesis and lungs may be responsible. Preterm newborns whose lecithin/sphingomyelin (L/S) ratio is less than 2, infants delivered by cesarean section, and those born of mothers with diabetes mellitus or after fetal distress are prone to RDS.

Cyanosis, increased respiratory rate, expiratory grunting, and retractions of the chest wall—generally the lower rib cage and sternum—are diagnostic findings in RDS.

Laboratory studies reveal acidemia, decreased P_{O_2}, and increased P_{CO_2}.

X-ray films of the chest may disclose a characteristic "ground glass" appearance of the lungs in RDS. However, roentgen studies are important also in the identification or exclusion of other causes of respiratory difficulty.

Therapy requires oxygen administration, but if excessive oxygen is given, retrolental fibroplasia may result. Correct acidosis, maintain fluid and electrolyte balance, assist ventilation (positive-pressure breathing), and maintain a thermoneutral state (37 ± 0.5 °C, or 98.6 ± 1 °F). Withhold oral feedings until the infant improves. Prophylactic antibiotic therapy may be warranted in severe cases.

If the infant can be successfully supported for 2–3 days, rapid improvement often follows without significant sequelae. Nonetheless, RDS is a major cause of neonatal death, particularly in infants under 36 weeks' gestational age.

NURSERY CARE OF THE NEWBORN

Immediate Care

A. General Measures: Place the infant supine on a flat surface or with the head slightly lowered in a heated crib. Avoid contamination. Irrigate the eyes with sterile normal saline solution. Administer vitamin K, 1 mg intramuscularly, if the mother has not received vitamin K during labor or as a dietary supplement. Aspirate mucus with a suction tube. Keep the infant in a slightly head-down position for evacuation of fluid from the nose and throat.

B. Observation: Examine the cord tie or clamp occasionally; retie or reclamp if oozing occurs. Record the infant's temperature hourly until it has stabilized. Keep the crib temperature at 24–25 °C (75–78 °F) or higher if the infant's temperature does not remain within the normal range. Record the time, relative amount, and character of urine and feces passed.

Fluid & Food

Do not feed the infant or offer water for 12 hours. Then give 5% dextrose solution according to the hospital schedule (every 3–4 hours). If the mother has been delivered at home or is a rooming-in patient, feedings may be on demand. After 24 hours, begin periodic breast or formula feeding.

Skin Care & Bathing

Wipe away excess vernix. Cleanse the skin daily (and when soiling occurs) with moist gauze and then dry. Avoid special creams or medicated soaps. Do not bathe the baby for at least 4–5 days. Avoid routine application of antiseptic preparations because of the danger of irritation or sensitization. Powders and oils are usually not necessary.

Medications

Consider prophylactic antibiotic therapy (1) if the membranes had been ruptured for over 24 hours before delivery (especially when frozen section of the cord reveals vasculitis or when clinical antepartal amnionitis is likely); (2) if laryngoscopy, intratracheal intubation, or prolonged resuscitation was required or if the infant has severe respiratory distress; and (3) when the stomach aspirate contains considerable numbers of bacteria at birth.

EXAMINATION OF THE FULL-TERM INFANT

The Infant at Birth

A. Position After Delivery: Attitude is determined largely by the infant's presentation in utero. Infants who presented by the vertex tend to assume the flexed "fetal position"; those delivered after face presentation maintain the extended head; and breech infants extend the legs for about a week.

B. Skin:

1. Vernix caseosa—a white, creamy material composed of sebaceous secretions, exfoliated cells, and lanugo—covers the skin of most term infants.

2. Slight initial cyanosis is common. With adequate oxygenation and normal cardiopulmonary function, the skin becomes ruddy within

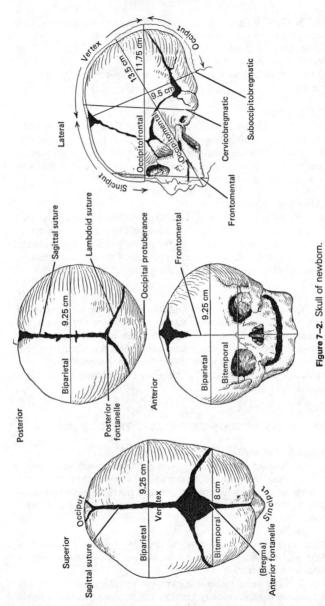

Figure 7–2. Skull of newborn.

moments after birth, although the extremities may remain dusky or mottled for the first day.

3. The skin is usually dry, with superficial cracks, especially in the folds of the body and over the hands and feet.

4. Milia (distended sebaceous glands) appear over the forehead, nose, and sides of the face as minute unpigmented papules.

5. Lanugo (downy hair) is often scattered over parts of the face, back, and extremities.

6. Petechiae, erythematous patches, and even frank port-wine stains (birthmarks) may be present. These most commonly occur on the face, the nape of the neck, and the scalp.

7. Abrasions, contusions, and persistent forceps impressions represent delivery trauma.

C. Head:

1. Size and bones–The head is obviously large in proportion to the body. "Molding" and even slight overlapping of the cranium may be noted in infants who presented by the vertex, especially after a difficult operative delivery. Nevertheless, the largest diameters of the infant are those of the skull. Two frontal, parietal, and temporal bones, one occipital bone, and the wings of the sphenoid bones compose the cranium. Only the bones of the base of the skull are firmly joined at term.

2. Caput succedaneum–Caput succedaneum is a soft, sometimes ecchymotic swelling of the scalp that represents the actual site of presentation at the cervix. A comparable edematous zone may develop over the sacrum or one buttock in complete breech presentation.

3. Craniotabes–Craniotabes, or thinning of the bones of the vault of the skull, is common and usually not significant.

4. Cephalhematoma–Cephalhematoma is blood between the periosteum and skull that does not cross a suture line. It needs no treatment. *Caution:* Do not aspirate—infection may develop.

5. Face–In striking contrast with that of the adult, the infant's face is much smaller than its cranium.

6. Fontanelles–Wide, unossified, slightly depressed areas over the cranium are called fontanelles. These are mainly at the juncture of the principal bones of the vault. The frontal or large fontanelle is between the parietal and frontal bones; the occipital, small, or posterior fontanelle is at the point of convergence of the 2 parietal bones with the single occipital bone. There are also 2 mastoid and 2 sphenoid fontanelles, but these are smaller and unimportant obstetrically. The fontanelles are small and slightly depressed at birth. If they are wide and full, suspect increased intracranial pressure.

7. Sutures–The fibrous unions between the bones of the head are called cranial sutures. The principal sutures are easily palpable: The coronal suture lies between the frontal and parietal bones in the anterior portion of the skull, and the sagittal suture lies between the parietal bones and extends from the frontal bone to the occiput. These sutures cause the anterior fontanelle to be diamond-shaped and the posterior fontanelle triangular.

8. Major diameters of the cranium–(Fig 7–2)

a. The occipitofrontal (OF) diameter is the distance from the prominence of the occipital bone to the frontal bone at the base of the nose. Average normal: 11.75 cm.

b. The biparietal (BP) diameter is the distance between the parietal bones at the widest point. It represents the greatest transverse diameter of the head. Average normal: 9.25 cm.

c. The bitemporal (BT) diameter is the greatest distance between the frontal bones and is measured from the midpoint of the coronal suture on each side of the head. Average normal: 8 cm.

d. The occipitomental (OM) diameter is the distance from the occipital prominence to the tip of the mandible. Average normal: 13.5 cm.

e. The circumference of the head is measured in the plane of the occipitofrontal diameter. Average normal: 34.5 cm.

9. Eyes–The iris is blue-gray in white infants but blue-brown in infants of pigmented races. Subconjunctival and even retinal hemorrhages may be noted. Minute retinal hemorrhages that do not involve the macula are not serious.

10. Mouth–Harelip or other nasolabial defects are obvious deformities. The gums are generally smooth except for an occasional small papule at the margin. These are retention cysts (Bohn's or Epstein's pearls). A few similar elevations may also be present over the central portion of the palate. Tongue-tie (short frenulum) may restrict the tongue. Cleft palate is often associated with harelip or other head and neck anomalies.

11. Ears–Maldevelopment of the ears or unusually lowset ears may accompany abnormalities of the genitourinary tract in both sexes.

12. Cheeks–The cheeks are rounded because of prominent sucking pads.

D. Neck and Trunk: At birth, the neck is very short; the head almost rests upon the infant's shoulders, which are not wide. The thorax is narrow and not deep, but the trunk is relatively long in proportion compared to that of the adult. The circumference of the shoulders is slightly less than that of the head.

1. Breasts–Breast tissue can be palpated easily in infants.

2. Lungs–Respirations are shallow at first, and abdominal breathing is the rule. The normal respiratory rate at rest is 38–44/min. Coarse breath sounds and harsh fremitus indicate incomplete inflation of the lungs. Unequal expansion or persistently limited excursions of the chest may indicate atelectasis or maldevelopment.

3. Heart–The average rate is 120–140 beats per minute. Sinus arrhythmia is often noted. Transient, soft murmurs without transmission are functional. The blood pressure (not easily obtained) is generally 80–85/50–55 mm Hg.

E. Abdomen:* The liver and kidneys are barely palpable. An experienced examiner will occasionally feel the tip of the spleen in a normal infant.

F. Genitalia: In males, the prepuce is long and completely covers the glans, to which it is adherent. The testes are usually within the scrotum at term. In females, the labia minora are prominent. A whitish mucoid discharge may be noted at the introitus.

G. Anus: The anus should be patent and the rectal sphincter competent at birth.

H. Extremities: The arms are relatively longer than the legs, unlike those of adults. Subcutaneous fat over the extremities obscures the musculature. The fingers and toes are short. The feet are stubby. Talipes (clubfoot) must be distinguished from mere relaxed flexion.

I. Reflexes: The following reflexes are normally present in the newborn: grasping, sucking, rooting, Moro, Chvostek, Babinski, tonic neck, deep tendon, abdominal, and cremasteric.

J. Temperature: The mature newborn's temperature ranges between 36.7–37.1 °C (98–99 °F); the premature infant's temperature is usually 1 degree, and often 3–4 degrees, lower.

K. Weight: Male infants outweigh females. White newborns weigh more than those of the darker races; second and subsequent infants are often heavier at birth than firstborn infants.

L. Blood: Normal values at birth are as follows:

> Red blood count: 4.1–7.5 million/μL (average: 5.9 million/μL).
>
> Hemoglobin: 14–24 g/dL (average: 19 g/dL), of which one-half to three-fourths is fetal hemoglobin.
>
> White blood count: 8000–38,000/μL (average: 17,000/μL)
>> PMNs: 60%
>> Lymphocytes: 20%
>> Monocytes: 10%
>> Immature white cells: 10%
>
> Platelets: 350,000/μL
> Nucleated red cells: < 500/μL
> Reticulocytes: 3%
> Sedimentation rate: Markedly accelerated
> Hematocrit: 54% ± 10%
> MCV: 85–125 fL

*For Umbilicus, see p 159.

MCHC: 36%

MCH: 35–40 pg

Levels of prothrombin (factor II), plasma thromboplastin component (factor IX), proconvertin (factor VII), and Stuart-Prower factor (factor X) are low. The level of proaccelerin (factor V) is either normal or slightly elevated.

M. Urine: About 30–60 mL of urine with low specific gravity is normally passed the first day. Protein and acetone are often present. Occasional casts, red cells, and white cells may be present. Uric acid crystals are often the cause of pink urine.

N. Stools: Meconium may be passed at birth or soon after.

Changes During the First Week
After Term Delivery

A. Position: Relaxed. Fetal position preferred.

B. Weight: Mature infants lose approximately 10% of their birth weight by the fourth to fifth day but regain it by the seventh day. Premature or sick newborns may lose 25% of their original weight despite therapy.

C. Skin: Color changes from ruddy to pink; petechiae and erythematous patches fade. Slight jaundice occurs on the second to fourth day in 40% of newborns but disappears by the seventh day. Earlier, more intense, persistent jaundice accompanies isoimmunization.

Peeling, especially of palms and soles, begins on about the fifth day. Transient fissures may form, particularly at the wrists. Fine-textured skin is soon notable.

Lanugo disappears from the face first (after the first week).

D. Head and Face: Molding and caput succedaneum are gone by the seventh day.

E. Chest: Slight breast engorgement, nipple prominence, and leakage of white, viscid "witch's milk" occurs on the second to third day in mature newborns of both sexes. Withdrawal of maternal steroid sex hormones at delivery is responsible.

F. Abdomen: The cord stump is dry and shriveled by the fifth day, off by the seventh day. Colic and vomiting on days 2–4 is due to swallowed air or blood or to overfeeding. Ileus occurs with passage of a meconium plug.

G. Genitalia: Vulvar engorgement, leukorrhea, and even slight pseudomenstruation (in 1 per 50–60 infants) during the first week are due to maternal estrogen accumulation followed by sudden depletion after birth.

H. Stools: Dark greenish, pasty, or tarry, slightly fetid stools change on the third or fourth day to softer, green-yellow stools. Stools are yellow and curdy with a slightly acid odor on about the sixth day, changing to brown after the seventh day. Large infants, those fed formula, or those delivered with difficulty have more numerous stools than other newborns. Foul-smelling, whitish, or dark, slimy, thin, or frothy stools suggest disease.

I. Laboratory Data: The hemoglobin level falls, that of bilirubin rises (to 13 mg/dL), and the icterus index is slightly elevated by the third or fourth day in mature newborns. Peak liver function is delayed 2–3 weeks (longer in premature infants). Urinary output increases to 200–300 mL/d by the seventh day.

Spinal fluid normally is slightly xanthochromic and contains a few white cells and slightly elevated levels of protein during the first week.

SURGICAL EMERGENCIES

Five serious congenital anomalies are responsible for over 90% of neonatal surgical emergencies.

Diaphragmatic Hernia

Diaphragmatic hernia is the most critical of neonatal emergencies. The time of onset of respiratory distress and the degree of diaphragmatic deficiency determine the seriousness of this abnormality.

Persistent marked cyanosis and dyspnea beginning at delivery are characteristic. Asymmetry and unequal movement of the thorax, absent breath sounds on the affected side, and a scaphoid contour of the abdomen are typical. Chest x-rays should reveal small bowel in the thorax and mediastinal displacement toward the unaffected side.

A. Emergency Measures: Insert an endotracheal tube (to avoid distention of the stomach) and give humidified oxygen at a positive pressure of less than 30 mm Hg. Higher pressure may cause alveolar rupture, pneumothorax, and death.

B. Medical Measures: Correct acidosis.

C. Surgical Measures: Insert a nasogastric tube and apply constant suction to decompress the stomach and intestines. Repair the hernia promptly.

D. Prognosis: The degree of pulmonary development and the success of the hernia repair are the major determinants in the outcome.

Esophageal Atresia

Esophageal atresia is an urgent problem. Hydramnios and cardiac and gastrointestinal defects may be associated abnormalities. There are numerous types of esophageal atresia depending upon the presence or absence of a concomitant tracheoesophageal fistula, the site of the fistula, and the point and extent of the esophageal obstruction.

The newborn will have increasing respiratory distress and excessive mucus production. Even a small amount of fluid will cause coughing and cyanosis.

A. Emergency Measures: Withhold fluids by mouth.

B. Medical Measures: Attempt to pass a catheter into the stomach and aspirate mucus. If this is impossible, esophageal atresia is the diagnosis. Frequent or continuous gentle suctioning of the upper pouch and pharynx will minimize tracheal aspiration of saliva. Check for congenital heart disease and other anomalies before surgery. Prescribe wide-spectrum antibiotic therapy.

C. Surgical Measures: Immediately correct the esophageal atresia (and tracheoesophageal fistula if this is present) and other digestive tract abnormalities.

Omphalocele, Gastroschisis

Omphalocele is a congenital intestinal hernia with protrusion of small bowel into the base of the umbilical cord. It may be accompanied by cardiac or other midline anomalies. Gastroschisis is herniation of viscera through an extraumbilical defect in the abdominal wall. In gastroschisis, the herniating bowel is not covered by skin—only by thin transparent membrane. Every effort must be exerted to preserve this membrane intact and to avoid infection.

A. Emergency Measures: Protect the hernia with sterile petrolatum dressings under a sturdy plastic or metal shield.

B. Medical Measures: Give broad-spectrum antibiotics.

C. Surgical Measures: Primary closure may be done if the hernia is smaller than 5 cm in diameter; larger defects require closure in stages.

D. Prognosis: The development of infection or the presence of other anomalies may seriously compromise the success of surgery.

Intestinal Obstruction

Abdominal distention and bile-stained fecal vomitus in the first 24–48 hours after delivery probably indicate congenital jejunal or ileal obstruction. Premature newborns or those with other anomalies are often afflicted.

A. Medical Measures: Pass a small catheter into the stomach of the newborn who vomits dark material and aspirate the gastric contents. If more than 25 mL is obtained, or if the fluid is bile-stained, assume intestinal obstruction until this diagnosis is disproved.

Obtain x-ray films of the abdomen. Dilatation of the small bowel and absence of gas in the colon are indicative of jejunal or ileal obstruction. A barium enema may rule out causes other than congenital obstruction, eg, megacolon.

B. Surgical Measures: Immediate exploratory laparotomy and relief of obstruction are mandatory.

Imperforate Anus

Imperforate anus is more prevalent in males than females, and many infants with this anomaly are preterm. Associated developmental abnormalities are common. There are 2 types of imperforate anus: low obstruction (eg, anal membrane) and high obstruction (eg, anal or rectal atresia). Attempts to pass a soft catheter (preferred) or insert a lubricated, gloved little finger will identify the obstruction.

Poorly executed or complicated surgery during the newborn period may result in fecal incontinence for the life of the individual. Hence, a surgeon experienced in pediatric surgery should be engaged. An anal membrane may only require simple incision to overcome the obstruction. Anorectal atresia will require a colostomy initially. Subsequent surgery, perhaps in childhood, will depend upon sacral or other abnormalities and the feasibility of sphincter control.

FETAL INJURY

Intracranial Hemorrhage

Intracranial hemorrhage is most commonly caused by birth trauma or hypoxia. Hemorrhage due to birth trauma is localized, and that due to hypoxia is diffuse within the brain substance. Those affected are usually undergrown or excessively large newborns. Intracranial hemorrhage may be categorized as follows: (1) Subdural hemorrhage: blood in the cerebrospinal fluid. (2) Subarachnoid hemorrhage: cerebrospinal fluid clear. (3) Interstitial hemorrhage: late discoloration of cerebrospinal fluid.

Difficult forceps operations, version and extraction, and complicated breech delivery often are associated with intracranial hemorrhage.

The signs of intracranial hemorrhage include reduced responsiveness or high-pitched cry, irritability, opisthotonos, twitching, and convulsions. A positive Moro reflex may be present at birth and disappear later, or the Moro reflex may be negative from birth. (Paralysis is a later observation in intracranial hemorrhage.) Elevation of the cerebrospinal fluid pressure may or may not develop after intracranial hemorrhage.

Subdural hemorrhage requires evacuation of the extravasated blood. Supportive therapy must be given as well. Elevate the infant's head, provide comfortable warmth (newborn's temperature to 38 °C [100.4 °F]), and give phytonadione (vitamin K), 5 mg intramuscularly. Repeated spinal taps to reduce increased pressure are not recommended. Consult a neurosurgeon or pediatrician.

The prognosis depends upon the site and extent of the hemorrhage, the degree of central nervous system damage, and associated problems such as immaturity.

Fracture of the Clavicle

The clavicle is the bone most often fractured at delivery, usually during breech extraction. Dystocia, especially failure of the breech to rotate or shoulder impaction with vertex presentation, may be the immediate problem. Limitation of motion of the arm, crepitus or irregularity of the bone, and absence of the Moro reflex on the affected side suggest fracture of the clavicle. X-ray films will identify the fracture. Immobilization of the shoulder and arm for several weeks should ensure a good prognosis.

Brachial Palsy

Traction or lateral extension injury to the brachial plexus, which often occurs during breech extraction or shoulder dystocia, may cause brachial palsy. The 2 principal types of brachial palsy are (1) high injury (Erb-Duchenne), which consists of damage to spinal nerves C4–6; and (2) low injury (Klumpke), which consists of damage to C7–8 and T1 or their trunks.

Edema or hemorrhage may cause temporary palsy; nerve laceration will cause permanent sensory and motor deficiency.

Splinting to prevent deformity is important. Surgery is not indicated. The prognosis depends upon the type, site, and degree of nerve damage.

Facial Palsy (Bell's Palsy)

Neonatal facial palsy or immobilization of the muscles of expression on the affected side is almost always due to misapplication of forceps and undue pressure of one blade against the seventh (facial) nerve during operative delivery.

There is loss of voluntary and involuntary contraction of facial muscles on the injured side. The eye fails to close, the forehead above does not wrinkle, and the mouth droops on the affected side.

Watchful expectancy is recommended. Improvement is slow, but permanent paralysis is rare.

FETAL MALDEVELOPMENT

Anencephaly, Microcephaly

Anencephaly and microcephaly are uncommon developmental anomalies in which the head is considerably smaller than normal.

In anencephaly, there is virtual lack of brain substance and absence of overlying skull. Very early antenatal viral infection or multifactorial inheritance may be causes. About 70% of anencephalics are female. In anencephaly, the pituitary gland is absent or vestigial, and lack of ACTH stimulation results in a diminutive, hypofunctional adrenal cortex. Amniotic fluid containing high levels of α-fetoprotein may indicate open neural tube defects, which may include anencephaly.

Most microcephalic individuals have a small but well-formed head, but the brain is diminutive and maldeveloped. The causes of microcephaly include infection (eg, rubella), maternal ingestion of antifolinic drugs, or exposure to excessive radiation—all during early pregnancy.

Anencephaly is incompatible with life. Microcephalics may live, but they are subject to cyanosis, apnea, vomiting, retraction of the head, and asymmetry of movements and reflexes. If they survive, they will have serious intellectual and motor handicaps.

Meningomyelocele

Meningomyelocele, herniation of the meninges containing cerebrospinal fluid through a defect in the vertebral column or skull, is occasionally seen in a newborn. Associated developmental abnormalities may be present. A rare case may be suspected antepartum if amniocentesis yields fluid strongly positive for α-fetoprotein. Meningomyelocele is a serious anomaly, but rarely is it responsible for dystocia. Infection may cause some cases of meningomyelocele, but if several cases occur in the same family, a genetic defect should be suspected.

Careful handling and protection of the herniation with sterile petrolatum gauze and sponge rubber is mandatory to avoid neurologic damage; meningitis develops promptly after contamination or rupture of the sac.

Surgical repair may be done in the neonatal period or delayed if other anomalies such as hydrocephalus require treatment.

The prognosis is poor. At least two-thirds of cases of meningomyelocele are operable, but many of these infants die or achieve only partial neuromuscular function.

Hydrocephalus

Hydrocephalus is an occasional congenital anomaly characterized by enlargement of the head due to excessive collection of cerebrospinal fluid in the cranial vault. Prominence of the forehead, weakness, convulsions, and atrophy of the brain are characteristic of hydrocephalus. Two types are recognized: (1) external hydrocephalus, an abnormal accumulation of cerebrospinal fluid between the brain and the dura mater; and (2) internal hydrocephalus, excessive accumulation of cerebrospinal fluid in the ventricular system of the brain.

Hydrocephalus, often a cause of dystocia, may be compounded by the injury sustained during the delivery process.

Individual nursing care, frequent turning of the newborn, and gavage feedings (if swallowing is deficient) may be required.

Surgical shunting may be necessary to avoid irreversible central nervous system damage, but this rarely is necessary during the neonatal period. The prognosis is good only in cases of slight hydrocephalus.

Cleft Lip or Palate

Cleft lip or palate is a congenital midline fissure or, more rarely, a double separation of the lip or palate. Lip and palate deformities may occur singly or in combination. Either or both anomalies are present in about one per 800 live births. Cleft lip and palate are polygenic disorders, ie, when the combination of genetic susceptibility and toxic environmental factors exceeds a developmental threshold, the abnormality becomes manifest.

Cleft lip or palate causes serious eating problems. In the latter, nasal regurgitation or aspiration of milk may occur. Special feeding techniques are required, eg, the infant is held in a sitting position for nursing; a cup or compression feeder is used.

Repair of these defects should never be attempted during the neonatal period. Cleft lip is best corrected when the infant weighs over 5450 g (12 lb); cleft palate repair is usually performed at about 18 months of age in order to permit normal speech development, which begins at about this time. Good function generally is achieved, but the cosmetic result may be less than desired.

Congenital Hip Dysplasia (Congenital Dislocation of the Hip)

In congenital hip dysplasia, the acetabulum is abnormally shallow, so that the head of the femur becomes dislocated superiorly and posteriorly to lie on the dorsal aspect of the ilium, where a false acetabulum may be formed. Congenital dislocation of the hip is an uncommon hereditary disorder, and 90% of cases occur in females. True dislocation may be present at birth if the presentation is breech. In other cases, dislocation may develop later. If hip dysplasia is not corrected, disability is compounded by the stretched joint capsule and delayed ossification of the head of the femur.

The signs of congenital hip dysplasia before dislocation are asymmetry, reduced movement, splinting, and limited abduction of the affected hip. After dislocation, all of the above signs are present and the leg is externally rotated and shortened. A click may be heard on cautious abduction of the leg, and a bulge of the femoral head should be felt.

X-ray is diagnostic.

Dislocation or dysplasia diagnosed in the first few weeks or months of life can easily be treated by splinting, with the hip maintained in flexion and abduction. Rigid plaster fixation is contraindicated, as this often leads to avascular necrosis of the femoral head.

With early diagnosis and proper treatment, the prognosis is good.

Talipes (Clubfoot)

Talipes is a congenital fixed deformity in which the foot is twisted out of shape or position. Talipes occurs in about one in 1000 live births. Any infant with a clubfoot should be examined carefully for associated anomalies, especially of the spine. Clubfoot tends to follow a hereditary pattern in some families or may be part of a generalized neuromuscular syndrome such as arthrogryposis or myelodysplasia.

Talipes most commonly involves plantar flexion of the foot at the ankle joint (talipes equinus). Other types include inversion of the heel (talipes varus) and forefoot abduction (talipes valgus).

Treatment consists of massage and manipulation of the foot to stretch the contracted tissues on the medial and posterior aspects, followed by splinting to hold the correction. When this is instituted in the nursery shortly after birth, correction is achieved much more rapidly. When treatment is delayed, the foot tends to become more rigid within a matter of days. As the child gets older, casting following manipulation and stretching is necessary. Special shoes and lower leg braces are usually necessary. About half of children with clubfoot eventually require surgery.

The prognosis depends upon the extent of the deformity and the response to progressive orthopedic treatment.

Diethylstilbestrol (DES) Related Abnormalities

Mothers who received diethylstilbestrol (DES) or one of its analogs during pregnancy may have offspring with developmental or functional genital problems. Single or multiple abnormalities may be noted; most have been recognized after puberty. Abnormalities are rare despite the fact that hundreds of thousands of pregnant women received DES between 1940 and 1970 in attempts to prevent abortion. Because most individuals exposed to DES antenatally are unaffected, an association rather than an actual cause and effect relationship may exist. A "trigger" factor is being sought.

In DES-exposed females, disorders include circumferential vaginal ridges, cervical deformity (eg, "coxcomb" cervix, hooding, cleft, pseudopolyps), cervicovaginal adenosis, dysplasia, and cervical incompetence. Hypoplastic or T-shaped uterus, constricting bands within the uterus, and tubal anomalies have also been reported. An increased frequency of oligomenorrhea and a lower incidence of pregnancy have been reported in these women also. More serious is the observation that 3–4 of 1000 women exposed to DES prenatally develop vaginal or cervical clear cell carcinoma.

In DES-exposed males, epididymal cysts, hypotrophic testes, and testicular capsular thickening are the most common gross lesions reported. Sperm analyses have revealed a low volume of ejaculate, oligospermia, and lower motile sperm counts. No equivalent of female clear cell carcinoma or increase in male genitourinary cancer has been noted, however.

INTRAUTERINE GROWTH RETARDATION
(Low-Birth-Weight or Small-for-Dates Neonate)

The characterization of newborns as term or premature on the basis of weight—ie, above or below 2500 g (5 lb 8 oz)—has little clinical significance and should be abandoned. Actually, many term infants

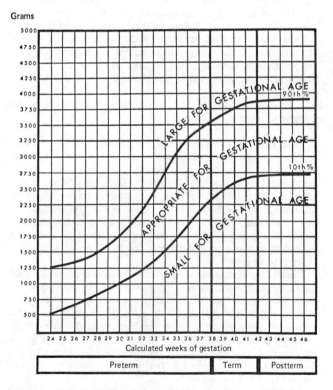

Figure 7–3. Classification of newborn infants by birth weight and gestational age. (University of Colorado Medical Center. Reproduced, with permission, from Battaglia FC, Lubchenco LO: A practical classification of newborn infants by weight and gestational age. *J Pediatr* 1967;**71:**160.)

(40% in some countries) weigh less than 2500 g, and in some areas many preterm infants weigh 2500 g or more.

To ensure optimal care, both weight and gestational age must be considered (Figs 7–3 and 7–4). The newborn should be weighed accurately at birth for proper drug dosage as well as for statistical purposes. The newborn weighing 2500 g or less is now termed a low-birth-weight neonate.

A small-for-dates, growth-retarded, or undergrown fetus is one considerably below the normal weight of offspring of the same gestational age. Moderately growth-retarded fetuses generally are identified as those below the tenth percentile, whereas those below the second percentile are considered severely undergrown. The type, severity, and duration of the problem (eg, preeclampsia) are the major determinants.

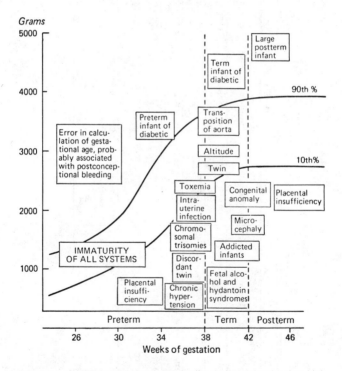

Figure 7–4. Conditions associated with intrauterine growth related to birth weight and gestational age classification. (Reproduced, with permission, from: *Nutricia Symposium.* HE Stenfert Kroese, BV. Leiden, Holland, 1968.)

Table 7–2. Postnatal estimation of fetal age on the basis of maturity (assuming normal growth). *

	27 Weeks	28–33 Weeks	34–37 Weeks	38–41 Weeks	42 Weeks or More
Anatomic maturity					
Sole creases	None.	Minimal—one or 2 creases.	Anterior third.	Extend to heel.	Deep creases over entire sole.
Scrotum	Testes undescended.	Testes high in scrotum; few rugae.	Testes above raphe; more rugae.	Testes bulge below raphe; rugae complete.	Pendulous, deep rugae, well pigmented.
Labia	Labia majora undeveloped.	Minora prominent.	Labia of equal prominence.	Majora covers minora.	Same.
Ear cartilage	Pinna soft and folded.	Still folded.	Returns from folded position.	Erect, with sharp ridges.	Same.
Breast tissue	None.	None.	Up to 4 mm.	5 mm or more.	Usually more than 10 mm; areolae very prominent.
Skin	Translucent and edematous.	Red.	Pink to red.	Pinkish white.	Thicker and white; often desquamated.
Nails	Visible; soft and small.	Soft and extending to fingertips.	Soft and extending to fingertips.	Extending to just beyond fingertips; not as soft.	Hard in consistency and extending well beyond fingertips.
Eyes	Closed.	Closed.	Opening.	Open eyes that fixate.	Open, good fixation.

Neuromuscular maturity					
Body flexion	None.	Flexes legs—froglike.	Flexes arms; knees under abdomen.	Same.	Same.
Moro reflex	Aimless.	Lateral extension.	Beginning embrace.	Embrace.	Same.
Neck tone	Limp.	Limp.	Head control on arm flexion (36–37 weeks).	Raises head in prone position.	Raises head in prone position; turns head from side to side.
Sucking and deglutition	Not synchronized.	Insufficient for total nipple feeding.	Adequate for normal intake.	Same.	Perfect.
Glabella tap (blink)	No response.	Develops (32–33 weeks).	Good response.	Same.	Same.
Pupil to light	No response.	Gradual contraction.	Good response.	Same—begins to follow.	Same.
Measurements					
Weight (g ± 1 SD)	1000 ± 350	1150–2000 ± 450	2200–2950 ± 450	3150–3600 ± 500	3300–4100 ± 500
Length (cm ± 1 SD)	37.5 ± 1.5	38.5–44 ± 1.5	45–47.5 ± 1.5	48.5–53 ± 2	50–54 ± 2
Head circumference (cm ± 1 SD)	25.5 ± 1	26–30 ± 1	31–33.5 ± 1	34–36.5 ± 1.5	35–37.5 ± 1.5

*Reproduced, with permission, from Babson SG et al: *Management of High Risk Pregnancy and Intensive Care of the Neonate,* 3rd ed. Mosby, 1975.

Gestational age should be determined from the records, ie, calculated on the basis of the menstrual history, date of quickening, fundal growth, and ultrasonographic findings. A further assessment of fetal age should be made after careful examination of the infant, including appearance, measurements, and neuromuscular function (Table 7–2).

Morbidity and mortality rates are highest among infants born before 33 weeks' gestational age and among those weighing under 2000 g regardless of gestational age. Studies also show that almost 3% of all infants dying in the neonatal period fall into these groups. Moreover, at least twice this number of high-risk infants are lost because of complications of pregnancy and delivery.

The prognosis is best (perinatal mortality rate < 0.5%) for infants who weigh 2750–4500 g (6 lb 1 oz to 9 lb 15 oz). Almost all of these are included within the 10th and 90th percentiles and have a gestational age of 38–42 weeks. These newborns seldom suffer serious complications during delivery.

The remaining newborns, approximately 15–20% of all live births, fall into a medium-risk category with a mortality rate of 0.5–10%. Be this as it may, this group does include occasional postterm infants (often clinically dysmature), some small-for-dates infants,* otherwise normal large-for-dates infants,* and numerous preterm infants who weigh over 2500 g but have a gestational age of 33 weeks or more. Consequently, small-for-gestational-age and large-for-gestational-age newborns should be identified as well as those who are preterm or postterm so that they will receive special care during the early newborn period.

Maternal factors commonly associated with intrauterine growth retardation include a hypoplastic or anomalous uterus, inadequate weight gain, unusually close spacing of pregnancies, drug abuse, and cigarette smoking. Maternal disease (eg, nephritis) often affects the maternal-placental relationship to the detriment of the fetus. Placental abnormalities such as small size, circumvallate placenta, or disordered function (eg, placental insufficiency or placental infarction) lead to undergrowth of the fetus.

The following are helpful in the anticipation or diagnosis of fetal growth retardation:

(1) A history of prior undergrown fetuses; repeated pregnancy in less than 1 year.

(2) Abnormal uterine enlargement as determined by increasing fundal height or maternal girth.

---

*A small-for-dates infant is a significantly undersized infant who, compared with age mates, is > 2 SD below the mean weight for that period of gestation. A large-for-dates infant is an oversized infant who exceeds the median weight for comparable newborns at that period of gestation by 2 SD.

(3) Laboratory or special tests–

(a) Ultrasonography–Less than a 2-mm increase in biparietal diameter per week from 13 to 34 weeks of pregnancy, or less than a 1-mm increase per week from 35 to 40 weeks of pregnancy.

(b) Low or falling serial plasma or urinary estriol determinations.

(c) Positive oxytocin challenge test.

(d) Meconium passage determined by amnioscopy or amniocentesis.

Treatment

A. Growth-Retarded Newborn: (Often with fetal asphyxia or meconium aspiration.)

1. Deliver early by the least dangerous means.

2. Aspirate the pharynx and trachea carefully and thoroughly, using a DeLee mucus trap catheter inserted transnasally, especially when meconium aspiration is possible.

3. Administer humidified oxygen to resuscitate; then give ultrasonic mist.

4. Maintain body warmth (skin temperature at 37 °C [98.6 °F]).

5. Correct acidosis if present. Check blood pH every 30 minutes and as necessary. Treat alkalosis with sodium bicarbonate solution intravenously.

6. Infuse 10% glucose, 80–100 mL/kg intravenously. Continue infusion until oral feedings are begun. Obtain blood glucose values every 12 hours and again 3 hours after infusion is stopped.

7. If infection is likely (premature rupture of membranes, aspiration of meconium), broad-spectrum antibiotics should be given until the infection is eradicated or specific antibiotic treatment can be instituted on the basis of cultures and sensitivity studies. Antibiotics that can be given initially include ampicillin, 200 mg/kg/d by intravenous infusion, plus moxalactam, 200 mg/kg/d in divided bolus additions to the ampicillin infusion; or ampicillin, 200 mg/kg/d by intravenous infusion, plus amikacin, 15 mg/kg/d in 2–3 divided doses either intramuscularly or as boluses added to the ampicillin infusion; or aqueous penicillin G, 50–100 thousand units intramuscularly daily, plus kanamycin, 15 mg/kg/d intramuscularly in divided doses every 12 hours for 5 days.

8. Obtain chest x-ray for evidence of aspiration syndrome (hilar opacities), pneumothorax (increased respiratory effort, cyanosis), or cardiomegaly (hypoglycemia or cardiac failure).

B. Undersized, Undernourished, or Dysmature Newborn: (Active and otherwise in good condition.)

1. Offer 10–15% glucose solution, 5–8 mL orally every 2–3 hours, as soon as acceptable.

2. Shift to full-strength formula (24–30 kcal/30 mL) after several glucose feedings have been tolerated.

3. Test blood with Dextrostix twice daily for the first 5 days as a screening test. If a faint blue color develops (possible low blood glucose level: > 30 mg/dL), obtain a quantitative blood glucose determination.

4. Add parenteral feedings if intake is unsatisfactory or if blood glucose level is less than 30 mg/dL.

THE LARGE-FOR-DATES, "LARGE," OR OVERSIZED NEONATE

The large-for-dates newborn has been defined arbitrarily as one weighing 4500 g (9 lb 15 oz) or more. Recently, the large-for-dates perinate has been defined as one over the 90th percentile (> 2 SD) for gestational age. Between 1 and 3% of neonates in the USA qualify.

The intranatal and postnatal morbidity and mortality rates of large-for-dates newborns are considerably higher than normal, the degree depending upon the fetopelvic dimensions, the presentation, and maternal complications.

Most oversized newborns are born of multiparas, many of whom are of large frame or obese, often with gestational or frank diabetes mellitus; some are 2 weeks or more overdue.

The large-for-dates fetus may suffer because of metabolic stress in maternal diabetes mellitus or may be exposed to more physical trauma during labor and delivery as compared with average-sized or smaller offspring. Hypoxia often develops during labor, and serious birth trauma may also jeopardize the large fetus. This is especially serious in breech presentation or when shoulder dystocia develops. Trauma during delivery may cause brachial or lumbar plexus injury or fracture of the clavicle. Central nervous system injury may occur during breech extraction or midforceps delivery.

Each successive fetus tends to be a bit larger. Women who are considerably overweight at the onset of pregnancy or who have gained excessively during gestation have appreciably larger progeny. Hence, the physician may anticipate a large fetus, particularly in diabetics. If fetopelvic disproportion is likely with prolonged or dystocic labor, or if fetal distress develops, cesarean section should be chosen over a probable difficult forceps delivery.

ISOIMMUNE HEMOLYTIC DISEASE OF THE NEWBORN
(Erythroblastosis Fetalis; Rh, ABO, or Other Incompatibility)

Isoimmunization is the development of antibodies against antigens from a genetically dissimilar individual. Antigens may be transferred by injection or transfusion of blood or by mingling of fetal blood with maternal blood during pregnancy or delivery.

Isoimmune hemolytic disease of the newborn is a disorder of the blood and blood-forming organs of the fetus and newborn that occurs when maternal plasma containing antibodies to the fetal red blood cells filters through the placenta into the fetal circulation. The antibodies destroy fetal red blood cells, causing the hemolytic anemia and hyperbilirubinemia characteristic of the disease.

The Rh antigen (Rh factor) is the most common cause of isoimmunization of the mother and isoimmune hemolytic disease of the newborn. Severe isoimmune hemolytic disease occurs in about 1 in 200 pregnancies in the USA. Blacks and Orientals are rarely afflicted. Similar but generally less serious problems may result from ABO or other red cell incompatibilities, eg, M, N, Kell, Duffy factors.

Pathologic Physiology

Individuals who carry the Rh factor are described as Rh-positive; those who lack this factor are called Rh-negative. The Rh factor is not antigenic for Rh-positive individuals, ie, they do not produce anti-Rh antibodies. Thus, Rh isoimmunization does not occur in Rh-positive women but can occur in Rh-negative women. If an isoimmune Rh-negative woman is carrying an Rh-positive fetus, isoimmune hemolytic disease of the newborn can occur.

Isoimmunization of the mother can result from transfusion of mismatched blood or from bleeding of cord blood into the maternal circulation when the placenta detaches during delivery or abortion. Once the mother is immunized, even minute amounts of Rh-positive fetal blood act as antigenic stimuli, causing a rise in maternal production of anti-Rh antibody (a rise in anti-Rh titer). The anti-Rh antibodies, which are agglutinins and hemolysins, are small enough to pass through the placenta to the fetus, where they clump and destroy (lyse) fetal red blood cells.

The destruction of fetal red blood cells by this process is called hemolytic disease of the newborn. The hematopoietic system of the fetus may not be able to compensate for the destruction of red cells; thus, hemolytic anemia occurs. The increased destruction of red cells also increases the level of unconjugated bilirubin, and because the immature liver does not conjugate bilirubin efficiently, hyperbilirubinemia occurs. Jaundice ensues, and as bilirubin accumulates in the plasma, it may cross the blood-brain barrier, be deposited in the nuclear zones of the midbrain and brain stem, and cause kernicterus.

Clinical Findings

A. Diagnosis of Isoimmunization of the Mother:

1. **First pregnancy, no previous transfusions or intramuscular**

injections of blood–Test as follows: A cell pool containing all of the common antigens is commercially available. If any agglutination occurs when the patient's serum and Rh testing sera are mixed, the patient has one or more antibodies that may present serious problems for the fetus. The antibodies usually can be identified by specific cell panel testing. The antibodies most frequently identified in this way are D, c, C, E, K, and Fy^a.

If this approach is used, routine ABO and Rh typing of the mother and father is no longer necessary. Instead, all antigens are sought and the patient's serum is tested against Rh testing sera at about the fifth month, when considerable antibody production is to be expected. If agglutination occurs, the antibody or antibodies are then identified.

If the Rh testing sera test is negative at the fifth month of pregnancy, the patient should be retested at 8–9 months.

2. Subsequent pregnancies (husband Rh-positive, or previous transfusions of possibly incompatible blood)–Test the mother's blood each month for antibody titer. Note the date of first appearance of antibodies; clinical hemolytic disease of the newborn does not usually develop for at least 10 weeks thereafter. Perform amniocentesis after the 26th week in definitely isoimmunized women (titer > 1:16) (see below).

B. Diagnosis of Isoimmune Hemolytic Disease of the Newborn:

1. Mild hemolytic disease–There may be only slight to moderate hemolytic anemia and early jaundice.

2. Moderately severe hemolytic disease–The placenta is large. Abnormal central nervous system signs consist of spasticity, inactivity, and stupor. Jaundice appears within the first 12–18 hours after delivery. Slight generalized edema is present. Moderate hepatomegaly and splenomegaly are noted.

3. Severe hemolytic disease–The fetus may be stillborn, or the above signs will be much more marked. Gross edema is present. Marked jaundice constitutes icterus gravis neonatorum.

C. Laboratory Findings:

1. The mother is Rh-negative and the infant Rh-positive. (Rh-positive infants are occasionally typed as Rh-negative initially because of blocking antibodies.)

2. Increased anti-Rh titer in mother's blood.

3. Amniotic fluid spectrophotometry–The condition of the fetus can be assessed by amniocentesis and spectrophotometric analysis of the amniotic fluid. First, the placental site should be determined and fetal abnormalities (eg, hydrops fetalis) identified by ultrasonography. The placenta must be avoided when the needle is inserted into the uterus. About 15 mL of amniotic fluid should be obtained and its optical density between wavelengths 375 and 525 nm determined and plotted on a graph as shown in Fig 7–5. Light absorption by bilirubin is maximal at 450 nm. A comparison of the values obtained, especially at 450 nm, with average

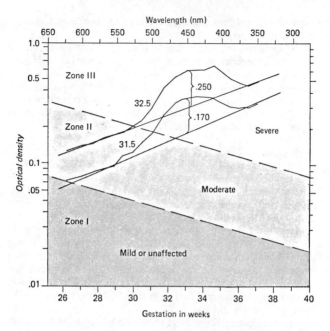

Figure 7–5. Transabdominal amniocentesis: spectrophotometric analysis of amniotic fluid surrounding an erythroblastotic fetus. Amniocentesis was performed at 31½ and 32½ weeks. The spectral absorption curve was obtained by plotting the optical densities at various wavelengths on 2-cycle semilogarithmic graph paper. A tangential line joining the lowest portions of this curve approximates the values for unstained amniotic fluid and is the baseline for calculations. The difference between the involved and uninvolved curves is measured at 450 nm (the wavelength at which maximum absorption by bilirubin or bilirubinlike products occurs) and plotted at the appropriate number of weeks of gestation (see dotted line). The case illustrated shows rapid progression from moderate to severe disease. Under such conditions, fetal death is often imminent. Immediate delivery is usually necessary if the gestational age will permit; otherwise, intrauterine fetal transfusion may be considered. (Reproduced, with permission, from Babson and Benson: *Clinical Perinatology.* Mosby, 1971.)

normal values during pregnancy will usually indicate whether it is safe to let the pregnancy continue or whether prompt delivery is indicated.

Liley plotted spectrophotometric determinants and established zones as guides to treatment and prognosis (Fig 7–5). Optical density values in zone I indicate an unaffected or mildly affected fetus; values in zone II indicate moderate isoimmunization; and those in zone III identify a severely affected fetus. If untreated, many severely affected fetuses die in the perinatal period.

If spectrophotometric readings fall in zone III on more than one occasion, intrauterine transfusion (before 32–33 weeks) or delivery (usually by cesarean section after 32–33 weeks) is imperative. If delivery is chosen, the mother should be given betamethasone (Celestone), 12 mg intramuscularly and the same dose 24 hours later (or its equivalent), to accelerate maturation of the fetal lungs and reduce the likelihood of respiratory distress syndrome.

Prevention

A. ABO Hemolytic Disease: Prevention of ABO hemolytic disease is not possible, but serious ABO hemolytic disease of the fetus is extremely rare. The fetus is usually only mildly anemic, and hyperbilirubinemia usually does not occur until after birth.

B. Rh Hemolytic Disease:

1. Do not give Rh-positive blood to an Rh-negative woman.

2. Rh_0 (D) immune globulin (RhoGAM) given up to 4 days after delivery, abortion, or amniocentesis will prevent Rh isoimmunization of the mother. (*Caution:* Do not immunize the infant. Do not administer intravenously.) Administer Rh_0 (D) immune globulin after abortion or amniocentesis without qualification or after delivery to all patients who meet the following criteria–

a. The mother is Rh-negative without Rh antibodies, ie, she has not received Rh-positive blood by transfusion or injection and the indirect Coombs test is negative.

b. The infant is Rh_0 (D)- or D^u-positive.

c. The cord blood is Coombs-negative.

Treatment

Note: Be prepared to give exchange transfusion to infants born of mothers whose histories indicate that ABO incompatibility is probable or certain or whose Rh antibody titers are persistently elevated.

A. ABO Hemolytic Disease: ABO hemolytic disease is less dangerous to the fetus than Rh hemolytic disease because the former rarely causes fetal death or severe anemia. However, both diseases are important concerns in the neonatal period because they both cause early jaundice in the newborn. Phototherapy and expectant management in the nursery are usually adequate treatment for jaundice due to ABO incompatibility. Exchange transfusion may be necessary if the serum bilirubin level exceeds 18 mg/dL.

B. Rh Hemolytic Disease:

1. Intrauterine fetal transfusion–A fetus considerably younger than 32 weeks of age may be too immature and anemic to survive even with the best care. In such cases, several fetal transfusions of group O,

Rh-negative blood, compatible with the mother's serum, should be given into the peritoneal cavity of the fetus at intervals of 10 days to sustain life until delivery and specific supportive care are possible—at about 32 weeks.

Trauma to or infection of the fetus and mother may be serious complications. The technical problems are such that intrauterine transfusion should only be attempted in medical centers where an experienced team is available.

2. Management of the infant with probable Rh hemolytic disease–

a. Administer oxygen to the mother during the second stage of labor and whenever fetal distress occurs. Withhold depressant drugs from the woman in labor.

b. Transfusions (generally into the umbilical artery)– Replacement transfusions are required in severe cases; no transfusions may be needed or small transfusions may be sufficient in mild or moderate cases. Use only Rh-negative, specific type or type O blood. Give 11–22 mL of blood per kilogram (5–10 mL/lb).

Consider exchange transfusion of the infant when any of the following are noted (in order of seriousness): (1) Evidence of severe isoimmune Rh hemolytic disease at birth, particularly when the duration of pregnancy is less than 37 weeks. (2) Serum bilirubin level of cord blood 3.5 mg/dL or more, or over 20 mg/dL in the first 24 hours or in the 24 hours after a transfusion. (3) Positive Coombs test on cord blood. (4) Jaundice in the first 12 hours of life. (5) Hemoglobin level less than 15 g/dL and reticulocyte count greater than 5%. (6) History of previous isoimmune hemolytic disease in infants born of the same parents, especially when the father is Rh-positive. (7) Consistently elevated maternal anti-Rh titer of 1:16 or more.

Prognosis

First-trimester abortion is almost never due to Rh incompatibility, because the anti-Rh antibody level during the first trimester is not high enough to cause severe damage to the fetus. Fetal death in utero or premature termination of pregnancy does occur later. Fetal death in utero near term or death in the neonatal period is the usual prognosis for infants with hydrops fetalis. Choreoathetosis often results if kernicterus develops in a newborn with icterus gravis.

If the infant with serious isoimmune hemolytic disease survives, there are no sequelae.

SEX DETERMINATION (INTERSEX)

Male and female are the only legal designations of sex. Sex determination requires an interpretive correlation of growth and development involving both morphologic and psychosocial criteria. Individuals with a congenital ambiguity of the external genitalia—one or more contradictions in the morphologic criteria of sex—present problems of intersexuality.

The morphologic criteria are (1) genetic sex, (2) chromosomal sex, (3) gonadal sex, (4) sex of the internal genitalia (duct system), (5) sex of the external genitalia, and (6) hormonal sex. The psychosocial criteria are (1) sex of rearing and (2) gender role.

Morphologic Criteria of Sex

A. Genetic Sex: This is established at fertilization. Normally, the mother (XX) and the father (XY) each contribute one of the 2 sex chromosomes to the offspring. Hence, the normal child bears either an XX or an XY sex chromosome combination. Occasionally, an abnormality such as an XO or XXY combination ensues because of "accidental" loss or gain of a chromosome, and gonadal maldevelopment and sterility may result.

B. Chromosomal Sex: This is an elaboration of the original genetic endowment. However, faulty chromosomal division—as in mosaicism (XX/XY) or in nondisjunction of sex chromosomes—may produce ambisexual incongruities.

C. Gonadal Sex: The early uncommitted embryonic gonad usually differentiates in accordance with the individual's genetic makeup. The Y chromosome, which contains a testis-directing gene, is a potent factor in determining male sex, perhaps mediated by the H-Y antigen. Individuals with a Y chromosome are male irrespective of the number of X chromosomes present. Males with an extra Y chromosome are identified occasionally. In adult life, these men are fertile and tend to be conspicuously tall. Nonspecific behavioral disorders, including aggression, are more common in multiple-Y individuals.

Absence of the Y chromosome results in an apparent (phenotypic) female. The X chromosome is female-directed, but it is a weak determinant in comparison with its Y counterpart. Two X chromosomes (XX) initiate ovarian development. In contrast, individuals with only one X chromosome (XO) have rudimentary gonads and reduced female characteristics; such persons are sterile. Extra X chromosomes in women—the "super-female" pattern (XXX)—rarely have a deleterious effect; in contrast, males with an extra X chromosome (XXY) develop male internal and external genitalia, but spermatogenesis, secondary sex characteristics, and mental capacity may be deficient and sterility is the rule.

D. Sex of the Internal Genitalia (Duct System): Abnormal development or atrophy of the gonads may alter sexual function, the characteristics of the sexual duct system, and external genitalia. Sex hormones administered to the mother between the sixth and eighth weeks of pregnancy do not affect gonadal differentiation in humans. However, development of the internal and external genitalia, which are basically formed by the 18th week, may be altered by androgens (exogenous or endogenous), resulting in the production of male ducts in a female fetus. Deficiency in Y chromosomal impetus, evident as a lack of the H-Y antigen, may result in anomalies or lack of male genital conduits.

E. Hormonal Sex: Differentiation of male external genitalia, which occurs between the eighth and twelfth week of pregnancy, requires adequate androgen stimulation. In most instances, once the gonad is committed to an ovarian or a testicular future, the intrinsic sex hormones develop the appropriate internal and external genitalia.

The individual's hormone moiety establishes and maintains the secondary sex characteristics. Normally, the ovaries predominantly produce estrogen and the testes androgen. In testicular feminization, an inborn insensitivity to androgen allows endogenous estrogen to dominate development. Excessive adrenal androgen, as in congenital adrenogenital syndrome, may masculinize the external genitalia of the fetus.

Psychosocial Criteria of Sex

A. Sex of Rearing: The sex of rearing is responsible for an individual's sexual orientation as a male or female, irrespective of gonadal development and chromosomal makeup. Hence, the gross appearance and functional capability of the external genitalia are much more important than the sex chromatin. Serious psychologic consequences may result from changing the sex of rearing after infancy. Therefore, it is seldom proper to advise social reorientation to the "true" somatic sex of an individual after infancy. Instead, the physician should exert efforts to complete the adjustment of the person to the sex role already assigned. Fortunately, most aberrations of sexual development are discovered in the newborn period or in infancy, when reassignment of sex causes few problems.

B. Gender Role: Personal feelings regarding one's sex role begin in infancy and are irreversibly established by about age 2. Deviant sex behavior (ie, homosexuality, transvestism, transsexualism) may be noted later, but there is no abnormal physical development associated with this change.

Classification of Intersexuality (Ambiguous Genitalia)

Classification may be anatomic or etiologic. Intersexuality may be divided into 4 major categories: (1) true hermaphroditism—a genuine combination of male and female gonadal elements; (2) gonadal dysgenesis, genetic male or female; (3) gonadal maldevelopment; and (4) extragonadal alteration of genitalia. Almost 50% of the newborns with anomalous genitals are females with (autosomal recessive) hyperadrenocorticism. True hermaphroditism is very rare.

Diagnosis

A. History: Mother's health; course of pregnancy and therapy in the pregnancy under study; genetic status of family; sibling abnormalities.

B. Physical Examination: Description of anomalies, including unusually tall or short stature, low hairline ("fur cap" distribution), Down's syndrome, web neck, wide arm span, abnormal breast development, inguinal hernia in females, anomalous genitalia, undescended testes, and edema of the feet and legs (only). **Note:** Suspect critical metabolic disorders in a newborn with ambiguous genitalia (eg, sodium loss in congenital hyperadrenocorticism).

C. Laboratory Tests:

1. A sex chromatin test (number of Barr bodies, the X chromatin bodies) should be performed on buccal cells in all instances of possible intersex. The number of Barr bodies is one less than the number of X chromosomes in the cell, eg, if there are 2 Barr bodies, the individual is XXX. XX females have over 50% chromatin-positive cells; males have less than 10% chromatin-positive cells. The results should be reported as a positive or negative Barr body test rather than as male or female in order to avoid arousing the concern of the patient or the family.

Y chromosomes can be identified by the characteristic "banding" of chromosomes produced by the Giemsa method of staining, by karyotyping, or by quinacrine staining and fluorescence microscopy.

2. Urinary 17-ketosteroid levels are markedly elevated, usually by the seventh day after delivery, in female and male intersex due to hyperadrenocorticism caused by an inborn enzyme deficiency. Such infants may develop critical sodium loss. Cortisone therapy conserves sodium and also suppresses the production of 17-ketosteroids except when a functional adrenocortical tumor is present.

3. The presence of pregnanetriol or pregnanetriolone in urine may identify congenital adrenogenital syndrome but not other causes of ambiguous genitalia.

4. Determine the gonadotropin level in a 24-hour urine specimen. This value is considerably elevated in adolescents with Turner's syndrome or Kleinfelter's syndrome.

D. Karyotyping: A karyotype should be done in all intersex cases except those related to the adrenogenital syndrome.

E. X-Ray Studies: When the vagina seems to be absent, a cystourethrogram may show the vagina and uterus to be above the urethra. A plain film of the abdomen and an intravenous urogram may disclose urinary tract abnormalities.

F. Special Studies:

1. Endoscopy may reveal urethrovaginal continuity.

2. Exploratory laparotomy and biopsy of the gonads may be done if a patient with anomalous external genitalia requires further evaluation.

Treatment

The objective of therapy is to make possible adequate sexual function and a good cosmetic result with as few psychosocial complications as possible. The sex of rearing is more important than gonadal and chromosomal sex in intersex decisions. In planning surgical reconstruction, however, consider the functional capacities of the external genitalia (to establish an adequate vagina is far easier than to reconstitute a diminutive penis) and the time of surgery. Since an infant can withstand alteration of sex and its psychologic impact far better than an older individual, plastic surgery ideally should be done before the child is 2 years old. However, because a neovagina does not increase in size as the child grows, operation should be postponed until full body growth has been achieved. Surgery should be done by early adolescence, because lack of a vagina is harmful to the adolescent girl's self-esteem and sense of physical adequacy. The girl who wants the corrective surgery will be properly motivated and will understand that she must use vaginal dilators after the operation to achieve a good result and keep the neovagina patent. Adrenalectomy and gonadectomy may be accomplished whenever indicated. Orchiopexy should be done before puberty if hCG therapy fails to cause descent of the testes.

Recommended management is as follows:

A. True Hermaphroditism: Urethrovaginogram, intravenous urogram, laparotomy, biopsy of gonads, removal of internal male or female genitalia (because of their tendency to become malignant), and appropriate revision of external genitalia, usually in accordance with sex of rearing.

B. Gonadal Dysgenesis, Male or Female: Long-term cyclic estrogen supplementation is required. Laparotomy and biopsy of "streak" gonads are rarely necessary. Rear as a female.

C. Gonadal Maldevelopment: This includes undescended testes, fused labia, and positioning of the vagina and uterus above the urethra. Urethrovaginogram, intravenous urogram, surgical exploration, orchiopexy, and reconstructive scrotal, labial, or vaginal surgery may be warranted. Individualize treatment. The sex of rearing may depend upon what can be accomplished surgically. Prosthetic testes may be required.

D. Extragonadal Alteration of Genitalia:

1. Male pseudohermaphrodite (testicular feminization)–Exploratory laparotomy and orchiectomy are indicated. The somewhat hypertrophic phallus requires no treatment.

2. Female pseudohermaphrodite (maternal virilization)–Rear as a female. The hypertrophic phallus should recede. Laparotomy is not justified.

3. Female pseudohermaphrodite (adrenogenital syndrome)–Maintain proper fluid and electrolyte balance. Provide early, prolonged corticosteroid therapy to inhibit production of ACTH. Rear as a female.

Correct gynatresia if present. Laparotomy and adrenal exploration are unwarranted unless the diagnosis of adrenal or functional ovarian tumor is supported by clinical and laboratory studies.

Prognosis

When the sex of rearing is contrary to morphologic sex, reassignment of sex is often successful in very early childhood. Later sex reassignment is rarely psychologically successful even when the results of surgical alteration of the genitalia and breasts are reasonably good. Fertility is likely only in the successfully treated pseudohermaphrodite.

Whether a true hermaphrodite has fathered a child is still debated. Fewer than 10 hermaphrodites have become pregnant.

Complications of the Third Stage of Labor | 8

POSTPARTAL HEMORRHAGE

Postpartal hemorrhage is the major cause of maternal deaths in the USA. Five to 8% of all patients delivered at term develop some degree of postpartal hemorrhage, which is defined arbitrarily as the loss of at least 500 mL of blood following delivery of the fetus. A more useful definition of postpartal hemorrhage is loss of blood in an amount equivalent to 1% or more of body weight, which relates readily to blood volume. However, this may be difficult to determine.

Blood loss must be measured (1 mL of blood = 1 g) or weighed accurately. Estimates are grossly inaccurate.

Postpartal hemorrhage may be sudden, massive, and exsanguinating or slow, continuous, and only slight to moderate in amount at any one time. Postpartal hemorrhage may be early, from delivery until 24 hours afterward; or late (secondary), from 24 hours to 4 weeks after delivery. About 2% of patients require hospitalization and often surgery or blood replacement (or both).

Uterine bleeding is normally controlled after delivery of the fetus by the ligature effect of the intertwining contracted myometrial muscle bundles.

Etiology

Many causes have been determined for postpartal hemorrhage: (1) mismanagement of the third stage of labor; (2) incomplete separation of the placenta; (3) uterine atony due to excessive analgesia or anesthesia, prolonged labor, retained adherent placental fragments (partial placenta accreta, adherent succenturiate lobe), or excessive uterine distention (as in multiple births, polyhydramnios); (4) laceration of the birth canal, eg, perineal-vaginal lacerations, cervical lacerations; (5) complications of pregnancy such as premature separation of the placenta, placenta previa, inversion or rupture of the uterus; (6) tumors of the cervix and uterus, eg, myomas, adenomyosis, choriocarcinoma, endometrial carcinoma, carcinoma of the cervix, hemangioma or aneurysm of a uterine vessel; (7) hematologic disorders, eg, disseminated intravascular coagulation, leukemia, thrombocytopenic purpura; (8) medical complications during

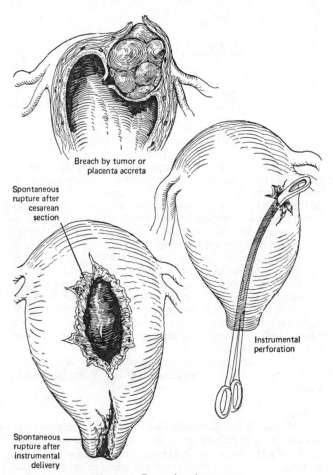

Figure 8–1. Types of uterine rupture.

pregnancy, eg, hypothyroidism, vitamin B complex deficiency, or vitamin K deficiency; (9) placenta accreta; (10) infections of the genital tract, eg, endometritis, parametritis.

Clinical Findings

Excessive bleeding can occur during any of the 3 phases of the third stage of labor. The type of bleeding varies according to the cause.

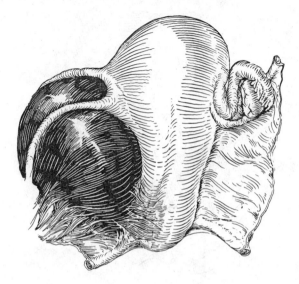

Figure 8–2. Rupture of lower uterine segment with bleeding into the broad ligament.

A. From Delivery to Separation of the Placenta:

1. Episiotomy, perineal or vaginal lacerations, or rupture of varices is usually accompanied by a steady ooze of dark red blood.

2. Cervical lacerations cause a free flow of bright red (arterial) blood.

3. Incomplete separation of the placenta or partial placenta accreta causes loss of dark blood in spurts that coincide with uterine manipulation or fundal contraction.

B. From Separation to Expression of the Placenta:
When expression of the separated placenta is delayed because the free placenta in the uterus covers the cervix, the fundus cannot contract well, bleeding continues, and blood is trapped. Large clots accompany the placenta when the afterbirth is finally expelled or extracted.

C. Following Recovery of the Placenta:

1. Atony of the uterus causes steady, persistent bleeding, with additional gushes during uterine contractions.

2. Prolapse of the uterus into the pelvis causes a profuse continuous flow of blood not related to uterine contractions.

3. Lacerations of the birth canal—particularly those of the uterus—cause continuous hemorrhage, principally of arterial blood.

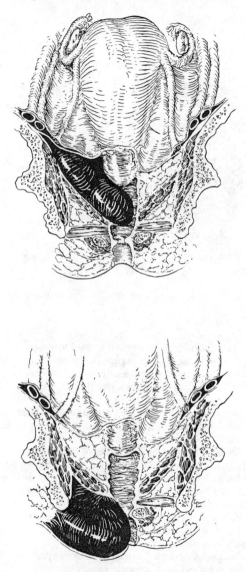

Figure 8–3. Hematoma in supralevator space (above) and infralevator space (below). (After Melody.)

Complications

Postpartal hemorrhage predisposes to shock, puerperal infection, embolism, and anemia.

Prevention

Faulty technique in expression of the placenta contributes to blood loss. The Pastore or Brandt-Andrews method of placental expression is preferred. The Credé maneuver is always contraindicated, and the fundus should never be used as a piston to push the placenta out.

It is essential to anticipate postpartal hemorrhage if possible so that preventive steps can be taken as outlined below. A history of postpartal hemorrhage in prior deliveries is an obvious indication for careful preventive management; other indications include multiple pregnancy, cesarean section, and infection of the uterus. Conditions that are often associated with postpartal hemorrhage but may be difficult or impossible to anticipate before the event are polyhydramnios, primary or secondary uterine inertia, desultory or prolonged labor, placenta previa, and premature separation of the placenta.

In the conditions mentioned above, postpartal hemorrhage may be prevented by the following measures:

(1) Near the end of the first stage of labor, begin a rapid intravenous infusion of 5% dextrose in water (500 mL) through a No. 18 needle.

(2) Immediately after delivery, add 0.5 mL (5 units) of oxytocin to the infusion bottle. (*Caution:* Do not inject oxytocin into the tubing; bolus administration will result.)

(3) On completion of the third stage, inject 0.2 mg of ergonovine (Ergotrate) directly into the tubing so that the patient will receive the drug promptly.

(4) Elevate the fundus out of the pelvis; massage the uterus until it becomes firm and remains so.

(5) Keep the patient in the delivery room (or recovery room) for at least 1 hour after delivery and until vital signs are stable.

Treatment

A. Emergency and Specific Measures: (See also Management of the Third Stage of Labor, Chapter 6.)

1. Repair episiotomy incisions; perineal, vaginal, or cervical lacerations (Fig 8–4); and ruptured varices promptly.

2. Incomplete separation of the placenta or partial placenta accreta accompanied by uterine bleeding–If bleeding is slight, wait about 10 minutes until the placenta separates. If bleeding is profuse, remove the placenta manually (without additional anesthesia, if possible), using the ulnar edge of the gauze-covered hand from above downward to avoid perforation of the uterus (Fig 8–5).

3. Delayed expression of separated placenta–Express the placenta

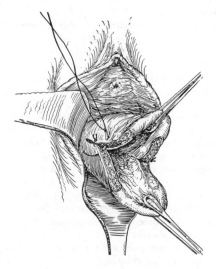

Figure 8–4. Repair of cervical lacerations. (After Edgar.)

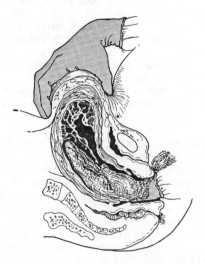

Figure 8–5. Finger and gauze curettement of uterus.

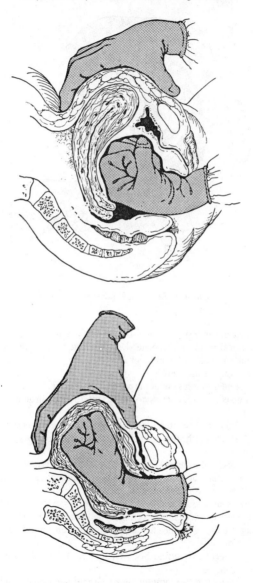

Figure 8–6. Bimanual compression of uterus.

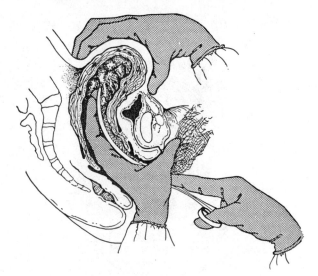

Figure 8–7. Packing the uterus with forceps.

when the signs indicate it is free. Do not delay recovery of the placenta until perineal repair is complete. Use the Pastore or Brandt-Andrews technique for placental expression.

4. Atony of the uterus–

a. Hold the uterus out of the pelvis and massage the fundus gently. If bleeding is profuse, give oxytocin, 0.5 mL (5 units) in an intravenous infusion.

b. Prolapse of the uterus into the pelvis–Lift the uterus and support the fundus. Elevate the cervix and uterus with gauze on a sponge-stick, if necessary.

c. Packing the uterus–This procedure (Fig 8–7) is now rarely done except as a temporary measure, eg, while preparations are being made for hysterectomy for rupture of the uterus.

Have available several jars of dry gauze, 1 yard wide and 5 yards long, previously folded into 4-inch strips and sterilized in wide-mouthed glass containers. A Holmes tubular packing instrument may be helpful but is not essential.

B. General Measures: See Management of the Third Stage of Labor, Chapter 6.

C. Treatment of Complications: Further hemorrhage and shock require emergency replacement of blood, correction of the bleeding problem, and antishock therapy. Death may occur from vasomotor or cardiovascular collapse.

Prognosis

The prognosis depends upon the cause of bleeding, the amount of blood lost, and the rapidity with which it is lost (in proportion to the patient's weight); the patient's general health; and the choice, speed, and completeness of therapy.

INVERSION OF THE UTERUS*

An inverted uterus is one that is partially or completely turned inside out. Inversion of the uterus is rare but very dangerous. Puerperal inversion is a critical emergency; it usually occurs just after delivery but may occur within 6 weeks after delivery. The incidence is about one in 15,000 deliveries and is lowest where obstetric care is of the highest quality. Nonpuerperal inversion, a less serious problem, occurs in one in 25,000 adult gynecologic or nonpuerperal patients.

Partial inversion (Fig 8–8) is herniation of the fundus into the

---

*For convenience, both puerperal and nonpuerperal inversion are discussed in this chapter.

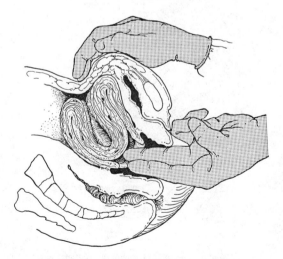

Figure 8–8. Partial inversion of the uterus.

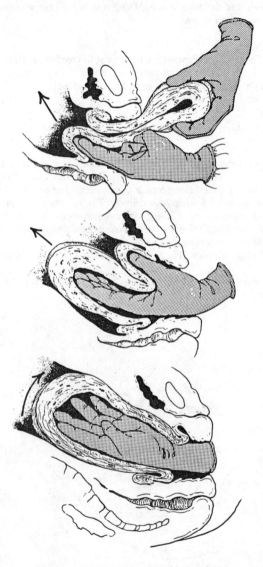

Figure 8–9. Manual replacement of inverted uterus.

uterine cavity. Complete inversion is extrusion of the corpus through the cervix into or beyond the vagina. Either type may be acute or chronic and spontaneous or induced.

Acute spontaneous puerperal inversion is due to straining by the patient after delivery or the weight of the infant on the cord and placenta (eg, when delivery is spontaneous and precipitous with the patient in a standing position and unattended).

Acute induced puerperal inversion is the result of (1) traction on the cord before placental separation, (2) severe "kneading" of the fundus (vigorous Credé maneuver) to induce placental separation and expulsion, (3) excessive pressure on the uterine fundus (Kristeller maneuver), (4) delivery of an infant with a short cord or one that has been shortened by coiling, or (5) hasty manual separation and extraction of an adherent placenta. Chronic induced puerperal inversion is due to the same causes as acute induced puerperal inversion but may not be recognized until more than 1 month after delivery.

Acute nonpuerperal inversion of the uterus may occur as a result of extrusion of a uterine tumor (most often a large pedunculated myoma) or as a complication of the extraction of a large, tesselated fibroid tumor. Chronic nonpuerperal inversion is due to the same causes but is not promptly recognized.

Clinical Findings

Acute complete inversion of the uterus causes sudden, agonizing pain combined with an explosive sensation of "fullness" extending downward into the vagina. Brisk bleeding and profound shock occur in over half of patients; death may result from exsanguination. If inversion is partial, pain and bleeding are less severe.

Bimanual examination is necessary. In the abdomen, the depressed fundus or absent corpus is revealed by "dimpling" or a craterlike depression. In the vagina, complete inversion is manifested by the presence of a large bleeding mass outside the introitus, often with the placenta attached; in partial inversion, a cup-shaped mass can be palpated just above or bulging through the cervix.

Chronic partial uterine inversion is characterized by persistent unexplained bleeding and discharge accompanied by discomfort.

Differential Diagnosis

A large submucous myoma at the external cervical os may cause the same symptoms as inversion, but the fundus is larger than normal and there is no craterlike depression in the abdomen.

Complications

Shock, hemorrhage, anemia, infection, and embolism may follow inversion of the uterus.

Prevention

Do not pull on the cord unless the placenta has separated; do not push on the fundus or use the Credé maneuver; do not leave the patient until the uterus is contracted and rounded. An abdominal binder is permissible, but do not place a pad or roll beneath it lest inversion recur.

Treatment

In acute puerperal inversion, the maternal mortality rate is high. Obtain consultation and assistance immediately.

A. Preparation of the Patient: Before attempting definitive treatment, control shock with intravenous fluids, plasma, whole blood, and oxytocin (Pitocin). Avoid giving ergot preparations, which cause continued tetanic contraction of the cervix and uterus, until the uterus is replaced (see below).

B. Manual Replacement: Replace the uterus by abdominovaginal manipulation (Fig 8–9), developing countertraction on the cervix while directing the inverted portion of the uterus upward. Deep general anesthesia (eg, halothane, ether) is required. Leave the placenta attached, compress the fundus in the anteroposterior diameter, and apply countertraction with a ring forceps grasping the anterior cervical lip. Cervical constriction may be relaxed with whiffs of amyl nitrite vapor or with 0.3–0.6 mL of epinephrine, 1:1000, intramuscularly. Retain the fist within the uterus until the corpus is well contracted by oxytocics (ergot) to prevent recurrence of inversion. Packs are not effective; they usually maintain uterine distention.

C. Surgical Replacement: If correction is not accomplished easily and quickly by manipulation, immediate surgery is mandatory.

1. Haultain technique (transabdominal)–Incise the posterior wall of the inverted uterus, replace the fundus with towel clamps placed hand-over-hand, and suture the uterine wall.

2. Spinelli technique (transvaginal)–Transect the cervix anteriorly, replace the fundus from below, and suture the cervix.

3. Küstner technique (transvaginal)–Incise through the cervix posteriorly, replace the fundus, and suture the cervix.

D. Hysterectomy: Chronic inversion of the uterus is treated by hysterectomy.

E. Postoperative Care: Administer broad-spectrum antibiotics; replace blood, fluid, and electrolytes; and decompress the stomach with a nasogastric tube.

Prognosis

Manual replacement of the uterus, when correctly performed, is successful in about 75% of patients with inversion. If the patient is not properly prepared for anesthesia or surgery, the mortality rate will be about 30%. Recurrence of inversion is possible but not likely.

The Puerperium | 9

The puerperium (arbitrarily designated as the 6 weeks following childbirth) is the period of adjustment after pregnancy and delivery when the mother's body is expected to return to its normal nonpregnant state.

PHYSIOLOGIC EVENTS OF THE PUERPERIUM

The height of the fundus and the size of the uterus decrease from delivery to 1–6 weeks thereafter (Fig 9–1). The uterus involutes rapidly

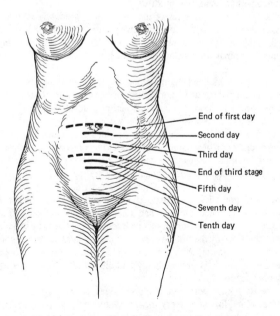

End of first day
Second day
Third day
End of third stage
Fifth day
Seventh day
Tenth day

Figure 9–1. Postpartal levels of uterine involution.

after delivery. Involution is complete by the sixth week postpartum, chiefly as a result of decrease in the size of individual myometrial cells. Because some connective tissue and an augmented vasculature persist permanently to some degree, the uterus remains slightly larger following a term pregnancy.

Regeneration of the endometrium is complete by the third week postpartum, but regeneration of the placental site is not complete until the fifth or sixth week.

Lochia rubra, the bloody discharge that follows delivery, usually becomes more serous and lighter in color (lochia serosa) after 2–3 days. In another week, the lochia normally becomes mucoid and yellowish because of the inclusion of leukocytes and disintegrating decidual elements. Discharge usually ceases about the fourth week after delivery.

The cervix gradually closes during the puerperium, and the external os is converted to a transverse slit about 3 weeks after delivery. The overdistended vagina gradually returns to its prepartum condition by the third week after vaginal delivery, although the rugae remain flattened and the torn hymen heals irregularly. These hymenal remnants are called carunculae hymenales (or myrtiformes).

The voluntary muscles of the pelvic floor gradually regain their tone, although tearing or overstretching during vaginal delivery may weaken the structures and predispose to genital hernias. Overdistention of the abdominal wall during pregnancy leads to diastasis of the rectus muscles.

The hypotonic and slightly elongated and dilated ureters and renal pelvis gradually revert to normal by the third month. Renal function returns to normal during the early puerperium, but nearly 50% of patients have mild proteinuria during the first week.

Following delivery, the average woman loses about 4 kg (9 lb) as a result of excretion of accumulated fluids and accompanying electrolytes. Most of the fluid changes occur within the first 2 weeks, after which time approximately normal nonpregnant values are the rule.

Changes in blood volume and hematocrit during the early puerperium are dramatic. The hematocrit rises about 5% above the predelivery value in patients who have had a normal vaginal delivery; in those who are delivered by cesarean section, there is a relative drop in hematocrit of about 5% by the fifth day postpartum. In contrast, a blood volume loss of approximately 20% can be expected by the fifth day in both the average patient delivered vaginally and the patient whose delivery by cesarean section was uncomplicated.

Most women with normal blood values during pregnancy and an average blood loss at delivery show a relative polycythemia during the second week postpartum. Iron supplementation is not necessary for normal nonlactating postpartum women if the hematocrit or hemoglobin concentration 5 days after delivery is about the same as the normal predelivery value.

Cardiac output peaks immediately after delivery, at which time it is 80% above the prelabor value in most normal patients. This is accompanied by elevated venous pressure and increased stroke volume. Bradycardia may be present. Rapid changes toward normal nonpregnant values occur thereafter, particularly during the first week, with a gradual decline during the next 3–4 weeks to prepregnancy values.

A hypercoagulable state is present during the puerperium and predisposes to thrombosis. By 3–5 days after delivery, platelet adhesiveness will have increased considerably, with lesser increases in platelet count and factor V and VIII values. However, fibrinolytic activity also increases. These values all diminish after the first week, returning to normal by about the fourth week.

Changes in lung volumes are rapid initially but slow later during the early puerperium. Expiratory residual volume and functional residual volume are decreased by the first month postpartum and return to normal by 6 months. The respiratory rate is increased during the puerperium but approaches normal in several months.

The hormonal changes immediately following delivery are abrupt. The hCG, estrogen, and progesterone titers fall to the normal nonpregnant range in 1 week. The prolactin level increases considerably during the first week, especially in patients who are lactating. A state of relative hypoestrinism occurs during the puerperium, especially in women who nurse their babies. Slight transient hypothyroidism may also develop.

Return of Ovulation & Menstruation

Nursing mothers neither menstruate nor ovulate. During breast feeding, greatly increased levels of prolactin are maintained by the anterior pituitary. Prolactin suppresses the release of LH but has no effect on the other gonadotropin, FSH. Nonetheless, as long as breast feeding is uninterrupted (not supplemented with bottle feedings), prolactin inhibits the ovarian response to FSH. Therefore, while prolactin levels are high, very little estrogen is released by the ovary, and uterine bleeding does not take place. With inhibition of the ovarian response to FSH, follicles do not develop; without an LH surge, ovulation does not occur. Thus, lactation, a natural method of contraception, does play a role in pregnancy spacing.

After abortion before the 15th week of pregnancy, the average time required for return of ovulation is 2–3 weeks, and menstruation should occur within 4–5 weeks. If the patient was 16–20 weeks pregnant, ovulation should occur within 4–6 weeks after abortion, and menses should resume within 6–7 weeks.

The time of the first ovulatory cycle after delivery is variable. In nonlactating women, ovulation may occur as early as the 25th–35th day postpartum. Menstruation resumes in about 40% of nonlactating women by the sixth week; by 12 weeks after delivery, 70–80% of nonlactating women will have begun to menstruate again.

CARE IMMEDIATELY AFTER DELIVERY

Transfer the patient to a recovery room or keep her in the delivery room for constant observation and treatment for at least 1 hour after delivery.

Uterine Massage & Management of Bleeding

After the third stage of labor, the uterus must be palpated frequently over several hours to make certain that the fundus remains firm and that vaginal bleeding is not excessive. Estimations of blood loss are inaccurate, especially when clots are passed; but the loss of about 300 mL or more of blood constitutes excessive bleeding, and if more than 500 mL is lost, frank hemorrhage has occurred.

When excessive bleeding occurs, treat as described on p 164.

Pulse & Blood Pressure

A. Pulse: Record the pulse rate and rhythm whenever the uterus is palpated—at least every 15 minutes for the first hour after delivery. The first warning of excessive blood loss may be an increase of 10–15 beats per minute in the pulse rate. If the pulse rate remains high, begin antishock therapy and treat for postpartal hemorrhage.

B. Blood Pressure: A fall in blood pressure may also presage shock. Elimination of placental circulation and contraction of the uterus after separation and delivery of the placenta restores at least 300 mL of blood to the maternal system. This normally causes a blood pressure elevation of 10–20 mm Hg and helps to support the diastolic pressure for several hours after delivery. The temporary rise then slowly dissipates.

Record the patient's blood pressure immediately when she arrives in her room and then every 12 hours for the first 24 hours and daily thereafter for several days. Preeclampsia-eclampsia, infection, or other complications may require more frequent determinations.

HOSPITAL (OR HOME) CARE DURING THE FIRST WEEK OF THE PUERPERIUM

Length of Hospitalization

All patients would benefit from at least 1 week of hospitalization after delivery, but the expense involved and the shortage of accommodations preclude a convalescence of this duration for many women. Most patients can return home safely 1–2 days after delivery.

Exercise & Early Ambulation

Caution: Early ambulation does not mean return to normal activity or work.

Early ambulation gives a psychologic lift and a sense of well-being, hastens involution of the uterus, improves uterine drainage, and may reduce the incidence of phlebothrombosis and thrombophlebitis by increasing circulation to the pelvis and lower extremities.

Rest is essential, and no patient should be compelled to get out of bed against her will; encourage but do not force the patient to be active. She should avoid lifting, straining, and pushing.

Diet

A regular diet is permissible as soon as the patient desires food and is free from the effects of analgesics, amnesics, and anesthetics. High-protein foods, fruits, vegetables, and milk products are recommended. A high fluid intake is recommended, especially for nursing mothers. The patient should not overeat; even lactating women probably require no more than 2600–2800 kcal/d. If necessary, continue the daily vitamin-mineral supplement for about 2 weeks for women who do not nurse and throughout the nursing period for those who do.

Vital Signs

Record the temperature, pulse, and respiration rate every 4 hours for 2–3 days at home or in the hospital.

Bladder Care

It is essential to avoid overdistention of the bladder, which is normally hypotonic in pregnancy and immediately after delivery. Normally, the marked polyuria notable for several days after delivery causes the bladder to fill in a relatively short time. If the bladder fills to 1000 mL or more, at least 2 days of decompression by catheter may be required to establish voiding without significant residual urine. If a woman requires catheterization 3 or more times per day during the first several days after delivery, insert a retention catheter for 2–3 days. Sulfisoxazole (Gantrisin) or a similar chemotherapeutic agent, 1 g orally 4 times daily, will usually prevent urinary tract infection while the catheter is in the bladder.

Bowel Function

The mild ileus that usually follows delivery can generally be reversed by administering a mild laxative such as milk of magnesia, 15–20 mL orally on the evening of the second postpartal day. If a bowel movement does not occur by the next morning, order a rectal suppository such as bisacodyl (Dulcolax) or administer a small tap-water enema. Occasional laxatives may be required subsequently, while the patient is sedentary. Avoid mineral oil because it absorbs fat-soluble vitamins.

Phenolphthalein, senna, and jalap laxatives should not be used if the patient is nursing because the infant may develop loose stools.

Oxytocics

Ergot products are valuable in the treatment of postpartal hemorrhage and endometritis, but they may be harmful as extended therapy after delivery.

Analgesics

Discomfort is easily controlled by simple analgesics, eg, aspirin, 0.6 g, with codeine, 30–60 mg, orally every 4 hours as necessary. Meperidine and morphine should be avoided.

Sedation

Hospital procedures, noise, and strange surroundings are not conducive to sleep at night. Sedatives such as phenobarbital, 30 mg orally at bedtime as necessary, will generally ensure a good night's rest.

Care of Episiotomy Incisions & Lacerations

Gently cleanse the area with medicated soap or detergent and water at least once or twice each day and after voiding or defecation. It is impossible to keep the pudendum sterile, but if it is kept clean and dry, healing should occur rapidly. Dry heat applied to the perineum with an infrared lamp for 20–30 minutes 3 times daily will relieve discomfort and promote healing.

Avoid applying greasy ointments or salves to the perineum because skin maceration may develop and infection is fostered by the protective oily film.

Inspect the episiotomy or repaired lacerations daily. Perform vaginal or rectal examination if hematoma or infection seems likely. Drain the sutured area if suppuration develops.

Baths

As soon as the patient is able, she may take a shower. Sitz or tub baths after the second postpartal day are probably safe if the tub is kept scrupulously clean.

POSTPARTAL EXERCISES

Restorative exercises will have no permanent effect on uterine position but will tone the skeletal muscles and improve the physique. Repeat each exercise 4 times twice daily and add another exercise each day. Continue daily for 1 month or longer.

First Day

Breathe in deeply; expand the abdomen. Exhale slowly, hissing; draw in abdominal muscles forcibly.

Second Day

Lie flat on back with legs slightly apart. Hold arms at right angles to the body; slowly raise arms, keeping elbows stiff. Touch hands together and gradually return arms to their original position.

Third Day

Lie flat on back with arms at sides. Draw knees up slightly. Arch back.

Fourth Day

Lie flat on back with knees and hips flexed. Tilt pelvis inward and contract buttocks tightly. Lift head while contracting abdominal muscles.

Fifth Day

Lie flat on back with legs straight. Raise head and one knee slightly. Then reach for, but do not touch, the raised knee with the opposite hand. Alternate with right and left hand.

Sixth Day

Slowly flex knee and then thigh on abdomen. Lower foot to buttock. Straighten and lower leg to the floor. Alternate with right and left leg.

Seventh Day

Raise one leg as high as possible. Keep toes pointed and knee straight. Lower leg gradually, using the abdominal muscles but not the hands. Alternate with right and left leg.

Eighth Day

Rest on elbows and knees, keeping upper arms and legs perpendicular with body. Hump back upward. Contract buttocks and draw abdomen in vigorously. Relax, and breathe deeply.

Ninth Day

Same as seventh day, but raise both legs at the same time.

Tenth Day

Lie flat on back with arms clasped behind head. Then sit up slowly. (If necessary, hook feet under furniture.) Slowly lie back.

POSTPARTAL CARE DURING THE FIRST
3 WEEKS AT HOME
(Postpartal Days 8–28)

Hygiene is essentially the same as practiced in the hospital. When the patient is dismissed from the hospital, tell her that she will note decreasing amounts of sanguineous vaginal discharge for about 3 weeks and possibly a "small period" during the fourth or fifth week after delivery (bleeding from the placental site). She should wear a brassiere constantly, especially if she is nursing, to preserve her figure but should wear a girdle only if necessary or if this is her custom. Vaginal douches should be used only upon specific indications. Coitus should not be resumed until an episiotomy or lacerations have healed.

Activity and responsibility should increase gradually during the recovery period at home. During the first 3–4 weeks after discharge from the hospital, a reasonable limited regimen is recommended.

Kegel Exercises

Active exercise involving the pubococcygeus muscle often will result in improvement of pelvic floor relaxation and urinary stress incontinence if no significant anatomic defects are present. Repeated contraction of the pubococcygeus muscle (as with attempts to stop voiding or a bowel movement in progress) for 5–10 minutes 3 or 4 times daily may restore tone and function.

POSTPARTAL EXAMINATIONS

First Postpartal Examination

Examine the patient during the fourth week or so after delivery if possible. It is advisable to begin therapy (eg, for cervicitis) as soon as possible and still have an opportunity for a second examination before the sixth week, when most patients can return to full activity or employment. The first postpartal examination should include the following:

A. Weight: The patient should have returned to her approximate prepregnancy weight by this time. A suitable diet may have to be prescribed. If she has performed her exercises faithfully, the muscles will be firm and fatty tissue distribution will have returned to its prepregnancy configuration.

B. Breasts: Note abnormalities of the nipples and lactation, the adequacy of support, and the presence of tenderness or mass formation.

C. Uterine Bleeding: Persistent uterine bleeding requires definitive investigation and treatment. A course of ergonovine (Ergotrate) may be required. In extreme cases, dilatation and curettage should be performed.

D. Vaginal Discharge: Leukorrhea ceases in about two-thirds of patients by the fourth or fifth week unless vaginitis, cervicitis, or chronic uterine subinvolution is present. Vaginitis will generally yield to specific treatment. For minimal cervicitis, daily acetic acid douches may be all that is required. Antibiotic therapy or coagulation is necessary when cervicitis is more extensive. Subinvolution may be the result of infection, retroposition, or retained products of conception; treatment must be directed toward correction of the specific problem, but douches and antibiotics are often helpful. Dilatation and curettage are occasionally required when subinvolution of the placental site or endometritis may be due to retained placental tissue. A vaginal pessary may support a retroposed uterus, improve the circulation, and enhance involution.

E. Pelvis: Do a complete rectovaginal evaluation. Perineovaginal support should be adequate. Examine the episiotomy incision and repaired lacerations.

If uterine malposition is present, review the record to determine if the patient had a uterine retroposition or descensus before or during early pregnancy. If so, and if there are no symptoms referable to the "tipped uterus," it is likely that this position is physiologic for her. About 20% of all women have a symptomless retroposition, and replacement of the organ is not necessary. If pain, abnormal bleeding, or other abnormal findings are present, insert a vaginal pessary as a trial procedure to encourage anteversion of the fundus. If uterine prolapse (descensus) is present, its degree should be noted and related to individual symptoms. Pessary support offers only temporary relief in such instances. If prolapse is marked, consider surgical correction.

Observe and, when necessary, treat cervical lesions until they are completely healed.

Repeat specific laboratory tests that were definitely abnormal during pregnancy.

F. Contraception: Discuss family planning. Prescribe the contraceptive method most suitable and acceptable to the couple if this is requested.

Further Examinations

Release the patient to full activity or employment if her recovery by the fourth week has been uneventful, or schedule another visit after appropriate therapy.

A gynecologic examination and cytologic vaginal examination should be performed 6 months after delivery. At that time, the above items and menstruation should be evaluated.

LACTATION

Lactation begins about 48–72 hours after delivery with sudden engorgement of the breasts when the milk "comes in." However, the infant can begin nursing almost immediately after birth, at which time the mother's breasts contain colostrum.

Physiology of Lactation

Estrogen and progesterone, present in large amounts during pregnancy, stimulate the ductal and alveolar systems of the breast, respectively. This causes proliferation and differentiation of the mammary glands and the production of clear, thin, serumlike colostrum as early as the second month of pregnancy. Colostrum continues to be secreted to term, but the high level of estrogen during pregnancy inhibits the binding of prolactin, an anterior pituitary hormone, in breast tissue, so milk is not produced. After delivery of the infant and the placenta, estrogen, progesterone, and hCS levels fall sharply, and prolactin stimulates the mammary alveoli to produce milk. Optimal levels of insulin and thyroid and adrenal hormones play a secondary but necessary role in lactation. Suckling is not needed to initiate lactation.

Suckling stimulates periodic prolactin secretion, but the prolactin level needed to maintain lactation is lower than that achieved during pregnancy.

Suckling also stimulates release of oxytocin from the posterior pituitary via a breast-to-pituitary neural reflex. In addition to its oxytocic effect, oxytocin is a galactokinetic hormone. It contracts the periacinar muscle fibers of the breast, causing ejection of milk into the major collecting sinuses that converge on the nipple. This is called the milk ejection or milk let-down reflex. Tension and fatigue inhibit the let-down reflex, but the infant's cry and nursing stimulate it.

Advantages of Breast Feeding

A. For the Mother: Breast feeding is convenient, costs nothing, is emotionally satisfying for most women, and speeds uterine involution.

B. For the Infant: Breast milk is digestible, readily available, at the right temperature, and free from bacterial contamination. The composition is ideal, and breast-fed infants have fewer allergy problems. The child receives passive antibodies and emotional satisfaction.

Disadvantages of Breast Feeding

A. For the Mother: Regular nursing restricts activities, and nipple tenderness or mastitis may develop.

B. For the Infant: There are no disadvantages if the mother is healthy and willing and the supply of milk is adequate.

Contraindications to Breast Feeding

Absolute contraindications to breast feeding are breast cancer; active pulmonary tuberculosis in the mother; severe mastitis; or maternal intake of antithyroid medications, cancer chemotherapeutic agents, or certain other drugs (see below). Hepatitis B antigen has been found in breast milk, but transmission by this route is unlikely to occur. Breast feeding is not usually possible for weak, ill, or very premature infants or those with cleft palate, choanal atresia, or phenylketonuria.

Drugs In Breast Milk

Innumerable drugs can be detected in a parturient's blood and milk. The drug level in milk depends on the concentration of the drug in the maternal blood, its solubility, its degree of ionization, and whether or not it is actively secreted into milk. If the mother has decreased renal function, drugs may be present in greater concentration in milk.

Nursing mothers should avoid unnecessary or excessive medication. Even in the usual dosage, the following drugs have been reported to be transmitted to the infant in sufficient quantities to cause apparent or potentially harmful effects: ampicillin, sulfonamides (antibiotics); chloral hydrate (sedative); propoxyphene (analgesic); morphine, heroin, methadone (narcotics); chlorthalidone (diuretic); diazepam, chlorpromazine, lithium (psychotropics); oral contraceptives, thyroid hormones; ^{131}I, uracils (antithyroid drugs); ^{131}I, cyclophosphamide (anticancer drugs); and pyrimethamine (antimalarial).

Principles of Breast Feeding

The normal, average mother's yield of breast milk is directly proportionate to the infant's demand, assuming that free secretion of milk has been established and feedings are given every 3–4 hours.

The infant does not nurse so much by developing intermittent negative pressure as by a rhythmic grasping of the areola; milk is "worked" into the mouth. Very little force is required in nursing because the breast reservoirs can be emptied and refilled independently of suction.

Nursing mothers develop a sensation of "drawing" and tightening—a "draught" or concentration—within the breast at the beginning of suckling after the initial breast engorgement disappears. They are thus conscious of the milk ejection reflex, which may even cause milk to spurt or run out.

The milk let-down phenomenon is inhibited by such factors as drugs, pain, breast engorgement, embarrassment, or adverse psychic conditioning. Milk production can be augmented by physical and emotional preparation during pregnancy as well as by good postpartal management.

For several days after the initial breast filling, the milk ejection reflex may be deficient. The breasts become so full and distended that the nipples appear retracted, the areolas are unyielding to the infant's efforts, and the infant obtains little or no milk. Manual expression of milk or the administration of oxytocin (or both) will usually start the flow and relieve the engorgement, whereupon nursing may be more successful.

The mother should nurse her infant at both breasts at each feeding, because overfilling of the breasts is the main cause of decreased milk production. Nursing at only one breast at a feeding leaves the other breast full, and the distention of the full breast inhibits the let-down reflex, causing a reduction in milk output in both breasts. Thus, alternating breasts from one feeding to the next may increase engorgement distress and reduce milk output. However, because infants suck most vigorously at the beginning of a feeding and tend to take the most milk from the breast offered first, alternating the breast *that is offered first* helps to ensure maximal milk production by both breasts.

Demonstrations of infant care and formula preparation are generally a part of the hospital nursing service program. Success or failure of breast feeding is related to the amount of factual information and emotional support available to the mother. Organizations such as the La Leche League, the Nursing Mothers of Australia, and the Plunkett Society in New Zealand have been very effective in promoting breast feeding.

Milk Production

With nursing, the average milk production on the second postpartal day is about 120 mL; on the third postpartal day, at least 180 mL; and by the fourth day, about 240 mL. A good rule of thumb for calculation of milk production for a given day during the first week after delivery is to multiply the number of the postpartal day by 60. This gives the approximate number of milliliters of milk secreted in that 24-hour period.

Assuming that all goes well, sustained milk production will be achieved by most patients after the first 10–14 days. A yield of 120–180 mL of milk per feeding is common by the end of the second week.

Early diminution in milk production may be due to failure to empty the breasts (weak efforts by the baby or ineffectual nursing procedures), emotional problems such as aversion to nursing, or medical complications (eg, mastitis, debilitation, Sheehan's syndrome). Late diminution in milk production results from too generous complementary feedings, emotional or other illness, or pregnancy. Hormones used in oral contraceptives interfere with optimal milk production.

Stimulation of Lactation

(1) During pregnancy, encourage the patient to breast-feed her infant. Explain the advantages of breast feeding and provide factual information and emotional support.

(2) The patient should prepare and "toughen" the nipples during the third trimester of pregnancy.

(a) The patient should wash the nipples daily with unscented mild soap and water, using a washcloth. After drying, she should apply liquid petrolatum. Scented soaps and skin or hand creams should not be used because they may contain irritants or allergens such as perfume. Alcohol should not be used because it dries and hardens the skin.

(b) Inverted or short nipples should be drawn gently outward every day to temporarily increase their length.

(c) The nipples should be protected with plastic film or nipple shields. Have the patient wear a well-fitted brassiere even at night to support the breasts, improve circulation, and avoid trauma.

(d) Teach the patient how to express colostrum gently from the breasts. This should be done several times a day during the last 4–6 weeks of pregnancy to open ducts blocked by inspissated secretions and to stimulate the flow of fluid. This will not cause premature labor.

(3) Beginning on the first postpartal day, if the mother's condition permits, allow the mature, normal newborn to nurse at each breast on demand or approximately every 3–4 hours for 3 minutes' total nursing time per breast per feeding. Increase the time by 1 minute each day, but never exceed 7 minutes per breast per feeding. The average infant obtains 60–90% of the milk in 4 minutes of nursing. Suckling for longer than 7 minutes may cause maceration and cracking of the nipples and mastitis.

(4) Have the mother drink a glass of cool water 5 minutes before nursing, or utilize other suggestions to strengthen the reflex of milk ejection. Beer, wine, or spirits will not increase milk production.

(5) Avoid engorgement and trapping of milk by gentle expression of excess milk before nursing with or without oxytocin, 0.5 units in 1 mL of normal saline intramuscularly, or 10 units in 0.25 mL of normal saline as a nasal spray, just before infant feeding.

Suppression of Lactation

If the patient does not choose to suckle her infant and wishes to "dry up" her breasts, estrogen or androgen (or combination estrogen-androgen) administration or mechanical inhibition of lactation may be effective. Hormones presumably suppress lactation by inhibiting the secretion of pituitary hormones. Hormonal suppression is effective only if started immediately after delivery. Late postpartum bleeding may be increased by estrogens, however.

A. Suppression With Hormones: See Table 9–1. Synthetic ergot preparations, eg, bromocriptine, are dopamine agonists that inhibit prolactin secretion. Prolonged treatment with these agents is necessary, and side-effects such as nasal congestion, headache, and nausea occasionally occur.

Table 9–1. Drugs commonly used to suppress lactation.

Drug	Dosage
Testosterone enanthate, 180 mg/mL, and estradiol valerate, 8 mg/mL (Deladumone)	2 mL IM before delivery.
Chlorotrianisene (Tace)	50 mg orally every 6 hours for 6 doses.
Bromocriptine (Parlodel)	2.5 mg orally twice daily for 14 days.

Note: Bromocriptine, which inhibits prolactin secretion, may be associated with earlier return of ovulation, a consideration in contraceptive counseling.

B. Mechanical Suppression: If the patient begins to nurse and later wishes to transfer her infant to formula feedings and dry up her breasts (eg, if mastitis develops or the infant is to be weaned), hormones will not be effective and mechanical suppression is indicated. The patient should cease nursing and should not express milk or pump her breasts. Apply a tight compression "uplift" binder for 72 hours and a snug brassiere thereafter. Ice packs and analgesics, eg, aspirin and codeine, may be used as necessary. Fluid restriction and laxatives are of no value.

The breasts will become distended, firm, and tender. After 48–72 hours, lactation usually ceases and pain subsides. Involution will be complete in about 1 month.

The uncommon but impressive occurrence of thromboembolic phenomena in parturients on high-dosage estrogen medication is reminiscent of similar problems ascribed to the oral contraceptives. When the likelihood of vascular occlusion is increased, as in post-cesarean section patients or those who have had a difficult vaginal delivery, a febrile course, etc, mechanical suppression of lactation is the logical choice when nursing is not elected.

Abnormal Lactation

Galactorrhea, the discharge of a milklike secretion from the nipple long after physiologic lactation or in a nonpregnant individual, is a sign, not a disease. Amenorrhea is an associated problem. Galactorrhea is seen more often now than formerly, probably because of the wider use of tranquilizers and oral contraceptives. The symptom is directly or indirectly related to hypothalamic-pituitary dysfunction.

Galactorrhea is associated with many abnormalities such as central nervous system tumors, breast or chest disease, endocrine dysfunction, and drug side-effects. Theoretically, galactorrhea may be due to (1) removal of the hypothalamic tonic inhibitory effect on the anterior pituitary (eg, tranquilizers or cessation of oral contraceptives); (2) inability of prolactin-inhibiting and releasing factors to reach the pituitary (ie, degenerative brain disorders); (3) production of prolactin associated with pituitary tumors; and (4) possible stimulation by TRH (thyrotropin-releasing hormone) in some patients with hypothyroidism. Breast manipulation, burns, or tumors of the chest probably involve sensory impulses to the central nervous system that cause increased prolactin production by the anterior pituitary. Functional ovarian or adrenal tumors produce hormones (eg, estrogen) that may influence the hypothalamus or pituitary. Even discontinuance of oral contraceptive medication may result in galactorrhea.

A discerning history and a thorough physical examination, including ophthalmologic, neurologic, and (perhaps) psychiatric evaluations, are required. Consider breast manipulation or medications including oral contraceptives, tranquilizers, and antihypertensive agents as causes of galactorrhea. In addition to the usual laboratory studies, obtain thyroid function studies to rule out hypothyroidism, plasma LH and FSH determinations, and CT scans of the pituitary. If the latter are abnormal and an adenoma is suspected, more extensive studies of anterior pituitary function are indicated. CT scan, carotid angiography, or pneumoencephalography may be necessary. A markedly elevated level of circulating prolactin suggests the presence of a pituitary tumor.

To treat galactorrhea, discontinue all previous medications. If a definitive diagnosis is possible (eg, pituitary tumor), specific treatment with bromocriptine or oral contraceptives may check the galactorrhea. Long-term follow-up employing CT scanning often will reveal a pituitary microadenoma. Surgery may be required if medical control is inadequate.

10 | Multiple Pregnancy

Twin pregnancy is the result of retarded segmentation of a single fertile ovum (identical, monovular, or monozygotic twins) or fertilization of 2 ova by 2 spermatozoa (fraternal or dizygotic twins). Triplets may develop from one, 2, or 3 fertilized ova. Multiple births occur in about one in every 90 confinements in the USA.

Slightly over 30% of twins are derived from one ovum, and nearly 70% develop from 2 ova (Fig 10–1).

An approximate estimate of the frequency of occurrence of multiple pregnancies can be given as follows:

Twins	1:90
Triplets	$1:90^2 = 1:8100$
Quadruplets	$1:90^3 = 1:729,000$, etc

In multiple births, males predominate over females, but to a lesser degree than with single births. The relative number of females increases as the number of fetuses increases in multiple births.

The parents' race and the mother's age and parity are important in

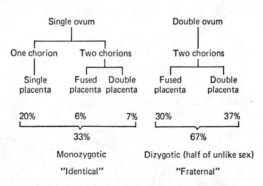

Figure 10–1. Placental variations in twinning. (After Potter.)

the incidence of double-ovum and triple-ovum pregnancies but not in single-ovum twinning, in which the rate is almost the same for all races. It is not known why older women who have had numerous children should produce more fraternal twins than young women of lesser parity do.

Multiple pregnancy is most common in blacks and least common in Orientals. Black couples have a 20–25% greater likelihood of conceiving twins, a 70–75% greater likelihood of conceiving triplets, and a 4 times greater likelihood of conceiving quadruplets than white couples do.

Identical twins result from fertilization of a single ovum by a single sperm: they are always of the same sex. Fraternal twins result from the fertilization of 2 or more ova by 2 or more single sperms. The 2 ova are released from separate follicles (or, very rarely, from the same follicle) at approximately the same time. Fraternal twins may be of the same or different sexes.

Single-ovum twinning results from temporary delay of development of the ovum prior to implantation.

Double-ovum twinning is in large part genetically determined; it is a recessive autosomal trait passed on via female descendants of mothers of twins. Therefore, there is no significant male contribution to twinning. Other causative factors of twinning are speculative.

Triplets may result from repeated twinning of one ovum (also called double twinning or supertwinning) and later death of one embryo, from twinning by 2 ova and elimination of one embryo, or from 3 simultaneously expelled and fertilized ova. Quadruplets arise from one, 2, 3, or 4 ova.

If segmentation of a fertilized ovum occurs early in the second week of pregnancy, conjoined (Siamese) twins develop; if cleavage is further postponed, incomplete twinning (2 heads, one body) occurs.

After the 30th week of pregnancy, each twin and its placenta generally weigh less than a singleton and its placenta, but near term the aggregate weight of twins and their placentas is almost twice that of a singleton. In the USA, the median weight of twins at birth is just over 2270 g (5 lb). Male infants weigh slightly more than females.

Double-ovum twins have 2 placentas (often fused to resemble one), 2 chorions, and 2 amniotic sacs. In contrast with single-ovum twin placentas, there is no anastomosis between the venous or arterial placental channels in fraternal twin placentas.

At delivery, the membranous septum between twins should be inspected and sectioned for evidence of the probable type of twinning. Roll a portion of the septum around a wooden applicator, fix, and send to the pathology laboratory for study. Single-ovum twins have a transparent (thin) septum made up of 2 amniotic membranes only (no chorion and no decidua). Double-ovum twins have an opaque (thick)

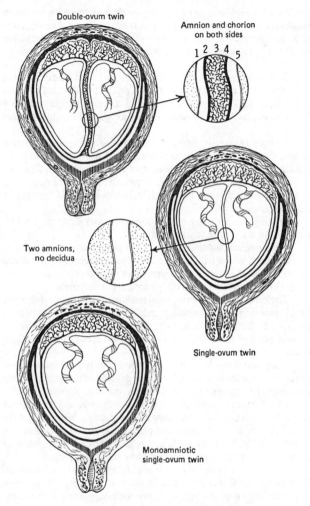

Figure 10–2. Amniotic membranes of twins.

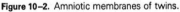

septum made up of 2 chorions, 2 amnions, and intervening decidua (Fig 10–2).

Almost two-thirds of twins can be identified as single- or double-ovum twins at birth by inspection of the placenta, study of the membranes, and finger-, palm-, and footprints. In the remainder, physical comparison and repeated psychologic testing over the years may be necessary to determine whether they are identical or fraternal twins. In some cases, it may be impossible to determine this with certainty. The problem is more than merely academic now that organ transplant surgery is possible. The exact relationship of triplets, quadruplets, or quintuplets to each other is often doubtful.

Single-ovum twins are smaller, have a higher incidence of congenital abnormalities, and succumb more often in utero than double-ovum twins. Crowding, competition for nutrition, cord compression and entanglement, very early birth, and operative delivery take a terrible toll in multiple pregnancy.

Injection studies of the placenta have revealed uncommon vascular anastomoses, almost exclusively in monozygotic twins, the most serious being an artery-to-vein shunt. Thus, twin-to-twin transfusion may occur. The recipient twin will be larger, plethoric, hypertensive, and edematous, with an enlarged heart, liver, and kidneys, and will have hydramnios resulting from polyuria. The donor twin will be smaller, growth-retarded, pallid, anemic, and hypovolemic and will have oligohydramnios secondary to dehydration. Both twins will be threatened with heart failure: one as a result of cardiac overload, the other as a result of anemia and hypovolemia.

The heart will not develop in a twin whose circulation is extremely deficient during the period of formation of the viscera. This fetus (acardius) then becomes parasitic and is nourished by whatever blood is pumped to it by its stronger sibling. Other deformities are also commonly present and depend upon the degree of deprivation.

Clinical Findings

A. Symptoms and Signs: The effects of multiple pregnancy on the mother include earlier and more severe abdominal distention, difficulty in breathing, nausea, pressure in the pelvis, backache, varicosities, and hemorrhoids. A ''large pregnancy'' (distended uterus) may be indicative of multiple pregnancy. Fetal activity is increased and more persistent in multiple pregnancy than in single pregnancy.

Manual diagnosis of multiple pregnancy is possible in about 75% of cases. The following signs should alert the physician to the possibility or definite presence of multiple pregnancy: (1) excessive maternal weight gain unexplained by edema or obesity; (2) polyhydramnios, manifested by uterine size out of proportion to the calculated duration of gestation (almost 10 times as common in multiple pregnancy); (3) outline or balottement of more than one fetus; (4) multiplicity of small parts; (5) uterus containing 3 or more large parts; (6) simultaneous recording of different fetal heart rates, each asynchronous with the mother's pulse and with each other and varying by at least 8 beats per minute (after irritation of the fetus mechanically, by pressure or displacement, to accelerate its

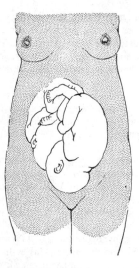

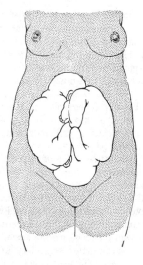

Figure 10–3. Both twins presenting by the vertex.

Figure 10–4. One vertex and one breech presentation.

heart rate); (7) palpation of one or more fetuses in the fundus after delivery of one infant.

B. Laboratory Findings: The hematocrit, hemoglobin level, and red cell count are usually considerably reduced. Maternal anemia is common in multiple pregnancy, beginning during the second trimester as the fetal demand for iron increases beyond the mother's ability to assimilate it.

C. Ultrasonography: Ultrasonographic examination will reveal the number of fetuses in plural pregnancy after the sixth to eighth week and their presentation after the 20th week. At the onset of labor, both twins will present by the vertex in almost 50% of cases (Fig 10–3); one will be a vertex and the other a breech in slightly over 33% of cases (Fig 10–4); both will be breech presentation in 10% of cases; and almost 10% will be single (or double) transverse presentations. (X-ray films in advanced pregnancy will also reveal the number and presentation of the fetuses, but because of potential genetic damage to mother and offspring, x-ray studies should be reserved for emergencies.)

D. Electrocardiography: Electrocardiography, utilizing electrodes placed on the mother's abdomen in midline positions, may be used to diagnose multiple pregnancy after the 20th week. Individual fetal electrocardiographic patterns will be superimposed upon the mother's.

Complications

A. Maternal:

1. Preeclampsia-eclampsia occurs 3 times as often in multiple pregnancy as in single-fetus pregnancies.

2. Premature labor and delivery–Three-fourths of all multiple pregnancies are delivered before term. The overdistended uterus finally reaches its limit of tolerance, and uterine contractions or premature rupture of the membranes (or both) occurs.

3. Uterine inertia and desultory labor–The myometrial fibers cannot contract well because they are overstretched by the greatly increased volume of the uterus.

4. Placenta previa–The surface of the placenta in multiple pregnancy is often greater than in single-fetus pregnancy and may reach the zone of the internal os.

5. Premature separation of the placenta occurs more often with rupture of the first bag of waters and the initiation of strong contractions, after delivery of one twin, and with preeclampsia-eclampsia.

6. Postpartal hemorrhage–Uterine atony is often accompanied by hemorrhage because of inability of the overdistended uterus to remain contracted after delivery.

B. Fetal:

1. **Antepartal complications**–Fetal death in utero is much more common in multiple pregnancy. Death may be due to cord compression, competition for nutrition, or developmental anomalies. The greatest hazard from cord compression is in single-ovum twins with only one amniotic sac; they may become entangled in their cords. Developmental anomalies are common with single-ovum twins and polyhydramnios. Almost twice as many single-ovum twins as double-ovum twins die in the perinatal period, many before delivery. Attrition is even greater for triplets, quadruplets, etc.

2. **Intrapartal complications**–These are the most common causes of fetal loss in multiple pregnancy. Delivery at least 1 month before term is often due to premature labor or premature rupture of the membranes, which occurs in about 25% of twin, 50% of triplet, and 75% of quadruplet pregnancies. Abnormal and breech presentation, circulatory interference by one fetus with the other, and operative delivery all increase fetal loss. Prolapse of the cord occurs 5 times as often as during a single pregnancy. Premature separation of the placenta before delivery of the second twin may cause death of the second twin by asphyxia. One twin may obstruct the delivery of both: in locked twins, the first is always a breech and the second a vertex presentation. The heads become impacted in the pelvis, and one or both fetuses may die despite operative intervention. Conjoined twins, united at the chest (thoracopagus), the sacrum (pygopagus), or the head (craniopagus), may be undiagnosed prior to labor. Dystocia occurs, and the twins may die during delivery.

3. Postpartal complications–Survival of multiple-birth newborns depends upon obstetric and pediatric difficulties and their solution. Twice as many twins as singletons are delivered before the 36th week of pregnancy. Intracranial injury is more common in premature infants— even those delivered spontaneously—and often leads to death in the neonatal period.

Differential Diagnosis

Multiple pregnancy must be distinguished from the following:

A. Single Pregnancy: Only one fetus can be palpated and only one fetal heart heard. Inaccurate dates may give a false impression of the duration of pregnancy, and the fetus may be larger than expected.

B. Polyhydramnios: Either single or multiple pregnancy may be associated with excessive fluid accumulation. Careful examination may distinguish one or more fetuses. Use ultrasonography or obtain x-ray films if the number and normality of the fetuses are still in doubt during the last trimester.

C. Abdominal Tumors Complicating Pregnancy: Fibroid tumors of the uterus are usually numerous and readily identified. Ovarian tumors are generally single and discrete.

D. Complicated Twin Pregnancy: If one double-ovum twin dies and the other lives, the dead fetus may become flattened and mummified (fetus compressus or fetus papyraceus). Its portion of the fused placenta will be pale and atrophic, but remnants of 2 sacs and 2 cords will usually be found.

E. Hydatidiform Degeneration: Hydatidiform degeneration of the placenta of one fetus of a double-ovum pregnancy may occur. The surviving fetus may be thought to be a primary single fetus until delivery.

Treatment

A. General Measures: The pregnant woman should maintain optimal weight during pregnancy: ideal weight for height and build plus about 16 kg (35 lb). Prevent anemia, preeclampsia-eclampsia, and vaginal infections, and treat them early when they do occur.

Reduced activity and prolonged rest periods (with the patient lying down) after the 28th week may reduce the incidence of prematurity in multiple births and, therefore, the unusually high incidence of perinatal morbidity and mortality in this gestational period. If the cervix is incompetent, consider cervical cerclage. Tocolytic drugs used in very early labor may prevent premature labor.

B. Delivery: A scrubbed, gowned, and gloved assistant should always be present for delivery of a patient with multiple pregnancy. Start an intravenous infusion of 1 L of 5% glucose in water through a No. 18 needle during the latter part of the first stage of labor, and continue it until the third stage is completed. Blood or specific medication can be administered through this line without delay when indicated. Type and cross match the patient's blood, and have several units of blood available in the delivery room for emergency transfusion.

Multiple pregnancy itself is not an indication for cesarean section, but breech presentation of either or both twins, disproportion (eg, conjoined twins), and twins known to be monoamniotic are.

1. Admit the patient to the hospital at the first sign of labor or leakage of amniotic fluid.

2. Anesthesia—Limit analgesia drastically during labor. The infants are usually premature, and operative intervention is often necessary. Use pudendal block anesthesia if possible; spinal, intravenous, and deep inhalation anesthesia may be dangerous. Give oxygen to the mother by face mask during the second stage of labor.

3. Check the presentations, using ultrasound. If the first fetus presents by vertex, deliver it in the usual manner. Avoid a difficult forceps or rapid breech delivery. If the second fetus is in transverse presentation, consider cesarean section if the fetus is small or perform an external version when the cervix is fully dilated. Make a deep episiotomy incision to minimize constriction of the head.

4. Clamp the cord promptly to prevent the second twin of a single-ovum pregnancy from partially exsanguinating through the first cord. Do not exert traction on the cord. Leave 4–6 cm of cord attached to each twin in case transfusion is required later. Label (A and B) the twins and the corresponding cords attached to the placenta.

5. Do not give ergot after the birth of the first twin. Reduction of the uteroplacental circulation will jeopardize the second twin.

6. Examine the patient vaginally immediately after delivery of the first infant to ascertain the presentation of the second. Rupture the second bag of waters. If there is no second amniotic sac (monoamniotic single-ovum twins), deliver the second twin at once to prevent asphyxia (premature separation of the placenta or cord entanglement). About half of such second twins die unless the delivery is expedited.

7. Avoid haste, but try to deliver the second twin within 10–15 minutes of the first to prevent hypoxia. Cautiously administer dilute oxytocin intravenously to stimulate uterine contractions when uterine inertia becomes a problem. If the second twin is in transverse presentation, attempt to guide it into the birth canal as a vertex by fundal pressure. If this is not possible, do a cesarean section if time permits; otherwise, do an internal version and breech extraction.

8. Manage the third stage of labor cautiously. Administer oxytocin, 1 mL intramuscularly immediately after delivery of the second twin, or start an intravenous oxytocin drip. Elevate but do not massage the fundus until after the uterus contracts and expels the separated placenta; then give an ergot preparation, eg, ergonovine, 0.1 mg intramuscularly, and gently massage and elevate the fundus for 15–30 minutes.

If separation of the placenta is delayed or bleeding is brisk, separate and extract the placenta manually. Use minimal inhalation anesthesia (trichloroethylene or nitrous oxide) for removal of the placenta.

9. Locked twins–With the patient under deep anesthesia, have an assistant support the twin already partially delivered as a breech. Push both heads upward out of the pelvis, and then try to deliver the head of the partially delivered twin. If this is not possible, apply forceps to the other twin and try to deliver both twins together. If this cannot be done, elevate the partially delivered twin, establish an airway, and protect the cord. When the undescended twin dies, decapitate it, deliver the first twin, and then deliver the body and head of the dead twin. Usually, both fetuses will die in the time needed to set up for a cesarean section.

10. Newborns with twin-to-twin transfusion syndrome generally require immediate treatment: phlebotomy and digitalization for the recipient; transfusion and possible digitalization for the donor.

C. Treatment of Complications: Preeclampsia-eclampsia, premature labor and delivery, etc, are managed as outlined elsewhere in this book. If dystocia occurs, use ultrasonography to rule out malpresentation or conjoined twins.

Prognosis

A. For the Mother: Maternal morbidity (infection) is 4–8 times higher with multiple pregnancy than with average vaginal delivery of a single term infant, but the mortality rate is only slightly increased. Preeclampsia-eclampsia, hemorrhage, and the complications of operative obstetrics increase the hazard to the mother.

B. For the Fetuses: The perinatal mortality rate for twins is 4–5 times that of single infants born at term. More single-ovum than double-ovum twins die in the neonatal period. The fetal mortality rate for triplets is twice that of twins. Rarely do quadruplets, etc, all live.

If the infant is delivered alive, its gestational age is the best criterion of survival. A twin or triplet weighing over 2500 g has a better prognosis than a singleton of the same weight because the former is more mature.

The best prognosis for twins is when both present by the vertex. Twins or other multiple infants delivered spontaneously do better than those extracted by forceps or after version.

The second twin is in greater danger than the first if it is smaller, because circulatory problems and the trauma of delivery may be more damaging.

The female twin of a male-female pair who survives twin-to-twin transfusion is not sterile (like a bovine freemartin).

Actual proof of monozygous twinning is successful skin grafting or organ transplantation, but there is a 95% probability of accurate zygosity diagnosis when the placenta is assessed and ABO, MNSs, Rh, Kell, Kidd, Duffy, and Lewis antigens are determined.

Obstetric Complications of Pregnancy, Labor, & Delivery | 11

ECTOPIC PREGNANCY

A fertilized ovum implanted outside the uterine cavity is an ectopic pregnancy. This occurs in one in 150–200 conceptions. Ninety percent occur in the uterine tube, and approximately 60% of these are on the right side. About 80% are diagnosed within the first 2 months after conception. Ectopic pregnancy may occur at any time from menarche to menopause, but at least 40% of cases occur in women between ages 20 and 29. The incidence of extrauterine pregnancy is inversely proportionate to parity, ie, it is higher in infertile (especially "one-child sterility") patients. There is no racial predisposition, but ectopic pregnancy occurs more frequently in lower socioeconomic groups and in women wearing an intrauterine device.

Ectopic pregnancy is classified as follows (sites of implantation are listed in decreasing order of frequency):

(1) Tubal: Ampullary, infundibular, isthmic, interstitial (angular, cornual), and bilateral.

(2) Ovarian.

(3) Cervical.

(4) Combined extrauterine and intrauterine (incidence is about one in 6000–7000 pregnancies).

(5) Abdominal.

Ectopic pregnancy may result from conditions that delay or prevent passage of a fertilized ovum through the uterine tube. At least 50% of cases are caused by tubal inflammatory lesions.

A. Tubal Factors: (In order of frequency.) Adherent luminal folds caused by inflammation, developmental abnormalities of the tube (congenital diverticula, accessory ostia, or atresia), peritubal adhesions, pelvic tumors, and excessive length or tortuosity of the tube.

B. Ovarian Factors: Fertilization of a trapped, unextruded ovum or one with an abnormally large adherent cumulus of granulosa cells; transmigration of the ovum; abnormally early implantation; and tubal abortion and reimplantation elsewhere (very rare).

C. Cervical Factors: In the rare cervical pregnancy, the site of implantation is by definition below the internal os. With such limited

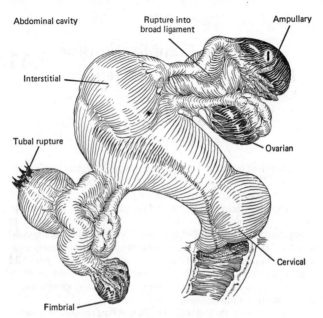

Figure 11–1. Sites of ectopic pregnancies.

space for development, spontaneous abortion with severe hemorrhage invariably occurs.

D. Abdominal Factors: Abdominal pregnancy may be primary, with the fertilized ovum implanting initially in the abdominal cavity, or, very rarely, secondary to rupture of a tubal pregnancy with the trophoblast maintaining its tubal attachment or the entire ovum implanting de novo elsewhere after the rupture. The incidence of abdominal pregnancy is one in 15,000 pregnancies; the fetal mortality rate is about 90%.

Pathology

Pregnancy becomes pathologic when a fertilized ovum implants outside the uterus because organs other than the uterus are not adaptable to pregnancy. The tissues into which the developing ovum is abnormally implanted lack resistance to the ovum, and no defense or barrier against the trophoblast develops. In a sense, the conceptus behaves like a malignant tumor. There may be little or no decidual reaction, and there is only slight muscular hypertrophy for accommodation. The trophoblast invades the muscle rapidly, with penetration of large blood vessels; internal hemorrhage then occurs.

In tubal pregnancy, distention and weakness of the tube predispose to rupture, especially with slight trauma. Extracapsular rupture occurs when a portion of the villous ovum extrudes through the tubal wall. In intracapsular rupture, the embryo, fluid, and blood are expelled from the fimbriated ostium of the tube after the amniotic and chorionic membranes tear. Bleeding may cease temporarily after either extracapsular or intracapsular rupture, but the embryo rarely survives. In occasional cases, pregnancy may continue if an adequate portion of the placental attachment is retained or if secondary implantation occurs elsewhere.

The corpus luteum of pregnancy continues to develop as long as the trophoblast is viable. The uterus becomes minimally enlarged and slightly softened; it contains decidua but no trophoblast. Decidual separation and bleeding occur when the conceptus dies. Only in interstitial ectopic pregnancy does blood from the tube drain via the uterus.

Termination of the Pregnancy

Ectopic pregnancy can terminate as follows:

(1) Tubal: Tubal abortion, missed tubal abortion, rupture into the broad ligament, rupture into the peritoneal cavity.

(2) Ovarian: Rupture into the peritoneal cavity.

(3) Cervical: Rupture into the vagina.

(4) Combined: Ectopic pregnancy almost always aborts; uterine pregnancy generally continues.

(5) Abdominal: Rupture into the lesser peritoneal cavity, rupture into the retroperitoneum, lithopedion, a viable infant.

Isthmic rupture usually occurs at about 6 weeks and ampullary rupture at 8–12 weeks. Interstitial rupture may occur at about 4 months, depending upon such factors as the size of the uterus and whether trauma occurs.

If intra-abdominal pregnancy occurs and a large fetus dies, it cannot be absorbed. It may become infected; it may become a mummified, calcified mass (lithopedion); or it may form a grayish, greasy object (adipocere).

Clinical Findings

No specific signs or symptoms are diagnostic. Ectopic pregnancy should be suspected when bleeding or abdominal pain occurs within the first 7–8 weeks after a missed period. The pregnancy may be acute (ruptured), chronic (threatened or atypical), or unruptured.

A. Symptoms and Signs: The following symptoms and signs (in the order noted) are present in 75% of cases: (1) Amenorrhea due to increasing hCG levels. (2) Uterine bleeding following failure of pregnancy, irrespective of its situation. (3) Abdominal pain due to rupture of the amniotic-chorionic sac, with local bleeding, or to bleeding manifested as an enlarging pregnancy, pulsion, and traction. (4) Pelvic mass caused by growth of the conceptus, hematoma from placental separation or host organ, adherence of bowel and omentum, or infection.

1. Tubal pregnancy–

a. Acute–(Almost 40% of tubal pregnancies.) Sharp pain in the abdomen and backache are the most common complaints. Scant but persistent uterine bleeding occurs in 80% of patients; 70% have a pelvic mass. A history of abnormal menstruation and infertility is present in about 60% of cases. Collapse and shock, often precipitated by vaginal examination, occur in 10%. Shock may follow sudden massive hemorrhage or severe pain and is characterized by weakness, thirst, profuse perspiration, "air hunger," vomiting, and oliguria.

b. Chronic–(About 60% of tubal pregnancies.) Blood escapes from the tube, pelvic discomfort increases, and a mass develops. Bluish discoloration around the umbilicus (Cullen's sign) may be present, indicating hematoperitoneum. Separation or extrusion of the pregnancy and hypotension reduce the bleeding area of the placental attachment. Clots compress the placental site, and the bowel and omentum become adherent. The hematoma often liquefies and is absorbed before infection develops.

c. Unruptured–(About 2% of tubal pregnancies.) Brief amenorrhea, tenderness, or adnexal fullness is present before the acute or chronic stage.

d. Advanced unilateral and bilateral tubal pregnancy is rare. Delivery of a viable fetus is exceptional.

2. Abdominal pregnancy–Because abdominal pregnancy may be secondary to rupture of a tubal pregnancy, a history of the rupture may be elicited. As the pregnancy progresses, there is often pressure and peritoneal irritation, causing nausea, vomiting, diarrhea, and abdominal pain, the latter especially notable with fetal movement. In late pregnancy, the fetal small parts are more readily palpable and the fetal heartbeat is louder than when the pregnancy is intrauterine. The position is abnormal because the fetus is high; transverse lies are common. Braxton Hicks contractions are not present, and the small (empty) uterus may be palpable.

The usual criteria for primary abdominal pregnancy are as follows: (1) Tubes, ovaries, and broad ligaments appear normal. (2) No evidence of penetration of the space between the broad ligament and the fimbriated extremity of the tube. (3) No intraligamentary rupture of the tube. (4) No evidence of escape of the ovum from the uterine cavity.

3. Combined extrauterine and intrauterine pregnancy is occasionally reported. Simultaneous pregnancies exist, one extrauterine and the other intrauterine. One or the other is usually diagnosed, but rarely both. The extrauterine fetuses usually die, and only approximately 60% of the intrauterine fetuses survive to viability.

4. Ovarian pregnancy is rare and is generally mistaken for early

tubal pregnancy or ovarian cyst. The exact diagnosis is not ascertained until after laparotomy.

5. Cervical pregnancy is very rare. Progression beyond 2–3 months is almost unknown. Termination is always acute, and the pregnancy is often misdiagnosed as advanced carcinoma of the cervix. Hemorrhage may be massive and can be fatal.

B. Laboratory Findings: Pregnancy tests using radioimmunoassay for the β subunit of hCG may be helpful, but they do not identify the site of pregnancy, and negative tests do not exclude an "old," aborted ectopic pregnancy with hematoma.

1. Blood–Anemia often develops suddenly and may be severe as a result of intraperitoneal bleeding. The white blood count is elevated if infection is present. The serum amylase level may be as high as 1600 Somogyi units/dL (normal: 80–180 units) if narcotics have not been given. Reticulocytosis (due to bleeding) is present; reticulocytes may increase to 2.2% (normal: < 1%). Hematin is detected by spectroscopy in peripheral blood 2 days after 100 mL or more of blood accumulates intraperitoneally.

2. Urine–Urine urobilinogen level is elevated, indicating decomposition of blood. Slight porphyrinuria is present with hematocele and hematoperitoneum but may also indicate a twisted ovarian cyst.

C. X-Ray and Ultrasonographic Findings: X-ray films may identify an established abdominal pregnancy. Ultrasonography rarely is diagnostic except to identify an intrauterine pregnancy in the differentiation of intrauterine from extrauterine pregnancy.

D. Special Examinations: Blood recovered by culdocentesis is evidence of hematoperitoneum if red cell rouleaux are absent; if red cells are crenated; if blood is dark and viscid and contains small clots; or if blood is noncoagulable (having already clotted and liquefied). Laparoscopy usually is diagnostic of ectopic pregnancy. D&C and endometrial biopsy may disclose decidual endometrium (without chorionic villi). If trophoblast is recovered, uterine pregnancy is established. Laparoscopy or exploratory laparotomy establishes the presence or absence of internal (not cervical) ectopic pregnancy. Laparotomy is indicated (1) when the diagnosis of ectopic pregnancy has been made or (2) when an acute abdominal emergency necessitates investigation.

A special test for abdominal pregnancy requires the intramuscular injection of 0.1 unit of oxytocin. Within 2 minutes, the uterus will contract; no change will be felt in the structures overlying an extrauterine fetus.

Differential Diagnosis

About 50 pathologic conditions are clinically similar to ectopic pregnancy: the most common are appendicitis, salpingitis, ruptured corpus luteum cyst or ovarian follicle, and uterine abortion (Table 11–1).

Table 11–1. Differential diagnosis of ectopic pregnancy.

	Ectopic Pregnancy	Appendicitis	Salpingitis	Ruptured Corpus Luteum Cyst	Uterine Abortion
Pain	Unilateral cramps and tenderness before rupture.	Epigastric, periumbilical, then right lower quadrant pain; tenderness localizing at McBurney's point. Rebound tenderness.	Usually in both lower quadrants, with or without rebound.	Unilateral, becoming general with progressive bleeding.	Midline cramps.
Nausea and vomiting	Occasionally before, frequently after rupture.	Usual. Precedes shift of pain to right lower quadrant.	Infrequent.	Rare.	Almost never.
Menstruation	Some aberration: missed period, spotting.	Unrelated to menses.	Hypermenorrhea or menorrhagia, or both.	Period delayed, then bleeding, often with pain.	Amenorrhea, then spotting, then brisk bleeding.
Temperature and pulse	37.2–37.8 °C (99–100 °F). Pulse variable: normal before, rapid after rupture.	37.2–37.8 °C (99–100 °F). Pulse rapid: 99–100.	37.2–40 °C (99–104 °F). Pulse elevated in proportion to fever.	Not over 37.2 °C (99 °F). Pulse normal unless blood loss marked, then rapid.	To 37.2 °C (99 °F) if spontaneous; to 40 °C (104 °F) if induced (infection).
Pelvic examination	Unilateral tenderness, especially on movement of cervix. Crepitant mass on one side or in cul-de-sac.	No masses.	Bilateral tenderness on movement of cervix. Masses only when pyosalpinx or hydrosalpinx is present.	Tenderness over affected ovary. No masses.	Cervix slightly patulous. Uterus slightly enlarged, irregularly softened. Tender with infection.
Laboratory findings	White cell count to 15,000/μL. Red cell count strikingly low if blood loss large. Sedimentation rate slightly elevated.	White cell count 10,000–18,000/μL (rarely normal). Red cell count normal. Sedimentation rate slightly elevated.	White cell count 15,000–30,000/μL. Red cell count normal. Sedimentation rate markedly elevated.	White cell count normal to 10,000/μL. Red cell count normal. Sedimentation rate normal.	White cell count 15,000/μL if spontaneous; to 30,000/μL if induced (infection). Red cell count normal. Sedimentation rate slightly to moderately elevated.

Complications

Without surgery, a ruptured ectopic pregnancy may hemorrhage and cause death. Infection often follows neglected ruptured ectopic pregnancy. Infertility develops in about 50% of patients who have undergone surgery for extrauterine pregnancy; approximately 30% of these become sterile. Chronic urinary tract infection and ureteral stricture may occur after infection. Intestinal obstruction and fistulas may develop after hematoperitoneum, peritonitis, or lithopedion formation.

Prevention

Avoid unperitonealized areas at surgery (adhesions form); treat salpingitis early and vigorously; perform D&C promptly for incomplete abortion.

Treatment

Operate immediately after the diagnosis is made. Delay is justified only to correct shock.

A. Emergency Treatment: Hospitalize the patient if ectopic pregnancy is suspected. Insert a large needle into a large vein and transfuse at least 2 units of blood, under pressure if bleeding is massive and facilities are available. Administer antishock measures as indicated, ie, keep the patient comfortably warm, give oxygen, and apply moderately snug tourniquets around the upper legs.

B. Surgical Treatment: *Control hemorrhage.* Remove the products of conception, but leave blood and clots (they will be absorbed and limit anemia). Use stimulant anesthetics (ether or cyclopropane); avoid depressants (spinal anesthesia, thiopental).

1. If the tube is grossly distorted, dilated, or damaged (as in pregnancy of over 3 months' duration), perform salpingectomy by cornual excision (not resection) to prevent repeat ectopic pregnancy and endosalpingosis of the stump.

2. If the pregnancy is early (small) or if tubal missed abortion has occurred, perform salpingostomy to enucleate the pregnancy and preserve the tube. Ligate bleeding points; suturing is not necessary.

3. Hysterectomy is usually required in ruptured interstitial or cervical pregnancy.

4. Oophorectomy is necessary in ovarian pregnancy.

C. Supportive Treatment: If symptoms and signs of infection are present, give broad-spectrum antibiotics; prescribe oral or intramuscular iron therapy (or both).

Prognosis

The maternal death rate due to ectopic pregnancy in the USA is 1–2%; the perinatal death rate is almost 100%. Ectopic pregnancy does not prevent subsequent normal pregnancy; most patients who have had one ectopic pregnancy later have normal pregnancies.

Ectopic pregnancy recurs in 10–12% of cases.

CAUSES OF THIRD-TRIMESTER BLEEDING

Obstetric bleeding is the major cause of maternal morbidity and mortality and is also a significant factor in perinatal morbidity and mortality. Vaginal bleeding occurs in late pregnancy in 5–10% of women. Multiparas are more commonly affected.

Antepartal bleeding may be classified as placental or nonplacental. It is essential to distinguish between these 2 large groups.

Placental bleeding, most often due to placenta previa or premature separation of a normally implanted placenta, often threatens the life of the mother or fetus.

Nonplacental bleeding is usually due to blood dyscrasia or lower genital tract disorders, including cervical or vaginal infections, neoplasms, and varices. Bleeding is generally slight; even carcinoma of the cervix or a ruptured vaginal varix usually does not cause hemorrhage. The same may be true of premature separation of the placenta and placenta previa, however, and vaginal examination (see p 267) is therefore necessary to make the differentiation. Rupture of the uterus, which occurs in about 1% of patients previously delivered by cesarean section, may cause vaginal bleeding; most of the blood loss will be concealed.

Diagnosis of the Cause of Bleeding

Because of the extreme hazard of uncontrollable antepartal uterine (placental) hemorrhage, it is vital to avoid an initial vaginal or even a "gentle rectal examination": either may cause critical bleeding. Only fragmentary and unreliable information is obtained in most cases by these procedures, and they usually must be repeated.

If the patient is seen at home, rectal or vaginal examination should be withheld and the vagina or cervix should not be packed. Transport the patient to the hospital, preferably by ambulance.

Procedure on admission to the hospital: (1) Place the patient at complete bed rest, flat in bed. (2) Do a complete, gentle abdominal examination. (3) Do not perform rectal or vaginal examination, but inspect the cervix to rule out carcinoma. (4) Cross-match the patient's blood and have 2–4 units of blood ready for immediate transfusion if necessary. (5) Give clear fluids only. (6) Reassure the patient and give mild sedation. (7) Identify the placental site by ultrasonography. (8) Observe closely for increasing or decreasing signs of bleeding or fetal distress.

Note: Over 90% of patients with third-trimester bleeding will cease to bleed temporarily in 24 hours with bed rest alone.

The abdominal examination should indicate the size and position of the fetus, the approximate duration of the pregnancy, the presentation and position of the infant, the presence or absence of tenderness, uterine resting tone and contractions, and the rate and regularity of the fetal heartbeat.

Save all perineal pads so that a reasonably accurate estimate of blood loss can be made.

Observe the patient for 24 hours if bleeding is not excessive or if hemorrhage ceases, assuming she is at or near term. If hemorrhage is profuse and persistent, however, prompt vaginal examination in an operating room readied for possible cesarean section ("double setup") should be done after preparation and blood replacement therapy.

If the patient is less than 33 weeks pregnant, the fetus is likely to be too small to survive if delivered. If the patient has placenta previa, avoid more than initial speculum examination. Penetration of the cervical canal may initiate hemorrhage that necessitates delivery.

At times, extended hospitalization or bed rest at home will be required for delivery of a viable infant. Recurrent, spontaneous, exsanguinating hemorrhage from placenta previa or premature separation is exceedingly rare. The calculated risk of later bleeding and the uncertainties of an incomplete or presumptive diagnosis are far outweighed by the decreased perinatal and maternal morbidity and mortality rates that accompany a conservative, nonaggressive program of management of antepartal bleeding.

PREMATURE SEPARATION OF THE PLACENTA
(Abruptio Placentae, Ablatio Placentae, Accidental Hemorrhage)

Premature separation of the placenta accounts for about 30% of all cases of antepartal bleeding before the delivery of the fetus. Two types are recognized: (1) concealed, painful hemorrhage (retroplacental bleeding without avenue of escape); and (2) external, painless hemorrhage (bleeding from the separated edge or lateral portion of the placenta with drainage of blood through the cervix).

Premature separation of the placenta occurs most often after the 28th week of pregnancy. If it develops earlier, it usually cannot be distinguished from other causes of abortion. The placenta detaches in about 50% of patients before the onset of labor and in 10–15% during the second stage of labor.

Vascular injury and vasodilatation are the major causes of premature separation of the placenta. This disorder is not influenced by race.

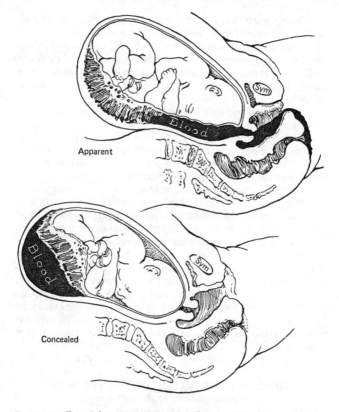

Figure 11–2. Types of premature separation of the placenta. Sym, symphysis. (Redrawn and reproduced, with permission, from Beck and Rosenthal: *Obstetrical Practice,* 7th ed. Williams & Wilkins, 1957.)

About 80% of patients are multiparas. Over two-thirds of women with premature separation of the placenta also have preeclampsia-eclampsia. Premature separation of the placenta occurs once in 175–200 pregnancies.

Predisposing factors include overdistention of the uterus, preeclampsia-eclampsia, renal disease, hypertension, short umbilical cord, vascular stasis, malnutrition, and multiparity. Precipitating factors include the following: (1) Sudden disturbance of the vascular equilibrium, as in vasodilatation secondary to shock. (2) Abrupt increase in blood pressure, as in paralytic vasodilatation or block or compression of the aorta. (3) Passive engorgement of the uterus and placenta, as in the "supine hypotensive syndrome," in which the vena cava is compressed by the enlarged uterus when the patient lies on her back, or due to torsion of the uterus by adnexal or uterine tumors. (4) Abdominal trauma, either due to a direct blow to the uterus or as a result of secondary transmission of force to the uterus. (5) Placental circulatory insufficiency, as in preeclampsia, chronic renal disease, or diabetes mellitus. (6) Rapid decrease in uterine volume, such as follows hasty delivery of the first twin or sudden drainage of hydramnios.

External hemorrhage is due to marginal or partial premature separation of the placenta. Further separation of the placenta, with labor and rupture of the membranes, may occur. Concealed hemorrhage may be associated with retroplacental bleeding when the margins are adherent or with complete separation of the placenta and laceration of the membranes following bleeding into the amniotic cavity.

The most serious type of premature separation of the placenta, concealed hemorrhage associated with adherent placental margins, occurs in about 15% of cases. The bleeding is within the decidua basalis, not the placenta itself; the extravasated blood infiltrates the uterine wall behind the placenta, forming a hematoma. Intramyometrial bleeding eventually results in uteroplacental apoplexy—the so-called Couvelaire uterus, a purplish or copper-colored, ecchymotic, indurated viscus that has lost its contractile force because of disruption of the muscle bundles. With uterine spasm, the blood pressure is increased in the intervillous spaces, and blood is forced into the uteroplacental vessels, bursting these channels and further enlarging the area of placental separation. Before delivery, the distended uterus cannot contract to control the bleeding. As the uterus loses its contractile force, blood from the retroplacental hematoma ruptures the decidual basal plate, completing the placental separation in that area.

Premature separation of the placenta causes colicky uterine pain, tenderness, and increased tone. Contractions are dysrhythmic and very painful; the patient may develop shock out of proportion to the amount of blood lost.

Disseminated intravascular coagulation and hypofibrinogenemia may develop in extreme cases of premature separation. Petechiae appear over the peritoneum, skin, and mucous surfaces; hemorrhage into internal organs occurs, and bleeding may occur in the gastrointestinal, respiratory, and genitourinary tracts.

A completely separated placenta may present before an unengaged (dead) fetus. This is called prolapse of the placenta.

Classification of Premature Separation of the Placenta

Grade 0: (About 30%.) No diagnostic signs or symptoms are present.

Premature separation is not recognized until the placenta is examined after delivery.

Grade 1: (About 45%.) There is external bleeding; uterine tetany and uterine tenderness may or may not be present. Shock does not occur, and there is no fetal distress. (Grade 1 rarely progresses to grade 2.)

Grade 2: (About 15%.) External bleeding may or may not occur. Uterine tetany and tenderness develop. Maternal shock does not occur, but fetal distress is always present and the fetus may die in utero. (Grade 2 frequently increases to grade 3.)

Grade 3: (About 10%.) External bleeding may or may not occur. Uterine tetany is marked. Maternal shock and fetal death in utero are the rule. A coagulation defect is usually present.

Clinical Findings

A. Maternal Symptoms and Signs: Patients with marginal premature separation of the normally implanted placenta who report external bleeding generally describe no unusual pain, only blood loss. Those with concealed hemorrhage have great pain when a retroplacental hematoma develops. If blood extravasates from the placental site, with blockage of the blood above the engaged presenting part, uterine discomfort may or may not be described.

The severity of the symptoms depends upon the degree of placental bleeding, the speed of separation, and the retention or pocketing of blood. If blood is retained, regional or generalized uterine pain or tenderness usually is progressive and severe. In extreme cases, agonizing generalized uterine pain and shock are reported. In mild cases, the discomfort may be localized, particularly if the placenta is implanted anteriorly; persistent, deep pelvic discomfort occurs if the placenta is implanted posteriorly. Other manifestations of premature separation with blood retention are a tender, firm (often ligneous or boardlike) uterus that fails to relax and constant lumbosacral backache of increasing severity. Uterine bleeding is rarely evident until advanced. The uterus may enlarge slightly if considerable blood is retained.

B. Fetal Signs: Electronic fetal monitoring may disclose fetal distress due to hypoxia. Tachycardia may be noted first; then bradycardia, and then fetal death.

C. Laboratory Findings: Anemia may occur (despite hemoconcentration); in concealed hemorrhage, anemia is often more severe than would be expected in view of the apparent blood loss. The capillary fragility test is positive when the coagulation time is increased. The coagulation time is frequently increased in patients with severe concealed hemorrhage. Plasma fibrinogen levels are often low. Fibrin degradation products should be identified.

Differential Diagnosis

A. Nonplacental Causes of Bleeding: Nonplacental bleeding is usually not painful. "Bloody show" due to cervical dilatation and effacement just before or during early labor may also be responsible for vaginal bleeding. Rupture of the uterus may cause vaginal bleeding but is associated with pain, shock, and death of the fetus.

B. Placental Causes of Bleeding: Placenta previa is associated with painless hemorrhage and is usually diagnosed by ultrasonography or by vaginal examination under a "double setup."

C. Undetermined Causes of Bleeding: In at least 20% of cases, the precise cause of antepartum bleeding during the last trimester is never determined. If serious problems can be ruled out, undiagnosed bleeding is rarely critical.

Complications

A. Maternal: Shock out of proportion to the degree of hypotension, disseminated intravascular coagulation (DIC), renal cortical ischemia followed by renal cortical necrosis, lower nephron nephrosis, and uteroplacental apoplexy.

B. Fetal: Premature separation of the placenta causes fetal hypoxia, which, if prolonged, results in cerebral damage that is often irreversible. Infants who survive may have cerebral palsy, mental deficiency, or both. More severe degrees of hypoxia cause fetal asphyxia and death.

Prevention

Improved obstetric care will reduce the incidence and severity of preeclampsia-eclampsia and associated premature separation of the placenta. The patient should be instructed to avoid lying supine. Prompt diagnosis and treatment of retroplacental (concealed) hemorrhage will usually reduce the seriousness of uteroplacental apoplexy. Rupture of the membranes often prevents the more serious complications of premature separation of the placenta. Although the danger of shock decreases after the uterus is emptied, postpartal hemorrhage may be a critical problem if disseminated intravascular coagulation is not treated properly.

Treatment

A. Emergency Measures: The clotting mechanism must be restored before any attempt is made to deliver the patient. Administer cryoprecipitate, frozen plasma, or fresh blood. Institute antishock therapy.

Rupture the membranes, if possible, irrespective of the probable mode of delivery.

B. Specific Measures: Premature separation of the placenta with external bleeding can usually be managed by rupture of the membranes to speed labor and vaginal delivery. If excessive, uncontrollable hemorrhage persists or if fetal distress is apparent, rapid cesarean section may be necessary.

An estimate of the magnitude or grade of premature separation (see p 269) is of great value in prognosis and therapy. Monitor the fetus carefully.

1. Grade 0–No specific measures are required. Premature separation is not recognized until after delivery.

2. Grade 1–When the patient is not in labor, watchful expectancy is indicated; bleeding ceases spontaneously in many cases. When labor begins, prepare for vaginal delivery in the absence of further complications.

3. Grade 2–Anticipate vaginal delivery if labor is expected within about 6 hours, especially if the fetus is dead. Cesarean section should be done if there is persistent evidence of fetal distress and the infant is likely to survive.

4. Grade 3–The patient is always in shock, the fetus has died, the uterus is tetanic, and a coagulation defect may be present. After correction of the coagulopathy, deliver the patient vaginally if this can be done within about 6 hours. (Vaginal delivery is probably best for the multiparous patient.) Otherwise, do a cesarean section.

C. General Measures: Prophylactic transfusion of patients who are slightly anemic and are actively bleeding often prevents shock; 3 or more units of bank blood must be available for immediate transfusion. Avoid excessive analgesia despite patient discomfort, since hasty delivery may be required. Give oxygen, 6 L/min, by nasal tube or face mask for fetal distress. Monitor the fetus electronically or keep a fetal heart chart.

D. Surgical Measures: If surgery is indicated, materials to control a coagulation defect must be on hand before the operation is undertaken, and correction of an existing coagulation defect must already have begun.

Cesarean section is indicated (1) when labor is expected to be of long duration (over 6 hours); (2) when hemorrhage does not respond to amniotomy and cautious administration of dilute oxytocin; (3) when early (not prolonged) fetal distress is present and the fetus is mature and likely to survive.

Hysterectomy for removal of a Couvelaire uterus, the source of hemorrhage, is rarely indicated. Such a uterus will contract and bleeding will almost always cease when the coagulation defect is corrected.

E. Treatment of Complications:

1. Disseminated intravascular coagulation (DIC, defibrination syndrome, consumption coagulopathy)–With premature separation of the placenta, gross clotting and destruction of endometrium and decidua occur behind the placenta. Clotting also occurs in small vessels in the uterus and elsewhere, causing uterine pain and tetany. This widely disseminated clotting consumes platelets and clotting factors. Fibrinolysis is a normal mechanism by which clotting is limited. In disseminated intravascular coagulation, however, considerable plasminogen (fibrinolysin) is converted to plasmin, and secondary fibrinolysis, an abnormally extensive and rapid process, quickly depletes many clotting factors. In addition, secondary fibrinolysis digests fibrinogen to smaller molecules that have a heparinlike anticoagulant action. With this sequence of events, the patient will begin to bleed from sites of needle punctures, the uterus, etc. The bleeding time becomes prolonged secondary to thrombocytopenia, and even though a delicate clot may form, it is soon lysed.

Shock, hypotension, and hypovolemia cause constriction of the microcirculation. Erythrocytes are damaged by being forced through a contracted vasculature partially blocked by clots. Hence, many broken, distorted red cell schistocytes ("helmet cells") in a smear of the peripheral blood are evidence of microangiopathic hemolytic anemia.

a. Laboratory indices of disseminated intravascular coagulation include (1) thrombocytopenia (apparent even in smear of peripheral blood), (2) depletion of factors I, II, V, and VIII (prolonged prothrombin time and activated partial thromboplastin time), (3) demonstration of fibrin degradation products in the plasma by prothrombin (3P) test, and (4) prolonged thrombin time.

b. Treatment of patient with premature separation of the placenta and disseminated intravascular coagulation–Correct the coagulation defect before attempting vaginal delivery or cesarean section. When bleeding is arrested and the coagulation defect is corrected, empty the uterus expeditiously.

(1) During active bleeding, the transfusion of platelets is often the best practical means of counteracting a clotting deficiency. A platelet pack contains about 20% fewer platelets than 1 unit of fresh blood. If the patient is bleeding severely, transfuse with *fresh* whole blood. If serious bleeding continues, administer cryoprecipitate, one bag/4 kg, to restore coagulation.

(2) If disseminated intravascular coagulation is diagnosed but the patient is not bleeding abnormally, administer heparin, 75–120 units/kg intravenously every 6 hours, to keep the clotting time at about 20 minutes. Persistent or delayed bleeding is unlikely if the uterus remains well contracted postpartum. If unusual bleeding ensues, protamine sulfate will counteract the effect of heparin.

Heparin has an antithrombin effect and also blocks intrinsic activation of thromboplastin. Since the consumption of clotting factors, including aggregation of platelets and release of granules of platelet components, is secondary to proteolysis of thrombin, heparin helps to correct disseminated intravascular coagulation.

(3) Fibrinolysins–Aminocaproic acid (Amicar) should *not* be given. This drug will complicate the problem by interfering with the mechanism of fibrinolysis.

2. Transfusion hepatitis–The risk of contracting hepatitis from a unit of whole blood is approximately 0.3%. It is only one-third as high when blood from donors negative for hepatitis B antigen (HBsAg) is used. The risk of hepatitis from fibrinogen may approach 25%; the risk from pooled plasma is about 10%. Cryoprecipitate packs are free of hepatitis B virus.

3. Renal cortical necrosis–Necrosis of the renal cortex is secondary to marked prolonged hypotension. Add a 50-mL bolus of 20% mannitol to the intravenous fluid line to reduce renal cortical ischemia.

4. Acute cor pulmonale–Cor pulmonale secondary to fibrin embolization to the lung reduces pulmonary ventilation. Oxygen therapy by face mask or tent is required. Avoid administration of excessive amounts of intravenous fluid or blood.

5. Lower nephron nephrosis and anuria–Most patients who develop premature separation of the placenta have preeclampsia-eclampsia, which may also be associated with lower nephron nephrosis and anuria. Daily fluid intake and output must be carefully monitored, and excessive amounts of sodium and potassium should not be given. Hemodialysis may be required in extreme cases when the serum potassium concentration rises above 7 mEq/L. Peritoneal dialysis or hemodialysis for the removal of excessive blood metabolites is also an established procedure for such problems in many hospitals.

Prognosis

External or concealed bleeding, excessive blood loss, shock, nulliparity, a closed cervix, absence of labor, and delayed diagnosis and treatment are unfavorable prognostic factors.

Worldwide maternal mortality rates are currently between 0.5 and 5%. Most women die of hemorrhage (immediate or delayed) or cardiac or renal failure. Early diagnosis and definitive therapy should reduce maternal mortality rates to 0.3–1%.

Fetal mortality rates range from 50 to 80%. About 30% of patients with premature separation of the placenta are delivered at term. Almost 20% of patients have no fetal heartbeat on admission to the hospital, and in another 20%, fetal distress is soon noted. When maternal transfusion is urgently required, the fetal mortality rate will probably be at least 50%.

Birth is premature in 40–50% of cases of premature separation of the placenta. Infants die of hypoxia, prematurity, and delivery trauma.

PLACENTA PREVIA

In placenta previa, the placenta develops within the zone of dilatation and effacement of the lower uterine segment, so that the placenta obstructs descent of the presenting part. The cause is not known, but decreased vascularity of the endometrium in the fundus due to tumors or scarring is assumed to be a factor. Tumors, atrophic changes, scars, and other conditions associated with impaired vascularization of the decidua are more commonly present with placenta previa. Almost 10% of cases occur in patients who have had cesarean sections, especially lower segment operations. Placenta previa is most common among older women and those who have borne many children. It occurs once in every 200–225 pregnancies that continue beyond the 28th week. The placenta completely covers the cervical os in only about 10% of cases.

The relative size of the placenta and its site of insertion are important factors in the development of placenta previa. The lower the insertion, the less suited is the uterine mucosa for nidation. The surface area

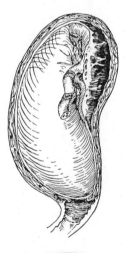
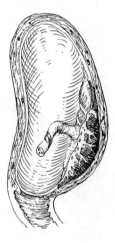
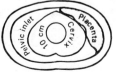
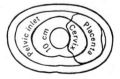

Figure 11–3. Normal placenta.   **Figure 11–4.** Low implantation.

of the placenta in placenta previa is generally 30–40% greater than that of a normal placenta. The placenta is inserted on the anterior wall of the uterus in 60% of cases (twice the normal incidence).

Bleeding in placenta previa may be due to either mechanical separation of the placenta from the uterus near the cervical os following dilatation or placentitis.

Placenta previa may be classified on the basis of the approximate area of the internal cervical os that would be covered by the placenta if the cervical os were permitted to become completely dilated (10 cm). The cervix, but not the placenta, will retract as the internal cervical os dilates and the lower uterine segment develops. This causes a shearing of the placental-cervical attachment.

In Fig 11–7, the internal os at term is represented at varying degrees of dilatation. Consider the internal os and the placenta as overlapping circles: If the edge of the placenta can be palpated at the center of the internal os, then about half of the area represented by the internal os will be covered by placenta when the internal os is completely dilated; this

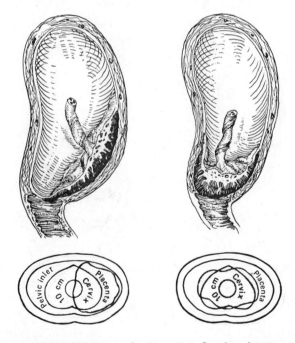

Figure 11–5. Partial placenta previa. **Figure 11–6.** Complete placenta previa.

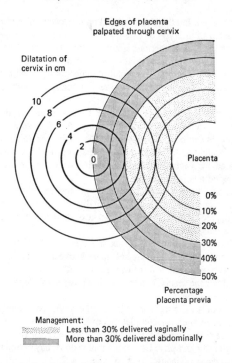

Figure 11–7. Relation of placenta previa to the cervix. (After Tatum.)

constitutes 50% placenta previa. If the placental edge can be palpated 3 cm laterally from the center of the internal os, 2 cm of the radius of the internal os should be covered on one side by the placenta at complete dilatation; this constitutes 20% placenta previa.

Caution: Do not try to determine any degree of placenta previa greater than 50% before delivery. This may produce uncontrollable placental hemorrhage.

Clinical Findings

A. Symptoms and Signs: Painless uterine bleeding is the principal symptom, but placenta previa rarely causes exsanguinating antepartal bleeding unless bleeding is initiated by pelvic or rectal examination before onset of labor. Although spotting may occur throughout the first and second trimesters of pregnancy, marked bleeding usually begins after the 28th week of gestation. Small gushes of dark blood and clots are frequently passed, but the character and time of occurrence of bleeding are not related to the type or extent of placenta previa.

Regional uterine tenderness is not present. Occasional contractions may be noted, but normal relaxation will occur.

Breech and abnormal presentations are common with placenta previa. Even a presenting vertex will remain unusually high and unengaged.

B. Sterile Vaginal Examination: If a vaginal examination is necessary, it should follow ultrasonography. A definitive diagnosis of placenta previa can be made only by sterile vaginal examination in the so-called "double setup" procedure. The patient should be hospitalized and prepared for vaginal or cesarean delivery, with typed and cross-matched blood available.

1. Inspect the lower genital tract for varicosities, ulcerative areas, tumors, or other sources of bleeding. Visualize the cervix and observe its apparent degree of dilatation, its thickness, and any bleeding from beyond the internal os.

2. Gently feel around the cervix and attempt to elicit ballottement of the presenting part. Note any soft mass between the presenting part and the cervix or in the lower uterine segment.

3. Palpate the cervix to determine its consistency, degree of dilatation, and effacement.

4. Carefully insinuate the finger into the cervical os. Gently feel for spongy tissue partially or completely covering the internal os.

5. Ascertain whether the membranes are intact or ruptured.

C. Ultrasonography: Ultrasonography alone may permit the diagnosis of placenta previa after the first trimester. This is a highly accurate method, but the degree of coverage of the os usually can only be approximated. It must be remembered that during the second trimester, the placenta will be observed by ultrasound to cover the internal os in 30% of cases. With development of the lower uterine segment, most of these low implantations will be carried to a higher station (placental migration); thus, a later confirmatory study is necessary before definitive action is taken.

D. X-Ray Studies: X-ray studies are potentially harmful and have been superseded by ultrasonography.

If ultrasonography is not available, radiography may be used. A crescent-shaped mass in the body of the uterus whose normal outlines are adjacent is probably the placenta. This finding almost completely rules out the possibility of placenta previa.

Placenta previa may be missed on soft tissue radiography with breech, transverse, or oblique presentation, polyhydramnios, abruptio placentae, bipartite placenta, placenta totalis, twins with 2 placentas, pelvic tumor, and lateral oblique malposition of the uterus.

E. Radioisotope Localization: Radioactive isotope localization of the placenta is a useful diagnostic procedure that has been supplanted by ultrasonography.

Differential Diagnosis

Extrauterine causes of bleeding may be revealed by vaginal and cervical inspection. Placental causes of bleeding other than placenta previa include premature separation of the normally implanted placenta and rupture of the ''marginal sinus'' of the placenta (a variation of placental separation). Premature separation of the margin of the placenta (rupture of the ''marginal sinus'') cannot be distinguished before delivery and inspection of the placenta.

Complications

A. Maternal: Maternal hemorrhage, shock, and death may follow severe antepartal bleeding from placenta previa. Death may also occur as a result of intrapartal and postpartal bleeding, operative trauma, infection, or embolism.

Premature separation of a portion of a placenta previa occurs in virtually every case and causes painless but excessive external bleeding. However, complete or wide separation of the placenta before full dilatation of the cervix is uncommon.

Intrapartal and postpartal endometritis, parametritis, and peritonitis commonly occur following placentitis.

Placenta previa accreta is a rare but serious abnormality in which the sparse endometrium and the myometrium of the lower uterine segment are penetrated by the trophoblast in a manner similar to placenta accreta higher in the uterus.

B. Fetal: Preterm delivery due to placenta previa is the major cause of fetal death, accounting for 60% of perinatal deaths. The fetus may die as a result of intrauterine asphyxia or birth injury. Fetal hemorrhage due to tearing of the placenta occurs with vaginal manipulation and especially upon entry into the uterine cavity at cesarean section done for placenta previa. About half of these infants lose some blood. The fetal blood loss is directly proportionate to the time lapse between laceration of a cotyledon and clamping of the cord.

Treatment

The type of treatment depends upon the amount of uterine bleeding; the duration of pregnancy and viability of the fetus; the degree of placenta previa; the presentation, position, and station of the fetus; the gravidity and parity of the patient; the status of the cervix; and whether or not labor has begun.

The patient must be admitted to the hospital to establish the diagnosis and ideally should stay in the hospital until delivery. Two or more units of bank blood should be typed, cross matched, and ready for transfusion. Be prepared to replace twice as much blood as the estimated loss. Occasionally, patients who have stopped bleeding before the 35th week of pregnancy may be sent home to bed rest, but they must be told that they will have to reenter the hospital if bleeding recurs.

There are 3 choices of therapy: (1) expectant treatment, terminating in either vaginal delivery or cesarean section; (2) artificial rupture of the membranes and vaginal delivery; and (3) cesarean section.

A. Expectant Treatment: Great improvement in the fetal survival rate can be achieved by postponing delivery. If at all possible, the infant should not be delivered before the 36th week. If severe hemorrhage occurs between 37 and 40 weeks, consider emptying the uterus. Earlier in pregnancy, a more conservative program is recommended. Maturity is a prime requisite for survival of the fetus.

About 85% of cases of placenta previa are now terminated artificially between the 36th and 40th week of pregnancy.

B. Mode of Delivery: *Caution:* Because uterine contractions are a major cause of hemorrhage, do not stimulate labor except by rupturing the membranes if this can be done easily. Because distention of the lower segment may rupture the uterus, avoid manipulative vaginal delivery; indications for cesarean section are liberalized with placenta previa.

Most multiparous patients with 20–30% placenta previa (marginal or minimally partial) probably can be delivered vaginally unless hemorrhage is excessive. If placenta previa is more than 30% (complete or extensively partial), delivery should be by cesarean section. Regardless of the degree of placenta previa, prompt abdominal delivery is indicated if the patient's status or that of a viable fetus deteriorates rapidly. Abdominal delivery will probably be necessary for breech, transverse, or oblique presentations.

1. Vaginal delivery–If vaginal delivery is decided upon, amniotomy should be done immediately. Although prolapse of the cord is a calculated risk, this probably will not occur if the patient is placed in the semi-Fowler position during drainage. Tamponade of the presenting part against the placental edge usually reduces bleeding as labor progresses.

If labor does not follow rupture of the membranes within 6–8 hours, give oxytocin (Pitocin, Syntocinon), 5 units (0.5 mL) in 1 L of 5% glucose, cautiously intravenously at a rate of 1–2 mL/min to stimulate labor.

Deliver the patient in the easiest and most expeditious manner as soon as the cervix is fully dilated and the presenting part is on the perineum. Monitor the fetal heartbeat continuously during the course of labor. If fetal distress develops, perform immediate cesarean section.

Bipolar (Braxton Hicks, internal podalic) version should not be attempted even if the infant is dead. Rupture of the lower uterine segment, cervical lacerations, and severe hemorrhage may occur.

2. Cesarean section–If cesarean section is decided upon, hypovolemic shock should be corrected by intravenous fluids and blood before the operation is started. Light, balanced general anesthesia or an epidural block may be the best choice of anesthesia.

The incision is important because of the placental location and the development of the lower uterine segment. If the incision passes through the site of placental implantation, the fetus may lose a significant amount of blood. With posterior implantations of the placenta, a low transverse incision is recommended if the lower uterine segment is well developed. Otherwise, a classic incision may be required to secure sufficient room and to avoid laceration of the placenta.

To avoid fetal hemorrhage during lower uterine segment cesarean section for placenta previa, separate the placenta gently, if at all; rupture the membranes; rotate the infant's face into the incision, aspirate the mouth and throat, and establish an airway; clamp the cord; deliver the infant and cut the cord.

If there is even a 1-minute delay after visible damage to the placental blood vessels, the infant may lose enough blood to require transfusion. If the infant's hemoglobin concentration drops to 12 g or lower 3 hours after delivery, transfusion is urgently required.

C. Treatment of Complications: Treat hemorrhage and shock promptly and adequately. Ample blood for transfusion is vital. Treat puerperal infection with massive doses of broad-spectrum antibiotics and correction of anemia. Placenta previa accreta is an indication for total abdominal hysterectomy.

Prognosis

Placenta previa is more common in repeat cesarean sections and occurs in at least 5% of such cases.

A. For the Mother: With proper management, the maternal prognosis in placenta previa is excellent. With modern therapy, the maternal mortality rate in the larger hospitals in the USA has dropped from over 1% to 0.5% during the past 20 years.

B. For the Infant: The perinatal mortality rate associated with placenta previa is about 15% in most medical centers, or about 10 times that of normal pregnancy. With expectant treatment to reduce the likelihood of preterm delivery and with ideal obstetric and newborn care, the perinatal mortality rate can probably be reduced ultimately to 10% (corrected for living viable infants without serious anomalies).

SPONTANEOUS & HABITUAL ABORTION

Abortion is the termination of pregnancy before the fetus is viable. Technically, viability is now considered to be reached at 23–24 weeks. With proper care in the neonatal period, an infant weighing slightly more than 600 g may survive.

Abortion may occur early, before the 16th week; or late, from the 16th to 28th weeks. About 75% of abortions occur before the 16th week; most of these before the eighth week.

The incidence of abortion is highest in early adulthood and just prior to the menopause. At least 12% of all diagnosed pregnancies terminate in spontaneous abortion.

Etiology

More than 60% of spontaneous abortions result from ovular or fetal defects; 15% are caused by maternal factors; the cause of the remainder is not known.

Random cases of spontaneous abortion occur without predisposition (10–15%); recurrent cases are the result of chronic germ plasm defects in ovum or sperm (0.5%). Habitual abortion (loss of 3 or more consecutive previable pregnancies) is usually secondary to persistent or recurrent causes.

A. Ovular and Fetal Factors: Organization of an early conceptus (even in a favorable site) may be faulty, and abortion ensues. This is especially true if implantation occurs outside the uterus.

1. First trimester–At least 60% of abortuses show anatomic abnormalities, but many pregnancies are expelled so early or are so degenerated that abnormalities cannot be determined accurately. Congenital absence of the embryo may occur. Cleavage defects of the ovum, absence of the chorionic cavity, and a hypoplastic trophoblast are found occasionally. Chromosomal anomalies are common: in studies of spontaneously aborted fetuses with chromosomal abnormalities, trisomy is the problem in about 50% studied, monosomy X accounts for almost 25%, and polyploidy is the next most common abnormality. Translocation is also noted in abortuses.

2. Second trimester–Worldwide, the major fetal causes of abortion during the second trimester are syphilis and shallow circumvallate implantation of the placenta. Fetal anomalies are less often responsible.

B. Maternal Factors Other Than Genetic Abnormalities:

1. Systemic disease–

a. Infections, eg, rubella, toxoplasmosis, cytomegalovirus disease, syphilis. Brucellosis is a questionable cause of human abortion.

b. Endocrine disorders, eg, severe hypothyroidism or diabetes mellitus.

c. Severe cardiac or hypertensive disease.

2. Undernutrition–Avitaminosis B or C or severely deficient protein or calorie intake.

3. Immunologic disease–Examples are Rh, ABO, or other blood group isoimmunization.

4. Toxic factors–Examples are folic acid antagonists, anticoagulants, lead poisoning (Table 4–2).

5. Uterine and cervical defects–Uterine anomalies may result in first- or second-trimester abortion. Incompetence of the cervix causes second-trimester abortion.

6. Trauma–

a. Direct–Penetrating wounds or concussion of the lower abdomen (eg, steering wheel or seat belt injury) after the fourth month of pregnancy may cause uterine abortion or placental separation. Abdominal surgery may cause uterine abortion.

b. Indirect–Medical or surgical shock, total body irradiation greater than 3000 R, or electrical shock (lightning or power-line contact). Coitus may excite abnormal uterine irritability and cause abortion.

7. Psychic or emotional causes–There is no good evidence to support the concept that abortion may be induced by psychic stimuli such as severe fright, grief, anger, or anxiety.

8. Other–Maternal hypoxia.

Clinical Findings

A. Symptoms and Signs: Abortion is classified clinically as (1) complete, (2) incomplete or inevitable, and (3) missed. In threatened abortion, the previable gestation is in jeopardy but the pregnancy continues.

1. Complete–In complete abortion, all of the conceptus is expelled. When complete abortion is impending, the symptoms of pregnancy often disappear and sudden bleeding begins, followed by cramping. The fetus and the rest of the conceptus may be expelled separately. When the entire conceptus has been expelled, pain ceases but slight spotting persists for a few days.

2. Incomplete or inevitable–In incomplete abortion, portions of the conceptus have already been passed; in inevitable abortion, evacuation of part or all of the conceptus is momentarily likely. Bleeding and cramps do not subside. Abortion is inevitable when 2 or more of the following are noted: (1) moderate effacement of the cervix, (2) cervical dilatation greater than 3 cm, (3) rupture of the membranes, (4) bleeding for longer than 7 days, (5) persistence of cramps despite narcotic analgesics, and (6) signs of termination of pregnancy.

Fever and generalized pelvic discomfort indicate infection. Retained tissue is evidenced by a patulous cervix, bleeding, and an enlarged, boggy uterus.

3. Missed–In missed abortion, the pregnancy has been terminated for at least 1 month but the conceptus has not been expelled. Symptoms of pregnancy disappear; the basal body temperature is not elevated. There is a brownish vaginal discharge but no free bleeding. Pain and tenderness are not present. The cervix is semifirm and only slightly patulous; the uterus becomes smaller and irregularly softened; and the adnexa are normal.

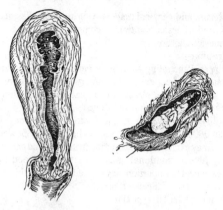

Figure 11–8. Complete abortion. At right: product of complete abortion.

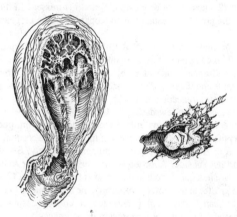

Figure 11–9. Incomplete abortion. At right: Product of incomplete abortion.

Fetal death at 18–26 weeks followed by missed labor and retention for more than 6 weeks may be associated with maternal fibrinogen depletion (''dead fetus syndrome''). Even though the mother's serum fibrinogen level is less than 100 mg/dL, she will not bleed spontaneously. However, cryoprecipitate should be given prior to evacuation of the uterus to prevent hemorrhage.

B. Laboratory Findings:

1. Urine–Pregnancy tests are negative or equivocally positive. On a stained smear of centrifuged sediment, the epithelial cells are similar in staining properties to those seen on smears of vaginal discharge.

2. Blood–If significant bleeding has occurred, blood studies will show anemia. If infection is present, the white blood cell count will be elevated (12,000–20,000). The sedimentation rate, already elevated by pregnancy, increases rapidly with infection and anemia. Pregnancy tests are usually negative.

3. Hormones–With the exception of hypothyroidism, it is unlikely that treatable abnormalities of hormone secretion cause abortion.

4. Cytology–The likelihood of spontaneous abortion is related directly to the percentage of karyopyknotic cells in the cytologic smear of vaginal cells obtained from the upper lateral vaginal wall. The karyopyknotic index (KI) is the number of karyopyknotic cells per 100 exfoliated cells counted. A normal KI is 10 or less. The incidence of abortion in patients whose KI is over 10 is approximately 20%.

C. Ultrasonography: Ultrasonography may disclose a total or partial collapse of the gestational sac, with fragmentation or separation of the placenta without a fetus or without a viable fetus.

D. X-Ray Findings: X-rays are useless in diagnosing early abortion. In advanced missed abortion, x-rays may reveal a distorted fetal skeleton and intrauterine gas.

Differential Diagnosis

(1) Ectopic pregnancy is the probable cause of menstrual abnormality, unilateral pelvic pain, uterine bleeding, and a tender adnexal mass.

(2) Unopposed estrogen stimulation causes abnormal uterine bleeding in the nonpregnant patient.

(3) Membranous dysmenorrhea is characterized by cramps, bleeding, and passage of endometrial casts. Decidua and villi are absent; amenorrhea does not precede membranous dysmenorrhea.

(4) Hydatidiform mole usually ends in abortion before the fifth month. Theca lutein cysts, when present, cause bilateral ovarian enlargement; the uterus may be unusually large. Bloody discharge may contain hydropic villi.

(5) Choriocarcinoma may cause abnormal bleeding after amenorrhea. Bilateral theca lutein ovarian cysts may be palpable in such cases.

Complications

Hemorrhage is a major cause of maternal death. Infection (septic abortion) is most common after criminally induced abortion; death results from salpingitis, peritonitis, and septicemia or septic emboli.

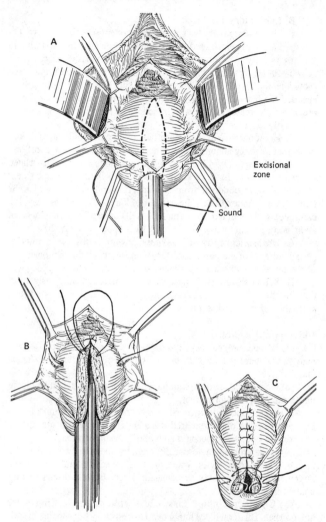

Figure 11–10. Correction of cervical incompetence in the nonpregnant patient (after Ball). *A:* Bladder displaced upward, exposing cervicouterine junction. *B:* Reapproximation of cervicouterine junction. *C:* "Crown suture" mucosal closure.

Perforation of the uterus, accompanied by injury to the bowel and bladder, hemorrhage, infection, and fistula formation, may occur during D&C because of the soft and vaguely outlined uterine wall. About three-fourths of cases of choriocarcinoma follow abortion. Infertility may result from inflammatory tubal occlusion or chronic cervicitis following uterine abortion.

Prevention

Many abortions can be prevented by study and treatment of maternal deficiencies or disorders before pregnancy, early obstetric care and adequate treatment of maternal disease, and protection of pregnant women from hazards to health in industry and from exposure to rubella or other viral infections. If an aborted fetus is found to be trisomic, amniocentesis for antenatal genetic assessment should be done during the second trimester of the next pregnancy. Cervical cerclage during the second trimester for closure of an incompetent cervix will prevent certain abortions.

A. Correction of Cervical Incompetence in the Nonpregnant Patient: Cervical incompetence is suggested by a history of repeated second-trimester abortion, usually following a traumatic vaginal delivery, and abnormal patulousness of the cervix (easy passage of dilators to No. 8 Hegar). Occult lacerations in the region of the internal os are a common cause of sequential second-trimester abortions. It is virtually impossible to locate the precise area of weakness, but excision of a segment of cervix and myometrium, including the area of the internal os, usually will correct the defect and improve function (Fig 11–10).

An incision is made anteriorly above the cervix and the dissection is continued anteriorly, with displacement of the bladder upward to expose the cervical canal and lower uterine segment. An arrow-shaped portion of tissue is removed with a sharp scalpel, and the margins are reapproximated, using interrupted medium-weight chromic catgut. The mucosal layer is closed with fine catgut sutures.

The operation is highly effective in preventing subsequent spontaneous second-trimester abortion.

B. Cervical Cerclage (Shirodkar Operation) in the Pregnant Patient: The placement, snug tie, and fixation of a nonabsorbable Mersilene or comparable strand, ribbon, or band beneath the mucosa and pericervical fascia at the cervico-uterine junction may be done during the pregnant state for correction of cervical incompetence (Fig 11–11). The physician must then decide whether to release the ligature during labor for vaginal delivery or to perform cesarean section near term.

Treatment

Successful management of abortion depends upon early diagnosis.

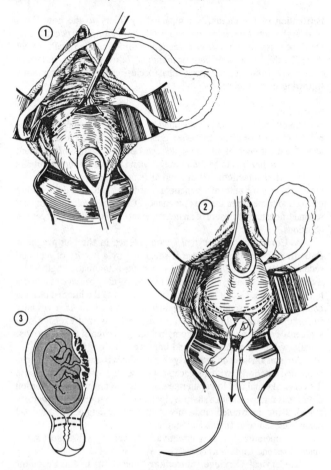

Figure 11–11. Cerclage of the cervix (Shirodkar) with incompetent os in pregnant patient.

A complete history should be taken and a general physical (including pelvic) examination done on every patient. Laboratory studies should include cultures of cervical mucus to determine pathogens in case of infection, antibiotic sensitivity tests, and a complete blood count. Thyroid or other endocrine studies should be made as appropriate.

A. Emergency Measures: If abortion has occurred during the second trimester, the patient should be hospitalized. In all cases, give oxytocics, eg, oxytocin (Pitocin, Syntocinon), 1 mL/500 mL of 5% dextrose in water intravenously, or 0.5 mL intramuscularly every 30 minutes for 2–4 doses, to contract the uterus and limit blood loss and aid in the expulsion of clots and tissues. Ergonovine (Ergotrate) should be given only if the diagnosis of complete abortion is certain. Give antishock therapy, including blood replacement, to prevent collapse after hemorrhage.

B. Specific Measures: Endocrine therapy has theoretical value in less than 5% of abortions (those due to maternal hormonal deficiencies), but treatment has rarely proved clinically useful.

C. General Measures: Place the patient at bed rest and give sedatives to allay uterine irritability and limit bleeding. Coitus and douches are contraindicated.

D. Surgical Measures: D&C should be performed for possible retained tissue. (Start an intravenous oxytocin drip before surgery to avoid uterine perforation.)

E. Treatment of Complications:

1. Uterine perforation–Observe for signs of intraperitoneal bleeding, rupture of the bowel or bladder, or peritonitis. Exploratory laparotomy and broad-spectrum antibiotic therapy may be necessary.

2. Pelvic thrombophlebitis and septic emboli may be critical sequelae. Consider antibiotics, anticoagulants, and clipping or ligation of the vena cava and ovarian veins.

Prognosis

A. For the Mother: The prognosis for the mother is good if all products of conception are removed and if choriocarcinoma and hydatidiform mole can be ruled out.

B. For Future Pregnancies: If an aborted fetus is found to be trisomic, amniocentesis for antenatal genetic assessment should be done during the second trimester of the next pregnancy.

Correction of maternal disorders may make future successful pregnancies possible. Unfortunately, little can be done to improve the prognosis when a serious genetic fault is heritable. If the genetic disorder is transmitted paternally, artificial insemination (AID) or adoption may be an acceptable alternative.

HYDATIDIFORM MOLE
(Trophoblastic Disease, Cystic
Degeneration of the Chorion)

Hydatidiform mole is a degenerative disorder of the chorion of unknown cause. It occurs as a complication of about one in 40,000 pregnancies in the USA, almost always during the first 18 weeks. It is more common among women under age 20 and over age 40 and is more than 5 times as prevalent in the Orient as in the West. In the USA, cancer (choriocarcinoma) is reported in about 2.5% of cases.

If hydatidiform mole occurs in a double-ovum twin pregnancy, one placenta is usually spared. In a single-ovum twin pregnancy, the entire chorion is diseased and both embryos are destroyed. Most or all of the villi show minute to gross swelling. The smaller blebs are pale, shiny, translucent, and yellowish-brown, resembling cooked tapioca; the larger hydatids resemble seedless white grapes. Some villi reach a diameter of about 1 cm. They contain small amounts of clear, pale amber fluid. A containing amniotic membrane may not be present. In most cases, no conceptus is found.

On microscopic examination, the villi are found to be greatly altered and enlarged. Although most are superficial, others are deep within the endometrium or even in the inner myometrium. The syncytial investment is complete. The cytotrophoblast is generally prominent, even proliferative, and persists well after the fourth month if evacuation of the mole does not occur. An edematous, avascular stroma is typical of hydatidiform mole. Bleeding and evidence of infection may also be observed.

Ovarian changes include theca lutein cysts and various degrees of luteinization of thecal elements caused by high levels of hCG produced by the trophoblast.

Clinical Findings

A. Symptoms and Signs: Excessive nausea and vomiting occur in over one-third of patients with hydatidiform mole. Uterine bleeding, beginning at 6–8 weeks, is observed in virtually all cases and is indicative of threatened or incomplete abortion. In at least 40% of cases the uterus is larger than would be expected in a normal pregnancy of the same duration; this is due to the great volume of the vesicular villi. Fullness, softness, and thinning of the entire lower uterine segment often occur in early pregnancy. Bilateral cystic ovarian enlargement develops in about 15% of cases as a result of gonadotropin stimulation of the ovaries. Preeclampsia-eclampsia, frequently of the fulminating type, may develop during the second trimester. Intact or collapsed vesicles often are passed through the vagina during episodes of spotting, since there may be no amniotic membrane to prevent evacuation. Vesicular changes may be noted in curettings from incomplete abortions not suspected of being molar pregnancies.

B. Laboratory Findings:

1. Routine urinalysis may reveal protein in the absence of significant formed elements, which, when accompanied by elevated blood pressure, suggests preeclampsia-eclampsia.

2. Reduced hematocrit, hemoglobin level, and red cell count as

well as increased white cell count and sedimentation rate are the result of bleeding and infection.

3. Hydatidiform mole, malignant mole, or choriocarcinoma is probably present when the hCG titer of a 24-hour urine collection exceeds 50,000 mIU/mL, the peak level of a normal pregnancy at 65 days after implantation. In proliferative trophoblastic disease, the hCG titer often is recorded at 1–2 million IU/24 h.

Radioimmunoassay of the β subunit of hCG is highly specific because it differentiates hCG from luteinizing hormone. In addition, it will detect persistent trophoblastic activity of such a low degree as to suggest a remission by less sensitive assays. Hence, it is highly sensitive and usually eliminates false-positive or false-negative reports.

4. The urinary 17-ketosteroid level is often twice that of normal pregnancy, but pregnanediol excretion is within the normal pregnancy range.

5. In some cases, thyroid hormone analogs (as estimated by the serum T_3 and T_4) may reach thyrotoxic levels because of a TSH-like hormone produced by the trophoblast. However, there is no clinical evidence of toxic goiter in such cases.

6. Identification of placental hydatids will establish the diagnosis.

C. X-Ray Findings: X-ray amniography should reveal the multitudinous vesicles of a hydatidiform mole. Chest x-ray may reveal lung metastases in malignant mole.

D. Ultrasonography: Ultrasound may identify a molar pregnancy ("snowstorm" effect) from the third month on.

Differential Diagnosis

Hyperemesis gravidarum or uterine bleeding may occur as a complication of any pregnancy. The fundus will also be larger than expected in multiple pregnancy, polyhydramnios, and uterine tumor complicating intrauterine pregnancy. Consider bilateral dermoid or other cystic enlargement of the ovaries during gestation as well as theca lutein cysts of hydatid mole.

Identify vesicles by microscopic examination of sloughed tissues to prove hydatidiform mole.

Complications

A. Nonmalignant Complications: Hemorrhage, especially in advanced molar pregnancy, is common before, during, and even after evacuation of the uterus by spontaneous or operative means. Infection is a major problem, since there may be no amnion barrier to cervical or vaginal contamination of the uterine cavity. Perforation of the thin-walled uterus during surgical evacuation may lead to infection. Spontaneous rupture of the uterus may occur with benign or malignant mole.

Hydatidiform moles are degenerative and benign and do not invade or metastasize; however, they may undergo malignant change (see below).

B. Malignant Complications: Invasive or malignant mole (also called mole destruens) may actually grow through the uterine wall and cause perforation and rupture of the uterus. It may also metastasize occasionally, usually to the lung, where it may cause chest pain, cough, or hemoptysis. Choriocarcinoma may be manifested by continued or recurrent uterine bleeding after evacuation of a mole or by the presence of an ulcerative vaginal tumor, pelvic mass, or evidence of distant metastatic tumor.

A distinction between invasive mole and choriocarcinoma is often difficult, and grading of the cancer usually is impossible. Half of all cases of choriocarcinoma occur as a complication of hydatidiform mole; about 25% follow abortion, and 25% complicate term pregnancies.

Initially, invasive moles may resemble those of the vesicular type grossly and microscopically. Others may reveal proliferation of both cyto- and syncytiotrophoblastic cells that invade the myometrium. Villi are occasionally seen in malignant moles but not in choriocarcinoma. Inflammation is frequently observed. Hemorrhage and necrosis are conspicuous.

Grossly, a choriocarcinoma is a dark purple, moderately well demarcated, soft tumor, often necrotic and hemorrhagic. Choriocarcinoma often involves the cervix or vagina, but in other instances only the uterine wall or other pelvic structures will be involved. This cancer metastasizes early via the bloodstream to involve lungs, liver, and brain. Ovarian lutein cysts are usually present.

Microscopically, sheets and strands of trophoblastic cells of variable size and maturity with hyperchromatism and numerous mitoses will be noted. Little or no stroma can be seen, and villi are never present. Inflammation may be minimal. Invasion of the myometrium, hemorrhage, and widespread coagulation necrosis are typical.

Following spontaneous evacuation of an early pregnancy, the uterus may remain boggy, and bleeding often persists. This may indicate retained products of conception, a hydatidiform mole, or even a choriocarcinoma. Similar symptoms may occur with subinvolution of an otherwise normal, empty uterus.

Treatment

Do not strive too long to support a questionable pregnancy; it may be a mole, even a malignant one.

A. Emergency Measures: Hemorrhage indicative of abortion requires immediate hospitalization. Type and cross match the patient's blood, and have at least 2 units of blood available for transfusion. Encourage spontaneous expulsion of most of the molar tissue by stimulation with intravenous oxytocin (see p 226) and use of suction curettage.

Manual curettage or use of a large blunt curet will probably be required for removal of adherent tissue. Bleeding will cease as soon as the uterine contents are evacuated and firm uterine contraction is established.

B. Specific (Surgical) Measures:

1. Evacuate the mole as soon as practicable after the diagnosis is established. Evacuation by suction curettage with concurrent intravenous administration of oxytocin to control bleeding is preferred. Then use blunt and sharp curettage to eliminate adherent molar tissue and obtain tissue from the decidua basalis for study by a pathologist. Give ergonovine (Ergotrate), 0.2 mg orally, every 4 hours after curettement until 4 doses have been given.

If the uterus is larger than a 5-month pregnancy, evacuate the mole by suction curettage. Perform a sharp curettage 4–6 weeks later.

Do not puncture or resect ovarian cysts; spontaneous regression will occur in most cases with elimination of the mole.

2. If cancer is suspected, consult other texts for details of treatment, or refer the patient to a gynecologic oncologist.

C. General Measures: Evaluate all products of conception for evidence of benign or malignant mole. Tissue obtained from the decidua basalis by sharp curettage should be submitted separately for pathologic study. Order a chest x-ray and examine for pulmonary or other metastases. Postmolar surveillance is necessary. The hCG titer should be determined once a month for 6 months after evacuation of the mole; a rising titer indicates choriocarcinoma or a new pregnancy. It is essential to use serum radioimmunoassays for the β subunit of hCG rather than commercial or biologic pregnancy tests.

The patient must avoid becoming pregnant again until at least 6 months after monthly determinations of the β subunit of hCG show negative results. Prescribe oral contraceptives if these are acceptable.

D. Supportive Measures:

1. Replace blood and administer iron if the patient is anemic. Ensure a proper diet.

2. Prescribe a broad-spectrum antibiotic if infection is suspected.

Treatment of Complications

A. Nonmalignant Complications: Hemorrhage is usually due to retained products of conception and is an indication for even a second D&C. If salpingitis or other infection develops, treat intensively with antibiotics. Rupture or perforation of the uterus is an indication for laparotomy and consideration of hysterectomy.

Subinvolution of the uterus will resolve. Prescribe ergonovine (Ergotrate), 0.01 g orally every 4 hours for 6 doses, and warm acetic acid vaginal douches daily for 1 week.

B. Malignant Complications: Cancer is rarely diagnosed from curettings alone. Continued or repeated bleeding after D&C; prolonged subinvolution of the uterus; visible, palpable, radiographic, or neurologic evidence of metastases; and a persistently elevated hCG titer (determined by radioimmunoassay for the β subunit of hCG) more than 2 months after uterine evacuation of a mole are presumptive evidence of malignant mole or choriocarcinoma.

Refer the patient to a gynecologic oncologist if cancer is suspected.

Prognosis

The prognosis after evacuation of hydatidiform mole is excellent, although surveillance is needed as outlined above. Mole recurs in about 1% of subsequent pregnancies. Choriocarcinoma develops in approximately 2.5% of all cases of malignant gestational trophoblastic disease.

The presence or absence of ovarian cystic enlargement is of no value in predicting malignant trends.

Most patients with malignant mole treated promptly and adequately will recover. Before the advent of cancer chemotherapy, almost 90% of patients with choriocarcinoma died in less than 1 year even with the best care. Now, the mortality rate is less than 10%.

VOMITING OF PREGNANCY & HYPEREMESIS GRAVIDARUM

Vomiting of pregnancy—including its most pernicious form, hyperemesis gravidarum—affects many expectant mothers. About two-thirds of these are primiparas. For unexplained reasons, vomiting of pregnancy is more common in women with multiple or molar pregnancy. Most cases of gastric upset are very mild, but rare patients require hospitalization. Intractable vomiting may be fatal, but therapeutic abortion is justified only in exceptional instances.

There are no proved causes of vomiting of pregnancy, although an elevated hCG titer has been suggested as a cause. When organic causes of vomiting are excluded by reasonable diagnostic study, it can usually be assumed that the symptom is emotional in origin. Fears of inadequacy, insecurity, and emotional conflicts lead to subconscious resentment and the figurative rejection of pregnancy symbolized by vomiting.

Most persons have different thresholds for vomiting and respond differently to the varied methods of treating emotional problems. Personal variations and degrees of disability are therefore to be expected.

Dehydration leads to fluid and electrolyte imbalances, particularly acidosis. Starvation causes hypoproteinemia and hypovitaminosis.

The results of excessive vomiting are dehydration, hypochloremia, acetonemia, hypokalemia, hypoglycemia, and hypoproteinemia. Liver and occasionally kidney damage occur, followed by hyperketosis, hyperbilirubinemia, nitrogen retention, vitamin deficiency, and jaundice. Death may occur from hepatic or adrenocortical failure; it is usually due to a combination of the 2.

Clinical Findings

A. Symptoms and Signs: Many patients have ambivalent feelings about the pregnancy.

The gastrointestinal symptoms vary in severity from occasional to protracted vomiting. Nausea and vomiting usually begin about 5–6 weeks after conception. In most cases, vomiting persists only until the 14th–16th week, though it may continue throughout pregnancy. Nausea and vomiting usually occur in the morning upon arising, but evening nausea and vomiting are almost as common and develop with fatigue, food odors as the evening meal is prepared, household confusion, or the husband's return home. In most cases, despite the severity of subjective complaints, there are few or no signs of nutritional deficiency.

B. Laboratory Findings: In severely ill patients, hemoconcentration will be reflected in a relative elevation of the hemoglobin level, red cell count, and hematocrit. A slight increase in the white cell count, a shift to the left in the differential count, and increased numbers of eosinophils may be noted.

Ketone bodies (acetone) often are found in the urine, which is usually concentrated. Slight proteinuria (trace to 1+) is a frequent finding.

In very ill patients, the serum proteins and alkali reserve are commonly depleted. If the patient is oliguric, the blood urea nitrogen, serum sodium, and serum potassium levels may be elevated.

With advanced secondary liver disease, the serum concentration of proteins, prothrombin, and fibrinogen will be decreased.

C. X-Ray Findings: If nausea and vomiting are severe, x-ray studies should be done to disclose possible hiatus hernia, peptic ulcer, or even gastric carcinoma.

D. Special Examinations: Periodic ophthalmoscopic evaluations will be required if the patient is seriously ill. Retinal hemorrhage and detachment of the retina are unfavorable prognostic signs.

Complications

Neuritis and bleeding due to hemorrhagic diatheses associated with vitamin deficiency may occur. Stress ulcers of the stomach may develop. Jaundice is a particularly ominous sign.

Treatment

A. For Slight to Moderate Nausea and Vomiting of Pregnancy:

1. General measures–Light dry foods and 6 small meals a day

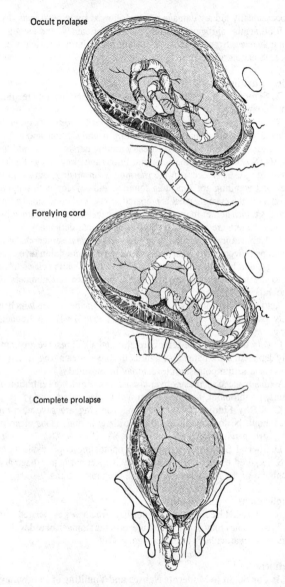

Occult prolapse

Forelying cord

Complete prolapse

Figure 11–12. Types of prolapsed cords.

may reduce nausea and vomiting. Increased fluid intake helps to prevent dehydration and acidosis. Ensure adequate rest. Provide explanation and reassurance, and relieve any fears related to pregnancy.

2. Medical measures–Sedation, eg, phenobarbital, 15 mg orally or rectally 2–3 times daily may be helpful. Antinauseants should be used only if necessary, because of their theoretically teratogenic effects. The antihistamines are beneficial in nausea and vomiting of pregnancy in proportion to their sedative effects. Narcotics have no place in the treatment of digestive problems during pregnancy. Vitamins are of no therapeutic value.

3. Psychotherapy–Seek to identify problems and conflicts and help the patient resolve them.

B. For Severe Nausea and Vomiting (Hyperemesis Gravidarum):

1. General measures–Insist upon complete bed rest without bathroom privileges until improvement occurs. Record fluid intake and output accurately. Give antiemetics rectally or parenterally.

2. Medical dietary measures–Permit nothing by mouth for the first 48 hours. Provide adequate parenteral fluids, electrolytes, carbohydrates, and protein by means of 10% glucose in water (2000 mL) and 5% glucose in normal saline (1000 mL) intravenously daily, with potassium added, plus vitamins. If the serum proteins are depleted, administer intravenous amino acid preparations, eg, Amigen, 500 mL twice daily. Vitamins—especially B complex, C, and K—should be added to the infusion.

Nasogastric tube feeding of a well-balanced liquid baby formula by slow drip should be instituted if the patient cannot retain food by mouth after 48 hours. If she responds to the above regimen after 48 hours, prescribe a dry diet in 6 small feedings daily with clear liquids 1 hour after meals.

3. Therapeutic abortion–Rarely, therapeutic abortion may be required in order to save the patient's life.

Prognosis

Vomiting of pregnancy is self-limited, and the prognosis is good. Intractable hyperemesis gravidarum is a serious threat to the life of the mother and the fetus.

PROLAPSE OF THE UMBILICAL CORD

A prolapsed umbilical cord may become compressed, resulting in fetal hypoxia.

Prolapse of the umbilical cord (Fig 11–12) can be classified as (1) forelying cord, in which the cord precedes the presenting part, is held within intact membranes, and can often be felt through the cervix; (2) occult prolapse, in which the·cord lies over the face or head of the fetus but cannot be felt on internal examination (membranes may be intact or ruptured); and (3) complete prolapse, in which the cord descends past ruptured membranes to extrude through the cervix into the vagina or even beyond the introitus.

With forelying cord or occult prolapse, the cord may be compressed intermittently by the presenting or other prominent fetal part, with resulting fetal hypoxia and possible permanent brain damage or even death of the fetus. With complete cord prolapse, the cord may be occluded longer and more completely, and the risk to the fetus is greatly increased. Complete prolapse of the cord occurs in about one in 200 advanced pregnancies.

Prolapse of the umbilical cord may be due to (1) abnormal presentation (breech, shoulder, face, brow, transverse, compound), (2) multiple pregnancy, (3) premature rupture of the membranes prior to engagement of the vertex or breech, (4) contracted pelvis (fetopelvic disproportion) or distorting pelvic tumor, (5) polyhydramnios, (6) low implantation of the placenta, and (7) abnormally long cord (over 75 cm).

Clinical Findings

A. Symptoms and Signs: In complete prolapse, the patient may feel the cord slide through the vagina and over the vulva after rupture of the membranes. Compression of the cord often causes violent fetal activity, obvious to the patient and even to the observer. The cord may be seen or felt by the patient or by a physician or nurse during external or internal examination, or it may be palpated during vaginal or rectal examination. Signs of fetal distress (eg, marked slowing of the fetal heartbeat) are often found on auscultation.

B. Special Examinations: Sterile vaginal examination will confirm the presence of complete cord prolapse and may confirm occult prolapse of the cord.

Complications

Mild or brief fetal hypoxia due to cord obstruction may cause no fetal damage. Marked or prolonged fetal hypoxia causes neurologic deficit or death.

Prevention

If the patient is in bed when the membranes rupture spontaneously and prematurely and if there is no extrusion of the cord, have the patient stand up at once despite gross leakage of fluid. The presenting part may gravitate over the inlet and prevent cord prolapse. If the patient remains in bed, the cord may slide down and out through the cervix.

Examine the patient vaginally promptly after rupture of the membranes, especially when a breech or transverse presentation is known to exist, to determine if prolapse is a possibility. Record the fetal heart rate at once and again within 30 minutes.

Treatment

A. Emergency Measures: For any type of prolapsed cord, place the patient in the knee-chest or deep Trendelenburg position and have her remain so. Administer oxygen by face mask. Using aseptic technique, try to push the cord back and loop it above a fetal ear. This may retain it inside the uterus. If this maneuver is successful, the patient should lie on one side in the Sims position with hips elevated and head and body at a lower level. If the presenting part then engages, the danger of recurrent prolapse of the cord may be over.

B. Delivery: Cesarean section usually is the best method of delivery. The following measures are to be condemned: manual dilatation of the cervix; incision of a rigid, thick cervix dilated less than 5 cm; and version and extraction.

Management depends upon the following factors:

1. Duration of pregnancy–If the pregnancy is of less than 26 weeks' duration, it is inadvisable to increase the maternal risk in an effort to salvage a very immature fetus. Abandon the fetus and allow labor and delivery to proceed.

2. Parity of the patient–Multiparous women have shorter labors than primigravidas, and fewer maternal complications usually result from operative delivery.

3. Quality of labor–The patient may not be in labor, or the labor may be desultory in contrast with strong labor close to delivery. The mode of delivery will depend upon the proximity of delivery.

4. Fetal presentation–A footling breech or a transverse presentation is less favorable than a vertex. The indications for cesarean section are liberalized in such cases.

C. Treatment of Complications: Lacerations of the birth canal must be repaired promptly. Blood transfusion may be required.

Resuscitation of the newborn is often a problem because of hypoxia, the trauma of delivery, and prematurity.

Prognosis

A. For the Mother: Infection or trauma associated with attempts at replacement of the cord or operative vaginal delivery of the fetus may complicate the puerperium. Anemia may result from excessive blood loss.

B. For the Infant: Brief (< 5 minutes), partial cord compression may not be harmful. Complete occlusion for the same period or partial occlusion for a longer time will cause severe central nervous system damage or death.

PUERPERAL SEPSIS
(See also Shock, p 303.)

Any infection in the genital tract that occurs as a complication of abortion, labor, or delivery is termed puerperal sepsis. Streptococci, staphylococci, clostridia, coliform bacteria, and *Bacteroides* are the pathogens most often identified. Debility (anemia, undernutrition), serious systemic disorders, premature or prolonged rupture of the membranes, protracted labor, and traumatic examinations or delivery predispose to puerperal infection.

The incidence of puerperal sepsis in hospitals in the USA is at least 10%. Puerperal sepsis is exceeded only by hemorrhage and preeclampsia-eclampsia as a cause of maternal death in this country.

Infection is acquired from hospital personnel in circumstances where scrupulous aseptic technique is not observed or from an endogenous source. Cellulitis resulting from vaginal or cervical lacerations may be the site of infection—as may the endometrium, particularly when endometritis occurs in the zone of placental attachment (the equivalent of a large surface wound). Endometritis, salpingitis, and peritonitis may then occur, and vasculitis in pelvic arteries and veins, thrombophlebitis, and embolization often ensue. Septicemia may develop, and local or distant abscesses may form.

Clinical Findings
Many genital tract infections are so mild as to cause few or slight symptoms. Others are violent, fulminating, and fatal within a short time.

A. Symptoms and Signs: Malaise, headache, anorexia, and remittent slight elevations in temperature and pulse generally begin 3–4 days after delivery. Vague discomfort in the perineum or lower abdomen and nausea and vomiting may follow. High fever (''childbed fever''), rapid pulse, ileus, and localization of pain and tenderness in the pelvis may be observed during the next 1–2 days. The lochia becomes foul or profuse. Bacteremic shock may occur. If improvement does not follow after 48–72 hours of antibiotic therapy, reexamine the patient: an abscess may be forming.

B. Laboratory Findings: Polymorphonuclear leukocytosis and an increased sedimentation rate indicate infection. Reduced hematocrit and hemoglobin levels indicate anemia. Identification of pathogens from cervical and uterine lochia by culture and sensitivity tests will require 36–48 hours.

C. X-Ray Findings: X-ray studies are not helpful except to exclude gastrointestinal, urinary, or pulmonary problems.

Complications & Sequelae
Genital tract infections commonly progress to peritonitis, pelvic

cellulitis and abscess formation, septicemia, pulmonary embolism, septic shock, and death. Other extremely serious problems secondary to such infections include dynamic or adynamic ileus, anemia, hepatitis, pneumonia, empyema, and meningitis. Any of these disorders may prove fatal.

If the patient recovers, chronic salpingitis may cause recurrent disability. Tubal occlusion may be the cause of "one-child sterility." Femoral thrombophlebitis ("milk leg") is often followed by chronic pain and swelling of the leg.

Differential Diagnosis

Febrile complications of the puerperium unrelated to genital tract infection include mastitis, urinary and respiratory infection, and enteritis, in that order of frequency.

Prevention

The prevention of puerperal sepsis consists of good obstetric care from the time the patient is first seen until she is discharged from the hospital, with particular emphasis on strict aseptic technique during manual examination and delivery. Obstetric trauma should be minimized, since injured, devitalized tissues are especially susceptible to anaerobic infection.

Treatment

A. **Emergency Measures:** Treat shock (see p 305).

B. **General Measures:**

1. Obtain specimens of cervical, uterine, and other discharges for culture and sensitivity studies. Strict isolation of the patient is necessary only if the causative organisms appear to be β-hemolytic streptococci or coagulase-positive staphylococci. For other infections, unit isolation is adequate.

2. Place the patient in the semi-Fowler position. Give a clear liquid diet for at least several days, and give intravenous fluids to maintain electrolyte and fluid balance.

3. Administer analgesics, sedative-hypnotic drugs, oxytocics, or laxatives as required.

C. **Specific Measures:**

1. Initially, give antibiotics in large doses, eg, penicillin G, 5 million units intravenously, plus kanamycin, 1 g intramuscularly, immediately followed by penicillin, 1.2 million units, with kanamycin, 0.5 g intramuscularly 4 times daily. In infections likely to be anaerobic, particularly if *Bacteroides* is thought to be present, substitute lincomycin, 1 g intravenously, for kanamycin. When the results of culture and sensitivity studies are known, continue therapy with the antibiotic of choice in large and repeated doses.

2. For treatment of disseminated intravascular coagulation, see p 273.

D. Surgical Measures: Hysterectomy is indicated for serious puerperal infections that do not respond to treatment. The site of infection may be the uterus, a postabortal uterine abscess, a hydatidiform mole, or a myoma. Clipping or ligation of the vena cava and ovarian veins may be lifesaving in case of repeated (often septic) pulmonary embolization. Pelvic drainage may be necessary. Abscesses may require surgical drainage.

Prognosis

The susceptibility of the pathogenic microorganism, the extent of involvement, the patient's resistance, and the promptness and adequacy of treatment determine the outcome. The maternal mortality rate due to puerperal sepsis in the USA is about 0.2%, but in some areas of the world, the mortality rate is vastly greater.

AMNIOTIC FLUID EMBOLISM

Amniotic fluid embolism is the sudden escape of amniotic fluid into maternal veins in the subplacental area after rupture of the membranes, usually during hard labor. Amniotic fluid embolism produces profound shock and often hemorrhage, disseminated intravascular coagulation, and death. About 5% of maternal deaths are attributed to this cause.

Most patients with amniotic fluid embolism are multiparas at term. However, the problem occasionally occurs during cesarean section after extraction of the fetus. In about one-third of cases of amniotic fluid embolism, the mother has some obstetric problem such as preeclampsia, fetal death, or infection. The membranes are always ruptured. Strong labor, often oxytocin-augmented, generally is in progress. Meconium may be present in the amniotic fluid.

Necropsy in fatal cases discloses amniotic cells, lanugo, and perhaps meconium in the pulmonary arterial system. Thrombi may be noted in the microcirculation (disseminated intravascular coagulation). Ecchymoses and other evidence of a bleeding diathesis may be present. Bile pigment often can be identified in the liver, spleen, kidneys, or brain, the result of red cell breakdown.

Clinical Findings

Sudden dyspnea, cyanosis, and profound shock occur, often followed by hemorrhage or death. If a massive amniotic fluid infusion has not occurred, the patient may be saved by prompt intensive therapy.

Complications

Generally, death is due to obstruction of the pulmonary circulation and right-sided heart failure. Hypofibrinogenemia and hemorrhage may develop as a result of disseminated intravascular coagulation.

Differential Diagnosis

The differential diagnosis includes other emboli, stroke, eclampsia, septic shock, cardiac failure, gastric aspiration, and toxic drug reaction. However, many of these bear only a superficial resemblance to amniotic fluid embolism when considered carefully.

Prevention

Artificial rupture of the membranes should be delayed or the membranes should be allowed to rupture spontaneously in patients in strong labor, especially when the fetus has died. Hyperstimulation of the uterus during labor (eg, use of oxytocics when labor is progressing satisfactorily) should be avoided. The uterus should be stimulated to contract before manual separation of the placenta.

Treatment

Treat for shock. Give 100% oxygen by mask, and apply moderately snug tourniquets to the legs or use military antishock trousers (MAST suit).

Administer the following intravenously: (1) Atropine, 0.4 mg, to overcome vagal cardiac depression and possible fibrillation. (2) Isoproterenol, 0.2 mg (slowly), to dilate the microcirculation. (3) Heparin, 0.05 g, to minimize the possibility of disseminated intravascular coagulation. (4) Papaverine, 100 mg, to dilate the pulmonary vasculature. (The action of papaverine is weak and unreliable.)

Insert a central venous catheter and record central venous pressure.

Deliver the infant without trauma if feasible.

Treatment of Complications

Digitalize the patient if cardiac failure is a possibility. For treatment of disseminated intravascular coagulation, see p 273.

Prognosis

The prognosis depends upon the severity of the insult and the rapidity of adequate therapy. Treatment is complicated and often ineffective. About half of patients with amniotic fluid embolism die rapidly, and half of those who survive the initial insult die within hours.

SHOCK

Shock is a syndrome characterized by prostration and hypotension due to diminished circulating blood volume of such a degree that perfusion of the vital organs is inadequate.

Elderly persons, acutely or chronically ill or severely injured individuals, and those who have had deep general anesthesia or major surgery are most susceptible to shock. Women with hypoadrenocorticism or those who have received regular therapeutic doses of corticosteroids (eg, for asthma or a collagen disease) may develop shock after physical stress because of reduced adrenocortical reserve. Pregnant women (particularly those with preeclampsia-eclampsia) have poor vascular tone and do not resist shock well. During pregnancy, endotoxin released in septic shock may provoke a generalized Shwartzman reaction without prior sensitization.

Classification

The shock syndromes encountered in obstetrics and gynecology may be classified clinically as follows:

(1) Hypovolemic shock most commonly follows hemorrhage, trauma, and dehydration. It is characterized by an absolute or relative decrease in blood volume.

(2) Cardiogenic shock may result from acute diminution of cardiac output and usually is associated with varying degrees of vasoconstriction (eg, myocardial infarction, heart failure, paroxysmal tachycardia, myocardial depressant drugs).

(3) Septic shock may complicate any significant systemic infection, but it most frequently occurs following bacteremia due to gram-negative organisms and their endotoxins.

(4) Toxic shock (see p 541) is often caused by an exotoxin produced by some coagulase-positive strains of *Staphylococcus aureus*. It is seen most often in menstruating women who use tampons and is characterized by fever, rash, hypotension, headache, vomiting, and diarrhea.

(5) Neurogenic shock, as seen in simple fainting, spinal anesthesia, and central nervous system injury, is usually associated with peripheral vasodilatation.

(6) Metabolic shock may occur in Addison's disease and other diseases due to adrenocortical insufficiency and in a wide variety of other disorders, including those listed above. Fluid and electrolyte and other chemical abnormalities in diabetic acidosis and in acute pulmonary, hepatic, or renal insufficiency may impair cardiovascular mechanisms and lead to shock.

(7) Anaphylactic shock is characterized by marked vasodilatation with relative hypovolemia. This may be due to allergy to drugs, sera, or other sensitizing agents.

(8) Drug shock may follow excessive administration of hypnotic drugs, anesthetics, vasodilators, vasoconstrictors, and other drugs.

(9) Vascular obstructive shock may occur as a result of blockage of major blood vessels by amniotic fluid, air, or blood clots. Supine hypotension in obstetric patients may be a contributing factor.

Clinical Findings

A. Impending Shock: A variable period of intense sympathetic activity generally precedes hypotension. Weakness; pallor; cool, moist skin; and tachycardia develop. (*Caution:* Do not confuse with simple fainting.) Fever and shaking chills precede collapse in septic shock. Marked orthopnea, arrhythmia, and severe chest pain are warning signs of cardiogenic shock.

B. Established Shock: Hypotension (systolic pressure < 100 mm Hg) is superimposed on the above early signs, and tachycardia (> 100) usually develops. Thirst, air hunger, severe prostration, and dulling of the sensorium are advanced signs. Coma, cardiac arrest, and death are imminent at this point.

C. Septic Shock: Chills, high fever, tachycardia, anorexia, and occasional nausea and vomiting are often preceded by a history of infected abortion, traumatic delivery, or recurrent pyelonephritis. Between 3 and 9 hours after the first shaking chill, a precipitous drop in body temperature to subnormal levels often heralds shock.

Treatment

Because multiple pathologic mechanisms are in operation, there is no simple and reliable physiologic pattern of a patient's response to shock. Survival of the patient depends upon early diagnosis, correct appraisal of physiologic abnormalities, monitoring of essential parameters, and a flexible plan of therapy based upon vital signs and laboratory data.

Act quickly. Shock is an acute emergency that takes precedence over all other problems except acute hemorrhage, cardiac arrest, and respiratory failure.

Determine the primary cause of shock promptly. A brief history (if available) and the gross physical findings will often permit the differentiation of hemorrhagic, cardiogenic, septic, or allergic shock. Except in neurogenic shock due to fainting—a self-limiting condition treated by placing the patient in the recumbent position and administering stimulants—proceed with antishock measures. Additional therapy may be required for specific problems.

A. General Measures:

1. Place the patient in the recumbent position. Avoid the Trendelenburg position, since it interferes with breathing. Disturb the patient as little as possible. Apply military antishock trousers (MAST suit), if available, to patients not bleeding vaginally.

2. Establish an adequate airway and ensure pulmonary ventilation. Administer oxygen by nasal catheter, mask, or endotracheal tube as required, especially when dyspnea or cyanosis is present.

3. Keep the patient comfortably warm with blankets. Do not apply external heat, since this will cause peripheral vasodilatation.

4. Control pain and relieve apprehension. Shock patients often have very little discomfort. A sedative such as pentobarbital sodium, 0.13 g intravenously, may be given. (*Caution:* Narcotics are contraindicated for patients in coma, those with head injuries or respiratory depression, and pregnant women who are likely to deliver within 1–2 hours.) Avoid overdosage of all drugs.

B. Fluid Replacement: The accurate determination of parenteral fluid requirements depends upon continuous clinical observation of blood pressure, temperature, pulse and respiratory rate, mental acuity, skin (color, temperature, and moisture), fluid intake, and urinary output. Frequent monitoring of central venous pressure and urine output and serial determination of blood pH and serum electrolytes, P_{O_2}, P_{CO_2}, and lactate are essential. Hemoglobin and hematocrit determinations may be useful but are not dependable guides to fluid replacement. Bacteriologic studies may be necessary (and are required in septic shock). Obtain blood for grouping, cross matching, hematocrit, coagulation time, complete blood count, and blood chemical determinations prior to starting an infusion.

If superficial veins have collapsed, puncture a large vein such as the femoral vein for temporary infusion prior to cutdown or perform percutaneous canalization of a major vessel such as the subclavian vein for central venous pressure determination. The latter procedure also provides a direct route for therapy to the heart in cases of extreme blood loss, septic shock, or serious electrolyte imbalance.

Restore adequate blood volume immediately. The most effective replacement fluid is usually whole blood, especially if the hematocrit is less than 35%. However, replacement of all blood loss with whole blood in complicated shock states is often harmful. Moreover, acid-base imbalances or dehydration may require correction, and solutions to correct specific problems (eg, mannitol for osmotic diuresis) may be necessary. Until whole blood can be given, consider intravenous administration of low-molecular-weight dextran, plasma, and plasma products (see below).

The normal central venous pressure (CVP) is 8–13 cm of water. If the central venous pressure is 8 cm of water or less, additional fluid replacement is essential, and very large amounts of blood or other fluids may be required, as judged by the initial estimate based on the patient's size. If blood volume replacement establishes normal cardiac function and adequate urine production (20–30 mL/h) with a central venous pressure of 10 cm of water, the problem probably was hypovolemia (corrected) regardless of cause. If shock, low arterial pressure, and poor circulation persist despite a central venous pressure of 10–13 cm of water, suspect cardiac insufficiency or fluid overload.

1. Whole blood–Whole blood must be correctly grouped and cross matched for possible transfusion. In dire emergencies, after initial resuscitation with crystalloid solutions (normal saline solution, lactated Ringer's injection), group O, Rh-negative blood may be used cautiously without cross matching. Treatment in cases of shock may require 4–5 L delivered under pressure in 30 minutes to restore central venous pressure to 10–13 cm of water. Use large needles and multiple venipuncture if transfusion is urgently needed.

2. Plasma–Plasma, serum albumin, and Plasmanate (a reconstituted blood product) are particularly valuable for the treatment of plasma loss. Posttransfusion hepatitis may occur in patients receiving pooled plasma; the risk is about 10%.

3. Plasma expanders–Dextran 40 (Rheomacrodex) is a low-molecular-weight dextran that is superior to other dextrans in reducing the viscosity of the blood and maintaining the microcirculation. Administer 1–1.5 g/kg in 10% solution in normal saline intravenously at a rate of 20–40 mL/min, but do not give more than required to sustain the blood pressure at 85–90 mm Hg. (*Caution:* Patients with cardiac or renal disease may develop pulmonary edema.) Since dextrans interfere with blood typing, blood samples should be obtained before dextran is administered. Dextrans can impair blood coagulation mechanisms and may cause infrequent (but serious) anaphylactoid reactions.

4. Saline, dextrose, mannitol* solutions–Normal saline solution, lactated Ringer's injection or 5% dextrose in saline (500–1000 mL intravenously) will expand blood volume for 1–2 hours until whole blood or blood products can be administered. Mannitol, 10% in normal saline solution, 200–300 mL intravenously, reduces renal vascular resistance, causes diuresis, and prevents lower nephron nephrosis. Saline is used as a diluent to avoid hyponatremia.

5. Correction of bicarbonate deficit–In shock therapy, severe acidosis, or hepatic insufficiency, sodium bicarbonate solution should be given to prevent or correct acidosis. The solution is available in vials containing 3.75 g (45 mEq) in 50 mL. The bicarbonate is given in 5% dextrose in water. The amount necessary to correct acidosis is determined by the blood pH (normal: 7.35–7.45) or serum or plasma P_{CO_2} (normal: 24–29 mEq/L). Serial determinations of these values should guide correction.

6. Adjustment of acid-base balance–Restore serum sodium, calcium, chloride, etc, to normal values, using periodic blood chemistry determinations as a guide.

C. Vasoactive Drugs: Vasopressors have almost no place in resuscitation if the patient is in shock. The only exception is cardiogenic shock, where a brief use of pressor drugs may increase myocardial contractility and thus improve cardiac function.

The vasodilator drugs are now in vogue in shock resuscitation. *The*

---

*Whether mannitol can be used safely in pregnancy is not definitely known.

vasoactive drugs should not be considered a primary form of therapy in shock. Volume replacement, correction of hypoxia and fluid and electrolyte imbalances, and a search for treatable causes should be done first. Unless volume replacement is adequate, the administration of vasodilators may result in prompt failure of the circulation due to a fall of blood pressure and circulatory collapse. Vasodilators are never indicated until the vascular volume has been restored to normal and the central venous pressure is in the high normal range. At that point, use of drugs that dilate the peripheral vasculature may decrease vascular resistance and thus decrease the work of the heart and improve cardiac output and tissue perfusion.

The drug of choice for cardiac resuscitation has been isoproterenol (Isuprel). This drug has 2 modes of action: it stimulates myocardial contractility and simultaneously lowers peripheral resistance. Give 1–2 mg in 500 mL of 5% dextrose in water intravenously at a rate that produces optimal circulatory benefit. Because of its inotropic effect, an increased incidence of cardiac arrhythmias precludes its use if the heart rate exceeds 120/min.

D. Corticosteroids: Corticosteroids may be beneficial in shock because they support the patient in a serious stress state, aid in the transfer of fluids from intra- to extracellular compartments, and, in septic shock, block intense sympathomimetic effects of endotoxin and restore vascular tone. They also have a beneficial antiallergic effect.

E. Treatment of Specific Types of Shock:

1. Cardiogenic shock–Convert arrhythmias. Digitalize for myocardial insufficiency. Relieve cardiac tamponade. Administer adrenergic drugs (see above).

2. Anaphylactic shock–

a. Give epinephrine, 1:1000 solution, 0.1–0.4 mL in 10 mL of normal saline solution slowly intravenously.

b. Give diphenhydramine hydrochloride or tripelennamine hydrochloride, 10–20 mg intravenously, if response to epinephrine is not prompt and sustained.

c. Give hydrocortisone sodium succinate (Solu-Cortef), 100–250 mg intravenously over a period of 30 seconds, as an adjunct to epinephrine and diphenhydramine. The dosage depends upon the severity of the condition. The drug may be repeated at increasing intervals (1, 3, 6, 10 hours, etc) as indicated by the clinical condition.

d. Inject aminophylline, 0.25–0.5 g in 10–20 mL of normal saline slowly intravenously for severe bronchial spasm. The duration of action is 1–3 hours, after which the drug may be repeated.

3. Hypovolemic shock–Replace volume, correct hypoxia and fluid and electrolyte balance, and seek treatable causes. Monitor treatment as discussed on p 306.

4. Septic shock–In addition to initial general shock therapy (see p 305), give specific treatment as follows:

a. Insert a central venous pressure line to monitor venous pressure and begin intravenous injection of plasma expander.

b. Give antimicrobial drugs aimed at the probable cause of sepsis: either of the following combinations may be used:

(1) Moxalactam, cefotaxime, or cefoperazone, 2 g every 4 hours into the intravenous infusion; plus an aminoglycoside, eg, amikacin, 15 mg/kg/d intramuscularly or intravenously.

(2) If the origin of sepsis is likely to be the female genital tract or the bowel, give clindamycin, 600 mg every 6 hours into the intravenous infusion, plus an aminoglycoside, as in (1).

c. Give methylprednisolone, 30 mg/kg intravenously twice. The interval between injections should be about 4 hours, and no more methylprednisolone should be given.

d. If organ perfusion appears to be poor, dopamine hydrochloride should be added into the intravenous line at a rate of 2–10 μg/kg/min.

e. Correct any electrolyte imbalances, and administer oxygen by nasal tube.

f. Continue search for a possible focus of infection and the source of sepsis (septic abortion, peritonitis, ruptured viscus, septic thrombophlebitis, etc).

g. If available, human globulin containing a high titer of antibodies to core glycolipid may markedly reduce the severity of shock and prevent death. (This is experimental.)

Evaluation of Antishock Therapy

Observe the patient continuously for clinical and laboratory signs of responses to therapy. Tachycardia subsides and the skin becomes warm and dry as blood pressure rises above 100 mm Hg.

(1) Record blood pressure, pulse rate, and respiratory rate every 15 minutes.

(2) Maintain a fluid intake and output chart, noting time and amount of replacement fluid given and measuring urine output every 30 minutes. Acute renal failure often is a sequela to deep, unresponsive, or prolonged shock.

(3) Monitor central venous pressure response, especially to initial rapid infusion or transfusion, as a guide both to diagnosis (hypovolemic versus cardiac shock) and to subsequent treatment. Try to rapidly achieve and maintain a normal central venous pressure (8–13 cm of water). Avoid under- or overreplacement of fluids.

(4) Auscultate the chest periodically for arrhythmia, rales, muffled tones (cardiac tamponade), or murmurs. Note the appearance of rales at lung bases (indicative of congestive failure). Obtain an ECG and appropriate medical consultation in severe cases.

(5) Determine CO_2 combining power; blood pH, Na^+, and K^+; hematocrit; and blood counts at intervals and compare with original values. Blood volume determinations (if available) may confirm the accuracy of estimates of fluid replacement needed. Nevertheless, these studies often are confusing because of regional blood pooling and fluid transfer between the intra- and extravascular spaces.

Anesthesia for the Shocked Patient

The choice of anesthesia for a major surgical or obstetric procedure for the patient in shock requires specific knowledge of the pharmacology and physiology involved. Ideally, the patient should respond to antishock therapy before operation. If the problem is critical, a calculated risk must be taken.

Preoperative medication should consist of atropine sulfate, 0.4 mg, well diluted in saline solution and given slowly intravenously. The following anesthetic methods are justified if the cause of shock has been accurately identified.

A. Hypovolemic Shock: Inhalation anesthesia with maximum oxygen concentration is preferable. Nitrous oxide and ethylene cause no electrolyte or metabolic impairment. Retention of CO_2 may occur if pulmonary ventilation is inadequate when cyclopropane, halothane, or fluroxene is used. Halothane often causes uterine relaxation, and further bleeding may occur. Regional anesthetic block may result in severe, uncontrollable hypotension. In vascular (caval) obstruction by the pregnant uterus, spinal or caudal anesthesia may further complicate the supine hypotensive syndrome. If this occurs, elevate the uterus; turn the patient to the semilateral position; place a support beneath the right hip to tilt the uterus to the left; and proceed with therapy.

B. Cardiogenic Shock: Local infiltration with the patient in Fowler's position is recommended.

C. Septic Shock: Cyclopropane probably is the best anesthetic, since vascular collapse, renal failure, and fever are present. Nitrous oxide and halothane administered in low concentration or minimal amounts of succinylcholine (the only muscle relaxant that is well hydrolyzed) is the second choice. (However, succinylmonocholine, produced during oliguria or anuria, may accumulate and retard dissipation of succinylcholine.)

D. Anaphylactic Shock: These patients rarely require surgery until improved. Use infiltration anesthesia when immediate operation is mandatory. Oxygen, vasopressors, and corticosteroids are of value. For bronchial spasm, give epinephrine by injection or inhalation (spray).

E. Neurogenic Shock: For replacement of uterine inversion (for example), any anesthetic with a rapid induction time (eg, cyclopropane or halothane) is the agent of choice.

Preeclampsia-Eclampsia (Eclamptogenic Toxemia; Toxemia of Pregnancy; Gestosis) & Other Hypertensive Disorders During Pregnancy

Preeclampsia-eclampsia is a disorder peculiar to pregnant women. The syndrome is characterized by hypertension, generalized edema, and proteinuria that usually occurs in the last trimester of pregnancy or the early puerperium (except when associated with hydatidiform mole). Eclampsia actually is the most fulminating degree of preeclampsia; it is characterized by convulsions and coma in addition to the other signs and symptoms of preeclampsia. Chronic hypertensive and renal disease may precede or be associated with preeclampsia-eclampsia and often predisposes to preeclampsia-eclampsia.

Primigravidas of all ages are most commonly affected. Preeclampsia-eclampsia is more prevalent among the nonwhite races, but this is probably due to economic factors and dietary deficiencies rather than racial susceptibility.

The importance of early recognition of preeclampsia-eclampsia cannot be overemphasized, especially since the patient is initially asymptomatic. Fulminating preeclampsia, usually diagnosed in the third trimester, probably could have been controlled earlier when symptoms were less serious. Uncontrolled preeclampsia may progress to eclampsia, permanent disability, or death and is a major cause (with hemorrhage and infection) of maternal death. Six to 7% of all pregnant women in the USA develop preeclampsia. About 5% of these cases progress to eclampsia, and about 5% of women with eclampsia die of the disease or its complications.

The cause of preeclampsia-eclampsia is not known, and speculation has been so extensive that this disorder has been called a "disease of theories." Predisposing factors include vascular and renal disease, diabetes mellitus, and malnutrition. A precipitating factor is probably interference with hormonal activity or metabolism by the placenta or decidua (eg, in diabetes mellitus), inasmuch as a fetus is not essential for the development of preeclampsia-eclampsia (which may occur in

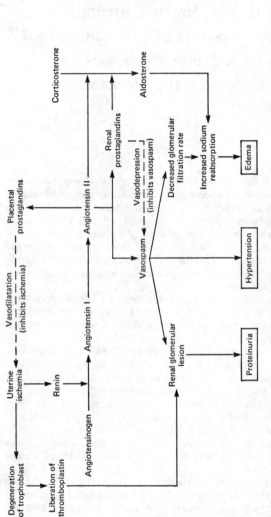

Figure 12–1. Preeclampsia-eclampsia may originate in relative ischemia of the uteroplacental unit, resulting in degeneration of trophoblastic tissue and release of thromboplastin. This may be followed by a compensatory response and then by aberration of the renin-prostaglandin system. Dashed arrows indicate inhibitory processes. (Modified and reproduced, with permission, from Speroff L: Toxemia in pregnancy. *Am J Cardiol* 1973;32:582.)

hydatidiform mole or after delivery). Uterine distention is not essential either, because preeclampsia-eclampsia has been associated with extrauterine pregnancy. No proximate toxic factor has been identified, though it has been suggested that hypersensitivity to angiotensin II, which activates the conversion of corticosterone to the pressor substance aldosterone, may be responsible for the abnormal vasospasm that occurs in preeclampsia-eclampsia. The importance of prostaglandins and angiotensin II in preeclampsia-eclampsia is suggested in Speroff's hypothesis of the mechanisms involved (Fig 12–1).

Pathologic Findings

In preeclampsia, there are no characteristic anatomic lesions; in eclampsia, definite gross and microscopic abnormalities are often seen. Although striking, the organic lesions generally are not sufficiently extensive to cause death. If the patient recovers from eclampsia, probably all of the morphologic abnormalities are reversible.

A. Brain: There may be edema with slight flattening of the convolutions. On section at necropsy, scattered focal hemorrhages may be found. Rarely, areas of infarction, eg, the pituitary, may be noted.

B. Lungs: "Wet" (edematous) congested lungs with multiple minute thrombi are commonly reported in patients who die of eclampsia.

C. Liver: Most patients have hepatic abnormalities. Usually the liver is pale, mottled, and firm, with small subcapsular hemorrhages. The capillaries around the portal spaces are dilated. Numerous small fibrin thrombi may be seen. Periportal hemorrhage, thrombosis, and necrosis are characteristic. The right lobe is usually more severely affected than the left.

D. Kidneys: The kidneys are usually slightly enlarged and pale. On section, the cortex is blanched and has numerous small hemorrhagic points. The glomerular vascular loop actually fills Bowman's capsule with large ischemic capillaries coiled in loops having ballooned tufts. The glomerular cells are swollen and prominent, but no evidence of proliferation is present. Adhesions between the thickened, wrinkled basement membrane and capillary rosette are typical. Vacuolization develops in the cells of the intercapillary space beneath the glomerular basement membrane. Scattered fibrin thrombi often are found. The tubules are often dilated with protein-containing urine. Few intraluminal red and white blood cells are seen. Hyaline degeneration and fatty infiltration of tubule cells are often found.

E. Placenta: No specific placental lesions are typical of preeclampsia-eclampsia. The placenta is often smaller than normal, however, and so-called red infarcts (intervillous fibrin deposits) are common. Premature aging or dysmaturity frequently occurs, as shown by increased and more severe endarteritis and periarteritis, a thinned and broken syncytium, and calcium and intervillous fibrin deposition.

F. Blood: Disseminated intravascular coagulation may develop as a result of patchy areas of placental degeneration and separation. Microfibrin emboli may be dispatched to the lungs, liver, or kidneys.

G. Fetus: Intrauterine growth retardation due to reduced uteroplacental perfusion may be marked. Fetal death may follow hypoxia or acidosis.

Pathologic Physiology

A. Arteriolar Spasm: Arteriolar spasm, consistently observed in the retinas, kidneys, and splanchnic region, promotes hypertension. A heightened pressor (and depressor) response indicates the lability of the vascular system.

B. Sodium and Water Retention:

1. Reduced glomerular filtration–A small volume of urine permits more efficient sodium reabsorption by the renal tubules. Sodium retention is an adjunct of growth and is normal during pregnancy, but sodium retention is exaggerated in preeclampsia-eclampsia. Nonetheless, retention of sodium does not cause this disorder.

2. Reduced serum levels of albumin and globulin resulting from proteinuria account for the diminished osmotic pressure of the blood despite hemoconcentration.

3. In certain patients, increased excretion of corticosteroids (including aldosterone) and vasopressin suggests increased tissue concentrations of these substances; this results in greater sodium and water retention.

C. Proteinuria: Degenerative changes in the glomeruli permit loss of protein via the urine. The albumin/globulin ratio in the urine of patients with preeclampsia-eclampsia is approximately 3:1 (in contrast with 6:7 in patients with glomerulonephritis). Renal tubular disease contributes only slightly to the leakage of protein. When the volume of urine is small, the protein concentration is high: excretion of less than 500 mL of urine per day is associated with a urine protein level of 1–4 g/dL (3–4+).

D. Hematology: Severe preeclampsia-eclampsia should be included with the disorders of coagulation because disseminated intravascular coagulation of varying degrees so frequently occurs. The severity of the coagulation defect does not always correlate with the severity of preeclampsia-eclampsia. Nonetheless, some hemolysis—eg, microangiopathic hemolytic anemia, deformed red blood cells, reduced fibrinogen, or increased fibrinogen degradation products—may be noted in patients with preeclampsia-eclampsia.

E. Blood Chemistry:

1. Elevated serum levels of uric acid, urea nitrogen, and creatinine are due to impaired renal clearance of these catabolites.

2. Some serum albumin and globulin are lost via the urine, but

blood proteins must also be lost or destroyed in other ways, because proteinuria alone is not sufficient to explain the abnormally low protein levels in severe cases of preeclampsia-eclampsia.

3. Low CO_2 combining power, especially after convulsions, is due to acidosis, caused in part by an increase in serum lactic acid.

4. Increased sulfobromophthalein retention and elevated levels of hepatic enzymes (eg, SGOT) indicate hepatic dysfunction.

Clinical Findings

A. Symptoms and Signs:

1. Preeclampsia–Preeclampsia is characterized by hypertension, generalized edema, and proteinuria in the absence of vascular or renal disease. The manifestations develop from the 24th week of pregnancy through the fourth week after delivery. Severe, persistent, generalized headache; vertigo; malaise; and nervous irritability are prominent symptoms due in part to cerebral edema. Scintillating scotomas and partial or complete blindness are due to edema of the retina, retinal hemorrhage, or retinal detachment. Epigastric pain, nausea, and liver tenderness are the result of congestion, thrombosis of the periportal system, and subcapsular hepatic hemorrhages.

a. Hypertension–Preeclampsia is diagnosed when persistent hypertension or a sudden rise in blood pressure, plus generalized edema and proteinuria, is observed during at least the last 3 months of pregnancy. If hypertension exists before the 20th week of pregnancy or for more than 6 weeks after delivery, it is due to hypertensive disease. If preeclampsia-eclampsia is superimposed on preexisting cardiovascular or renal hypertensive disease, there is an additional elevation of blood pressure, and management is more difficult and the prognosis more grave for both mother and infant. Ninety-five percent of cases of preeclampsia-eclampsia occur after the 32nd week, and about 75% of these patients are primigravidas. The incidence (6–7% of all pregnant women in the USA) is at least doubled with multiple pregnancy, hydatidiform mole, and polyhydramnios.

The blood pressure normally rises slightly with increasing age. Adult nonpregnant women are considered to be "normotensive" (ie, not hypertensive) with a systolic blood pressure less than 140 mm Hg or a diastolic blood pressure less than 90 mm Hg (or both). In pregnant women of any age, hypertension exists (1) when the systolic pressure is 140 mm Hg or more or the diastolic pressure is 90 mm Hg or more or (2) when there is a rise of 30 mm Hg or more above the patient's prepregnant systolic level or 15 mm Hg or more above the prepregnant diastolic level (for 2 or more days). Hypertonicity of the vasculature is responsible.

Roll-over test: The roll-over test, which may identify women likely to develop preeclampsia-eclampsia, should be done at each visit from the 24th week on. The test is performed as follows: (1) Allow the patient to rest on her left side for at least 5 minutes. (2) Determine the blood pressure once it is stable. (3) Roll the patient onto her back; measure the blood pressure again. (4) Measure the blood pressure again in 5 minutes. If the diastolic pressure rises by 20 mm Hg or more when the patient turns from the lateral recumbent to the supine position, the test is positive (even though the blood pressure remains within the normal range), and the woman has approximately a 60% chance of developing preeclampsia. If the test is negative, the likelihood of the patient developing preeclampsia is about 1 in 100.

b. Edema–The generalized edema of preeclampsia must be apparent *above* the waist. Such patients usually have a weight gain of 1.8 kg (4 lb) or more during any 1- to 2-week period from the 24th through the 35th week of pregnancy or a gain of 0.9 kg (2 lb) or more per week from the 35th week to term.

Swelling due to fluid accumulation is first noted in the lower extremities and soon becomes generalized. Edema involving the upper part of the body is always a pathologic finding; it may be an early indication of preeclampsia. Tightness of finger rings and puffiness of the face are danger signs. Oliguria accompanies edema in many patients; anuria is a grave sign.

c. Proteinuria–Any grossly detectable protein in a urine specimen obtained by catheterization or the clean-catch method is abnormal. If urine output is normal, proteinuria exists when proteinuria of 1+ or more is found with a qualitative test or when quantitative analysis of a 24-hour urine collection shows a minimum of 100 mg/dL. Increased glomerular permeability is the cause. (Pyuria or hematuria is due to other causes.)

Note: Many believe it is illogical to designate mild and severe preeclampsia as different categories, because such designations detract from a proper appreciation of the seriousness of the disorder.

2. Eclampsia–A patient with signs of preeclampsia who has at least one convulsion or episode of coma between the 24th week of pregnancy and the end of the second week after delivery (including the third stage of labor) must be presumed to have eclampsia if other causes can be excluded. Eclampsia is classified according to the time of occurrence of the first convulsion with respect to the time of delivery: (1) Prepartal eclampsia denotes convulsions before delivery. In intercurrent eclampsia, the patient is free of convulsions for at least 24 hours during the antenatal period; this designation is continued until the patient is delivered or has another convulsion. Patients in this group tolerate labor much better and can be delivered with greater safety than most intrapartal eclamptics. (2) Intrapartal eclampsia denotes one or more convulsions during labor or delivery. (3) Postpartal eclampsia denotes one or more convulsions after the third stage of labor and through 4 weeks after delivery. Almost 90% of convulsions during the early puerperium occur on the first day.

Preconvulsive symptoms may be noted in severe preeclampsia. Eclampsia is further characterized by generalized tonic-clonic convulsions; coma after convulsions, followed by amnesia and confusion; marked hypertension preceding a convulsion, with hypotension thereafter (during coma or vascular collapse); stertorous breathing, rhonchi, and frothing at the mouth; twitching of muscle groups (face, arms, etc); nystagmus; and oliguria or anuria.

B. Laboratory Findings:

1. Preeclampsia–Only urinalysis (revealing proteinuria without hematuria or pyuria) is helpful in diagnosis. The hematocrit rises in proportion to the severity of preeclampsia. Blood chemistry values are usually slightly elevated. Serial blood urea nitrogen and serum uric acid determinations often show a gradual increase concomitant with reduction of creatinine clearance as preeclampsia becomes more severe.

2. Eclampsia is associated with proteinuria of 3+ to 4+, hemoconcentration, a greatly reduced blood CO_2 combining power, and increased serum uric acid, blood nonprotein nitrogen, and blood urea nitrogen levels.

C. Special Examinations: Ophthalmoscopic examination may reveal papilledema, retinal edema (increased "sheen"), retinal detachment, vascular spasm, arteriovenous "nicking," and hemorrhages. Repeated examination is helpful in determining improvement or failure of treatment in preeclampsia-eclampsia.

Differential Diagnosis

Hypertensive disease and renal disease are discussed here because it is important to differentiate them from preeclampsia and because preeclampsia-eclampsia is frequently superimposed upon them. Atypical disorders associated with hypertension or proteinuria should be reevaluated 4–6 months after delivery.

A. Chronic Hypertensive Cardiovascular Disease or Essential Hypertension: Hypertension is a significant sign in essential hypertension, arteriosclerosis, glomerulonephritis, pyelonephritis, and preeclampsia-eclampsia. A history of persistent blood pressure elevation before pregnancy is the most valuable clue to the diagnosis, but if hypertension is detected before the 20th week (when normotension or hypotension is the rule), it is safe to conclude that it was present before pregnancy. Preeclampsia and eclampsia occur before the 24th week only in hydatidiform mole.

Chronic hypertensive disease complicates 10–15% of all pregnancies. A family history of hypertension is recognized in 75% of all pregnant women with essential hypertension. Multiparas or women over 35 years of age are most commonly affected. The blood pressure is labile to activity, heat and cold, sedation, and emotional stress. Slight proteinuria may be noted. Blood chemistry and renal function studies show

Table 12–1. Differential diagnosis of chronic hypertensive cardiovascular disease and preeclampsia.*

Features	Hypertensive Disease	Preeclampsia
Onset of hypertension	Before pregnancy; during first 20 weeks of pregnancy.	After 20th week of pregnancy (exception: trophoblastic tumors).
Duration of hypertension	Permanent. Hypertension persists beyond 3 months postpartum.	Hypertension usually absent at 6 weeks postpartum; always by 3 months postpartum.
Family history	Often positive.	Usually negative; may be positive.
Past history	Recurrent "toxemia."	Psychosexual problems common.
Age	Usually older.	Generally teenage, early 20s.
Parity	Usually multigravida.	Usually primigravida.
Habitus	May be thin or brachymorphic.	Usually eumorphic.
Retinal findings	Often arteriovenous nicking, tortuous arterioles, cotton wool exudates, hemorrhages.	Vascular spasm, retinal edema; rarely, protein extravasations.
Proteinuria	Often none.	Usually present (see definition); absent at 6 weeks postpartum.

*Reproduced, with permission, from de Alvarez RR: Chapter 34 in *Current Obstetric & Gynecologic Diagnosis & Treatment,* 4th ed. Benson RC (editor). Lange, 1982.

normal results unless the disease is severe. The changes in the retinal arterioles (eg, narrowing), cardiac enlargement, electrocardiographic changes, arrhythmias, and other findings are proportionate to the severity of the disease. Sudden, excessive weight gain and generalized edema are not present unless toxemia is superimposed.

B. Primary Renal Disease: Chronic glomerulonephritis, chronic pyelonephritis, and polycystic kidney disease account for only about 5% of all instances of hypertension during pregnancy but are accompanied by preeclampsia in almost 50% of cases. Renal disease almost always antedates the pregnancy. A history of glomerulonephritis after scarlet fever or pyelonephritis—or a family history of polycystic kidney disease—is of great value in the diagnosis. Gross proteinuria and cellular elements and casts in the centrifuged sediment (with or without hypertension) are usually noted at the first visit. The specific gravity of the urine is of narrowed range or fixed. Retinal damage may be present.

C. Convulsive Disorders: Convulsions may be due to hypertensive encephalopathy, epilepsy, thromboembolism, drug intoxication or withdrawal, trauma, hypoglycemia, hypocalcemia (of parathyroid or renal origin), hemolytic crisis of sickle cell anemia, or the tetany of alkalosis as well as eclampsia.

D. Coma: Coma usually follows the convulsions of eclampsia, but it may occur instead of convulsions. Other causes of coma (in descending order of probability) are epilepsy, syncope, alcohol or other drug intoxication, acidosis or hypoglycemia (diabetes), stroke, and azotemia.

Complications

A. Early: About 5% of preeclamptic patients develop eclampsia. The more marked the symptoms, the greater the likelihood of convulsions and coma and the higher the fetal and maternal mortality and morbidity rates. Convulsions increase the maternal mortality rate 10-fold and the fetal mortality rate 40-fold. The causes of maternal death due to eclampsia are (in descending order of frequency) circulatory collapse (cardiac arrest, pulmonary edema, shock), cerebral hemorrhage, and renal failure. The fetus usually dies of hypoxia or acidosis.

Blindness (due to retinal detachment or intracranial hemorrhage) or paralysis (due to cerebrovascular accident) may persist in patients who survive eclampsia.

About 30% of patients who develop premature separation of the placenta have one of the hypertensive disorders. Approximately half of such patients will be found to have hypertensive disease and about one-fourth preeclampsia-eclampsia. So-called "toxic separation of the placenta" (abruptio placentae) is almost always associated with severe preeclampsia or eclampsia.

Renal or hepatic failure and disseminated intravascular coagulation are rare complications.

Postpartal hemorrhage is common in patients with hypertensive syndromes during pregnancy.

Toxic delirium in patients with eclampsia, either before or after delivery, poses serious medical and nursing problems.

Injuries incurred during convulsions include lacerations of lips and tongue and fractures of the vertebrae. Aspiration pneumonia may also occur.

B. Late: Fifteen to 20% of patients with severe preeclampsia or eclampsia (without known preexisting hypertensive or renal disease) suffer a recurrence of preeclampsia-eclampsia with subsequent pregnancies. This is probably due to the initial problem, ie, undiagnosed chronic hypertensive cardiovascular disease.

Permanent hypertension, the result of vascular damage, does not occur as a result of preeclampsia-eclampsia (see below).

Preeclampsia is superimposed upon chronic hypertensive disease in at least 50% of cases; the seriousness of the preeclampsia-eclampsia is directly related to the severity of the underlying cardiovascular disorder. Fetal growth may be retarded, probably because of reduced uterine blood flow and placental dysmaturity (premature aging). The perinatal mortality rate is much higher than that in normal pregnancies or in preeclampsia-eclampsia not associated with chronic hypertensive cardiovascular disease.

In women with mild hypertensive disease who do not develop preeclampsia, repeated pregnancies will not cause a progression of the hypertensive disease.

It is usually impossible to determine the vascular and renal status of the patient before pregnancy. Therefore, some patients who are assumed to have post-preeclampsia-eclampsia hypertension probably have chronic hypertensive disease that was not apparent before pregnancy but has continued without relation to the pregnancy.

Prevention

Since there are no known specific causes of preeclampsia-eclampsia, prevention can be achieved only in a general way by providing the highest quality prenatal care whenever the possibility of preeclampsia is suggested by the history and initial examination (eg, patients with diabetes mellitus or hypertensive or renal disease). Frequent prenatal examinations are essential, and every effort must be made to obtain the confidence and cooperation of the patient. The diet during pregnancy should be high in proteins and contain adequate vitamins and minerals. The patient should be permitted to gain about 12 kg (25 lb) more than her ideal nonpregnant weight; if she is overweight, she should be helped to lose cautiously. A moderate salt intake is reasonable. Diuretics should not be used. Alert diagnosis and effective management of prodromal symptoms prevent clinical preeclampsia in the third trimester.

Patients with severe cardiovascular and renal disease should be advised to avoid pregnancy. (However, unless hypertension or infection supervenes, pregnancy or preeclampsia-eclampsia will not impair renal function due to primary renal disease.)

Treatment

The objectives of treatment include (1) prevention or limitation of convulsions and coma, (2) avoidance of cardiovascular and renal complications, (3) reduction of general vasospasm, (4) correction of fluid and electrolyte imbalances and hematologic abnormalities, and (5) delivery of a normal fetus that will survive.

Treat preeclamptic patients vigorously. Monitor the fetus by fetal activity determination (FAD) and estriol determinations before labor and by electronic monitoring during labor. Deliver by the means that is most expeditious and least harmful to the patient and fetus. After the 34th week, cesarean section may be indicated for patients who do not respond to therapy or who are not good candidates for induction of labor. Fetal death may occur if delivery is delayed more than 2 weeks in preeclampsia.

Eclampsia must be treated by appropriate palliative measures. Conservative treatment is indicated initially. Pregnancy should not be terminated until the patient has definitely recovered from the convulsive episode. Monitor eclamptic patients and their fetuses as indicated above.

A. Preeclampsia: The objectives of treatment are to prevent eclampsia and vascular accidents, to preserve the pregnancy until the fetus is known to be viable, and to deliver a normal, viable infant.

Treatment consists of palliative measures and termination of pregnancy at the appropriate time.

1. Home management–Most patients with early preeclampsia can be managed at home. A patient who has not responded to the following program of treatment after 48 hours must be hospitalized for more intensive care.

a. General measures–Place the patient at bed rest; allow few visitors for brief periods. Bed rest should increase uterine blood flow, lower blood pressure, and improve fetal well-being.

b. Examinations and procedures–Determine blood pressure daily when the patient is awake; determine protein levels daily in clean-catch morning urine specimens.

c. Diet and fluids–Allow a normal diet with 100 g of protein. Record fluid intake and output. If urine output is within the normal range (1000 mL or more daily), encourage a fluid intake of 2500 mL/d.

d. Medications–Give sedatives, eg, diazepam, 5 mg orally 3 times daily.

2. Hospital care–Any patient who does not respond to home management (as above) after 48 hours must be hospitalized; complete rest is mandatory.

a. Examinations and procedures–If blood pressure rises above 165/100 mm Hg, especially if the patient is hyperreflexic, give magnesium sulfate or other antihypertensive drug (see below). Measure protein quantitatively each day in a 24-hour urine collection. (If possible, obtain urine by the clean-catch method to avoid admixture with vaginal mucus.) Determine serum concentrations of nonprotein nitrogen, creatinine, and protein. Uric acid levels may be useful but are not essential. Perform daily ophthalmoscopic examination, noting in particular arteriolar spasm, edema, hemorrhages, and exudates.

b. Diet and fluids–Prescribe a high-protein diet (1800 kcal). Record fluid intake and output. If urine output exceeds 500 mL/d, give fluids to replace this amount. Fluids should be neither specifically limited nor forced.

c. Sedatives and anticonvulsants–Give sedatives in adequate doses (eg, phenobarbital, 60 mg orally 3 times daily) to calm the patient. Prevent or control convulsions with magnesium sulfate, never with morphine, thiopental, phenytoin, or diazepam. The latter drugs impair cerebral oxygenation and renal function and depress fetal circulation and metabolic exchange.

The dosage of magnesium sulfate is 4–6 g in 5% dextrose in water given slowly intravenously over a period of 10–20 minutes, followed by

1 g/h to achieve a blood level of 6–7 mEq/L. Magnesium sulfate is excreted only in the urine; therefore, the dosage should be reduced for oliguric patients. If diuresis develops, the dosage can be increased. For severe convulsions, give magnesium sulfate intravenously for 12–18 hours after delivery.

In addition to preventing convulsions, magnesium sulfate also causes splanchnic vasodilatation, with resultant lowering of blood pressure. Urine output is increased.

Magnesium depresses the central nervous system. The normal serum magnesium concentration is 1.5–3 mEq/L. Deep tendon reflexes—particularly knee jerks—decrease when the magnesium level is above 4 mEq/L and disappear at magnesium levels near 10 mEq/L; at levels of about 12.5 mEq/L, respirations are slowed or absent and cardiac arrest may occur. Consequently, a repeat parenteral dose is contraindicated by any of the following findings: (1) urine output less than 100 mL/h in the preceding 4 hours, (2) respiratory rate below 16/min, or (3) absent or very sluggish knee jerk. Marked slowing of respiration or hyporeflexia in the newborn infant of a mother who has been receiving magnesium sulfate also suggests the possibility of a toxic serum level of magnesium. In cases of overdosage or unexpected reduction of urine output, give a calcium salt such as calcium gluconate, 20 mL of 10% aqueous solution slowly intravenously, and repeat every hour until urinary, respiratory, and neurologic depression has cleared. (Do not give more than 8 injections of a calcium salt within 24 hours.)

d. Diuretics–Diuretics are contraindicated in the treatment of preeclampsia-eclampsia.

e. Antihypertensive drugs–Diazoxide may be the most effective drug for the treatment of severe hypertensive crises in which an immediate effect is essential. Diazoxide is packaged in ampules containing 300 mg/20 mL. When diazoxide is given in 30-mg boluses (diluted) intravenously every 1–2 minutes with continuous monitoring of the blood pressure, a rapid effect may be expected. The drug should be discontinued when the diastolic pressure reaches 100 mm Hg. The duration of effect is 4–12 hours; therapy may be repeated after that time.

Hydralazine causes vasodilatation and increases cerebral, coronary, and renal circulation and function. Give 20–40 mg in 250 mL of 5% dextrose in water slowly intravenously for a potent hypotensive effect. After the blood pressure has been reduced gradually to normal levels, 150 mg of the drug orally 4 times daily will often control marked hypertension, although one-tenth of this dose administered in dilute solution intravenously 3–4 times daily may be more effective. The most common side-effects are tachycardia, nausea, and vomiting.

f. Anticoagulants–If clinical disseminated intravascular coagulation develops, heparinization prior to delivery may improve the prognosis, but a reversal of the heparin effect with protamine sulfate during early labor is recommended.

g. Fetal assessment–Determine fetal maturity (L/S ratio or rapid surfactant test) and monitor the fetal status closely by means of serial plasma or 24-hour urinary estriol levels so that delivery can be properly planned. Fetal activity determination and an oxytocin challenge test may be important because reduced uterine blood flow and placental function may become critical factors in preeclampsia-eclampsia. Monitor the fetal heart rate carefully.

B. Eclampsia:

1. General measures–Hospitalize the patient in a single, darkened, quiet room, at absolute bed rest with bed rails in place for protection during convulsions; and provide special nurses around the clock. Allow no visitors (not even the husband).

Do not disturb the patient for unnecessary procedures (eg, enemas, tub baths), and leave the blood pressure cuff on her arm. Turn the patient on her side to prevent inferior vena cava syndrome and aspiration of vomitus. The following should be kept at hand: a padded tongue blade to be placed between the patient's teeth during convulsions; a bulb syringe and catheter or suction machine to aspirate mucus or vomitus from the mouth, glottis, or trachea; and an oxygen cone or tent (masks and nasal catheters produce excessive stimulation). Typed and cross-matched whole blood must be available for immediate use because patients in eclampsia often develop premature separation of the placenta with hemorrhage and are susceptible to shock.

2. Laboratory tests–Insert a retention catheter so that the amount of urine passed can be accurately measured. Determine quantitatively the protein content of each 24-hour urine specimen until the fourth or fifth postpartal day. Nonprotein nitrogen, CO_2 combining power, and serum protein levels should be determined (for evidence of nitrogen retention and acidosis) as often as the severity and progression of the disease indicate. Creatinine clearance tests may indicate impending renal failure; sulfobromophthalein retention and greatly elevated levels of hepatic enzymes may presage liver failure. Coagulation studies may suggest disseminated intravascular coagulation.

3. Physical examination–Check the blood pressure hourly during the acute phase and every 2–4 hours thereafter. Evaluate fetal heart tones every time the mother's blood pressure is obtained. Perform ophthalmoscopic examination once a day. Examine the face, extremities, and especially the sacrum (which becomes dependent when the patient is in bed) for signs of edema.

4. Diet and fluids–If the patient is convulsing, give nothing by mouth. If she can eat and drink, give a low-sodium (1 g of sodium chloride per day), high-carbohydrate, high-protein, low-fat diet (1500 kcal). Provide potassium chloride as a salt substitute. Measure and record fluid intake and output for each 24-hour period. If the urine output exceeds 700 mL/d, replace the output plus invisible fluid loss (approximately 500 mL/d) with salt-free fluid (including parenteral fluids). Give 200–300 mL of 20% dextrose in water 2–3 times a day during the acute phase to protect the liver, to replace fluids, and to aid in nutrition. (Do not give 50% glucose; it will sclerose the veins.) Use no sodium-containing fluids (eg, physiologic saline, Ringer's injection).

Give 25–50 mL of salt-poor albumin or 250–500 mL of plasma or serum if oliguria is present or if the serum protein concentration is less than 5 g/dL. Since serum contains sodium, it should be used only if salt-poor albumin is not available.

5. Sedatives–Administer a mild sedative upon admission and maintain reasonable sedation thereafter.

6. Anticonvulsant–Magnesium sulfate is by far the best anticonvulsant. This drug is toxic even at slight overdosage. Dosage, precautions, contraindications, and antidote are discussed on pp 321–322.

7. Delivery–The most direct method of treatment of eclampsia is termination of pregnancy. Control eclampsia before attempting induction of labor or delivery. Determine the relative maturity and well-being of the fetus by amniocentesis and serial estriol measurements. Use electronic fetal monitoring. Deliver the infant by the safest, most expeditious method. Cesarean section is preferred for primigravidas, but induction by rupture of the membranes and vaginal delivery may be appropriate for some multiparas. The method of delivery should be individualized; indications for cesarean section have been liberalized. However, cesarean section may be lethal for a patient with continuing convulsions or coma; convulsions and coma should be absent for a period of 12 hours before elective cesarean section is performed.

For cesarean section, well-controlled epidural or caudal anesthesia may be employed. Spinal anesthesia is contraindicated because it may cause sudden, severe hypotension. After delivery, give thiopental anesthesia during abdominal closure. If an anesthesiologist is not available, procaine, 0.5 or 1% (or its equivalent), can be used for local infiltration of the abdominal wall. For vaginal delivery, pudendal block is preferred.

Obstetric patients with chronic hypertensive cardiovascular or renal disease should be managed in a manner similar to those with preeclampsia. Many of the former will have superimposed preeclampsia, and it may not be possible to decide what the basic problem actually was until at least 3–4 months after delivery, when appropriate tests and studies should be ordered.

Prognosis

Preeclampsia subsides following delivery, but in severe cases, eclampsia may occur 1–4 weeks postpartum.

The hypertensive syndromes of pregnancy, including preeclampsia-eclampsia, rarely cause maternal death unless eclampsia occurs, but these disorders are a major maternal cause of perinatal death (at least 20% in the USA). The maternal mortality rate in eclampsia is 10–15%. The prognosis for the mother and fetus in preeclampsia-eclampsia depends upon the adequacy of prenatal care, the time of onset and duration of the disorder, the occurrence of eclampsia, the development of premature separation of the placenta, and the adequacy of treatment. Most patients with preeclampsia-eclampsia improve strikingly in 24–48 hours with modern therapy. However, because hypertension and proteinuria usually persist and very few patients are cured, early termination of pregnancy is usually required.

Conservative therapy will benefit the fetus more than delivery before the 34th week. After this time, if medical therapy is unsuccessful, delivery must be considered. Cesarean section offers the best hope of delivering a viable infant.

Although infants of mothers with preeclampsia-eclampsia are small for their gestational age (mainly because of placental dysfunction), these newborns fare better than premature infants of the same weight born of nonhypertensive mothers. If the duration of pregnancy can be accurately determined, the fact that the fetus is small is an added incentive to early delivery.

Eclampsia in the first pregnancy does not result in chronic hypertension. However, many multiparas who have had preeclampsia-eclampsia may later be found to have hypertensive disease. In such cases, chronic hypertensive cardiovascular or renal disease probably was present but undiagnosed during the pregnancy.

Medical & Surgical
13 | Complications
During Pregnancy*

DERMATOLOGIC COMPLICATIONS

Pregnancy has a sparing effect on most dermatoses; with a few exceptions, skin disorders during pregnancy and the puerperium are similar to those in nonpregnant women.

Dermatologic disorders induced by pregnancy include abnormalities of pigmentation (eg, chloasma), herpes gestationis, noninflammatory pruritus of pregnancy, angiectids or vascular spiders, and erythema palmare. Dermatologic disorders usually aggravated by pregnancy include candidal vulvovaginitis, acne vulgaris (early in pregnancy), erythema multiforme, dermatitis herpetiformis, granuloma inguinale, condylomata acuminata, pemphigus, neurofibromatosis, and systemic lupus erythematosus. It is unlikely that malignant melanoma is aggravated by pregnancy. Pregnancy is likely to have a beneficial effect on acne (late in pregnancy), psoriasis, and seborrheic dermatitis.

Chloasma (Melasma)

Chloasma consists of blotchy, petal-shaped, yellowish-brown pigmented patches symmetrically distributed over the forehead, nose, and malar prominences. These become confluent to form the "mask of pregnancy." Chloasma usually fades soon after delivery. Only cosmetic treatment is required. Hydroquinone cream (Eldoquin), 2%, applied nightly, may limit the development or speed the clearing of chloasma, but skin may develop a grayish color.

Herpes Gestationis

This serious but rare disease, which occurs only during pregnancy, may be a variation of dermatitis herpetiformis, a disease of unknown cause. It is an intensely burning, itching, occasionally painful, urticarial, papulovesicular eruption that involves the buttocks, legs, back, upper abdomen, and extensor surfaces but rarely affects the mucosa. Grouped vesicles on inflammatory bases are typical. The lesions leave small

*Carcinoma of the breast during pregnancy is discussed in Chapter 20.

pigmented scars on healing. This disease usually begins after the fifth month of pregnancy. A high eosinophil count in blood and vesicle fluid is usual. Biopsy shows subepidermal bullae and increased numbers of eosinophils in tissue. Herpes gestationis almost always disappears after pregnancy.

Treat first with sulfonamides, 1 g orally 3 times daily for 1 week and then 0.5–1 g daily. If this is unsuccessful, give corticotropin repository injection (gel), 50 units intramuscularly daily for 3 days, followed by prednisone (or equivalent), 20–30 mg orally daily in divided doses for 10–14 days. If improvement occurs, reduce the dose of prednisone to the lowest amount that will control the disorder.

Termination of pregnancy may be justified in severe, unresponsive cases of herpes gestationis.

Herpes gestationis may recur in subsequent pregnancies.

Noninflammatory Pruritus of Pregnancy

The cause is not known. No cutaneous lesions can be seen, but the patient experiences intense itching all over the body. Areas excoriated by scratching may become infected.

A papular pruritic dermatosis of pregnancy with a high fetal mortality rate has been described recently. Abnormally elevated hCG levels are reported with this dermatologic problem but not with noninflammatory pruritus of pregnancy. Symptomatic therapy is advised for the latter.

Erythema Palmare

This benign disorder is a dusky thenar and hypothenar vascular engorgement of the skin of the hands noted 4–6 weeks after the onset of pregnancy. The erythema disappears during the early puerperium. It is based upon genetic predisposition and provoked by hyperestrogenism (as are vascular spiders also; see below).

Vascular Spiders or Spider Angiomas

These are small, red, pulsating (arteriolar) telangiectatic points in the skin over the face, neck, thorax, and arms. Most vascular spiders develop during the second and third trimesters of pregnancy and fade almost to invisibility after delivery. They reappear during later advanced pregnancies. In most instances, these angiomas have only minor, temporary cosmetic significance, but the possibility that cirrhosis and hereditary hemorrhagic telangiectasia (and their complications) may be related must be kept in mind.

Pruritic Urticarial Papules & Plaques of Pregnancy

This recently described, intensely pruritic cutaneous eruption of late pregnancy is of unknown origin. Symptoms include numerous erythematous urticarial papules and myriads of minute plaques that first appear on the abdomen and then spread to involve the thighs and, at times, the buttocks and arms. Tissue biopsy of the lesions aids in the differential diagnosis, which includes herpes gestationis, prurigo gravidarum, and papular dermatitis of pregnancy. Corticosteroid therapy is moderately beneficial, but the dermatitis improves rapidly after delivery. Occasional patients have slight subsequent itching of the hands, sometimes during menses. The infants are free of skin abnormalities. Because of the small number of patients followed, the probability of recurrence of the disorder in subsequent pregnancies is uncertain.

HEART DISEASE

Congenital heart disease now is the principal cardiovascular problem complicating pregnancy in the USA. Rheumatic heart disease is less of a problem today than a generation ago because of better rheumatic fever prophylaxis, improved health care, and advances in cardiovascular surgery. Syphilitic carditis still occurs. Reported incidences of heart disease vary from 0.5 to 2% of obstetric patients.

Heart disease is a major cause of maternal death, but maternal and perinatal mortality rates are only slightly increased if the disability is minimal. With marked degrees of cardiac disease, the maternal mortality rate is 1–3% and the perinatal mortality rate may reach 50% even in large medical centers.

Functional Classification of Heart Disease*

For practical purposes, the functional capacity of the heart is the best single measurement of cardiopulmonary status.

Class I: Ordinary physical activity causes no discomfort.

Class II: Ordinary activity causes discomfort and slight disability.

Class III: Less than ordinary activity causes discomfort or disability; patient is barely compensated.

Class IV: Patient decompensated; any physical activity causes acute distress.

Eighty per cent of obstetric patients with heart disease have lesions that do not interfere seriously with their activities (classes I and II) and usually do well. About 85% of deaths ascribed to heart disease complicating pregnancy occur in patients with class III or IV lesions (20% of all pregnant patients with heart disease). Nevertheless, much can still be

*New York Heart Association, 1964.

done to improve the prognosis for the mother and infant in these unfavorable circumstances.

Pathologic Physiology

The effects of pregnancy on certain circulatory and respiratory functions are summarized in Table 13–1.

Three major burdens on the heart are associated with pregnancy: cardiac output is increased by more than one-third; the heart rate is accelerated by 10 beats per minute; and the blood volume is expanded by one-third. These unavoidable stresses must be considered in appraising the patient's ability to undergo pregnancy, delivery, and the puerperium.

In addition to these unavoidable physiologic burdens, there are avoidable or treatable medical liabilities, eg, anemia, obesity, hyperthyroidism, myxedema, infection, and emotional and physical stresses.

Youth, adequate functional cardiac reserve, stability of the cardiac lesion, and an optimistic, cooperative attitude are important assets that do much to improve the cardiac patient's chances for a successful confinement.

Labor, delivery, and the early puerperium impose the following specific physiologic burdens on the maternal heart:

A. During Labor and Delivery:

1. The heart rate increases with the beginning of each contraction in response to intermittent physical stress, slows at the end of each contraction, and returns to the resting level between contractions.

Table 13–1. Effect of pregnancy on maternal circulatory and respiratory functions.

Function	Change
Heart rate	Slow increase of 10–20 beats/min between 14 and 30 weeks. Rate maintained at this level to 40 weeks.
Arterial blood pressure	Systolic unchanged or slightly decreased until 20th week, then rises to prepregnancy levels. Diastolic slightly reduced (period of maximal pulse pressure).
Venous blood pressure	Arms: No change. Legs: Gradual marked increase between 8 and 40 weeks.
Cardiac output	Increases from about 4.5 L/min before pregnancy to 6–7 L/min by the tenth week, then plateaus until delivery.
Total body water	Increases by 1–2 kg by term.
Plasma and blood volume	Rises 25% between 12 and 34 weeks, then declines slightly to 40 weeks.
Red cell mass	Augmented 10–15% between 8 and 40 weeks.
Vital capacity	Rises 15% by 20th week; decline of 5% by 40 weeks.
Oxygen consumption	Increases 15% between 16 and 40 weeks.
Circulation time	Decreases from 13 to 11 seconds by 32nd week, returns to 13 seconds by 40th week.

2. Oxygen consumption increases intermittently with uterine contractions, approaching that of moderate to severe exercise.

3. Tachycardia during the second stage may result from distention of the right atrium and ventricle by blood from the uterus and from the effect of straining.

B. During the Puerperium:

1. Cardiac output increases slightly for about 1 week after delivery. Elimination of the placenta, contracture of the uterus, and reduction of the pelvic circulation suddenly makes more blood available to the heart.

2. The decrease in plasma volume (and increase in hematocrit) for about 12 hours after delivery is due primarily to readjustments in venous pressure. A second marked decrease in plasma volume, with an accompanying reduction in the amount of total body water, persists for 7–9 days. These changes are due to postpartal diuresis.

Treatment

Determine the functional cardiac status (class I–IV) before the third month if possible and again at 7–8 months. Obtain consultation with a cardiologist for all class II–IV patients early in pregnancy. Restrict physical activity to necessary duties only, with fatigue as a limiting factor. Make certain that the patient obtains assistance with essential household duties (child care, laundry, cleaning, and marketing). Help the patient and her family to understand the medical problem, and allay her fears, anxiety, and tension. Periods of maximal cardiac stress occur at 14–32 weeks, during labor, and, particularly, during the immediate postpartal period. Especially good rapport and medical control must be maintained at these times.

A. Medical Measures: Correct anemia, hyperthyroidism, and obesity as indicated. Treat cardiac complications such as congestive failure, pulmonary edema, infective endocarditis, and arrhythmia as in the nonpregnant patient. Prevent and treat preeclampsia-eclampsia. Treat all infections specifically, promptly, and vigorously. Intercurrent respiratory, gastrointestinal tract, or urinary tract infections can be serious. Restrict sodium intake and use diuretics, but not to the point of hyponatremia. Avoid hypokalemia.

B. Obstetric Measures:

1. Prevent complications in labor, delivery, and the puerperium.

2. Administer full doses of analgesics as necessary, but do not give scopolamine, because it may cause excitement and overactivity.

3. Delivery should be under local or regional anesthesia if possible. Administer oxygen freely during labor and in the early puerperium, when tachycardia, dyspnea, and chest pain are most severe.

4. Shorten the terminal stage of labor by elective low forceps delivery to spare the patient the effort of bearing down in the second

stage. Do not intervene too early, however, or lacerations, excessive blood loss, and shock may occur.

5. Manage the third stage of labor carefully to limit postpartal bleeding. Do not administer ergot preparations (which have a pressor effect), and give oxytocin only if necessary after delivery for uterine atony.

6. Lower the patient's legs promptly after delivery to reduce drainage of blood into the general circulation.

7. Anticipate the possibility that some women who have experienced no cardiac symptoms during pregnancy or labor sometimes go into shock or acute cardiac failure immediately after delivery because of sudden engorgement of the splanchnic vessels. Treat for hypovolemic shock and acute cardiac failure.

8. Class I or II patients may breast-feed if they wish to do so.

9. Prescribe cautious, brief, early ambulation for class I–III patients provided the medical course is otherwise uncomplicated. Class I patients may be sent home at the same time as patients without complications.

10. Class II–IV patients should remain in the hospital after delivery until cardiovascular function is stable. Class IV patients must remain in bed for as long as necessary to recover from the effects of labor and delivery.

11. Before discharge, make certain that the patient is returning to a controlled home situation where adequate rest in a nonstressful milieu will be possible. Recommend contraception and discuss sterilization, particularly for class II–IV patients.

C. Surgical Measures:

1. Therapeutic abortion may be indicated in 5–8% of cases of heart disease complicating pregnancy. Patients who have had cardiac failure in a previous pregnancy will usually have failure again with another pregnancy and so should be aborted. Abortion is seldom beneficial after the fourth month but may be considered (see Chapter 16).

2. If the cardiac lesion is severe enough to warrant abortion and if surgical treatment is not available and there is little prospect that therapeutic advances will alter the situation favorably, sterilization may be indicated. If the patient is not sterilized, strict pregnancy prevention must be employed.

3. Mitral valvotomy is indicated only in patients with severe stenosis of the mitral valve who have insufficient cardiac reserve, even with ideal supportive therapy, to withstand the stress of pregnancy. In general, such patients will have had cardiac decompensation in a previous pregnancy despite the best care.

Open-heart surgery is extremely dangerous for the fetus because of hypoxia despite a well-functioning heart-lung bypass.

4. Cesarean section is not recommended for the pregnant cardiac

patient unless it is performed for primarily obstetric reasons. A woman who can withstand a major operation almost always can undergo vaginal delivery.

Prognosis

When heart disease complicates pregnancy, the prognosis for the mother and the infant depends upon the severity of the heart disorder; the availability of medical and obstetric care; medical and surgical complications; the patient's emotional, socioeconomic, and environmental status; and local policy regarding therapeutic abortion and sterilization. Although rheumatic heart disease is not exacerbated by successive pregnancies, the increased load of pregnancy and infant care on a cardiac patient frequently will cause a downhill course. Data are not available regarding the long-range prognosis for other types of heart disease.

Cardiovascular disease has continued to be the fourth leading cause of maternal death (after infection, preeclampsia-eclampsia, and anesthesia complications) over the past 50 years. The maternal mortality rate for all types of heart disease is 0.5–3% in large medical centers in the USA, and heart disease accounts for 5–10% of all maternal deaths.

The perinatal mortality rate (including fetal deaths due to therapeutic abortion) largely depends upon the functional severity of the mother's heart disease. Rates are as follows:

Mother's Functional Disability	Perinatal Mortality Rate
Class I	About 5%
Class II	10–15%
Class III	About 35%
Class IV	Over 50%

The incidence of congenital defects is greater among infants delivered of women with congenital and syphilitic heart disease than among those delivered of women with normal hearts, but rheumatic and other types of heart disease do not increase the incidence of fetal anomalies.

POSTPARTUM CARDIOMYOPATHY

Postpartum cardiomyopathy is a disorder of the heart muscle of unknown, possibly viral, origin that presents clinically with onset of cardiac failure. This serious, even critical complication is most often seen in older multiparas and women who have had preeclampsia-eclampsia or a multiple pregnancy. These women have no evidence of prior heart disease. The disorder usually develops in the first month postpartum but may occur as late as 3–5 months postpartum.

The initial symptoms are moderate respiratory distress and chest pain. The holosystolic murmur of mitral insufficiency and evidence of cardiomegaly and left heart failure aid in the diagnosis. Focal myocardial degeneration and fibrosis of muscle fibers with mural thrombi develop, but coronary artery disease is not present. There is low-output cardiac failure with ventricular dilatation and pulmonary and systemic hypertension but no pericardial effusion.

Obtain medical consultation. Digitalize the patient and treat pulmonary edema. Consider anticoagulant therapy to minimize pulmonary or systemic emboli. Extended bed rest accelerates recovery.

Patients whose heart size returns to normal within 6 months and who can resume their usual routine have a good prognosis. Postpartum cardiomyopathy may recur after a later pregnancy, however.

CARDIAC ARREST

Cardiac arrest is cessation of heart action as a result of acute myocardial hypoxia or alteration in conduction. Ventricular standstill (asystole) and ventricular fibrillation are the immediate causes. Cardiac arrest occurs most commonly during induction of anesthesia and during operative surgery or instrumental delivery. Cardiovascular disease increases the risk of cardiac arrest; hypoxia and hypertension are contributory causes. Cardiac arrest may follow shock, hypoventilation, airway obstruction, excessive anesthesia, drug administration or drug sensitivity, vagovagal reflex activity, myocardial infarction, air and amniotic fluid embolism, and heart block.

Cardiac arrest occurs about once in 800–1000 operations and is apt to occur during minor surgical procedures as well as during major surgery. It occurs about once in 10,000 obstetric deliveries—usually operative, complicated cases. Fortunately, it is possible to save up to 75% of patients when cardiac arrest occurs in the well-equipped operating or delivery room.

Clinical Findings

Premonitory signs (especially during induction of anesthesia, intubation or extubation, moving the patient, deep or prolonged anesthesia, hypoxia or hypotension with vagotonal effect) consist of irregular cardiac rhythm, bradycardia, and sudden or marked hypertension. Absence of a palpable pulse in a major artery (aorta, carotid, femoral), absence of heart sounds over the precordium, and dilatation of the pupils are diagnostic of cardiac arrest. Emergency treatment should not be withheld for electrocardiographic confirmation of the diagnosis.

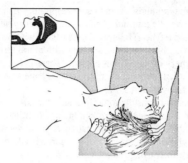

(1) Open airway by positioning neck anteriorly in extension. Inserts show airway obstructed when the neck is in resting flexed position and opening when neck is extended.

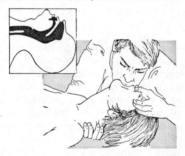

(2) Rescuer should close victim's nose with fingers, seal mouth around victim's mouth, and deliver breath by vigorous expiration.

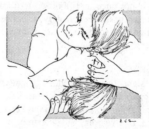

(3) Victim is allowed to exhale passively by unsealing mouth and nose. Rescuer should listen and feel for expiratory air flow.

Figure 13–1. Technique of mouth-to-mouth insufflation.

Prevention

Ensure a constant, generous oxygen supply during induction of anesthesia and throughout surgery and delivery.

Avoid undesirable vagal effects: (1) Give atropine sulfate before surgery or delivery. (2) Give atropine sulfate, 0.4–0.6 mg intravenously, for bradycardia, atrioventricular dissociation, or atrioventricular nodal rhythm. (3) Avoid placing excessive traction on the viscera during surgery or on the fetus during delivery. (4) Do not administer vasopressors such as epinephrine or ephedrine during cyclopropane or trichloroethylene anesthesia.

Prevent and treat hypotension promptly and effectively.

Cardiopulmonary Resuscitation (CPR)* (For treatment of asphyxia or cardiac arrest.) (See Fig 13–1.)

Phase I: First Aid (Emergency Oxygenation of the Brain)

Basic life support must be instituted within 3–4 minutes for optimal effectiveness and to minimize permanent brain damage. *Do not wait for confirmation of suspected cardiac arrest.* Call for help but do not stop preparations for immediate resuscitation.

Step 1: Place patient supine on a firm surface (not a bed). (A 4 × 6 foot plywood board should be available in emergency aid stations.)

Step 2: Determine whether the patient is breathing. If the patient is not breathing, take immediate steps to open the airway. In unconscious patients, the lax tongue may fall backward, blocking the airway. Tilt head backward and maintain in this hyperextended position. Keep mandible displaced forward by pulling strongly at the angle of the jaw.

If Victim Is Not Breathing:

Step 3: Clear mouth and pharynx of mucus, blood, vomitus, or foreign material.

Step 4: Separate lips and teeth to open oral airway.

Step 5: If steps 2–4 fail to open airway, forcibly blow air through mouth (keeping nose closed) or nose (keeping mouth closed) and inflate the lungs 3–5 times. Watch for chest movement. If chest movement does not occur immediately and if pharyngeal or tracheal tubes are available, use them without delay. Tracheostomy may be necessary.

*Modified after Safar.

Step 6:   Feel the carotid artery for pulsations.

a. If Carotid Pulsations Are Present:

Give lung inflation by mouth-to-mouth breathing (keeping patient's nostrils closed) or mouth-to-nose breathing (keeping patient's mouth closed) 12–15 times per minute—allowing about 2 seconds for inspiration and 3 seconds for expiration—until spontaneous respirations return. Continue as long as the pulses remain palpable and previously dilated pupils remain constricted. Bag-mask techniques for lung inflation should be reserved for experts. If pulsations cease, follow directions in 6b, below.

b. If Carotid Pulsations Are Absent:

Alternate cardiac compression (closed chest cardiac massage; Fig 13–2) and pulmonary ventilation as in 6a, above. Place the heel of one hand on the sternum just above the level of the xiphoid. With the heel of the other hand on top of it, apply firm vertical pressure sufficient to force the sternum about 4–5 cm (2 inches) downward (less in children) about once every second. After 15 sternal compressions, alternate with 3–5 quick, deep lung inflations. Repeat and continue this alternating procedure until it is possible to obtain additional assistance and more definitive care. Resuscitation must be continuous during transportation to the hospital. Open heart massage should be attempted only in a hospital. When possible, obtain an ECG, but do not interrupt resuscitation to do so.

Phase II: Restoration of Spontaneous Circulation

Until spontaneous respiration and circulation are restored, there must be no interruption of artificial ventilation and cardiac massage while steps 7–13 (below) are being carried out. Three basic questions must be considered at this point: (1) What is the underlying cause, and is it correctable? (2) What is the nature of the cardiac arrest? (3) What further measures will be necessary? The physician must make plans for the assistance of trained hospital personnel, cardiac monitoring and assisted ventilation equipment, a defibrillator, emergency drugs, and adequate laboratory facilities.

Step 7:   Provide for adequate prolonged oxygenation by intubation, administration of 100% oxygen, and mechanically assisted ventilation. A cutdown for long-term intravenous therapy and monitoring should be established as soon as possible.

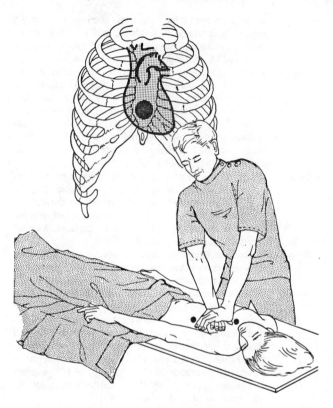

Figure 13-2. Technique of external cardiac massage. Heavy circle in heart drawing shows area of application of force. Circles on supine figure show points of application of electrodes for defibrillation.

Attach electrocardiographic leads and take the first of serial specimens for arterial blood gases and pH. Promote venous return and combat shock by elevating legs, and give intravenous fluids as available and indicated. The use of firmly applied tourniquets or military antishock trousers (MAST suit) on the extremities may be of value to occlude arteries in order to reduce the size of the vascular bed.

Step 8: If a spontaneous effective heartbeat is not restored after 1–2 minutes of cardiac compression, have an assistant give epinephrine (adrenaline), 0.5–1 mg (0.5–1 mL of 1:1000 aqueous solution) diluted to 10 mL, intravenously every 5 minutes as indicated. Epinephrine may stimulate cardiac contractions and induce ventricular fibrillation that can then be treated by DC countershock (see below).

Step 9: If the victim is pulseless for more than 5 minutes, give sodium bicarbonate solution, 1 mEq/kg intravenously, to combat impending metabolic acidosis. Repeat no more than one-half the initial dose every 10 minutes during cardiopulmonary resuscitation until spontaneous circulation is restored. Monitoring of arterial blood gases and pH is required during bicarbonate treatment to prevent alkalosis and severe hyperosmolar states.

Step 10: If asystole and electromechanical dissociation persist, continue artificial respiration and external cardiac compression, epinephrine, and sodium bicarbonate as above. Give also calcium chloride, 5–10 mL (0.5–1 g) of 10% solution intravenously every 5–10 minutes as indicated. Monitor blood pH, gases, and electrolytes.

Step 11: If electrocardiography demonstrates ventricular fibrillation, maintain cardiac massage until just before giving an external defibrillating DC shock of 200–300 J for 0.25 second with one paddle electrode firmly applied to the skin over the apex of the heart and the other just to the right of the upper sternum. Monitor with electrocardiography. If cardiac function is not restored, resume massage and repeat 3 shocks at intervals of 1–3 minutes. If cardiac action is reestablished but remains weak, give calcium chloride or calcium gluconate, 5–10 mL (0.5–1 g) of 10% solution intravenously; it probably should not be used in patients who have been taking digitalis.

Step 12: Thoracotomy and open heart massage may be considered (but only in a hospital) if cardiac function fails to return after all of the above measures have been used.

Step 13: If cardiac, pulmonary, and central nervous system functions are restored, the patient should be carefully observed for shock and complications of the precipitating cause.

Phase III: Follow-Up Measures

When cardiac and pulmonary function have been reestablished and satisfactorily maintained, evaluation of central nervous system function deserves careful consideration. Decisions about the nature and duration of subsequent treatment must be individualized. Physicians must decide if they are "prolonging life" or simply "prolonging dying." Complete recovery after appropriate treatment has been reported in a few patients unconscious up to a week.

Step 14: Support ventilation and circulation. Treat any other complications that may arise. Do not overlook the possibility of complications of external cardiac massage (eg, broken ribs, ruptured viscera).

Step 15: If circulation and respiration are restored but there are no signs of central nervous system recovery within 30 minutes, hypothermia at 30 °C for 2–3 days may lessen the degree of brain damage.

Step 16: Meticulous postresuscitation care is required, particularly for the first 48 hours after recovery. Observe carefully for possible multiple cardiac arrhythmias, especially recurrent fibrillation or cardiac standstill.

HEMATOLOGIC DISORDERS

ANEMIA

Physiologic and pathologic changes in the mother during pregnancy make the determination of anemia difficult. Not only do blood values during pregnancy differ from those in the nonpregnant patient, but these factors also vary with the course of pregnancy.

In every evaluation of clinical and laboratory data, the following questions must be answered: (1) Is anemia present? (2) Is there evidence of iron deficiency? (3) Are megaloblasts present in the blood smear? (4) Are there signs of hemolysis? (5) Is there bone marrow deficiency?

1. IRON DEFICIENCY ANEMIA

Iron deficiency anemia must be considered in all cases of anemia of uncertain cause—regardless of cell morphology. Iron deficiency in women is usually due to blood loss resulting from excessive menses, postpartal hemorrhage, or iron deprivation from previous pregnancies. About 95% of pregnant women with anemia have the iron deficiency type. Iron deficiency anemia occurs in at least 20% of pregnancies in the USA. Severe iron deficiency anemia is associated with definitely increased perinatal morbidity and mortality rates.

Iron stores are small, and absorption of iron is limited. A normal diet contains 12–15 g of iron, or approximately 6 mg/1000 kcal, of which 5–10% (0.6–1.5 mg) is absorbed. (However, more iron is absorbed in iron deficiency anemia.) Because less than 1 mg of iron normally is excreted per day, normal individuals are in positive iron balance. Chronic bleeding of as little as 2–4 mL/d may lead to negative iron balance and iron deficiency anemia. Unfortunately, there is no way to estimate iron reserves while the hemoglobin concentration remains within the normal range. If the hemoglobin concentration is reduced, however, the storage iron is depleted.

Pregnancy increases the woman's total iron requirements. Of the approximately 1 g (4–5 mg/d) of elemental iron required by a normal pregnancy, 300 mg is needed by the fetus and placenta and 700 mg augments the maternal hemoglobin mass. About 200 mg of iron is lost in bleeding during delivery and the puerperium, and about 500 mg of iron from maternal erythrocytes is returned to iron stores postpartum. Thus, the mother loses about 500 mg of iron per pregnancy. Repeated pregnancies, especially when there is a short interval between them, may result in severe iron deficiency. Many women who are anemic before pregnancy never "catch up" during pregnancy or after delivery.

An increase of about 30% in total blood volume is necessary to meet the demands of the pregnancy and the associated enlargement of the vascular system. If the plasma increases considerably more than the red cell mass, an apparent "physiologic" anemia of pregnancy will be evident because the hematocrit and hemoglobin concentration are low. Nonetheless, when the hemoglobin concentration is less than 12 g/dL or the hematocrit is below 35%, true anemia exists.

Clinical Findings

A. Symptoms and Signs: The symptoms may be vague or long-standing. Pallor, easy fatigability, palpitations, tachycardia, and dyspnea are described. Inquire about a history of blood loss or dietary inadequacy.

B. Laboratory Findings: A stool guaiac test may demonstrate occult gastrointestinal bleeding. A stained smear of bone marrow should be examined for hemosiderin, which is always absent in iron deficiency anemia but present in normal or increased amounts in all other anemias.

The hemoglobin level may fall to as low as 5 g/dL, but the red cell count is rarely below 2.5 million/μL. The red cells are usually microcytic and hypochromic (although in approximately 20% of adults, the red cells are normocytic and nearly normochromic). Reticulocytes and platelets are present in normal or increased numbers. The white cell count is normal. The serum iron level usually is below 30 μg/dL (normal: 90–150 μg/dL); total iron-binding capacity is elevated to 350–500 μg/dL (normal: 250–350 μg/dL). Only in iron deficiency is the serum iron level low and the total iron-binding capacity elevated. The percent saturation is 10% or less.

Differential Diagnosis

Iron deficiency anemia must be distinguished from other hypochromic, microcytic anemias (eg, anemia of infection, intestinal parasitosis, hemoglobinopathy, and anemia with intramedullary hemolysis).

Prevention

If iron is given prophylactically, the great majority of patients will maintain a hemoglobin concentration greater than 12 g/dL.

Treatment

Iron is curative for this type of anemia. Prompt, adequate treatment is necessary, but transfusions are rarely required.

A. Oral Iron Therapy: The maximum absorption is about 25 mg/d. Give either ferrous sulfate, 0.2 g, or ferrous gluconate, 0.3 g, 3 times daily after meals.

B. Parenteral Iron Therapy: The indications for parenteral administration are intolerance or refractoriness to oral iron (poor absorption). Parenteral iron should be given only in the amounts necessary to correct the deficiency. The total dosage should be 250 mg for each gram of hemoglobin below normal (normal in women: 12–16 g/dL).

Iron dextran injection (Imferon) for intramuscular use contains 5% metallic iron (50 mg/mL). Give 50 mg (1 mL) immediately and then 100–250 mg intramuscularly twice a week until the total dosage has been given. Inject deeply with a 2-inch needle into the upper outer quadrant of the buttock, using the "Z" technique (pulling the skin and superficial musculature to one side before inserting the needle) to prevent leakage of the solution and tattooing of the skin. Imferon may also be given intravenously in doses of 250–500 mg. A test dose of 0.5 mL should be given first; if the patient experiences no unusual reaction, the entire amount may be given over 3–5 minutes.

Prognosis

Signs and symptoms of iron deficiency anemia will clear with correction of the anemia. Improvement following the use of parenteral iron therapy is usually only slightly more rapid than with oral medication.

2. FOLIC ACID DEFICIENCY ANEMIA
("Pernicious" or Megaloblastic Anemia of Pregnancy)

"Pernicious" anemia of pregnancy is caused by folic acid—not vitamin B_{12}—deficiency. This disorder is most common in multiparas over age 30. The reported incidence varies from one in 40 to one in 200 deliveries. Folic acid deprivation is most common where dietary resources are inadequate, although some women on apparently adequate diets may be deficient. Curiously, only a small percentage of women with low serum folic acid levels have folic acid deficiency anemia. Folic acid deficiency anemia follows malnutrition and is often associated with alcoholism or protracted vomiting. It may be associated with multiple pregnancy or preeclampsia-eclampsia and may accompany sprue or sickle cell disease. It often occurs in epileptic patients who have received prolonged primidone (Mysoline), phenytoin (Dilantin), or barbiturate medication.

Clinical Findings

A. Symptoms and Signs: Lassitude, progressive anorexia, mental depression, and nausea are the principal complaints. Pallor often is not marked. Glossitis, gingivitis, vomiting, and diarrhea often occur. There are no abnormal neurologic findings.

B. Laboratory Findings: Folic acid deficiency results in hematologic findings similar to those of true pernicious anemia (vitamin B_{12} deficiency), which is very rare during the reproductive years. With folic acid lack, blood changes appear sooner. The hemoglobin concentration may be as low as 4–6 g/dL. The red cell count may be less than 2 million/μL in severe cases. Extreme anemia often is associated with leukopenia and thrombocytopenia. The mean corpuscular volume (MCV) is normal or increased. The peripheral white cells are hypersegmented. The bone marrow is hyperplastic and megaloblastic. Free gastric hydrochloric acid is present in normal amounts. Serum iron levels are high and serum vitamin B_{12} levels normal.

Complications

Secondary infection, placental separation bleeding, and fetal and maternal death may occur. Nevertheless, the fetus does surprisingly well even when the mother's anemia is severe.

Treatment

Give folic acid, 5–10 mg/d orally or parenterally, until a hematologic remission is achieved. Megaloblastic anemia of pregnancy does not usually respond to vitamin B_{12} even in large doses. Administer iron orally or parenterally (or both) as indicated. Prescribe a high-vitamin, high-protein diet. Transfusions are rarely necessary except when anemia is extreme.

Therapeutic abortion and sterilization are not indicated for folic acid deficiency anemia.

Prognosis

Folic acid deficiency anemia during pregnancy is not apt to be severe unless it is associated with systemic infection or preeclampsia-eclampsia. If the diagnosis is made at least 4 weeks before term, treatment can often raise the hemoglobin level to normal or nearly normal. The outlook for mother and infant is good if there is adequate time for treatment. Spontaneous remission usually occurs after delivery. Anemia usually recurs only when the patient becomes pregnant again.

3. APLASTIC ANEMIA

Aplastic anemia is rare, but it may be devastating during pregnancy. The anemia may be a toxic sequela to administration of drugs such as chloramphenicol, phenylbutazone, mephenytoin, or alkylating agents. Hair dyes, insecticides, and cleaning fluids may be implicated also. In about half of cases, the cause cannot be identified.

The rapidly developing anemia causes pallor, fatigue, and tachycardia. Pancytopenia is usually present.

The red cell count may be less than 1 million/μL, and the cells usually are slightly macrocytic. The reticulocyte count may be low, although variability is the rule. The white cell count may be less than 2000/μL and the platelet count less than 30,000/μL. The icterus index is usually low. The bone marrow is fatty, with few red cells, white cells, or megakaryocytes. Hemosiderin is present in normal amounts on a stained smear.

Fetal death or premature labor may ensue. The mother may die from infection or hemorrhage.

Treatment, in addition to discontinuing exposure to the toxic agent (if known), consists of giving prednisolone (or equivalent corticosteroid), 10–20 mg orally 4 times daily, and transfusions of fresh packed red cells as necessary. Platelet-rich fresh blood may check abnormal bleeding. Treat infection with appropriate antibiotics, but do not give antibiotics prophylactically.

4. DRUG-INDUCED HEMOLYTIC ANEMIA

Drug-induced hemolytic anemia often occurs in individuals with inborn errors of metabolism. Blacks frequently are affected, and deficiency of glucose-6-phosphate dehydrogenase, a red blood cell enzyme, is the most common cause. A catalase and glutathione deficiency is associated with this disorder. The trait is sex-linked and of intermediate dominance. While it is far more common in American black males, at least 2% of American black females are afflicted also. The fetus as well as the mother may suffer from this disorder.

Red cell values are normal for individuals with the African variant of the disorder until they are exposed to certain (oxidant) drugs such as primaquine, nitrofurantoin, and sulfonamides; then they develop an acute, moderately severe but self-limited hemolytic anemia. Hemolysis may also be precipitated by certain viral or bacterial infections and by diabetic acidosis. The Mediterranean variant, found especially in Sardinians, Sicilians, Greeks, Sephardic Jews, Iranians, and Arabs, is more severe; some of these individuals have chronic hemolytic anemia, and their white cells also lack the enzyme. Following infections or upon exposure to drugs or (in some cases) fava beans, a profound hemolytic anemia may develop. Other variants of the enzyme defect have been observed in northern Europeans and Chinese.

Specific laboratory tests to identify susceptible individuals include a glutathione stability test, a cresyl blue dye reduction test, a methemoglobin reduction test, and a commercially available dye reduction spot test.

Treatment of the infection or discontinuation of exposure to the drug or toxic material generally leads to recovery.

5. SICKLE CELL ANEMIA
(Sickle Cell Disease)

Sickle cell anemia is a heritable disorder that occurs almost exclusively in blacks. The abnormal hemoglobin (S, C, or D) is transmitted as a dominant trait. Heterozygous carriers have mixtures of normal and S (or C or D) hemoglobin in their red cells (sickle cell trait). These individuals have few or no problems. Homozygous individuals have only hemoglobin S (or C or D) and have sickle cell anemia. Because sickle hemoglobins are less soluble in deoxygenated form, the red cells sickle at low oxygen tension, especially at a low pH. The viscosity of whole blood increases, resulting in stasis and obstruction of blood flow in small blood vessels, perivascular edema, and pain and swelling in the involved organs. A crisis—often precipitated by respiratory infections, exposure to cold, or fever—is manifested by attacks of abdominal, head, joint, or bone pain lasting for hours or days.

Most patients have moderately severe anemia, but the sickling, not the anemia, is usually the major problem. The hemoglobin level is often about 8 g/dL. The red cell count is 1.5–4 million/μL. Sickling is usually apparent on the blood smear, but the distortion becomes very marked a few minutes after a drop of fresh 2% solution of sodium metabisulfite is added to the blood. Numerous nucleated red cells may be present. Leukocytosis occurs during a crisis.

Sickle cell tests (sodium metabisulfite or Sickledex) do not differentiate between sickle cell trait and sickle cell anemia. Hemoglobin electrophoresis will identify sickle cell disease due to other hemoglobinopathies.

Bone and joint pains may resemble rheumatic fever. A rigid, tender abdomen may suggest an acute surgical problem, but persistence of normal bowel sounds may be a helpful differentiating sign. Headache, convulsions, and paralysis due to cerebral thrombosis may be mistaken for eclampsia. The spleen is not enlarged in sickle cell anemia but may be in other hemoglobinopathies.

In sickle cell anemia, the red cell count is always low; the finding of a low hemoglobin level and a normal red count in a black patient with sickling suggests iron deficiency anemia plus sickle cell trait rather than sickle cell anemia.

Complications include hematuria, pyelonephritis, leg ulcers, bone infarction, osteomyelitis, cardiopathy, and cholelithiasis. An aplastic crisis may follow a severe infection. Almost half of all pregnancies in women with sickle cell anemia end in perinatal death.

Pregnancy is very deleterious to sickle cell disease. Almost half of these pregnancies are complicated by anemia (often with folic acid and iron deficiency overlay), pyelonephritis, thrombosis, and bone and joint pain. Iron and folic acid supplements should be given to all pregnant patients with sickle cell disease. Replacement transfusions may be lifesaving during sickle cell crises. The maternal mortality rate may be as high as 5–10%. Cesarean section should be done on obstetric indications.

The fetus is at considerable increased risk because of the complications but will suffer no specific adverse effects. It will inherit sickle cell trait or disease.

Treatment is symptomatic. For sickle cell anemia during pregnancy, consider partial exchange transfusion to bring the hemoglobin level to 10–12 g/dL in the third trimester. Bed rest and analgesics are helpful. Meperidine, sodium bicarbonate (3.5 mEq/kg/h intravenously), or 2.5% glucose with 0.45% sodium chloride intravenously may relieve pain. Elimination of infection and transfusion are required for an aplastic crisis.

Avoidance of pregnancy—by sterilization if necessary—is indicated. Oral contraceptives are contraindicated in patients with sickle cell disease because they may induce thromboembolic phenomena.

Genetic counseling is indicated for individuals with sickle cell trait or sickle cell anemia.

HEMORRHAGIC DISORDERS

The incidence, types, diagnosis, and treatment of hemorrhagic disorders complicating pregnancy are in most respects the same as in nonpregnant women. Anemia due to blood loss, postpartal hemorrhage, and development of bleeding diseases in the fetus may at times have a significant influence on the morbidity and mortality rates of both mother and infant.

Idiopathic thrombocytopenic purpura, when it has its onset during pregnancy, may be very serious. The maternal mortality rate in this condition is 1–2%, but the fetal mortality rate may be as high as 20%. If the mother fails to respond adequately to medical treatment, including corticosteroids and blood transfusions, splenectomy may be necessary. Particularly in early pregnancy, abortion may follow surgery. Cesarean section should be elected for obstetric reasons only.

Disseminated intravascular coagulation (see p 272) may occur in cases of premature separation of the placenta, amniotic fluid embolism, and intrauterine retention of a dead fetus. Bleeding in such instances may be very severe. Treatment is discussed on pp 271–274.

LEUKEMIA, LYMPHOMA, & HODGKIN'S DISEASE

Leukemia, lymphoma, or Hodgkin's disease complicating pregnancy is uncommon. The incidence of myelocytic leukemia is 5–6 times that of lymphocytic leukemia. Chronic myelogenous leukemia is 3 times more common than acute myelogenous leukemia.

Lymphoma and Hodgkin's disease usually are chronic, whereas most lymphatic leukemias are acute. While the chronic varieties may persist for years, patients with acute leukemia die within a few months of its onset.

Pregnancy has no specific effect on leukemia, lymphoma, or Hodgkin's disease. Consequently, the patient should receive good obstetric care and specific treatment of the malignancy, provided that the treatment will not harm the pregnancy.

The debilitating effect of leukemia on the mother is the main problem and is dependent upon the type and stage of the disease and the duration of pregnancy. Normochromic, normocytic anemia occurs in leukemia and Hodgkin's disease. Moderate thrombocytopenia and marked leukocytosis must be expected. Bleeding and premature delivery are very common. The perinatal mortality rate is very high. Several cases of possible transfer of leukemia or Hodgkin's disease to the offspring have been reported, but these are exceptional.

Little can be done for the patient with acute leukemia, but much can be done for the comfort of the patient with chronic leukemia, lymphoma, or Hodgkin's disease. Radioisotopes must be avoided during pregnancy, but local radiation therapy to the liver, spleen, or lymphatic masses may be given provided the uterus is shielded from radiation. Irradiation, antimetabolite drugs, and alkylating agents are hazardous to the fetus, especially during the first trimester. However, anticancer drugs have been given during the last half of pregnancy without deleterious effect to the fetus. Therapeutic abortion may be indicated if extensive specific anticancer treatment is indicated.

GASTROINTESTINAL DISORDERS

PEPTIC ULCER

Although pregnancy generally exerts an ameliorating effect on peptic ulcer, hemorrhage or perforation may occur during or shortly after pregnancy. During late pregnancy, a flare-up of peptic ulcer may be due to aggravation by anxiety. Exacerbation of peptic ulcer may occur in the puerperium in response to the stress of labor and delivery or as a result of a rise in gastric acidity during lactation and the anxieties and obligations of motherhood.

Medical treatment is the same as for the nonpregnant woman, but cimetidine and other histamine receptor antagonists have not been approved in the USA for use during pregnancy or lactation. Surgery should be reserved for emergencies.

HIATUS HERNIA

Hiatus hernia, or partial protrusion of the stomach or esophagus (or both) through the diaphragm, develops in patients with a weakened or congenitally widened diaphragmatic crux because of increased intra-abdominal pressure during pregnancy and progressive enlargement of the uterus with elevation of the stomach by the uterine fundus. It occurs more frequently in multiparas and in older or obese pregnant women. About 15% of all pregnant women develop hiatus hernia.

Persistence of nausea and vomiting beyond mid pregnancy and progressive pyrosis, eructation, and regurgitation of food and acid contents during recumbency are typical findings. The sensation of substernal pressure may be quite severe and is relieved by erect posture but aggravated by lying down.

Conservative treatment is usually adequate to carry the patient through pregnancy and delivery. Prescribe a bland diet, small meals, antispasmodics, and antacids; and caution the patient against lying down or exercising immediately after eating or drinking. Prevent unnecessary increases in intra-abdominal pressure by prescribing laxatives for constipation, by restricting lifting and straining, and by the use of low forceps delivery so that the patient will not have to bear down during the second stage of labor. The patient should sleep in a semireclining position. Obese women should be encouraged to lose weight.

Postpartal surgery should be considered only if the symptoms are persistent and marked. Excessive blood loss should be replaced by means of transfusions, and iron should be given for chronic anemia.

The great majority of hiatus hernias are resolved soon after delivery, and the relief of symptoms is usually dramatic.

DYNAMIC ILEUS

Mechanical obstruction of the intestine (most frequently the small bowel) occurs about once in 6000 pregnancies. About half of cases occur during the second trimester, when the enlarging uterus displaces the bowel sufficiently to stretch adhesions. Mechanical obstruction is often due to adherence of an ileal loop and the cecum after appendectomy or of the small intestine and uterus or broad ligament after myomectomy, uterine suspension, or adnexectomy. Mechanical obstruction should be considered as a cause of ileus in women with one or more abdominal scars. Other causes of obstruction include incarceration of a loop of intestine in an external or internal hernia, volvulus, and intussusception.

Surgical relief of the obstruction is indicated without delay. Pre- and postoperative gastric suction is required. Fluid and electrolyte imbalance must be corrected early. (**Note:** Hypokalemic alkalosis can cause convulsions that may be confused with eclamptic seizures.) Broad-spectrum antibiotics should be given parenterally if infection occurs.

The maternal mortality rate may be as high as 20% if treatment of septic closed-loop obstruction is delayed.

ADYNAMIC ILEUS

Adynamic (paralytic) ileus, diminished or absent contractility of the bowel, is a cause of intestinal obstruction. Mild adynamic ileus is present for 1–3 days even after normal delivery; brief moderate paralysis of the bowel is a secondary consequence of laparotomy, including cesarean section. Other obstetric and gynecologic conditions that may cause adynamic ileus are intraperitoneal and retroperitoneal hemorrhage and infection, pyelonephritis, nephroureterolithiasis, torsion of the adnexa, bladder atony, and hypokalemic acidosis. Older women seem more prone to adynamic ileus than young ones.

Adynamic ileus in obstetric and gynecologic patients almost always responds to withholding oral food and fluids, correction of fluid and electrolyte imbalance by means of parenteral fluids, intestinal decompression, and evacuation of the rectosigmoid colon by means of enemas. If mechanical obstruction can be ruled out, vasopressin, 1–2 units subcutaneously or intramuscularly (*not* intravenously) every 30 minutes for 6–8 injections, may be helpful. (*Caution:* Vasopressin is contraindicated in preeclampsia-eclampsia, epilepsy, and cardiac and renal disease.) Gastric suction usually will suffice. If ileus is marked, a long intestinal tube (Werner, Miller-Abbott) should be inserted to decompress the small bowel.

APPENDICITIS

Appendicitis occurs about once in 1200 pregnancies. Management is more difficult than when the disease occurs in nonpregnant persons because the appendix is carried high and to the right, away from McBurney's point; hence, the traditional localization of pain does not usually occur. The distended uterus displaces the colon and small bowel; uterine contractions prevent abscess formation and walling-off; and the intestinal relationships are disturbed. In at least 20% of obstetric patients with appendicitis, the correct diagnosis is not made until the appendix has ruptured and peritonitis has become established. Delay may lead to premature labor or abortion.

Early appendectomy is indicated. If the diagnosis is made during labor or near term, cesarean section and appendectomy should be done to minimize peritonitis. Therapeutic abortion is never indicated. If drains are necessary, they should be transabdominal, never transvaginal.

With early diagnosis and appendectomy, the prognosis is good for the mother and infant.

ULCERATIVE COLITIS
(Nonspecific or Idiopathic Colitis)

The cause of ulcerative colitis is not known. Young women are most commonly affected, and the peak incidence is in the second and third decades. Girls occasionally develop the disorder prior to adolescence, and sexual development is often delayed.

In severe, fulminating cases, colitis induces intractable bloody diarrhea, fever, fluid and electrolyte imbalance, collapse, toxicosis, and death. When the disease becomes chronic, malnutrition and invalidism are associated with remissions and exacerbations of diarrhea.

Ulcerative colitis in mature women has little or no effect upon fertility or pregnancy, but pregnancy may have a profound effect on this disease under certain circumstances. When pregnancy occurs while the colitis is inactive, an exacerbation is unlikely; but when conception coincides with active ulcerative colitis, 50–75% of patients will suffer a severe relapse during pregnancy and in the puerperium. When colitis has its onset during pregnancy, more than half of the patients will suffer a hectic course and a few will die. When colitis has its onset during the puerperium, most patients will have a very severe, often protracted course. Pregnancy almost never exerts a favorable effect on the course of ulcerative colitis.

There is no specific treatment. Symptomatic and supportive medical measures, corticosteroids, and the sulfonamide and antibiotic drugs are usually employed during pregnancy, and ileostomy may occasionally be done in emergencies.

Therapeutic abortion is justified in rare cases of acute, fulminating, treatment-resistant colitis exacerbated by pregnancy or when uncontrollable colitis is first noted during early pregnancy.

COLON & RECTAL CARCINOMA

Pregnancy increases the likelihood of spread of carcinoma of the colon or rectum. Malignant tumors of the lower bowel are often neglected or treated palliatively during pregnancy, with tragic results. The prognosis is extremely poor for the pregnant patient with carcinoma of the colon or rectum unless prompt radical surgery is possible.

The symptoms of rectal and colon carcinoma include constipation of increasing severity, often alternating with transient diarrhea, and rectal bleeding or blood-streaked stools. Anemia and weight loss are late signs.

In almost two-thirds of cases, the lesion can be reached by the examining finger and biopsied through the sigmoidoscope even during pregnancy. Barium x-ray studies may reveal the site and extent of the lesion.

The treatment of apparently resectable carcinoma of the rectum and colon during pregnancy depends upon the duration of the pregnancy at the time of the diagnosis as well as the extent of the malignancy. From the 4th to the 20th week, radical resection and colostomy via the abdominoperineal approach is indicated, avoiding the pregnant uterus. In the absence of obstetric contraindications, vaginal delivery at term should be permitted. From the 21st to the 28th week, the pregnancy should be sacrificed by hysterectomy and abdominoperineal resection and colostomy performed. After the 28th week, cesarean section should be done as soon as fetal viability seems likely; 3–4 weeks after delivery, the cancerous bowel should be resected and a colostomy constructed.

For incurable cases, cesarean delivery is indicated as soon as the fetus is viable. Palliative resection should be done at delivery or afterward to prevent intestinal obstruction.

CHOLEDOCHOLITHIASIS & CHOLECYSTITIS

Severe choledocholithiasis and cholecystitis are uncommon during pregnancy despite the fact that women have an increased tendency to form gallstones (one-third of all women over age 40 have gallstones). When acute gallbladder inflammation or biliary colic does occur, it is usually in late pregnancy or, more often, in the puerperium. Pregnancy is considered a predisposing cause of gallstones; although mechanical stasis and altered blood cholesterol metabolism have been considered as contributing factors, the true relationship remains unknown. About 90% of patients with cholecystitis have stones.

Symptomatic relief may be all that is required. Meperidine or atropine is effective in alleviating pain and ductal spasm.

Gallbladder surgery in pregnant women should be attempted only in extreme cases (eg, obstruction), because it greatly increases the perinatal mortality rate (up to about 15%). Cholecystostomy and lithotomy may be all that is feasible during advanced pregnancy, with cholecystectomy deferred until after delivery. On the other hand, withholding surgery when it is definitely needed may result in necrosis and perforation of the gallbladder and peritonitis. Intermittent high fever, jaundice, and right upper quadrant pain may indicate cholangitis due to impacted common duct stone. In such cases, surgical removal of gallstones and establishment of biliary drainage are essential.

Therapeutic abortion or early delivery (by induction or cesarean section) is not warranted.

CHOLESTATIC JAUNDICE OF PREGNANCY
(Recurrent or Idiopathic Jaundice of Pregnancy, Hepatosis)

Cholestatic or recurrent jaundice of pregnancy is an uncommon disorder of successive pregnancies that is caused by an inherited deficiency in liver metabolism. Hepatic excretory insufficiency, apparently provoked by estrogen, may be a distressing and confusing complication of pregnancy.

Cholestatic jaundice of pregnancy is characterized by itching, gastrointestinal complaints, and jaundice during the last trimester of pregnancy; the symptoms disappear within 2 weeks following delivery but tend to recur in subsequent advanced pregnancies. The levels of most liver enzymes are only slightly elevated, and the results of hepatic function tests are normal.

The diagnosis of cholestatic jaundice of pregnancy requires the exclusion of other liver disorders, eg, viral hepatitis, drug toxicity, cholecystitis. A history of jaundice during a previous pregnancy or with use of oral contraceptives is most helpful diagnostically.

Treatment is symptomatic. Jaundice and itching may be reduced by administration of ion-exchange resins, which absorb bile salts. The phenothiazines frequently used to relieve itching are contraindicated because they will increase the jaundice. Management should include careful fetal surveillance; in cholestatic jaundice of pregnancy, maternal urinary estriol levels are poor indicators of fetal compromise. The offspring is rarely affected except in severe cases, when chronic fetal distress may develop. Abortion is not indicated, but early delivery may be warranted.

Combination oral contraceptives will activate cholestatic jaundice, but progestogen alone should be well tolerated for birth control.

INTRA-ABDOMINAL SURGERY

Elective major surgery should be avoided during pregnancy. However, normal, uncomplicated pregnancy has no debilitating effect and does not alter operative risk except as it may interfere with the diagnosis of abdominal disorders and increase the technical problems of intra-abdominal surgery. Abortion is not a serious hazard after operation unless uterine manipulation is necessary or peritoneal sepsis or other significant complications occur.

During the first trimester, congenital anomalies may be induced in the developing fetus by hypoxia. It is best to avoid surgical intervention during this period; if surgery does become necessary, the greatest precautions must be taken to prevent hypoxia and hypotension.

The second trimester is usually the optimal time for operative procedures.

VIRAL HEPATITIS
(Hepatitis A, Infectious or Epidemic Hepatitis;
Hepatitis B, Serum Hepatitis)

Viral hepatitis affects females of all ages (see also p 535). Pregnancy has been said to increase resistance to viral hepatitis, but, paradoxically, the manifestations may be more severe and prolonged when the disease occurs in advanced pregnancy. When viral hepatitis develops during the first trimester, the likelihood of fetal anomalies is increased about 2-fold. The incidence of abortion is not increased, but that of premature delivery is.

Treatment consists of supportive medical measures as for the nonpregnant patient. Avoid operative obstetric intervention. Anesthetics, analgesics, and sedatives may be hepatotoxic. A low prothrombin concentration may lead to hemorrhage, which should be treated with oral or parenteral vitamin K. No major surgical procedures should be performed unless the need is great. Therapeutic abortion is almost never advisable. The maternal and fetal risks are low if adequate nutrition is maintained.

Terminate pregnancy only in case of impending or actual hepatic coma. Deterioration may justify cesarean section if the infant is viable.

Administration of immune serum globulin USP, 0.02–0.04 mL/kg body weight intramuscularly, to all contacts may prevent or reduce the severity of hepatitis A. For prevention of hepatitis B, see p 536. Do not allow a pregnant patient to lose too much weight during periods when hepatitis is prevalent in the community (usually in the winter). Poor nutrition may make the patient more susceptible to viral hepatitis.

If obstetric care is good, the maternal mortality rate is approximately that of nonpregnant women with viral hepatitis.

It is wise to allow more than 1 year to elapse between hepatitis and subsequent pregnancy. Late in this interval, there must be no clinical abnormality related to liver dysfunction; no alterations in total blood proteins, serum albumin and globulin, albumin-globulin ratio, serum alkaline phosphatase, and serum transaminases (SGOT and SGPT); and no abnormal results of other liver function tests. All tests should be done in the same laboratory and repeated at 3, 6, and 9 months after delivery and early during the next pregnancy.

Liver Function Test Values in Pregnancy

Liver function test values in pregnancy are the same as in the nonpregnant state with the following exceptions: (1) Serum albumin decreases slowly during pregnancy from about 4.2 to 3.5 g/dL, with a gradual rise to normal in 6–8 weeks after delivery. (2) Alpha and β globulin levels increase slightly and γ globulin decreases very slightly in pregnancy. (3) Cephalin flocculation is elevated in 25% of pregnancies. (4) Serum alkaline phosphatase increases gradually during pregnancy; at term, average values are 6.3 Bodansky units and 19 King-Armstrong units.

ABDOMINAL HERNIAS
(Intestinal)

As pregnancy advances, the enlarging uterus tends to fill the abdomen and displace the intestines, so that nonadherent bowel may recede from an inguinal aperture. The uterus also shields incisional and other "weak points" from herniation. Hence, many abdominal hernias reduce spontaneously during pregnancy. A few irreducible (adherent) ones become incarcerated. Pregnancy permanently enlarges umbilical and incisional hernial rings. Femoral and pelvic hernias are uncommon, but they are important because they are often overlooked in obstetric patients.

The patient must not be permitted to strain in the second stage of delivery; low forceps should be employed after full dilatation of the cervix.

Emergency operation for the relief and correction of an incarcerated hernia may be required during pregnancy. Delay elective surgery for repair of an abdominal hernia until after delivery; the need for herniorrhaphy is not an indication for cesarean section.

CONNECTIVE TISSUE DISORDERS

RELAXATION OF THE PELVIC JOINTS
(Pregnancy Pelvic Arthropathy)

Slight relaxation of the pelvic joints, the result of increased circulating steroid sex hormones and relaxin, is normal during pregnancy. The degree of relaxation is variable, but considerable separation of the pubis and instability of the sacroiliac joint occur occasionally, causing pain and difficulty in walking. Obesity and multiple pregnancy contribute to the disability of pregnancy pelvic arthropathy. About one patient in 100 suffers from pelvic joint pain; about one in 1500 is seriously incapacitated.

Joint relaxation is progressive in most obstetric patients during the second trimester and early part of the third trimester. Undue mobility persists until after delivery. Joint stability may not return to normal until several months postpartum.

Pelvic arthropathy is presumed to be due to an exaggerated elasticity of connective and collagen tissue in response to the hormones of pregnancy. However, the extent of disability is not always directly related to the degree of play in the joints concerned.

Pain in the sacroiliac and pubic joints on standing, walking, and turning may be extreme. With the index finger in the vagina and the thumb above the symphysis, the examiner can feel abnormal movement of the pubic bone when traction is placed on one of the patient's legs while the other thigh is held firmly. Ultrasonograms of the patient's pelvis, taken while she is standing on the right leg and while she is supported by the left, will usually reveal the magnitude of pelvic joint relaxation. Ultrasonic evidence of separation of the pubic bone of more than 2 cm is abnormal. X-ray studies should be avoided, if possible, to limit radiation to the fetus.

Prolonged sacroiliac backache may be a sequela to sacroiliac arthropathy of pregnancy.

Treatment consists of limitation of activities, analgesics, and a sturdy, fitted girdle that gives support by snug encirclement of the sacrum, symphysis, and greater trochanters.

To prevent extended disability, every precaution must be taken to avoid exaggerated positions, marked traction, and sudden movement of the patient while she is under general anesthesia during delivery.

RHEUMATOID ARTHRITIS

Rheumatoid arthritis occurs rarely during pregnancy, but it may be extremely serious, especially during the puerperium.

Pregnancy suppresses rheumatoid arthritis, probably as a result of increased adrenocorticosteroid production. In general, patients with this disease are considerably improved during the last trimester, presumably because of an elevated cortisol level. Following delivery, however, and for as long as 2–4 months thereafter, there is a likelihood of serious relapse and rapid progression of the disease. For obscure reasons, lactation appears to prolong remission. The fetus is never adversely affected.

Treatment is directed toward reduction of inflammation and pain, preservation of joint function, and prevention of deformity. Adequate rest, analgesic drugs, and physical therapy are the mainstays of treatment. Pregnancy is not a contraindication to use of corticosteroids in the treatment of rheumatoid arthritis, although they should be used cautiously during the first trimester.

The prognosis is unpredictable but generally discouraging.

SYSTEMIC LUPUS ERYTHEMATOSUS (SLE)

Systemic lupus erythematosus affects principally females and develops most frequently during the childbearing years. It is a rare but often extremely serious complication of pregnancy.

Pregnancy does not consistently influence the course of this disorder. In over half of patients with SLE, the disease remains unchanged, and in a few cases it improves during pregnancy; but the number and severity of exacerbations may increase during pregnancy and especially during the puerperium. In contrast with nonpregnant patients with acute SLE, the probability of an exacerbation is 1–3 times greater in the first half and 1–2 times greater in the second half of pregnancy. The probability of a flare-up during the puerperium is 6–7 times that during the nonpregnant period.

Spontaneous abortion, usually before the 14th week, occurs in about 20% of patients with acute SLE. The incidence of premature labor and delivery and of preeclampsia-eclampsia is also increased. An association between maternal SLE and congenital heart block in the newborn has been described.

Corticosteroids may relieve the symptoms and reduce the number and intensity of acute exacerbations. Salicylates are beneficial.

Prednisone, 30–50 mg (or equivalent) daily orally in 4 divided doses, may be required for the treatment of an acute attack. After improvement has occurred, the drug dosage may be gradually reduced to withdrawal or to a maintenance dose of about 10 mg/d that may be given for a prolonged period during pregnancy and the puerperium.

Patients must avoid overactivity and exposure to the sun and other sources of ultraviolet light. Pigmented, emollient cosmetic lotions opaque to ultraviolet light may be applied over facial lesions. Analgesics and physical therapy may be given for musculoskeletal discomfort.

Pregnancy rarely exacerbates SLE so severely that therapeutic abortion is justified. Cesarean section should be done only for clear-cut obstetric indications.

The maternal mortality rate is approximately 20% and the perinatal mortality rate about 30% in acute disseminated SLE. The mortality rates in chronic SLE depend upon the duration and severity of the disease. The postdelivery period may be the most critical; thus, corticosteroids should not be discontinued too early.

Corticosteroid therapy before or during pregnancy probably does not influence the number of patients going to term or the fetal outcome.

Recommend barrier type contraception. Hormones of the oral contraceptives may induce antinuclear antibody formation and trigger an exacerbation of SLE. Avoid intrauterine devices because the likelihood of infection is increased with steroid therapy. If sterilization is desired, the husband is the better candidate, because surgery may be deleterious to a woman with SLE.

RENAL DISEASES

URINARY TRACT INFECTION

The urinary tract is especially vulnerable to infection during pregnancy because increased levels of steroid sex hormones and the pressure exerted by the gravid uterus upon the ureters and bladder cause hypotonia and congestion. This predisposes to ureterovesical reflux and urinary stasis. Cervicitis and vaginitis also lead to urinary infection. The trauma of labor and delivery and urinary retention after delivery may initiate or aggravate infection in the urinary system. *Escherichia coli* is the offending organism in about 80% of cases.

Almost 10% of pregnant women suffer from urinary tract infection. Asymptomatic bacteriuria occurs in about 5% of all pregnant women, and intercurrent pyelonephritis can be expected in approximately 30% of these patients if prophylactic treatment is not initiated. Urinary tract infection will develop in only 1–2% of pregnant women without antecedent bacteriuria. Serious antepartal infection occurs in 5–8% of pregnant women. An additional 5% develop urinary tract infections after delivery. Chronic pyelonephritis, a major cause of death in older women, often follows recurrent acute urinary tract infections during successive pregnancies. Symptomatic urinary tract infection is responsible for a considerable increase in the incidence of premature delivery and perinatal death. Whether asymptomatic bacteriuria is associated with early birth is debatable at present.

Patients with asymptomatic or symptomatic bacteriuria during pregnancy require investigation after the puerperium. Most will be found to have important upper urinary tract abnormalities.

The diagnosis should be based upon stained smear and culture of a catheterized or clean-catch specimen of urine. An acid-fast stain of the urinary sediment should be performed if tuberculosis is suspected. If the culture reveals more than 100,000 colonies per milliliter, treatment is required. Sensitivity tests to determine response to the various anti-infective agents are desirable. An initial urinary infection should be treated first with sulfisoxazole, 2 g orally immediately and then 1 g 4 times daily for 2 weeks; or nitrofurantoin, 100 mg orally 4 times daily for 2 weeks. If after 4–5 days of treatment a repeat culture discloses significant infection, sensitivity tests and appropriate re-treatment for a similar period are indicated. Recurrent or fulminating infections require ampicillin, 250 mg 4 times daily. Change to other drugs as dictated by the results of laboratory studies, but treat for 2 weeks. Do not give tetracyclines to a pregnant woman, because the fetus is apt to develop yellow deciduous teeth of poor quality.

Three successive negative urine cultures taken at weekly intervals are necessary before the patient can be considered cured.

If urine cultures are not available, a stained smear of the centrifuged sediment of a catheterized or clean-catch specimen may be examined for bacteria each week for 3 weeks. If no bacteria or pus cells are seen and the patient is asymptomatic, she is presumed to be cured.

For urgency and frequency, give one Levamine (butabarbital and hyoscyamine) capsule every 2 hours as necessary.

Force fluids (if indicated) and alkalinize the urine. Give analgesics, laxatives, and antipyretic drugs as indicated.

If obstruction is present, urethral or ureteral catheterization may be necessary. Ureteral obstruction usually resolves after delivery, but if it is permanent, surgical repair may be required. If response to chemotherapy and ureteral catheterization is inadequate, nephrostomy may be necessary, particularly during the second trimester and prior to fetal viability. Induce labor at term by amniotomy. Therapeutic abortion is rarely warranted except perhaps for severe urinary tract tuberculosis.

Routine urinalysis during pregnancy must include microscopic examination and stain for bacteria (and cultures) to discover asymptomatic bacteriuria.

Avoid urethral catheterization whenever possible; when catheterization is necessary, sterile technique is essential. Eradicate genital and urinary tract infections promptly. Study and treat patients before or early in pregnancy when there is evidence or a history of a previous urinary tract infection, especially during pregnancy. Even if a "cure" is achieved, suppressive long-term antibiotic therapy continued throughout pregnancy and the puerperium may be warranted.

If initial treatment proves ineffective, the patient should be referred to a urologist.

GLOMERULONEPHRITIS

An initial attack of acute glomerulonephritis is rare during pregnancy; most obstetric problems relating to glomerulonephritis involve transitional chronic forms of the disease. There is no evidence that pregnancy aggravates glomerulonephritis.

Infertility, abortion, premature delivery, fetal death in utero, premature separation of the normally implanted placenta, and placental dysmaturity occur more frequently in women with glomerulonephritis than in normal women. Nephritis causes hypertension, predisposes to preeclampsia-eclampsia, and is associated with a high incidence of perinatal mortality and morbidity. Fetal growth and activity must be carefully monitored.

The medical treatment of glomerulonephritis is the same whether or not the patient is pregnant. Corticosteroids may be harmful, and antibiotics are ineffective. Therapeutic abortion may be justified for acute, severe exacerbations of glomerulonephritis with renal insufficiency.

Glomerulonephritis may be an indication for cesarean section when placental dysmaturity or preeclampsia-eclampsia occurs.

URETERAL STONE

Ureteral stone is more common during pregnancy than otherwise because hypercalciuria occurs during pregnancy and calcium and vitamin D are supplemented; because the renal pelvis and ureter dilate in response to high levels of steroid sex hormones; and because minor (physiologic) obstructive uropathy is characteristic of pregnancy. Small, previously retained stones are thus permitted to enter the proximal ureter. Most ureteral stones are passed in the urine, albeit painfully; others become impacted. Sudden, agonizing pain in the costovertebral angle and flank with radiation to the lower quadrant and vulva, urinary urgency, and hematuria without (initially) pyuria or fever are characteristic of ureteral stone. Intravenous urography may demonstrate partial obstruction and the stone.

Symptomatic therapy with analgesics and antispasmodics is always indicated and may be best given parenterally. Retrograde catheter manipulation may dislodge the stone and permit it to pass, or the stone may be extracted transurethrally. If such efforts are unsuccessful and progressive hydronephrosis develops, remove the stone by extraperitoneal ureterolithotomy irrespective of the patient's obstetric status.

NEUROLOGIC DISEASES

The effect of neurologic diseases on pregnancy is rarely critical. Certain neurologic diseases may be aggravated by pregnancy (eg, chorea gravidarum [Sydenham's chorea], severe nonspecific polyneuritis, and herniation of an intervertebral disk).

GENERAL COMMENTS REGARDING NEUROLOGIC DISEASE DURING PREGNANCY

Pregnancy is not an absolute contraindication to urgent neurosurgery for the evacuation of a subdural hematoma, removal of an intracranial tumor, or treatment of an intracranial aneurysm. However, neurologic disorders are only rarely so serious as to require interruption of pregnancy.

Consider sterilization only when the woman's life and health will be jeopardized by subsequent pregnancy or when there is a significant likelihood of transmission of serious hereditary disorders.

Childbearing by individuals with serious hereditary neurologic diseases should be discouraged.

HEADACHES

The patient with a constant, throbbing, "splitting" headache, usually of the bilateral type, either frontal, sincipital, or occipital, should be examined for generalized edema, hypertension, and proteinuria, which may indicate preeclampsia-eclampsia. Tension headaches, functional in origin, are likely to occur for the first time or to be severely exacerbated during pregnancy. Tension headaches are much more common than vascular (migraine) type headaches.

VERTIGO & SYNCOPE

Vertigo and syncope occur occasionally during pregnancy on sudden change of position or station. Weakness due to low blood glucose concentration, postural hypotension, or cerebrovascular insufficiency may be interpreted as "unsteadiness." Dizziness and faintness during pregnancy are usually brief sensations; the patient rarely falls and almost never injures herself.

EPILEPSY

Convulsive seizures may be associated with disturbed physiology: edema, alkalosis, fluid and electrolyte imbalance, cerebral hypoxia, hypoglycemia, or hypocalcemia. Recurrent attacks of grand mal or petit mal epilepsy and psychomotor seizures may be activated or intensified during pregnancy. They are more frequent during the last trimester in women who are hypertensive, proteinuric, and edematous.

Epilepsy has no demonstrable effect on the clinical course of pregnancy. The effect of pregnancy on epilepsy cannot be predicted.

It may be difficult to differentiate epilepsy from eclampsia. An accurate history of seizures in the nonpregnant state is most helpful in the diagnosis of epilepsy. The burden of proof is on the physician who claims that convulsions in the third trimester of pregnancy do not indicate eclampsia.

If preeclampsia-eclampsia can be ruled out, grand mal seizures generally can be controlled by slow intravenous administration of 2.5% sodium amobarbital or 10 mL of 50% magnesium sulfate. Rapidly administered intravenous sodium amobarbital may cause fatal pulmonary edema and right heart failure because of vascular instability of patients with severe preeclampsia or eclampsia.

Phenytoin (Dilantin) may be toxic to the fetus. Other sedative drugs that are safer for the offspring include phenobarbital, diazepam (Valium), and chlordiazepoxide (Librium).

Fluid retention must be avoided in epileptic patients, and they must be kept on adequate anticonvulsant therapy during pregnancy and after labor. Acetazolamide (Diamox) is especially effective for pregnant epileptics.

Prevent aspiration of gastric contents by placing the patient on her side (never on her back). Extend the head and hold the tongue out to ensure a clear air passage. Restrain the patient gently to prevent injury. Slip a soft mouth gag between her jaws so that she will not bite her tongue. If convulsions are prolonged or severe, give diazepam (Valium), 0.5–1 g intravenously, or phenytoin (Dilantin), 150–250 mg intravenously at a rate not exceeding 50 mg/min. (*Caution:* Because of their depressive central nervous system effects, do not administer narcotics or general anesthetics unless absolutely necessary to control repeated seizures.) When seizures occur for the first time in a woman during pregnancy, careful neurologic examination, including electroencephalographic studies, is indicated.

Therapeutic abortion is not medically indicated for epilepsy, because this disorder may or may not constitute a problem during pregnancy. The risk of having an infant with epilepsy is 2–3% if one parent has epilepsy; it is 20–25% if both parents are afflicted.

POLYNEURITIS OF PREGNANCY

Polyneuritis of pregnancy is due to lack of thiamine (vitamin B_1). Polyneuritis is rare where the socioeconomic level of the population is high. In the USA, the disorder generally results from pernicious vomiting or chronic alcoholism in early pregnancy. Signs and symptoms of polyneuritis develop first in the lower and then in the upper extremities. Cardiorespiratory and central nervous system problems follow.

Treatment consists of thiamine hydrochloride, 20–25 mg orally, intramuscularly, or intravenously daily in divided doses for 2 weeks, and then 10 mg orally daily. Ensure a high-calorie, well-balanced diet.

With early and adequate treatment, the prognosis is favorable.

CEREBROVASCULAR ACCIDENTS

The higher incidence of vascular accidents during pregnancy than in the nonpregnant state may be partially explained by collagen changes in the blood vessels during pregnancy. Subarachnoid hemorrhage from all causes is more common during pregnancy. Recurrent subarachnoid hemorrhage may be an indication for cesarean section. Hypertension of preeclampsia-eclampsia, intravenous administration of ergot (pressor) preparations, and increased intracranial pressure with straining during the second stage of labor may account for rupture of congenital cerebral aneurysms, arteriovenous malformations, or thrombosed cerebral veins.

MULTIPLE SCLEROSIS

The cause of this disorder is unknown. The incidence is 2–3 per 1000 pregnancies. The dominant pathologic feature is patchy demyelinization of the brain and spinal cord.

Pregnancy cannot be implicated in the onset of multiple sclerosis. Hence, exacerbations and remissions must be coincidental. Physiologic changes during pregnancy do not influence the development or the course of multiple sclerosis; thus, therapeutic abortion is not medically indicated. However, because care of the child will impose an additional burden on the woman, early therapeutic abortion in severe cases may be warranted. Whenever pregnancy is interrupted on such an indication the patient should also be sterilized.

Multiple sclerosis does not affect the course of labor. Spinal anesthesia should be avoided when spinal cord disease is present. Vaginal delivery is preferred.

Pregnancy is not contraindicated after a remission of several years.

CHOREA GRAVIDARUM

Sydenham's chorea (St. Vitus' dance) that recurs or develops for the first time in young women during pregnancy is believed by many to be a form of encephalitis, often associated with acute rheumatic fever. Although very rare, it may be a serious complication of pregnancy. It usually appears early after the first missed period and, curiously, often vanishes following termination of pregnancy. Treatment is similar to that of Sydenham's chorea in the nonpregnant patient.

MYASTHENIA GRAVIS

Myasthenia gravis, probably a metabolic disorder involving acetyl-choline utilization at the myoneural junction, affects motor function, causing muscle weakness, particularly of the face, tongue, throat, neck, arms, and respiratory muscles. The peak prevalence of myasthenia gravis is at about age 25. Pregnancy may complicate the disorder, although some patients undergo remission during pregnancy. With proper management, most myasthenic patients complete pregnancy safely, and congenital myasthenia gravis is rare; thus, therapeutic abortion is not indicated.

The physician should be alert to specific symptoms—easy fatigability, intermittent double vision, drooping of the upper eyelids, facial muscle weakness, and, in more serious cases, upper arm weakness and breathing difficulty. Infections may precipitate the onset or relapse and must be treated aggressively during pregnancy. Neostigmine (Prostigmin) is beneficial. If edrophonium chloride (Tensilon) is used, it should be given cautiously intravenously. Since edrophonium may precipitate uterine contractions, it is best avoided altogether.

Myasthenic patients usually tolerate labor well because they already have some degree of muscle relaxation. Meperidine is the obstetric analgesic of choice. Local anesthesia is preferred. If general anesthesia is required, nitrous oxide, oxygen, and cyclopropane is usually the best combination. Oxytocin may be given, but scopolamine and muscle relaxants are contraindicated.

Myasthenic patients must be carefully supervised postpartum, because relapses often occur during the puerperium.

An occasional newborn may have myasthenia gravis and require neostigmine treatment for 1–2 months. Complete recovery is the rule.

HERNIATED INTERVERTEBRAL DISK

Herniation of the nucleus pulposus of an intervertebral disk in the lumbar region may occur during pregnancy. The estrogens, progestogens, and relaxin cause weakening of the fibrous rings of the interverte-bral disks and swelling of the nuclei pulposi. Hypervascularization of the nonosseous tissue of the back and pelvis contributes to the relaxation of back support. Moreover, the equilibrium of the lumbosacral joint is disturbed during pregnancy because of an increase in the volume and weight of the abdominal contents.

There are no obstetric complications due to disk hernia, but disability and even paralysis may occur in extreme, neglected cases.

Prescribe bed rest and traction. Sedatives and analgesics are benefi-cial. Back strain or injury should be avoided during pregnancy and the puerperium, and obese patients should lose weight. Temporary or per-manent relief usually follows medical management. Severe, recurrent, or progressive pain and incapacity may require surgery, but this is rarely necessary during pregnancy.

ENDOCRINE & METABOLIC DISEASES

THYROTOXICOSIS

Toxic goiter is extremely serious for the pregnant patient and, indirectly, for her offspring. Overtreatment of thyrotoxicosis during pregnancy may result in maternal and fetal hypothyroidism and may cause maldevelopment and goiter in the infant.

Toxic goiter does not increase the hazard of spontaneous abortion or fetal anomalies but does increase the incidence of premature delivery, postpartal hemorrhage, cardiovascular complications secondary to myocardial strain, psychosis, liver damage, and thyroid "storm." Preeclampsia-eclampsia may occur slightly more often in women with toxic goiter.

Most of the complications and sequelae relate to overtreatment, particularly when overtreatment results in the development of hy-pothyroidism during pregnancy.

Treatment

A. Emergency Measures: All pregnant patients with moderate or marked thyrotoxicosis should be hospitalized at bed rest and given sedatives.

B. Specific Measures: Individualize treatment according to the degree of toxicity and the duration of pregnancy.

Toxic goiter during pregnancy may require antithyroid drug therapy, eg, propylthiouracil (or equivalent), 0.1 g orally 3 or 4 times daily. In order to avoid resultant hypothyroidism, T_4 (levothyroxine, Synthroid) should be given.

Subtotal thyroidectomy must not be attempted until the patient has become euthyroid following medical treatment. Iodides may be used for a few days before subtotal thyroidectomy in the second trimester, but long-term use of iodides can damage the fetal thyroid gland. Premature termination of pregnancy is less likely to occur if surgery can be deferred until after the first trimester.

Therapeutic abortion is almost never required. Toxic goiter is not an indication for induction of labor or cesarean section. These procedures are done only on obstetric indications.

C. Treatment of Complications: Thyroid or T_4 (levothyroxine, Synthroid) should be administered whenever hypothyroidism develops, immediately before and for several weeks after thyroidectomy, or when the patient receives a thiourea compound.

If a congenitally athyreotic or markedly hypothyroid infant does not receive thyroid or one of its analogs promptly, followed by continuation of the maintenance dose to ensure euthyroidism, normal mental and physical development cannot be expected.

Prognosis

The prognosis is excellent for mother and fetus if normal thyroid function can be achieved promptly and then maintained.

HYPOTHYROIDISM

Slight thyroid deficiency is common among obstetric patients, and replacement therapy is indicated in such cases to maintain the mother's health and to ensure uneventful continuance of pregnancy. More severe deficiency causes abortion, premature labor, and congenital fetal anomalies. Women with moderate to severe degrees of hypothyroidism are relatively infertile, and sterility is the rule in myxedema.

Treatment

A. For The Mother: Pregnant women with early hypothyroidism may be treated initially with relatively large doses of thyroid supplement. T_4 (levothyroxine, Synthroid), 0.05–0.3 mg/d, probably is better than desiccated thyroid because its action is more rapid and more predictable than that of crude thyroid. Begin T_4 in doses of 0.05–0.1 mg/d, and increase the dose weekly to the limit of tolerance, adjusting the dosage to maintain optimal effect. Desiccated thyroid may be given in doses of 30 mg/d initially and the dosage increased weekly up to a total of 60–200 mg/d for maintenance. The optimal dosage may be estimated on the basis of the serum T_3 and T_4, but clinical judgment is often very accurate. Thyroid overdosage causes nervousness, tremors, tachycardia, insomnia, sweating, vomiting, diarrhea, and weight loss.

The nonspecific use of thyroid medication is to be condemned.

B. For The Infant: Give T_4 (levothyroxine, Synthroid) 0.025–0.05 mg (or equivalent of desiccated thyroid) orally daily for 1–2 weeks, and then increase the dose gradually to 0.1 mg/d or more depending upon response. Reduce dosage if irritability, tachycardia, fever, or diarrhea occurs.

Prognosis

With prompt, adequate, and continued thyroid replacement, the prognosis is excellent for mother and infant. If a hypothyroid infant does not receive prompt replacement therapy, irreversible mental and physical retardation is to be expected.

DIABETES MELLITUS

Pregnancy is a diabetogenic state. This is manifest in the development of gestational diabetes, in the intensification of overt diabetes, and in the occurrence of metabolic complications such as ketoacidosis. Pregnancy places an additional strain on carbohydrate metabolism even in healthy women without diabetes, and pregnant diabetics will usually require increased amounts of insulin.

The changes in carbohydrate metabolism and insulin during pregnancy are discussed on p 42. Reduced insulin production or decreased sensitivity to insulin seriously affects carbohydrate metabolism: underutilization of glucose results in postprandial hyperglycemia and excessive glycogenolysis and gluconeogenesis followed by hyperglycemia and glycosuria. Associated alterations in lipid metabolism lead to ketonuria and metabolic acidosis. Insulin deficiency also results in decreased protein synthesis and increased protein degradation and nitrogen excretion.

There are 2 major types of diabetes mellitus. Type I, insulin-dependent diabetes, is usually of juvenile onset and is associated with deficient insulin secretion. The pathogenesis is multifactorial, with genetic predisposition. Type II diabetes is non-insulin-dependent. This disorder has a strong hereditary component and usually develops in adults who are overweight or pregnant. Serum insulin levels are elevated, and the tissues are insensitive to insulin.

Diabetes mellitus occurs as a complication of one in every 325–350 pregnancies in the USA and is an important cause of maternal and perinatal morbidity. Although maternal death is rare with modern treatment, the perinatal mortality rate is 10–30%.

Classification of Pregnant Diabetics. (After White et al.)

Class A: Diabetic status based only on an abnormal glucose tolerance curve.

Class B: Onset of diabetes after age 20; duration of diabetes 10–19 years; no vascular disease.

Class C: Onset of diabetes between ages 10 and 19; duration of diabetes 10–19 years; no vascular disease.

Class D: Onset of diabetes under age 10; duration of diabetes 20 or more years; vascular disease, including calcification of leg vessels.

Class E: Same as group D, plus calcification of pelvic vessels.

Class F: Same as group E, plus nephropathy (often Kimmelstiel-Wilson intercapillary nephrosclerosis).

Class H: Coronary artery disease.

Class R: Malignant proliferative retinopathy.

Effect of Diabetes Mellitus on Pregnancy & Delivery

Infertility and abortion are increased in poorly controlled diabetes only. Maternal fluid and electrolyte balance is easily disrupted. Both the mother and the infant may be edematous. The incidence of polyhydramnios is 10 times the general incidence. Preeclampsia-eclampsia is much more frequent (30–50%), especially with prepregnancy vascular sclerosis and hypertension. Congenital anomalies of all types are 5–6 times more frequent. The risk of fetal death is heightened, particularly after the 36th week, because of maternal acidosis and placental insufficiency. Premature labor and delivery are common. The likelihood of an excessively large fetus (> 4000 g) is greater. Dystocia and operative delivery are more frequent, and fetal mortality and morbidity rates are consequently increased.

The incidence of early neonatal death from respiratory distress syndrome or hypoglycemia (due to hyperplasia of fetal islets of Langerhans) is increased.

Clinical Findings

A presumptive diagnosis of diabetes mellitus is based upon symptoms and signs, but the diagnosis depends upon results of laboratory tests. Laboratory results showing persistent glycosuria, hyperglycemia, and a reduced glucose tolerance during pregnancy are diagnostic.

Diabetic screening is required in any pregnant woman with a history of diabetes, a previously unexplained premature stillbirth or hydramnios, a prior newborn weighing more than 4500 g (9 lb 15 oz), 2 small newborns without known cause for their small size, or a previous term-sized infant with respiratory distress syndrome. Obesity or glycosuria before the 20th week or recurrent glycosuria after the 20th week should be investigated.

Glycosuria in the fasting specimen suggests diabetes, but this test is less reliable during pregnancy because many patients have a lowered renal threshold for glucose after the first trimester. Moreover, other substances—notably lactose—that may give false-positive tests for glucose may be excreted in the urine during the last 4–6 weeks of pregnancy and particularly during the postpartal period. For these reasons, glycosuria is of less concern than significant hyperglycemia, especially hyperglycemia with ketosis.

A normal fasting blood glucose level does not rule out diabetes. Moreover, fasting blood glucose levels may be slightly elevated or the postprandial blood glucose may be elevated in other diseases besides diabetes (eg, liver disease). A glucose tolerance test is required if the 2-hour postprandial blood glucose level exceeds 120 mg/dL.

The generally accepted normal values for whole blood glucose in the oral glucose tolerance test are as follows: fasting level, 90 mg/dL; 1 hour, 165 mg/dL; 2 hours, 145 mg/dL; 3 hours, 125 mg/dL. A glucose tolerance test containing 2 or more above-normal values is abnormal.

Before glucose tolerance testing, place the patient on a high carbohydrate intake for at least 48 hours, because carbohydrate restriction decreases tolerance.

In pregnancy, the fasting blood glucose level is often slightly low, yet the oral glucose tolerance curve may be of the diabetic type. These changes are most marked after the sixth month. However, following oral administration of glucose, blood glucose levels do not rise as high during as after pregnancy.

Immediately after delivery, most normal patients' glucose tolerance test curves begin to approach nonpregnant values. Many return to normal in 48–72 hours, and all readjust during the early puerperium.

Caution: It is unnecessary and possibly harmful to perform a glucose tolerance test on a patient whose initial fasting blood glucose level is 200 mg/dL or more.

Treatment

Treatment goals during pregnancy include a well-balanced diet, weight control, and maintenance of 2-hour postprandial blood sugars at 150–200 mg/dL, with insulin if necessary. Frequent observation of the patient for complications such as preeclampsia, urinary tract infection, and polyhydramnios is essential.

A. Emergency Measures:

1. Diabetic acidosis and coma–Admit the patient to a hospital and obtain medical consultation. Determine blood glucose, CO_2 combining power, and, if possible, serum sodium and potassium levels. Treat with insulin as for any patient with diabetic acidosis or coma.

2. Insulin shock–If the patient is comatose and it is not possible to rapidly differentiate between diabetic coma and insulin shock, treat first for insulin shock by giving 20–40 mL of 50% glucose in water slowly intravenously. Determine the cause and make the necessary adjustments of insulin or food.

B. Antenatal Care: Evaluate the patient as a candidate for pregnancy before conception if possible.

1. Obtain a fasting blood glucose level and a 2-hour glucose tolerance test on all obstetric patients with glycosuria, and inquire about any previous fetal deaths in utero, previous large babies at birth, or fetal disproportion. If the patient is known to have diabetes or is a diabetes suspect or asymptomatic subclinical diabetic, obtain consultation with an internist. The patient, internist, and obstetrician should work in close cooperation, but the obstetrician must assume primary responsibility. Admit the patient to the hospital if necessary.

2. Adjust diet to the ideal nutritional state depending upon the patient's height, weight, and build. Prescribe vitamin and mineral supplements as indicated.

3. Overt diabetics usually require insulin, and the insulin requirement is usually greater during pregnancy. Diet and insulin must be regulated by blood glucose determinations (never urine glucose). Check urine frequently for ketosis. It is rarely possible to control diabetes in a pregnant woman with oral hypoglycemic agents, which may be teratogenic.

4. The patient must be seen by both the obstetrician and the internist at least every 2 weeks to maintain control of diabetes and weight gain and to prevent preeclampsia-eclampsia and infection. Avoid hyperglycemia and glycosuria. The fasting blood glucose level should remain at 110–150 mg/dL. Prevent acidosis and ketosis or sustained hypoglycemia. Check carefully for possibile urinary tract infection.

C. Diabetic Management:

1. Management of class A diabetic patients–

a. Diet–The patient should be placed on a diabetic diet modified for pregnancy, ie, 30–35 kcal/kg ideal weight; 50–60% carbohydrate, 20–25% protein, and 20% fat. Calories are distributed over 3 meals and 3 snacks. The goal of therapy is not weight reduction but prevention of both fasting and postprandial hyperglycemia.

For example, a woman whose ideal weight is 55 kg (120 lb) should have a daily diet of 1925 kcal (35 × 55). The caloric value of carbohydrate and protein is 4.1 kcal/g, and that of fat is 9.3 kcal/g; thus, the composition of the diet is as follows:

> 60% carbohydrate = 1150 kcal ÷ 4.1 kcal/g = 280 g
> 20% protein = 385 kcal ÷ 4.1 kcal/g = 95 g
> 20% fat = 385 kcal ÷ 9.3 kcal/g = 40 g

b. Monitoring–

(1) Use ultrasonography to determine gestational age at 18 and 22 weeks.

(2) Obtain fasting blood glucose level and 2-hour postprandial blood glucose level at 18 and 22 weeks (limits: fasting, 105 mg/dL; postprandial, 150 mg/dL).

(3) Test urine daily for glucose and acetone.

(4) Determine plasma estriol levels after 40 weeks; do fetal activity determinations and oxytocin challenge test if indicated.

2. Management of class B-H diabetics–

a. Diet–Similar to class A.

b. Insulin dosage–The NPH/regular ratio should be 2:1 in the morning and 1:1 in the evening, and the morning total should be twice the evening total. **Example:** 40 units NPH and 20 units regular in the morning; 15 units NPH and 15 units regular in the evening.

c. All patients with severe diabetes should have periodic retinoscopy to identify progressive diabetic retinopathy or signs of preeclampsia.

d. Monitoring–

(1) Determine gestational age by ultrasonography at 18–22 weeks, and repeat ultrasonogram every 3–4 weeks to measure fetal growth.

(2) Determine plasma estriol levels weekly during the 28th–32nd weeks, 3 times a week during the 33rd–34th weeks, and daily after 34 weeks.

(3) Do fetal activity determinations and oxytocin challenge test (if indicated) weekly after the 34th week.

D. Delivery:

1. Consider elective delivery if the L/S ratio indicates pulmonary maturity at 38 weeks. Consider vaginal delivery if the vertex is presenting and other details are favorable. Cesarean section is indicated if the fetus is estimated to weigh more than 3800 g or if presentation is by the breech. Give insulin by infusion during induction or cesarean section.

2. Terminate pregnancy by the most expeditious means if there is a significant sustained fall in plasma estriol concentration or a positive oxytocin challenge test. (If the L/S ratio does not indicate fetal maturity, the decision to deliver the infant or continue observation is a calculated risk.)

E. Obstetric Measures: Therapeutic abortion may be justified in certain instances of diabetic retinopathy or retinitis proliferans or in Kimmelstiel-Wilson disease.

Neonatal Care

A pediatrician should be present at delivery. If possible, special nurses should be engaged for 24-hour care of diabetic babies in the premature nursery.

A. At Delivery:

1. Clamp the cord immediately after delivery to avoid hypervolemia.

2. Obtain blood for glucose determination at birth and every 3 hours for 12 hours. If the glucose level is less than 30 mg/dL, give glucose, 65 mg/kg in 0.25 N saline slowly intravenously. After resuscitation, instill 10 mL of 20% glucose into the stomach and remove the tube.

B. In the Nursery:

1. Give 4 mL of 20% glucose in water orally through a rubber-tipped medicine dropper every hour for at least 12 hours; then start hourly feedings of 5% glucose in water; follow in 12 hours by milk formula feedings.

2. Administer phytonadione (vitamin K_1), 1 mg intramuscularly.

3. Observe for tremor and convulsive movements. These may be due to hypocalcemia, in which case give 10% calcium gluconate, 5 mL intravenously, after a blood specimen is drawn for calcium and glucose determinations.

4. Keep warm in a heated isolette or crib.

5. Administer oxygen at 30–40% concentration, 55% humidity, and a temperature of 80–85 °F (26.6–29.4 °C).

6. Observe respirations; turn the infant frequently; stimulate breathing when necessary.

7. If signs of respiratory distress syndrome develop, give glucose solution intravenously (as above) whether the blood glucose level is low or not. Give a broad-spectrum antibiotic (but avoid the tetracyclines because dental dysplasia results from their use). Discontinue oral feedings temporarily. Obtain pediatric consultation.

Postpartal Management

Carefully evaluate the mother's diabetic status during the puerperium, since changes may occur.

Prognosis

Joint management by an internist, obstetrician, and pediatrician will result in lower maternal and perinatal mortality and morbidity rates. The maternal mortality rate with modern therapy should be less than 0.2%. Deaths are due to diabetic coma, preeclampsia-eclampsia, infection, nephropathy, cardiac complications, dystocia, and embolism. Neglect and improper treatment are the main contributory causes of virtually all maternal deaths. An irreversible increase of diabetic retinopathy and nephropathy occurs in most patients during pregnancy.

Factors influencing fetal survival are the severity of diabetes, control of diabetes during pregnancy, placental function, placental bleeding, preeclampsia-eclampsia, polyhydramnios, and interruption of pregnancy before the 34th week or after the 39th week of gestation. The perinatal mortality rate even with modern therapy is 10–30%. Fetal anomalies occur in 5–6% of infants and are very frequent with polyhydramnios. Abnormalities cannot be correlated with the severity of the mother's diabetes, however.

In general, vaginal delivery is safer than cesarean section for the fetus.

PARATHYROID DYSFUNCTION & TETANY

Pregnancy normally causes a slight (secondary) hyperparathyroidism. Severe, chronic hyperparathyroidism causing osteitis fibrosa cystica is rare during pregnancy except in patients with long-standing renal disease. The most serious problems relating to parathyroid dysfunction during pregnancy are hypoparathyroid tetany and muscle cramps. Tetany is usually associated with a calcium deficiency or phosphate excess (eg, due to intake of calcium phosphate prenatal capsules), or lack of vitamin D and parathyroid hormone. In established hypoparathyroidism, hypocalcemia is a dilutional phenomenon during pregnancy. The requirements for vitamin D and calcium may be greater than in nonpregnant women.

Tetany may follow infection or the hypocalcemia that sometimes occurs during lactation, or it may be seen during the latter months of pregnancy if calcium supplements are inadequate. Hyperventilation during labor may precipitate tetany.

Tetany of the newborn is unusual in breast-fed infants, but it may occur transiently if the infant's phosphate intake is excessive, eg, if too much cow's milk is given or as a result of relative hypoparathyroidism in the neonatal period.

INFECTIOUS DISEASES

All systemic infectious diseases of the mother, if severe enough, can complicate pregnancy by causing death of the fetus or premature labor and delivery. High fever, septicemia, and toxicosis are usually responsible. With the exceptions discussed in detail below, however, most maternal diseases such as pneumonia, scarlet fever, and typhoid fever are not responsible for fetal anomalies. The so-called TORCHES infections (*to*xoplasmosis, *r*ubella, *c*ytomegalovirus disease, *her*pes simplex, and *s*yphilis) may be devastating to the fetus.

TOXOPLASMOSIS

Toxoplasmosis, a multisystem disease caused by the protozoon *Toxoplasma gondii*, is a serious threat to the fetus. Cytologic evidence of *T gondii* infection is present in almost 25% of women in the USA. Most cases are chronic. Cats who hunt rodents harboring the parasite excrete infective oocytes in feces. Human infection follows hand-to-mouth contact after disposal of cat litter or after ingestion of rare meat from cattle or sheep grazed in contaminated fields. Cats are therefore considered undesirable pets for pregnant women, and meat should be well cooked to avoid toxoplasmosis.

Parasitemia can result in fetal infection, which is far more likely and serious when acute toxoplasmosis occurs during pregnancy. However, transmission of the disease also occurs in asymptomatic, chronic cases when trophozoites are similarly released into the maternal circulation.

Toxoplasmosis resembles cytomegalovirus disease in the mother and the infant. Severe toxoplasmosis is associated with growth retardation, micro- or hydrocephalus, microphthalmia, chorioretinitis, central nervous system calcification, thrombopenia, jaundice, fever, and death.

The Sabin-Feldman dye test and the indirect immunofluorescence test are diagnostic of toxoplasmosis. Both tests give positive results 2–3 weeks after infection and for years thereafter. Thus, without sequential tests, an acute infection cannot be distinguished from a chronic one. A recent *T gondii* infection is probable if, when 2-fold dilutions of both acute and chronic convalescent sera are tested at the same time, the dye test titer increases 8-fold or more or the indirect immunofluorescence antibody titer rises 4-fold or more. The diagnosis of toxoplasmosis in a newborn is supported by elevated IgM in cord blood. Culture of the organism in experimental animals is possible but difficult. Routine antenatal screening for antibodies to *T gondii* should be done; if negative, repeat tests during pregnancy are recommended.

Treatment of toxoplasmosis during pregnancy is problematic. Pyrimethamine currently is the drug of first choice against *T gondii*. However, this drug may be teratogenic, especially during the first trimester. Sulfonamide therapy is effective but must be discontinued prior to delivery. Sulfonamide drugs have a greater albumin-binding affinity than bilirubin, which may rise after delivery to critical levels, and even exchange transfusion of the newborn may be necessary to avoid kernicterus. If the newborn is treated with pyrimethamine, folinic acid supplementation will be required to reduce the toxicity of the drug. Sulfadiazine often is used additionally.

In congenital toxoplasmosis, treatment will not affect developmental and neurologic damage, but progression of the disease can be controlled. Encysted (intramuscular) forms of *T gondii* cannot be eradicated by any therapy and may cause recrudescence of the disease.

EXANTHEMATOUS DISEASES

Most of the exanthematous diseases are caused by viruses, which invariably gain access to the fetus via the placenta. The effect on pregnancy and the fetus depends upon the virulence of the virus, the mother's resistance to the disease, and the stage of fetal development. Fetal immunity depends largely on maternal active immunity (eg, rubella) or passive immunity (eg, immune serum globulin administration). High fever or toxicosis may cause increased uterine contractility and loss of the pregnancy; viral placentitis and viremia followed by fetal death in utero may lead to abortion or premature delivery.

Rubella (German Measles)

Rubella virus is extremely teratogenic. Many infants are abnormal and maldeveloped if the mother contracts rubella during the first trimester of pregnancy. Excluding patients affected during epidemics, the risk of congenital anomalies occurring during the first 3 months of pregnancy declines from 50% (first month) to 10%. After the first trimester, the danger of anomalies is negligible.

Fetal defects include cataracts, congenital heart disease, dental dysplasia, deafness, and mental retardation. It may take 1–2 years to be certain of the extent of infant defects. There is some evidence that an abnormal child may be born of a mother who has previously had rubella but contracts a subclinical form of the disease when reexposed during pregnancy years after the first infection.

Prophylactic immune serum globulin may prevent the rash but not the viremia of rubella, even when given before exposure to the disease. Therefore, though immune serum globulin may obscure the sign (rash) that the mother has been exposed to a teratogenic agent, the virus may still be a significant threat to the fetus.

In the event that a woman develops rubella in the first trimester of pregnancy, the question of whether or not to perform therapeutic abortion is invariably raised. There is no unanimity of opinion. Many insist

Table 13–2. Exanthematous diseases in pregnancy.

Disease	Effect of Disease on Pregnancy	Effect of Disease on Offspring
Rubeola (measles)	Abortion; premature labor if disease is severe.	May be born with rash.
Varicella (chickenpox)	Severe, disseminated epidemic type may be fatal to mother due to necrotizing angiitis.	Virulent infection may cause fetal death in utero. Newborn may be born with pocks.
Rubella (German measles)	Occasional early abortion.	Congenital anomalies if disease occurs during first trimester.

that even a 10–15% risk of a seriously damaged fetus is justification for a therapeutic abortion. However, this does mean sacrificing 9 normal fetuses out of 10 fetuses at risk in order to prevent the unwanted survival of one abnormal infant. Moreover, the malformations may be so slight that good health and function and a normal life span are possible.

Susceptibility to rubella can be demonstrated by the absence of specific serum hemagglutinating antibody. Attenuated rubella virus vaccine will confer active immunity for a prolonged but uncertain period. Because the vaccine can infect the fetus, immunization should be carried out in women *only* if they are not pregnant and pregnancy can be avoided for 3 months after vaccination. This may require a negative pregnancy test—or administration of vaccine during a menstrual period or immediately after childbirth—and effective contraception. Reactions to the vaccine may include mild fever, local soreness at the site of injection, and arthralgia. Spread of the virus to others is not a problem.

CYTOMEGALOVIRUS DISEASE

Most cases of cytomegalovirus (cytomegalic inclusion) disease are clinically inapparent. In some cases in adults, the symptoms are like those of infectious mononucleosis. The disease is usually sexually transmitted; cytomegalovirus (CMV) is recovered from 15–20% of women examined in public health clinics and from the semen of men who have had numerous sexual partners. During pregnancy, often the only sign is mild leukorrhea. The virus can be cultivated from the salivary glands of 10–25% of healthy individuals, from the cervix of 10% of healthy women, from the urine of 1% of all newborns, and sometimes from breast milk. This carrier state probably explains subsequent cases occurring in the same family. A specific virus-neutralizing and complement-fixing antibody reaction indicates that most women have at some time sustained infection by this virus. About 20% of adults do not have neutralizing antibody to cytomegalovirus and thus are considered susceptible.

It was formerly thought that cytomegalovirus disease occurred only occasionally during pregnancy, but there is now evidence that the disease is much more prevalent than was thought and causes severe anomalies in about 10,000 infants in the USA per year.

Cytomegalovirus disease is usually acquired by the fetus during early intrauterine life. In the newborn, the disease produces erythroblastosis and thrombocytopenia that lead to scattered hemorrhages. Chorioretinitis, periventricular necrosis with calcification, microcephaly, and sclerosis of the bones are often noted at birth. Early jaundice beginning on the first or second day, melena, hematemesis, and hematuria develop. The antemortem diagnosis can be made by identification of cytomegalic inclusion cells in the gastric washings, cerebrospinal fluid, or fresh urine. Culture of the cytomegalovirus is proof of the diagnosis. The direct and indirect serum bilirubin are elevated, but the Coombs test is negative. Death usually occurs soon after birth as a result of interstitial pneumonitis, focal hepatitis, or adrenocortical failure.

No specific cure is known. Corticosteroids and supportive therapy together with immune serum globulin may be helpful. Therapeutic abortion is not justified because there is no means of making the diagnosis prior to delivery. An occasional infant survives, but marked developmental and psychomotor deficiencies and hepatosplenomegaly are usually present.

HERPES SIMPLEX
(See p 537.)

SYPHILIS
(See p 524.)

GONORRHEA
(See p 521.)

POLIOMYELITIS

Poliomyelitis has been virtually eradicated in the USA, but it is still a serious problem in developing countries. Poliomyelitis exerts an unfavorable effect on pregnancy and the puerperium. The incidence of poliomyelitis is greater in pregnant patients than in nonpregnant women of comparable ages. Approximately 67% of women who contract poliomyelitis during pregnancy are between the ages of 20 and 29, and about 75% are parous.

Pregnancy aggravates poliomyelitis, and the disease in turn increases the risk of abortion and fetal loss. Rare congenital anomalies are ascribed to poliomyelitis. The fetus may contract poliomyelitis during its passage through the birth canal.

The infant may show growth retardation if the mother contracts poliomyelitis in the early months of pregnancy. Give immune serum globulin to protect the infant against poliomyelitis. If the newborn survives, flaccid paralysis may be present.

Salk vaccine contains killed virus; Sabin vaccine is an attenuated live virus preparation. Either can be given whether the patient is pregnant or not, but it is preferred to give the vaccine to nonpregnant women.

The maternal mortality rate in pregnancy complicated by poliomyelitis is 5–10% higher than in normal women. The later in pregnancy the disease is contracted, the higher the morbidity and mortality rates for both mother and infant.

PULMONARY TUBERCULOSIS

Tuberculosis of the bronchi, lungs, and pleura is not directly affected by pregnancy. Tuberculous pregnant women are slightly more prone to spontaneous abortion and premature delivery than other women. Tuberculous endometritis and placentitis occur in advanced cases, but congenital tuberculosis is exceptional. Interruption of pregnancy because of pulmonary tuberculosis is almost never justified now that antituberculosis drugs are available. Pneumothorax, pneumoperitoneum, and thoracic surgery are not contraindicated. Infants born of tuberculous mothers are no more likely to develop the disease than others provided they are separated from the infected mother and unfavorable environment at birth.

However, it is important to discourage pregnancy in women with active tuberculosis and to maintain close medical supervision of those tuberculous women who do become pregnant. Institute follow-up study of all women with a history of treated tuberculosis, and be alert to the possibility of reactivation of tuberculosis during each pregnancy. Advise deferring pregnancy (and prescribe contraception, if acceptable) until tuberculosis has been inactive for at least 2 years, if minimal; 3 years, if moderately advanced; and 5 years, if far-advanced. Obtain chest x-rays of all obstetric patients as soon as pregnancy is diagnosed. In patients who have had tuberculosis, order chest x-rays during the third month, at term, and 6 months after delivery. The management of the pregnant patient with tuberculosis requires the collaboration of the pulmonary physician and the obstetrician. The treatment of tuberculosis includes rest (physical and emotional), hospitalization if the disease is moderate or advanced, and chemotherapy. The reader is referred to other texts for details of treatment.

MALARIA

Malaria may cause abortion or premature labor and delivery. Infants of mothers with malaria are often smaller than average. Approximately 10% of infants born of women with demonstrable parasitemia will have plasmodia in cord blood films.

Malaria may cause infertility; it also complicates pregnancy. Malarial relapses often occur during pregnancy for unknown reasons. A renewal of attacks is common during the puerperium or after hemorrhage and infection.

Labor is frequently prolonged and hazardous for obstetric patients with malaria. These women become fatigued sooner, and operative delivery is required more often. The parasite is not transmitted in the milk, but lactation should be discouraged in women with clinical evidence of malaria. The severity of maternal malaria is reflected in the stillbirth rate, which rises as pregnancy approaches term; and the vitality of newborns who do survive is temporarily reduced.

No antimalarial drug is completely safe for use during pregnancy. If a pregnant woman must be treated for malaria, other texts should be consulted for details of treatment.

LISTERIOSIS

Maternal listeriosis may be responsible for abortion and fetal disease or death depending upon the severity of the infection and the duration of pregnancy. Encephalitis and granulomatosis of the newborn are described also. Pregnant women suffering from a septic form of this disease have only malaise, but they may transmit the infection to the fetus either transplacentally or when the fetus is exposed to the organisms in the lower genital canal during birth.

A diagnosis of listeriosis during pregnancy is difficult but can be made by complement fixation or fluorescent antibody tests of leukorrheic discharges. A positive complement fixation test in high dilution is almost invariably present in acute maternal infection. Gram-positive rods should be sought in the meconium of the newborn to diagnose listeriosis early.

Treat the mother and child with large doses of penicillin or erythromycin.

14 | Dystocia (Difficult Labor)

PELVIC DYSTOCIA

Pelvic dystocia occurs when there is significant shortening of any of the internal dimensions of the bony pelvis. Unfavorable alterations in the structure and dimensions of the pelvis may be congenital or may be due to malnutrition, tumors, injuries, or disorders of the spine and lower extremities. About 15–20% of women in the USA have pelves that may cause complicated delivery.

Growth of the pelvic bones is complete in adolescence, when the pelvic epiphyses fuse. The causes of abnormal human pelvic configuration generally relate to prepuberal disease, but fractures and tumors are also responsible. The causes may be classified as follows:

(1) Congenital and hereditary disorders: Congenital dislocation of the hips, chondrodystrophy.

(2) Disease of the pelvic bones: Rickets, osteomalacia, fracture with misalignment, tumor.

(3) Disorders of the spine: Lumbar kyphoscoliosis, causing abnormal transmission of force to the pelvis.

(4) Abnormality of one extremity: Unilateral equinovarus or paralysis of one leg, causing unequal force to be transmitted to the sides of the pelvis.

The birth canal is a series of rigid spaces or areas bounded by bony walls or prominences that act as baffles. They limit or guide the presenting part largely by deflection. Descent and internal rotation are markedly influenced by the characteristics of the virtually unyielding bony pelvis.

Clinical Pelvimetry

The basic measurements useful in clinical appraisal of the pelvis are described on pp 121–125. Normal and abnormal values are listed in Table 14–1. Other useful pelvic measurements are the following:*

*The interspinous and intercristal diameters of the inlet and the intertrochanteric and external conjugate (Baudelocque) diameters have been abandoned as reliable guides to pelvic capacity.

Table 14—1. Measurements in clinical pelvimetry.

Measurement	Normal Value	Abnormal Value (Possibly Inadequate)
Biischial diameter (BI)	$\geqslant$ 8 cm	< 8 cm
Posterior sagittal diameter of outlet (PS)	8—9.5 cm (direct)	< 8 cm
Anteroposterior diameter of outlet (AP)	$\geqslant$ 11.9 cm	< 11.8 cm
Interspinous diameter of mid pelvis	$\geqslant$ 10.5 cm	< 8.5 cm
Diagonal conjugate (DC)	> 11.5 cm	< 11.5 cm
True conjugate (CV)	> 10 cm	< 10 cm
Angle of pubic arch	110—120°	< 90°

A. External: The anterior obstetric sagittal dimension (normal: 7–9 cm) provides important information about the forepelvis and the outlet, since it is an estimation of the subpubic angle and the length of the symphysis. It is the distance from the midpoint of an 8-cm bar (the minimal biischial distance) placed beneath the pubic arch to the top of the symphysis as measured with a McDermott pelvimeter. The fetal head must curve around the sacral promontory as it descends. For further descent and internal rotation, the head must hug the inner aspect of the symphysis and then its lower surface. The longer the symphysis and the narrower the subpubic angle, the deeper the pelvis and the wider the retropubic curve must be for vaginal delivery. Prominent ischial spines and a narrow mid pelvis may also cause dystocia. If the anterior obstetric sagittal dimension is 7–9 cm, midpelvic difficulties are not likely; if the measurement is 9–10 cm, slight difficulty may be expected; and severe dystocia should be anticipated and cesarean section may be required when the measurement is more than 11.5 cm.

B. Internal:

1. The obstetric conjugate (normal: at least 10 cm) is measured from the sacral promontory to the nearest point on the symphysis, which usually is one-third of the distance below the superior margin. The obstetric conjugate is actually the shortest diameter of the pelvic inlet.

2. The transverse diameter of the inlet is normally about 12 cm. Pelvic contraction exists if this measurement is less than 11.5 cm.

Dystocia occurs when any significant pelvic dimension is markedly small unless other dimensions compensate by being larger than normal. Relative disproportion will impede and absolute disproportion will prevent the safe vaginal delivery of a normal infant.

Obstruction may develop at the plane of the pelvic inlet, the mid pelvis, the pelvic outlet, or all 3.

Actually, because the outlet is not truly a plane but a shallow space—an extension of the midplane of the pelvis—the midplane and the outlet should be considered as one in the management of the patient with a contracted pelvis.

Any pelvic measurement is important only in relation to fetal size. Disproportion may occur with "normal" or even spacious pelvic measurements if the infant is relatively large or presents abnormally (see Fetal Dystocia, below).

Clinical Classification

The clinical classification of pelvic contraction is based principally upon pelvic measurements. The measurements are used to estimate pelvic adequacy with reference to the present pregnancy.

Note: A pelvis is classified as contracted when the DC is 11.5 cm or less or when the BI is 8 cm or less. Pelvic contraction almost invariably causes narrowing of the subpubic angle and lack of roundness of the pubic arch. A BI less than 8 cm and a direct PS less than 7 cm—ie, the sum of the BI and the PS is less than 15 cm—may cause difficulty in labor and delivery (Thoms's rule).

If small dimensions or gross distortions are recorded initially, repeat the pelvic measurements during the third trimester when greater muscular relaxation and patient cooperation may give more favorable results. Confirmed contracture usually requires x-ray pelvimetry and consultation regarding the management of labor and mode of delivery.

Three levels of pelvic dystocia are recognized: inlet, mid pelvis, and outlet dystocia.

A. Inlet Dystocia: Inlet dystocia occurs in about 5% of patients at term. Lack of engagement of the vertex before or during early labor may indicate cephalopelvic disproportion. In addition to an adequate inlet (DC > 10.5 cm, etc), other factors influencing engagement are the diameters and malleability of the fetal head, pseudo-overriding at the pelvic brim due to uterine anteversion, low-lying placenta, malpresentation of the fetus, and fetal anomalies. Inlet dystocia is suggested when attempts to maneuver the head into the inlet by applying fundal pressure (DeLee-Hillis maneuver) are unsuccessful.

B. Mid Pelvis Dystocia: Contraction of the mid pelvis alone is 4–5 times as frequent as isolated inlet contraction. Insufficient space in the mid pelvis should be suspected, even before the head has engaged, in the presence of a contracted outlet, prominent or close spines, a masculine physique, a flattened or irregular sacrum, or premature rupture of the membranes with a high vertex or malposition of the fetus. Midpelvic dystocia may be due to funneling of the pelvis (convergence of the side walls and lateral bore, flattening of the sacral concavity) or abnormal projections into the pelvic canal by bony protuberances (prominent ischial spines or genital tumors).

Distortion of the birth canal at the mid pelvis prevents rotation of the fetal head and may even direct the vertex toward the sacrum rather than toward the outlet. In other instances, only rotation to the transverse may be permitted. The vertex is commonly deflected.

C. Outlet Dystocia: Isolated outlet dystocia is rare; outlet dystocia is almost always associated with mid pelvis dystocia.

X-Ray Pelvimetry

The internal pelvic architecture cannot be precisely evaluated by clinical examination alone, since it is difficult to obtain reliable midpelvic measurements manually. However, clinical pelvimetry provides adequate information in most cases. Most of the important pelvic diameters can be measured using ultrasound, but considerable skill and experience are required for accurate mensuration. X-ray visualization is necessary for complete appraisal of the pelvis. Its use should be limited to cases in which proper diagnosis cannot be made by other means or the mode of delivery or conduct of labor will depend on the information obtained by this method. However, radiologic measurements are only ancillary guides and should not be used to forecast the outcome of delivery. Descent and rotation may not occur until the cervix is fully dilated and the membranes have ruptured. The final decision to resort to cesarean section should rest on x-ray pelvimetry alone only in extreme cases of pelvic contracture.

The major dimensions of the superior strait influence the diameter and ease of engagement of the presenting part. The mechanism of labor depends upon the relative size and shape of the mid pelvis and outlet.

A. Indications: X-ray pelvimetry may be indicated at term in 5–8% of obstetric patients, particularly in the following cases:

1. A high social premium on the infant–First pregnancy late in childbearing years or a history of difficult delivery, eg, stillbirths, birth injury, dystocia, or midforceps delivery.

2. Unusual physical findings–Short stature, especially with stigmas of rickets or the short, squat "dystocia dystrophy" build; marked lordosis or kyphosis; unusual gait; history of injury or disease likely to distort the pelvis.

3. Obstetric problems before labor–Contracted inlet or outlet, or narrowing of the interspinous diameter; unengaged vertex at term in a primigravida; large infant (over 4000 g), especially in a diabetic mother; fetal malpresentation, including breech presentation, when vaginal delivery is contemplated.

4. Medical indications–Severe diabetes mellitus, etc.

5. Complications of labor–Failure to progress in labor despite frequent strong, sustained contractions; primary or secondary uterine inertia.

B. Methods: The most popular methods include the following:

1. Isometry or positional method (Thoms, Torpin)–Two films are required:

a. A lateral film of the pelvis is obtained after placing a graduated, notched metal rod in the patient's gluteal fold. The pelvic dimensions may be measured directly from the film by using a centimeter rule.

b. An anteroposterior film of the pelvic inlet is taken with the plane of the superior strait and the film parallel and separated by a known distance. A second exposure of the film is made with a metal grid placed in the plane of the inlet after the patient leaves the x-ray table. Proportionate or isometric diameter values may be obtained directly from the film.

2. Parallax or precision stereoscopic method (Caldwell-Moloy)—An anteroposterior film is obtained; then the tube is moved a slight measured distance laterally and a second film is taken. With stereoscopic viewer, the dimensions of the virtual image may be measured accurately using a centimeter rule held at the same span as the tube distance (infinity). The pelvic shape and capacity may also be evaluated 3-dimensionally.

3. Orthometric method (Hodges)—The pelvic planes are reproduced in either lateral or anteroposterior views as accurate scale tracings using a calibrated instrument similar to the camera lucida. Precise measurements of the pelvis at all levels may be made in this manner.

4. Triangulation method (Ball)—Exact measurements of the pelvic diameters can be calculated using pairs of anteroposterior pelvic roentgenograms taken at 90-degree angles to one another.

Determination of Fetal Head Size

The size of the fetal head can be determined by ultrasonography or x-ray studies. Ultrasonography gives slightly more accurate results and does not expose the fetus and mother to radiation.

X-ray fetal cephalometry requires a lateral and, usually, an anteroposterior inlet and outlet view using one of the methods outlined above. The aim of such studies is to compare the fetal head size and the diameters and contour of the birth canal. The mother should be erect so that the presenting part will drop as far as possible into the true pelvis.

The biparietal diameter and the slightly larger suboccipitobregmatic diameter are the significant fetal cephalic dimensions in engagement. The biparietal diameter has important implications for pelvic "fit" at all levels. The occipitofrontal diameter is a good index of fetal maturity. Serious technical difficulties in cephalometry always occur when the fetus is in abnormal presentation (head in the uterine fundus with breech presentation, floating vertex presentation, obliquity of the fetal head at any level, or transverse presentation).

Pelvic Types

The following is the obstetric classification of pelvic types developed by Caldwell and Moloy: (1) Gynecoid or human female type,

Table 14—2. Pelvic types. (After Caldwell and Moloy.)

	Gynecoid	Android	Anthropoid	Platypelloid
Inlet	Rounded or slightly heart-shaped. Ample anterior and posterior segments.	Wedge-shaped or rounded triangle. Posterior segment wide, flat; anterior narrow, pointed.	Anteroposterior ovoid with length of anterior and posterior segments increased. Transverse diameter reduced.	Transverse ovoid; increased transverse AP diameter of both segments.
Sacrum	Curved, average length.	Straight with forward inclination.	Normally curved but long and narrow.	Curved, short.
Sacrosciatic notch	Medium width.	Narrow.	Wide, shallow.	Slightly narrowed.
Side walls (AP view)	Straight, divergent, or convergent.	Usually convergent.	Straight.	Straight or slightly divergent.
Side walls (lateral view; "lateral bore")	Straight, divergent, or convergent.	Usually convergent.	Often straight.	Straight or divergent.
Interspinous diameter	Wide.	Shortened.	Shortened.	Increased.
Pubic arch	Curved.	Straight.	Slightly curved.	Curved.
Subpubic angle	Wide.	Very narrow.	Narrow.	Wide.
Biischial diameter	Wide.	Shortened.	Often shortened.	Wide.

with a circular or slightly heart-shaped inlet (40–45%). (2) Android type, which simulates the male pelvis including the rounded or triangular superior strait (15–20%). (3) Anthropoid, apelike, or anteroposterior ovoid pelvis (20–30%). (4) Platypelloid or flat pelvis, with a transverse oval inlet (2–5%). The important features of each pelvic type are shown in Table 14–2.

Most pelves are not pure types but incorporate features of 2 varieties. For example, a pelvic inlet with a rounded (gynecoid) posterior segment and an elongated and ovoid (anthropoid) anterior portion is classified as a gynecoid-anthropoid inlet. Other variations or combinations of the 4 types are possible in the configuration of the inlet. The mid pelvis and outlet are not designated as gynecoid, android, etc. Nevertheless, significant distortion and contracture at these levels may prevent spontaneous or even safe operative vaginal delivery.

Among American black women, android pelvis is only about half as frequent as in white women and platypelloid pelves are seen only occasionally, but anthropoid pelves account for almost half. Great varia-

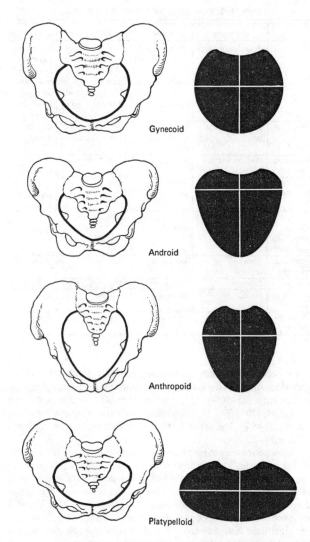

Figure 14–1. Pelvic types. White lines in the diagrams at right show the greatest diameters of the pelves at left.

tions in the heredity and environment of foreign populations make other generalizations regarding pelvic configurations futile.

Clinical Implications of Pelvic Types (See Fig 14–1.)

A. Gynecoid Pelvis: The inlet is rounded with open anterior and posterior segments. Unless the pelvis is smaller than normal (the generally contracted variety) or the fetus is large, a normal birth is likely.

1. Antepartum–Engagement of the vertex occurs at term or early in labor in the transverse diameter of the inlet in over two-thirds of patients.

2. Intrapartum–Normally, with good labor, descent of the vertex through the midplane of the pelvis is rapid, and internal rotation to an occiput anterior position takes place when the biparietal diameter of the head is at or slightly below the spines. Unless an extremely narrow pubic arch, anterior beaking of the sacrum, or other abnormality obstructs the outlet, further descent and extension of the head beneath the symphysis are unimpeded and the infant is delivered normally.

B. Android Pelvis:

1. Antepartum–Engagement is delayed by the encroachment of the sacral promontory into the posterior segment of the superior strait and the narrowness of the anterior segment of the inlet. Occiput transverse presentation occurs in almost three-fourths of cases.

2. Intrapartum–Convergent pelvic side walls and lateral bore, with contracted sacrosciatic notches and a narrow subpubic arch, predispose to a posterior position and require descent of the vertex as a posterior almost to the pelvic floor. Funneling at the mid pelvis wedges the presenting part and restricts its progress, and lack of space between the prominent spines and outlet contraction increase dystocia. Molding of the occiput often leads to its arrest in descent because it cannot rotate easily. Because of difficulty in rotation, the head may have to be delivered by forceps as an occiput posterior presentation despite possible damage to the mother's soft tissues.

C. Anthropoid Pelvis:

1. Antepartum–This pelvic conformation is characterized by an elliptical inlet with a long anteroposterior diameter and a short transverse diameter. The sacral promontory is not prominent and does not impede engagement. The sacrosciatic notches are wide. The vertex usually enters the inlet in either the anterior or posterior position. The former occurs only slightly more often.

2. Intrapartum–Because the ischial spines are often prominent or close-set, the head descends in the position of engagement to the outlet. Rotation usually must be accomplished below or above the spines. If this is not possible, the head will have to be delivered as an occiput posterior presentation.

D. Platypelloid Pelvis: Rickets during childhood is often the cause of flat pelvis and sacral flattening with ridging or bossellation. This combination is extremely serious for the mother and infant during labor. Nonrachitic pelves are often merely foreshortened in the anteroposterior dimension; others are generally contracted. Each presents individual problems.

1. Antepartum–A contracted inlet causes malpresentation or delayed engagement of the vertex at term. A rachitic patient is often short in stature and may have a pendulous abdomen. At term, the high, unengaged presenting part exaggerates the anteflexion of the uterus. Premature rupture of the membranes and prolapse of the cord are frequent complications of flat pelvis. If and when the vertex does enter the pelvis, it engages in the transverse position.

2. Intrapartum–Delivery may be difficult if the CV is 8 cm or less even though the transverse diameter of the inlet is normal (13.5 cm).

In a flat pelvis, engagement may occur with moderate extension of the head, because the bitemporal diameter is 1 cm less than the biparietal diameter. Asynclitism (lateral flexion of the head) may aid engagement, since the vertex must hug either the symphysis or the sacral promontory to enter the superior strait at all. Descent will be slow; the parietal bone may present with the sagittal suture far anterior or posterior depending upon whether anterior or posterior asynclitism (respectively) is present. Pelvic dystocia and failure of application of the presenting part to the cervix may result in secondary inertia, or poor labor may be observed from the start. Expect molding of the head with a large caput succedaneum.

Fortunately, the flat pelvis is often shallow. However, the sacrum may be flattened and irregular, especially if it is rachitic. The arch is usually widened (unless the pelvis is generally contracted or has a funnel tendency). However, forceps application and downward traction in the transverse position with eventual rotation may bring the occiput beneath the symphysis for delivery.

Differential Diagnosis

Lack of engagement may be due to abnormal fetal presentation or position, fetal anomaly, poor labor, placenta previa, pendulous abdomen with uterine anteflexion, or pelvic tumor rather than to fetopelvic disproportion. Failure of descent or rotation of the vertex may be due to ineffectual labor, bowel or bladder distention, or pelvic tumor.

Complications

A. Maternal: Pelvic dystocia may cause prolonged labor (slow progress with relative disproportion), secondary uterine inertia (myometrial fatigue), contraction ring formation (exaggerated retraction), rupture of the uterus (dissipation of force), infection (premature rupture of membranes, long labor, trauma to the birth canal), hemorrhage (lacerations of the birth canal), separation of the symphysis (rupture of the symphyseal ligament during forceps delivery or malrotated vertex), fistula formation (bladder, bowel), and levator or sphincter damage and may necessitate operative delivery (forceps, cesarean section).

B. Fetal: Common fetal injuries with any type of pelvic dystocia are intracranial hemorrhage, depressed and other types of skull fracture, hypoxia, infection, and cervical and brachial plexus damage.

Prevention

The avoidance of pelvic dystocia requires accurate clinical pelvimetry early in each pregnancy. If the findings are unusual or if obstructed labor ensues, x-ray pelvimetry and cephalometry may be indicated.

Treatment of Inlet Dystocia

A. Emergency Measures: If fetal distress occurs, give the mother oxygen and turn her on her side. Monitor the fetus. Immediate cesarean section may be required with cord prolapse, marked fetal distress, or maternal complications.

B. Specific Measures:

1. Measurement of DC–The DC only helps to detect marked inlet contracture. However, if the DC is 11 cm or less in the average Caucasian patient at term, cesarean section will be required.

2. Trial of labor–In borderline cases of pelvic contraction, a trial of labor permits observation of labor for a reasonable period of time to determine whether vaginal delivery may be accomplished with safety for both mother and infant. It should be undertaken only upon consultation, preferably with an experienced obstetrician or radiologist. The safety of a trial of labor is judged according to the maternal and fetal conditions before, during, and after labor, not by the number of hours elapsed.

If the CV is less than 8.5 cm, cesarean section probably will be required. In vertex presentations in which the radiologist reports below-average pelvimetry values with a "small" fetus (approximately 3000 g), a trial of labor is indicated. If the values obtained by pelvimetry are above the mean and the infant is not excessively large (< 4000 g), allow a trial of labor (even with slow progress), since pelvic dystocia is unlikely. Because the fetal head represents the largest diameter of the infant at term, there is no trial of labor for breech presentations. Instead, the decision to attempt vaginal delivery of an average-sized or small infant presenting by the breech is based on the quality and intensity of labor, dilatation and effacement of the cervix, and descent of the presenting part. X-ray pelvimetry and cephalometry should be done in questionable cases. The method of delivery should be decided before labor progresses too far.

In a trial of labor, observe the strength, frequency, and character of uterine contractions; effacement and dilatation of the cervix; and descent of the fetal head. Await the onset of spontaneous labor, and avoid heavy analgesia. Rupture the membranes artificially only when the cervix nears full dilatation. If advancement of the head does not occur within 4–6 hours of strong labor (or 6–8 hours of moderate labor), prepare for cesarean section.

3. "Test" of labor–The test of labor (not to be confused with a trial of labor—see above) is an appraisal of the patient's ability to engage the fetal head with strong labor for 1 hour after complete dilatation of the cervix and rupture of the membranes. A test of labor is rarely performed today, since the decision to operate or continue labor should be (and is) made earlier.

C. Surgical Measures: If cesarean section is necessary, the low cervical type is preferred. (*Caution:* Never attempt vaginal delivery by version or breech extraction or high forceps delivery in cases of inlet disproportion. The fetus—and perhaps the mother also—may die. If the infant dies during labor, embryotomy and vaginal delivery are usually feasible.)

Treatment of Mid Pelvis Dystocia

A. Emergency Measures: Give oxygen for fetal distress. Monitor the fetus. Immediate cesarean section may be required for severe fetal distress or maternal exhaustion during labor.

B. Specific Measures:

1. Obtain x-ray pelvimetry and cephalometry when an abnormal presentation (including breech) complicates midplane contracture. Determine the course of action before the onset of labor. Elective cesarean section is justified in the uncommon instance of marked midplane (or outlet) contraction.

2. Ascertain that engagement has occurred. Excessive molding together with caput succedaneum may give the false impression that the head is engaged. If the fetal head obliterates the available retropubic space and the greatest diameter of the skull has passed through the inlet, engagement is certain.

3. Reevaluate the mid pelvis and outlet clinically when engagement is followed by desultory labor (secondary uterine inertia) or lack of satisfactory progress after good labor. Consider the depth and regularity of the sacrum, the prominence of the ischial spines, the interspinous diameter, the width and depth of the sacrosciatic notches, and the BI and PS of the outlet. If one or more of these indices are significantly abnormal in relation to the size of the fetus, x-ray pelvimetry and cephalometry are indicated. Permit a trial of labor when the interspinous diameter (observed by x-ray) is 9.5 cm or more and the anteroposterior diameter of the midplane is 10.5 cm or more, provided that outlet measurements are adequate and the fetus is small or average-sized.

Mengert determined that the product of the anteroposterior and transverse diameters of the midplane is normally 125 (100%) for women in the USA (Mengert index). When the Mengert index is less than 85%, perform cesarean section if a brief trial of labor is unsatisfactory.

A trial forceps delivery—gentle traction or gradual rotation toward an anterior position (or both)—after a second stage of 1–2 hours may be elected by an experienced obstetrician when an infant of average size is arrested by a borderline midplane contraction in the absence of outlet contracture. If this is unsuccessful, the diagnosis is abandoned trial forceps (failed forceps), and cesarean section is required.

C. General Measures: Encourage the patient and avoid tension. Do not stimulate labor with oxytocics if disproportion is likely. Monitor the fetus. Limit sedation; do not perform caudal or spinal block until the fetal biparietal diameter is well below the ischial spines. Maintain fluid and electrolyte balance.

D. Treatment of Complications: Suture lacerations (especially cervical), replace excessive blood loss, and give appropriate antibiotics for infection. Consider laparotomy if rupture of the uterus is likely.

Treatment of Outlet Dystocia

A. Emergency Measures: Give oxygen for fetal distress. Cesarean section is required if fetal distress complicates a severe but previously unrecognized outlet disproportion during labor.

B. Specific Measures:

1. Perform elective cesarean section when the sum of the BI and PS is less than 15 cm. (See Thoms's rule, p 122.)

2. A trial of labor is not possible in outlet dystocia, because of the hazard to the fetus.

3. If an incurved, ankylosed coccyx obstructs the presenting part, fracture it at the sacrococcygeal articulation after induction of anesthesia and then deliver the fetus with forceps.

C. General Measures: As for mid pelvis dystocia.

D. Treatment of Complications: Suture lacerations, replace excessive blood loss, and prescribe appropriate antibiotics for infection.

Prognosis

In general, the size of the pelvis is more significant to the outcome of labor than its shape.

An experienced physician can accurately predict the course of labor in about two-thirds of patients before or early in labor. The remainder will require trials of labor and x-ray or other consultation.

The diagnosis of pelvic adequacy is generally easy and accurate; the diagnosis of pelvic inadequacy is difficult and inaccurate. The price of error in either case is increased fetal and maternal mortality and morbidity.

SOFT TISSUE DYSTOCIA

Soft tissue tumors or a rigid pelvic floor may be responsible for dystocia. Vaginal and rectal examinations or ultrasonography may identify a cervical, ovarian, or other tumor impeding labor.

DYSTOCIA DUE TO UTERINE DYSFUNCTION

Dystocia may occur when the myometrial contractions are irregular, too weak or strong, too frequent or infrequent, or too brief or prolonged. The tone of the uterine wall is perhaps even more important than the character of the contractions to the progress of labor. A hypertonic uterus relaxes poorly between contractions and is unusually firm during contractions; a hypotonic uterus is flaccid between contractions and not firm even at the height of contractions. Neither a "tight" nor a "loose" uterine wall is efficient during labor.

Cervical effacement and dilatation depend upon frequent strong, sustained, regular uterine contractions, with good relaxation between contractions. Normally, a uterine contraction begins near one cornu and spreads over the uterus to the lower segment. When contractions are inefficient—especially in hypertonic uterine states—contraction begins in the lower segment and spreads upward (reversed polarity). The so-called colicky uterus is characterized by general irritability and many ectopic contractions; inadequate cervical dilatation and effacement result. Failure of the cervix to dilate and efface, coupled with inefficient labor, leads to prolonged labor.

Uterine dystocia complicates 2–3% of labors at term. At least 90% of cases occur in primigravidas.

Any of the following may cause uterine dystocia: uterine anomalies and tumors (eg, bicornuate uterus, myomas), uterine distention (eg, polyhydramnios), delayed or missed labor (eg, fetal death), cervical abnormalities (eg, scarring, fibrosis, tumors), and maternal disease (eg, ventral hernia, chronic illness). Some cases classed as idiopathic are perhaps due to psychogenic factors. In many cases of uterine dystocia, minor degrees of fetopelvic disproportion or resistance of the soft parts within the pelvis appear to reduce the efficiency of contractions. When there is lack of engagement, labor is further compromised.

Uterine dysfunction may complicate all stages of labor. Prompt diagnosis and appropriate treatment are essential in order to avoid dire consequences for the mother and fetus. Trauma and infection are the principal dangers for both mother and fetus. Violent labor may result in fetal distress, precipitate delivery, and injury to both mother and fetus. The incidence of infection during delivery is directly related to the length of labor, particularly when the membranes are ruptured. The necessity for operative delivery is increased in prolonged labor. Even if delivery is accomplished eventually, postpartal atony of the uterus may cause exsanguinating hemorrhage.

In evaluating the quality of labor, the presentation, position, and size of the fetus and the dimensions and configuration of the pelvis must be considered. The expulsive forces work against the resistance of the soft and firm tissues of the pelvis. Resistance is overcome slowly or not at all in dystocia due to uterine dysfunction.

A. Hypotonic Contractions: In most instances of dystocia due to uterine dysfunction, hypotonic contractions prolong the acceleration phase of labor. Hypotonic contractions occasionally occur during the latent phase of labor also. The term uterine inertia is synonymous with hypotonic uterine dystocia and implies ineffectual labor. There are 2 types, primary and secondary.

1. Primary uterine inertia–In primary uterine inertia, contractions are ineffectual from the start of labor. This may be due to induction of labor or spontaneous rupture of the membranes before the uterus is "ready" to contract normally, congenital anomalies of the uterus, unengaged presenting part, malpresentation, or malposition.

2. Secondary uterine inertia–In secondary uterine inertia, good contractions give way to poor ones. This may be caused by overdistention of the uterus (due to polyhydramnios, multiple pregnancy, or a large fetus), which stretches and thins the myometrium; excessive analgesia and anesthesia, which obliterates uterine contractions; emotional tension and release of catecholamines, which may reduce the stimulatory effect of oxytocin on the myometrium; or fetopelvic disproportion, which causes uterine fatigue.

B. Hypertonic Contractions: Hypertonic contractions usually occur during the active phase of labor and become more severe as labor progresses. They are more serious than hypotonic contractions.

Clinical Findings (See Fig 14–2.)

A. Hypotonic Uterus: In a flaccid uterus, cervical dilatation and effacement are usually normal; pain is slight and complaints are minor; and contractions are weak but fundal dominance is maintained.

B. Hypertonic Uterus: There are 2 basic types, and fetal distress may develop in both; hence, the fetal heart tones should be monitored.

1. The fundus and lower uterine segment are tense; the cervix may be normal or spastic. Pain is extreme and seems to the observer to be out of proportion to the force of the contractions. Backache is persistent. Ileus and urinary retention are common. Uterine polarity is reversed, with lower segment dominance. A contraction ring often forms with uterine fatigue.

2. In "colicky uterus" (occasionally with a septate or bicornuate fundus) with a normal or spastic cervix, the uterus is irritable and prone

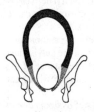

Normal

Colicky

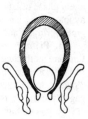

Asymmetric
and colicky

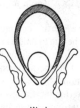

Weak

Hypertonic lower
segment

Hypertonic
internal os

Figure 14–2. Normal and dysfunctional uterine contraction types. (After Jeffcoate.) Black, strong contraction; shaded, slight contraction; white, atonic areas.

to asynchronous action. The patient complains of almost constant pain that is worse with contractions. Restlessness and aerophagia are common. Variable polarity and incoordinate contractions are apparent. A contraction ring may eventually form.

Differential Diagnosis

False labor is usually a sequence of irregular, slightly crampy uterine contractions that do not increase in frequency or intensity. The uterus is generally hypotonic. The cervix does not dilate or efface, and the presenting part does not descend. False labor actually consists of strong Braxton Hicks contractions.

Cervical dystocia is due to either scarring and stenosis of the cervix, usually as a result of surgery or infection, or functional spasm, in which case hypertonic uterine inertia is often an associated factor.

Retraction ring (Bandl's ring) is a narrow but viselike, unyielding zone of myometrial contraction between the upper and lower uterine segments—an exaggerated, pathologic retraction ring. This disorder only occurs after long labor against a mechanical obstruction, ie, it is a complication of malpresentation or fetopelvic disproportion. Constant, agonizing uterine pain and tenderness precede rupture of the lower uterine segment. Rupture is inevitable unless cesarean section is done or the obstruction is relieved. The markedly thickened uterine wall above the ring makes palpation of the fetus difficult.

Constriction ring is a persistent contraction of all or part of a segment of the uterus around a narrowed portion of the fetus. The ring is the result of dysrhythmic uterine contractions and may occur at any level during any stage of labor. Constriction ring often is associated with prolonged (never obstructed) labor, especially after the membranes have been ruptured for some time. Characteristically, colicky pains persist well after the uterine contraction ceases. On examination, the flaccid cervix is observed to hang loosely, even during a contraction, so that the presenting part remains abnormally mobile. Vaginal palpation often reveals that the ring is compressing the fetus considerably above the relaxed cervix. Medication may relax the ring (see p 394); however, no drug is dependable. Operative intervention is often required. The fetus is endangered by hypoxia, asphyxia, and delivery trauma.

Missed labor is very rare. Labor begins at or near term but soon ceases. The fetus dies before or soon after failure of labor and is retained. Amniotic fluid is reabsorbed. The products of conception then disintegrate, and infection often develops.

Uterine anomalies are discussed on p 579.

Prolonged labor (ie, labor that continues for 24 hours or more) may be due to failure of the expulsive forces, fetopelvic disproportion, or abnormal presentation or position of the fetus.

Precipitate labor (ie, delivery occurs in 3 hours or less) may be due to excessively strong, frequent contractions or reduced resistance of soft tissues in the pelvis.

Complications

The incidence of prolonged labor, operative delivery (and possible injury), and intrapartal and postpartal infection is increased in uterine dystocia.

Prevention

Antepartal conditioning of the patient does much to allay her fears and anxieties and seems to improve the quality of labor if other factors are favorable. Avoidance of induction and limitation of heavy analgesia early in labor will ensure the quality of labor. Early recognition and proper treatment of dystocia due to uterine dysfunction will usually prevent serious complications.

Treatment

A. Specific Measures:

1. Hypotonic uterus–Unless fetopelvic disproportion is present, stimulate labor by amniotomy and by giving oxytocin, 1–2 mU/min intravenously, with an increase of this dosage every 15–20 minutes if necessary, provided that no fetal or maternal complications develop.

2. Hypertonic uterus–In the absence of fetopelvic disproportion, give morphine sulfate, 15 mg intramuscularly, to relieve pain; and phenobarbital, 60 mg intramuscularly, for sedation. Catheterize as necessary to avoid painful bladder distention. Correct fluid and electrolyte imbalance if indicated. When labor resumes (in 2–4 hours), apply an abdominal binder if the uterus is pendulous and the direction of force of the uterine contraction is not in the axis of the birth canal. Maldirection of force may be the basic cause of poor engagement and failure of descent.

3. "Colicky uterus"–Treat as for hypertonic uterus (see above). Paracervical anesthesia may relax the cervix sufficiently to permit effacement and dilatation.

B. General Measures: Reassure the patient and maintain fluid and electrolyte balance. Broad-spectrum antibiotics should be given to all patients with signs or symptoms of intrapartal infection and to those in prolonged labor.

C. Surgical Measures:

1. If fetal distress and desultory labor occur despite stimulation of the hypotonic uterus, proceed to cesarean section.

2. Cesarean section is indicated in prolonged labor, especially prolonged labor associated with borderline cephalopelvic disproportion or constriction ring, and in retraction ring.

D. Treatment of Associated Problems:

1. False labor–Reassure the patient and await the onset of true labor.

2. Cervical dystocia–

a. If dystocia is due to scarring and stenosis of the cervix, incise the cervix—perhaps at the 2-o'clock and 4-o'clock positions—when it becomes effaced. Perform cesarean section only if incision and vaginal delivery are not feasible.

b. If cervical spasticity and hypertonic uterine inertia are present, sedate the patient adequately during labor. Use regional anesthesia in the late first stage and during the second stage of labor. Dührssen's incisions should be used only when absolutely necessary. Cesarean section may be necessary.

3. Constriction ring–

a. In the first stage of labor–Give intravenously 10% glucose in water containing 0.5 g of calcium gluconate and 2.5 g (5 mL of 50% solution) of magnesium sulfate per liter.

b. In the second stage of labor–Give amyl nitrite, one pellet inhaled, or epinephrine, 1:1000 solution, 0.5 mL intramuscularly, and ether anesthesia.

4. Missed labor–Prevent cervico-uterine contamination (avoid artificial rupture of the membranes). Stimulate the refractory uterus repeatedly (but not continuously) by intravenous administration of oxytocin, 1–2 mL (10–20 units) per liter of 5% glucose in water, after topical application of prostaglandin (PGF_2 in a gel) to the cervix. If intrauterine infection occurs and attempts to evacuate the uterine contents are not successful, consider total abdominal hysterectomy with drainage. Laparotomy is indicated only for treatment of perforation of the uterus or intraperitoneal complications.

5. Precipitate labor–Give analgesics in minimal doses and use regional anesthesia. Consider cautious elective induction of labor at term when the patient gives a history of repeated episodes of precipitate labor.

E. Treatment of Complications:

1. Prolonged labor–Determine the cause and give appropriate treatment; give broad-spectrum antibiotics in full doses; and maintain fluid and electrolyte balance. Consider delivery by cesarean section.

2. Postpartal hemorrhage–See p 226.

3. Postpartal infection–Administer broad-spectrum antibiotics and ergot preparations.

Prognosis

The prognosis is good for both mother and fetus if the diagnosis is made early and appropriate treatment is given. Prolonged labor, intrapartal infection, and trauma are particularly dangerous to the fetus.

DYSTOCIA OF FETAL ORIGIN

Anomalous development, large size, or abnormal presentation or position of the fetus often retards or obstructs the process of labor and delivery. This occurs in approximately 0.5% of labors at term. With large fetuses, the incidence of shoulder dystocia may approach 20%.

Dystocia due to fetal abnormalities is caused by nonengagement or arrest of the presenting part. In vertex presentations with disproportion due to a large or hydrocephalic fetus, the head may never enter the pelvic inlet. Lack of engagement is notable also in malpresentation. If the fetus is deformed or enlarged, the head may be able to traverse the superior strait, but the body may then obstruct to prevent further descent. Shoulder dystocia is impaction of the fetal shoulders after the head is delivered in cephalic presentations. In breech presentations, engagement with obstruction by a following part may prevent or retard vaginal delivery.

The site of arrest will depend upon the presentation and the severity and location of the fetal deformity in relation to the maternal pelvic dimensions and architecture.

Previous uncomplicated pregnancy is no guarantee of safe delivery in subsequent pregnancies. A woman who has been delivered of one or more average-sized infants without difficulty may produce one no larger that may present abnormally and fail to engage or may arrest deep in the pelvis because of malposition. Such a woman may also develop a larger, disproportionate fetus.

Causes of Fetal Dystocia

The size of the infant in relation to the mother's pelvis and the shape and consistency of the presenting part determine the "fit" of the infant in the birth canal. Fetal causes of dystocia include the following:

A. Large Size: (> 4000 g.) Heredity, maternal diabetes mellitus, and parity of the mother (the size of infants tends to increase with parity) influence the size of the fetus.

B. Anomalous Development: Monsters (conjoined twins), hydrocephalus.

C. Abnormal Girth:

1. Internal abnormality–Hydrops fetalis, ascites, abdominal tumor (congenital cystic disease of the kidney, teratoma).

2. External abnormality–Myelomeningocele, sacral tumor.

D. Malpresentation: Transverse, oblique, shoulder, breech, or compound presentation. Shoulder dystocia is more likely to occur in obese patients or those with diabetes mellitus; those with a history of oversized (> 4000 g) postdate or macrosomic infants; those who require midforceps delivery after a prolonged second stage of labor; and those who receive epidural anesthesia too early in labor, with the result that the fetal head does not descend and rotate normally.

Clinical Findings

A. Symptoms and Signs: If labor is good, with adequate uterine tone and strong, sustained, regular uterine contractions, slow progress may be due to fetal factors. When the head is abnormally large, progress may be slowed by abnormal presentation, failure of the presenting part to engage, or unusual position. When the body is distended or deformed, engagement of the vertex may occur with arrest of descent after the thorax passes through the pelvic inlet. Hydrocephalus will occasionally deter engagement in vertex presentations, or there may be stoppage at the inlet if the infant presents by the breech. An unusual contour of the uterus may be noted on palpation in extreme cases of fetal anomaly near term.

Delivery will be impossible unless the fetal shoulders can traverse the pelvic inlet. In the normal course of events, the shoulders (the bisacromial diameter) enter the pelvis in an oblique diameter and then shift during descent and internal rotation to the anteroposterior diameter (which is shorter than the oblique in gynecoid, android, and platypelloid pelves). This permits the shoulders to enter the inlet. The anterior shoulder then stems beneath the symphysis, and first one shoulder and then the other shoulder and the thorax are delivered. In shoulder dystocia, the bisacromial diameter of the fetus usually obstructs in the anteroposterior diameter of the pelvis (except when the pelvis is anthropoid, in which case obstruction occurs in the transverse or oblique diameter); one or both shoulders overhang the margin of the symphysis and fail to engage. Impaction of both shoulders is rare. Arrest of the anterior shoulder is more serious than arrest of the posterior shoulder.

The diagnosis of shoulder dystocia can be made only after the head has been delivered. Then the following are diagnostic: (1) The head recoils back against the perineum and remains immobile because spontaneous restitution is restricted. (2) Even moderate traction with fundal pressure fails to deliver the infant. (3) No fetal abnormality (eg, tumor) or maternal problem (eg, uterine contraction ring) capable of arresting delivery is found on vaginal examination.

B. Ultrasonographic Findings: Ultrasonography may reveal an anomaly and is preferred to roentgenography.

C. X-Ray Findings: X-ray films, if feasible during the first stage of labor, may disclose a skeletal anomaly.

D. Special Examinations: Vaginal examination may reveal unusual cranial configuration (as with anencephaly, meningocele).

Differential Diagnosis

Malpresentation or faulty engagement may be due to a maternal disorder or placental abnormality rather than a fetal anomaly. Abdominal or vaginal examination may disclose pelvic tumors or exostoses that arrest the presenting part after its engagement and partial descent. Ultrasonography or x-ray films may disclose a low-lying placenta. Abnormal position or even incomplete rotation of the fetus during the birth process may occur without obvious cause.

Complications

Operative delivery may be necessary, and maternal injury may occur. Fetal death usually follows cerebral or abdominal decompression upon delivery. In delivery complicated by shoulder or breech dystocia, traction injury to the brachial plexus may result in brachial palsy, or the humerus or clavicle may be fractured; hypoxic brain damage or intranatal death may result unless the impaction is quickly resolved.

Prevention

Early diagnosis of the fetal anomaly (preferably before labor begins) is important. Although shoulder dystocia cannot be predicted, it occasionally may seem likely on the basis of the history, physical examination, or progress of labor. Ultrasonographic measurement of the fetal chest and maternal pelvic diameters may identify problems that could lead to arrest of the shoulders. Liberalization of indications for cesarean section for women at risk for shoulder dystocia will reduce its incidence. Elective termination of pregnancy, usually by induction and vaginal delivery, is recommended when the fetus obviously cannot survive (eg, anencephaly).

Treatment

A. Emergency Measures: Immediate sterile vaginal examination, with the patient under deep inhalation anesthesia, may be required when delivery is difficult or impossible after the birth of a part of the body. Rotate the fetus so that its shoulders are in the anteroposterior diameter of the pelvis; this may allow palpation of an anomaly or may facilitate delivery in shoulder dystocia.

B. Specific Measures for Shoulder Dystocia: If shoulder dystocia is suspected, first perform a generous episiotomy. If the first attempt to deliver the anterior shoulder fails, it is highly imprudent to repeat the maneuver. When the head is subjected to sharp lateral flexion or moved downward in a jerky manner, great tension is put upon the brachial plexus, and Erb's palsy may result. A number of maneuvers capable of freeing the shoulder or shoulders must be tried, preferably after anesthesia has been rapidly induced. None is easy, but the author prefers the following sequence:

1. Cautiously draw the head downward and backward until the anterior shoulder impinges against the symphysis. Then lift the head upward. This will aid in delivery of the posterior shoulder.

2. Slip a hand behind the fetus, and hook the posterior axilla with a finger. Exert the heaviest possible downward traction in an effort to advance the posterior shoulder into the hollow of the sacrum. It is difficult to exert enough traction in this fashion to do any damage. If the posterior shoulder can be advanced more deeply into the hollow of the sacrum, a little more room will be provided, and the anterior shoulder may engage for prompt delivery.

3. Using the same approach as above, grasp the posterior fetal arm and sweep it across the abdomen. Flex the fetal elbow; then loop a finger around the forearm and draw the hand and arm down and out. Engagement of the anterior shoulder should follow.

4. The operator's hand may be insinuated behind the anterior shoulder to rotate the shoulders into an oblique pelvic diameter, after which moderate traction on the head, aided by suprapubic pressure, should bring the shoulders into and through the pelvic inlet.

5. Fracture or disarticulation of a clavicle, although difficult and traumatic, will shorten the bisacromial diameter and thus simplify extraction.

6. Rotate the fetal shoulders through an arc of 180 degrees, from LOT to ROT (or the reverse) (screw principle of Woods). Since the posterior shoulder is already engaged relatively low in the pelvis, rotation of this shoulder to the anterior causes it to stem beneath the symphysis anteriorly in a manner similar to that encountered when one disengages a screw. The formerly impacted (anterior) shoulder, rotating in the opposite direction while fundal pressure is applied, comes into the hollow of the sacrum and is easily delivered. (*Caution:* This procedure should not be attempted without practice on a mannequin or considerable obstetric experience.)

7. Cleidotomy is appropriate if the fetus is dead.

C. General Measures: Attempt vaginal delivery, but avoid giving the patient heavy analgesia until the cause of the dystocia is known. If the hazard to the mother seems too great, perform cesarean section after first informing the husband or closest adult relative about the fetal deformity and the chances that the infant will survive.

D. Surgical Measures: Operative intervention is almost always required. Drainage of cerebrospinal fluid from a hydrocephalic infant or paracentesis for abdominal decompression may be required for delivery. Embryotomy may be necessary for delivery of a dead fetus. Cesarean section is justified in the rare instance of living conjoined twins or for other gross abnormality when vaginal delivery might jeopardize the mother's life or health.

E. Treatment of Complications: Birth canal injury (see p 167), postpartal hemorrhage (see pp 226 and 272), and puerperal infection (see p 301) are common sequelae of delivery of malformed fetuses or those that present abnormally. For treatment of fracture of the clavicle and injury of the brachial plexus, see p 202.

Prognosis

If a complicated, traumatic delivery can be avoided, the prognosis for the mother is good. The prognosis for the infant with developmental anomalies ranges from guarded to very poor depending upon the seriousness of the anomaly. A large infant safely delivered does just as well as an infant of normal size, although large infants born of diabetic mothers require special care. If the infant's clavicle or humerus is fractured during delivery, the prognosis is good when the arm and shoulder are immobilized for several weeks. When brachial palsy results from injury of the brachial plexus, the prognosis depends on the type, site, and degree of nerve injury. The prognosis with fetal hypoxia varies (see p 98).

DYSTOCIA OF PLACENTAL ORIGIN

Placenta previa may prevent delivery of the fetus because of its situation near or over the internal os or because of excessive bleeding, often secondary to examination or instrumentation during labor. Also, a placenta implanted posteriorly in the lower uterine segment, opposite the promontory of the sacrum, may prevent descent of the presenting part, suggesting bony dystocia.

Painless ante- or intrapartal bleeding may suggest placenta previa. A low-lying, posteriorly implanted placenta generally is symptomless.

No pelvic contractures, tumors, or fetal abnormalities are identifiable with a low, posteriorly implanted placenta; and the pattern of labor is normal. Soft tissue dystocia (eg, uterine myoma) or fetal malpresentation or malposition must be considered.

Ultrasonography or x-ray studies are diagnostic only if the placenta can be identified. Amniography may be very revealing.

Emergency measures consist of management of placenta previa (see p 279). Cesarean section probably will be required for patients presenting with over 30% placenta previa. Except when a small infant can descend past the point of placental obstruction, cesarean delivery will be necessary in cases of low-lying posterior placental insertion.

The prognosis is good with early recognition of the problem and cesarean section.

Operative Delivery | 15

FORCEPS OPERATIONS

Forceps operations, providing traction or rotation of the fetal head (or both), are used to expedite labor or to actually deliver the fetus. There are both fetal and maternal indications for the use of obstetric forceps; today, forceps are occasionally mandatory but more often elective. Forceps procedures are classified principally according to the situation of the head within the bony pelvis (see p 407). Some type of forceps operation is used in 20–30% of births in most large hospitals in the USA.

Properly performed forceps operations will frequently save the life

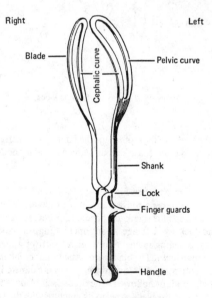

Figure 15–1. Simpson forceps.

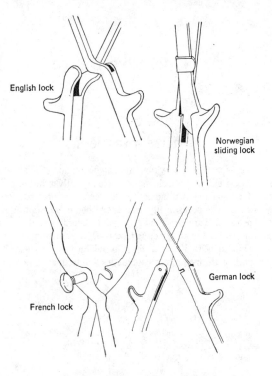

English lock

Norwegian
sliding lock

French lock

German lock

Figure 15–2. Types of forceps locks.

or preserve the health of the mother and the infant; improperly performed forceps operations often cause serious permanent injury or death of one or both.

The Obstetric Forceps (See Figs 15–1, 15–2, and 15–3.)

The obstetric forceps consists of a pair of metal blades each connected to a shank and the shank to a handle. The blades are crossed, like scissors, and lock by a flange arrangement (English lock), a screw (French lock), a sliding device (Norwegian lock), or a notch and pin coupling (German lock). The blades are named right or left according to the side of the patient's pelvis toward which they are directed. They may be fenestrated, solid, or hollowed. The tip of each blade is the toe; and the inferior curve of the blade, toward its juncture with the shank, is the heel. Most forceps blades are fixed to the shank at an angle that will correspond to the pelvic axis when they are applied to the fetal head. Thus, in the classic forceps, the dorsal contour describes a pelvic curve. The cephalic curve is the lateral rounding of each blade that permits the forceps to "fit" the fetal head.

Axis traction is the correct forceps guidance of the head through the most favorable areas of the pelvis. It is actually a duplication of the mechanism of labor.

Types of Forceps (See Figs 15–3 and 15–4.)

Hundreds of modifications of forceps have been designed, and all have their advantages and disadvantages. The choice of whether to use forceps—and which forceps to use—always depends on the specific problem faced and the physician's experience with delivery problems and obstetric instruments. No forceps design can be "the best" for all problems.

There are at least 6 basic types of forceps:

A. Classic Forceps: This forceps is derived directly from the original Chamberlen forceps. It has fenestrated blades with good cephalic and pelvic curves and usually a flange lock. There are 2 subdivisions of the classic forceps: (1) Forceps with overlapping shanks and considerably rounded cephalic curves. (The Elliot forceps, the prototype, is considered by many to be a multipurpose forceps.) This instrument is ideal for the unmolded head. (2) Forceps with separated shanks that provide a flattened cephalic curve. (The Simpson forceps is the prime example.) A molded head is well accepted by this instrument. Modifications of both of these subtypes are now available with solid blades.

B. Tarnier Forceps: The Tarnier forceps, the first practical axis traction instrument, has fenestrated blades, partially closed shanks with an extended but shallow cephalic curve, and a fair pelvic curve. A French screw lock and an additional screw clamp ensure purchase on the head. Rods from the heel of each blade connect with a traction bar via 2 swivel joints. The Tarnier forceps permits excellent adjustment of the direction of force. Although moderately heavy, this instrument is an excellent tractor for large, molded heads in the mid pelvis. When it is used as a rotator, the long, extended blades may be hazardous to maternal soft parts and may also dangerously compress the fetal head.

C. Kielland Forceps: This forceps is light in weight and fenestrated. It has an intermediate cephalic curve but no pelvic curve, a long shank, and a sliding lock bracket (on the left blade only). Buttons on the handle finger guards indicate the backs of the blades (which must always be directed toward the fetal occiput). The Kielland forceps is most useful for transverse and posterior position arrests, but a good application can often be obtained on even the aftercoming or asynclitic head. This forceps is exceptionally well suited to rotation of the fetal head.

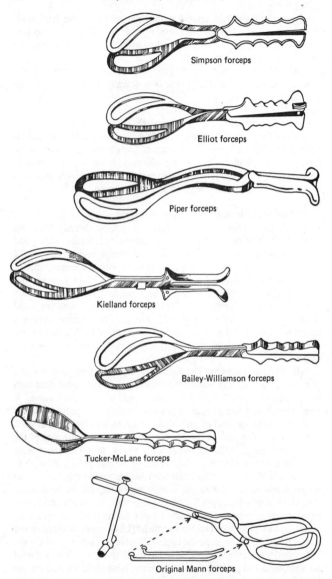

Figure 15-3. Types of forceps.

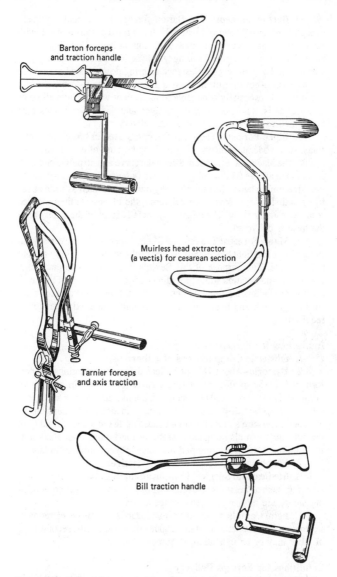

Barton forceps
and traction handle

Muirless head extractor
(a vectis) for cesarean section

Tarnier forceps
and axis traction

Bill traction handle

Figure 15–4. Types of forceps with traction handles and a head extractor for cesarean section.

D. Barton Forceps: The Barton forceps has a light, uniquely hinged, fenestrated anterior blade. The fenestrated posterior blade, with its deep cephalic curve, is heavy in comparison. Coupling is accomplished with a restricted sliding type lock. The blades have no pelvic curve. The Bartonforceps is designed to bring down a head arrested in the transverse position in mid pelvis and then rotate it to the anterior position. It is especially applicable to the patient with a platypelloid or android pelvis. It is a poor tractor, however, and classic type blades must be applied as a low forceps for actual delivery.

E. Piper Forceps: The Piper forceps is used in breech presentations. It is moderately heavy and very long because of its curved, open shank. The blades have a flattened cephalic curve and no pelvic curve. A flange lock allows fixation of the parts. In order to apply this forceps to the aftercoming head, the infant's body must be elevated as soon as the trunk and shoulders have been delivered; the blades are then inserted from beneath the body. The infant may actually straddle the shanks until the head is delivered.

F. Mann Forceps: The original Mann forceps has a universal joint in the shank and light blades with a deep cephalic curve but only a slight pelvic curve. The purpose of this flexible instrument is to encourage normal internal rotation while providing traction for descent of the head; it is used to facilitate normal descent. Two light rods, one on each side, fix to the shank and blades to provide rigidity when axial traction is required.

Indications for Forceps Delivery

A. Obstetric Complications of Labor:

1. Dystocia–About 75% of indicated forceps operations are performed because ineffectual uterine contractions result in prolonged, desultory labor. Prolonged or desultory labor may also be due to slight or relative fetopelvic disproportion. Although inadequate dimensions of the bony pelvis are a more important cause of disproportion, rigidity of the soft parts can also impede passage of the infant. Poor flexion or malrotation of the presenting part may also prevent progress in labor.

2. Prophylactic forceps delivery (elective).

B. Medical and Surgical Complications of Labor: These include disorders such as heart disease (class III or IV), appendicitis complicating labor, and intracranial hemorrhage at term.

C. Fetal Complications of Labor: Established late deceleration or severe variable deceleration of the fetal heart rate during the second stage of labor may be an indication for forceps delivery.

Conditions for Forceps Delivery

The use of forceps is permissible only when *all* of the following conditions prevail, regardless of the urgent need for delivery:

(1) The head must present correctly (vertex presentation, face presentation with chin anterior, or aftercoming head in breech presentation) and must be engaged.

(2) There must be no clinically demonstrable cephalopelvic disproportion.

(3) The cervix must be dilated and effaced.

(4) The membranes must be ruptured.

(5) The bladder and rectum must be empty.

(6) An episiotomy (generally a mediolateral incision for forceps operations other than outlet) must have been performed.

(7) There must be maternal or fetal indications (see above) for use of forceps.

Classification of Forceps Deliveries

(1) Low forceps is the application of forceps when the head is visible during contraction, with the bony portion of the head resting on the perineal floor and the sagittal suture in the anteroposterior or oblique diameter.

(2) Mid forceps is the application of forceps before the criteria for low forceps are met but after the plane of the greatest cephalic diameter (biparietal) has passed the inlet.

(3) High forceps is the application of forceps before engagement has taken place. Floating forceps delivery is accomplished by applying the blades to a high, "floating" (unengaged) head. High or floating forceps has been abandoned because of the dire injuries that it almost always inflicts on both mother and infant. If the biparietal diameter has not passed through (below) the inlet, forceps delivery is contraindicated.

The foregoing definitions refer only to the station of the head at the time the operation is begun. Four additional definitions apply to special circumstances:

(4) Trial forceps is the application of cautious traction after apparently satisfactory mid forceps application, with the intention of abandoning attempts at forceps delivery if undue resistance is encountered.

(5) Abandoned forceps is the elective resort to cesarean section after trial forceps.

(6) Failed forceps is the continued attempt to accomplish forceps delivery (usually mid forceps) in spite of problems resulting in injury to the mother or fetus.

(7) "Prophylactic forceps" (DeLee) is the use of outlet forceps (not low or mid forceps) and episiotomy to reduce maternal stress by shortening the second stage of labor, prevent injury to the pelvic floor and viscera, limit blood loss, and prevent injury to the fetal head.

Only experienced operators should be permitted to perform even prophylactic forceps operations. For the inexperienced physician, prophylactic forceps delivery is meddlesome midwifery.

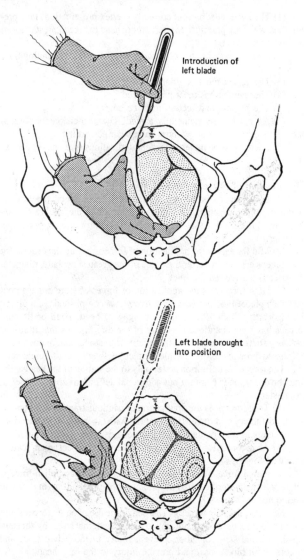

Introduction of
left blade

Left blade brought
into position

Figure 15–5. Forceps application.

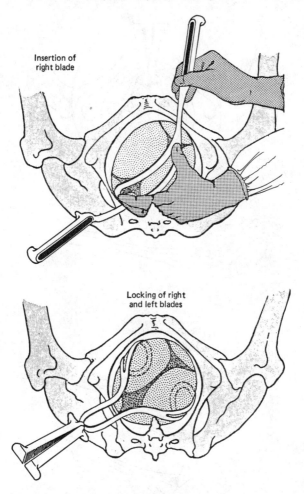

Figure 15–5 (cont'd). Forceps application.

The Technique of Use of Obstetric Forceps (See Fig 15–5.)

The use of the obstetric forceps proceeds in the following steps:

A. Insertion: Classically, the left forceps handle is held like a violin bow in the operator's left hand, and the blade is directed toward the left side of the patient's pelvis and the left side of the fetal head. The

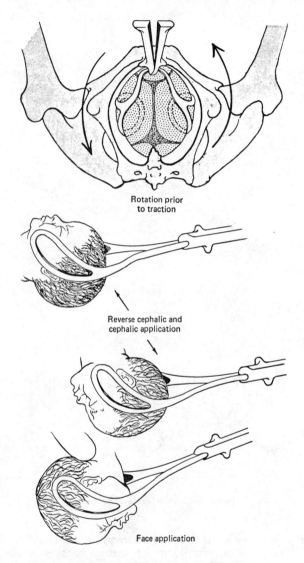

Rotation prior
to traction

Reverse cephalic and
cephalic application

Face application

Figure 15–5 (cont'd). Forceps application.

right forceps handle is held in the right hand, and a similar procedure is followed on the right side.

B. Application: With the left handle in the left hand, insert 2 or 3 fingers of the right hand into the vagina and guide the blade to its optimal position on the fetal head. Repeat with the right blade, using the left hand to guide the blade.

C. Articulation: Couple the blades at the shank only if this can be done without using force. Properly applied forceps should articulate easily. Check the position of each blade by noting its relation to the fetal ear. If the blades are not properly applied, revise the application. The first blade is more apt to be applied correctly; therefore, the second blade should be readjusted initially and a second attempt made to couple the forceps. If articulation is still not easily accomplished, remove both blades, check the position of the head, and reinsert and reapply the forceps properly.

D. Rotation and Traction: Turn the fetal head with the forceps or draw it outward, simulating the mechanism of labor in that particular pelvis. Apply traction only in the axis of the pelvis. Use steady traction with arm force only (never body weight). Simulate labor contractions: gradually apply traction, sustain its maximum intensity for not more than 25 seconds, then gradually release it; repeat after 15–20 seconds. Extraction of the head may be possible with the same pair of forceps, or it may be necessary to rotate with one pair and deliver with another.

E. Disarticulation: Disengage the forceps when its purpose has been accomplished, or desist if this cannot be done easily and safely.

F. Removal: Extract the blades in reverse order of their insertion.

Forceps Delivery: Vertex Presentations

(1) Kneel on one knee or sit on a low stool in front of the patient. Be braced to avoid slipping and to maintain steady, controlled traction.

(2) Insert forceps. Hold each blade lightly, and slip it into the introitus along the posterior vaginal wall. As the forceps is advanced, carry it to the correct side of the pelvis.

(3) Apply each blade to the proper side of the fetal head between the eye and the ear from the parietal prominence to the malar ridge or the maxillary ridge. The posterior fontanelle will be just anterior to the plane of the shanks. The posterior fontanelle and the sagittal suture must be in a plane bisecting the angle of the forceps blade and shank, and the fenestration of the blade should be scarcely palpable (if at all).

(4) Articulate or lock the forceps (see above).

(5) Apply traction only in the axis of the pelvis. The forceps design often allows a degree of axis traction (Piper and Hawks-Dennen forceps), but an axis traction arrangement built into the forceps (Tarnier, DeWeese) or an attachment to the shank of the forceps (Bill traction bar) will provide much more effective direction of force. Grasp the handles

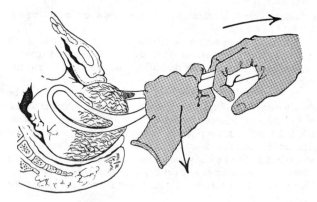

Figure 15–6. Axis traction (Pajot's maneuver).

with the right hand, palm upward, and insert the index or second finger
between the shanks. Hold the shank near the blades with the left hand and
gradually exert downward force in the direction of least resistance.
Apply outward traction with the right hand, using the handles, but avoid
compressing the head. This combined effort (Pajot's maneuver, Fig
15–6), which simulates axis traction will generally draw the head away
from the symphysis and downward. Alter the degree and direction of
traction as the head descends in the birth canal. Avoid excessive force.
Simulate labor contractions (see above). It may be necessary to rotate the
head back to an oblique position to bring it past an angulated, ankylosed
coccyx. Check the fetal heart rate and rhythm after each pull.

(6) Rotation:

(a) Oblique position to anterior (ROA or LOA to OA)–Apply the
classic forceps without the axis traction attachment in the usual manner.
After forceps articulation, rotate the occiput to the anterior and apply
traction downward in the axis of the pelvis.

(b) Transverse position to anterior (ROT or LOT to OA)–Digitally
or manually rotate the head to the oblique or anterior position if possible.
Do this in the mid pelvis where the pelvic diameters are greatest. Rotate
left-sided positions with the right hand, and vice versa. After rotation,
have an assistant exert counterpressure on the uterine fundus to hold the
head in its new position.

(i) Digital rotation–Gently insert the tips of the first 2 fingers of one
hand into the posterior fontanelle. When the head is lifted slightly toward
the side of the occiput, it will generally turn to the anterior position. Fix
by fundal pressure.

(ii) Manual rotation–Insert the fingers and thumb of one hand into

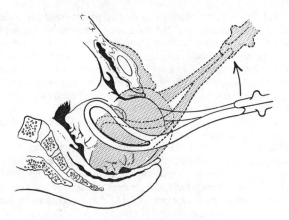

Figure 15–7. Upward traction with low forceps.

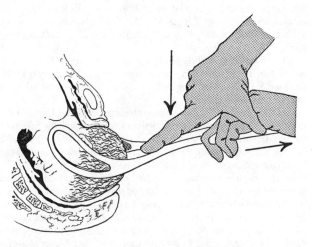

Figure 15–8. Modified Pajot's maneuver.

the vagina with the palm up. Grasp the head with the tips of the fingers behind the posterior parietal bone and the thumb over the anterior malar bone. Flex the head and rotate it to the transverse position or farther, but do not let it disengage. Retain the vertex in its new position by fundal pressure.

(iii) Forceps rotation using classic forceps–Introduce the anterior blade first. Do not insert the blade too far posteriorly into the vagina, but move it gently over the face to the anterior ear beneath the symphysis. Insert the posterior blade and adjust the application so that the forceps locks easily. Compress the blades to hold the head, and bring the vertex anteriorly. Rotate the forceps handles in a wide arc, almost sweeping the thigh, to avoid gouging the fornices with the toe of the forceps. Deliver the infant by traction applied in the axis of the pelvis.

(iv) Forceps rotation using Kielland forceps (ROT or LOT to OA)–

(a) Classic application–Insert the first 2 fingers of the free hand into the vagina anterior to the head. Cautiously insert the anterior blade into the vaginal canal along the hand, past the symphysis and cervix, and into the cavity of the uterus until only the handle and shank distal to the lock are visible. Depress the handle gently so that the toe of the blade can be seen or felt above the symphysis. "Flip" or quickly turn the blade over so that the button is directed toward the occiput. This can be done with remarkable ease. Insert and apply the posterior blade and lock the forceps, at this point with LOT or ROT. (Disregard asynclitism, because this will correct itself with rotation due to the sliding lock.) Rotate at the optimal level while applying slight downward traction. Recheck the application after rotation. Correct for deflection before continuing traction.

(b) Wandering method of application–Insertion, application, and articulation are approximately as described for the classic forceps rotation (see ¶ [iii], above). The buttons on the handles of the Kielland forceps aid in orientation.

(v) Forceps rotation using Barton forceps (ROT or LOT to OA)–Insert the hinged anterior blade posterior to the head, with the fingers of the opposite hand within the vagina as a guide. Move the blade over the face (or occiput) to apply the forceps to the anterior aspect of the head behind the symphysis. While an assistant holds the handle of the anterior blade upward, insert the heavier, curved posterior blade along the head in the midline. Draw the handle of the posterior blade upward and lock it with the anterior blade. Apply downward traction in the axis of the pelvis (not in the axis of the forceps). Once the head is below the point of arrest, rotate it to the anterior position. Sweep the handles toward the opposite thigh to facilitate rotation, or use the axis traction bar attachment to turn the head in the proper arc. Disarticulate and remove the blades. Apply classic forceps for delivery.

(c) Forceps rotation of posterior to anterior position (LOP or ROP to OA)–

(i) Manual rotation of a posterior position to a transverse position should usually be attempted first, whereupon a classic or Kielland forceps (or even Barton forceps in unusual cases) may be applied for further rotation to the anterior position.

(ii) Scanzoni maneuver (double application of forceps)—Apply the blades as for an LOA, even though the true position is ROP. Move the more anterior blade into position; insert the posterior blade more directly. Rotate the head clockwise to an anterior position for an ROP and counterclockwise for an LOP. Rotation is best made in the shortest arc, provided the turning process goes easily; otherwise, attempt rotation in the opposite direction. An axis traction bar will usually aid in rotation and extraction. Remove the blades and then reapply them for an anterior position (now achieved) and accomplish delivery by gradual traction.

(iii) The DeLee "key-and-lock" maneuver is ideal for rotation of posterior occiput positions. This is actually a stepwise rotation by simple multiple reapplications of the forceps, preferably of the Simpson type.

(iv) Kielland forceps rotation (single application of forceps)—If the position is ROP, apply the Kielland forceps "upside down" (buttons down, ie, toward the occiput). After locking, rotate the head through the shorter arc and recheck the position of the blades but do not remove them. Correct the application, if necessary, and proceed to deliver the infant by traction in the axis of the pelvis.

(v) Occasionally, it is safer for mother and infant to slowly deliver as a posterior presentation a large, markedly molded head that has been brought down to low forceps level by natural forces. Use a classic forceps applied for an anterior position and a generous mediolateral episiotomy.

(7) Disarticulate and remove the forceps by reversing the motions used in applying and articulating the blades. Unlock the forceps gently, and carry the handle of the top blade over the symphysis toward the opposite flank. Repeat the process with the other blade. The blades disengage easily because they follow the cephalic curve of the head. If there is resistance to removal of the blades, deliver the head with one or both blades still applied.

Forceps Delivery: Face & Brow Presentations

Forceps delivery for face and brow presentations is hazardous for the fetus. In most instances, cesarean section is required on a fetal indication.

Complications of Forceps Operations

A. For the Mother: Perforation of the uterus, separation of the symphysis, fistula formation, laceration of the cervix and sulcus, third- or fourth-degree lacerations, uterine prolapse.

B. For the Fetus: Skull fracture, intracranial injury.

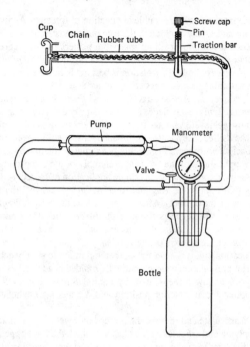

Figure 15–9. Modified Malmström vacuum extractor.

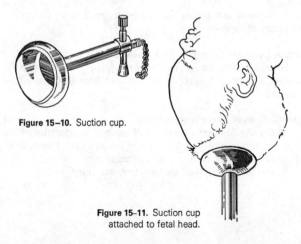

Figure 15–10. Suction cup.

Figure 15–11. Suction cup
attached to fetal head.

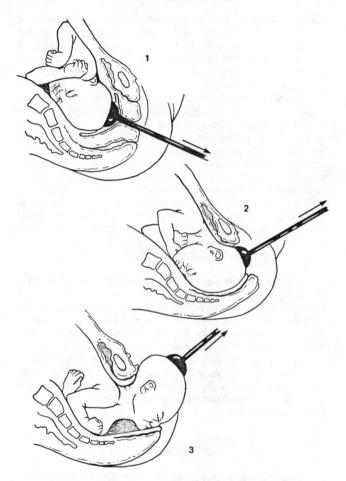

Figure 15–12. Application of vacuum extractor. Extractor may be applied at any station of fetal head. The applications shown are (1) high, (2) mid-high, and (3) low outlet application. Arrows indicate direction of traction.

THE VACUUM EXTRACTOR

The vacuum extractor, or ventouse (Figs 15–9, 15–10, 15–11, and 15–12), is an effective traction device for use instead of the obstetric forceps in expediting delivery of the fetus in vertex presentation. The indications for its use are the same as for the use of forceps, except that the vacuum extractor cannot be used for rotation. It is essentially a suction cup applied to the infant's scalp for traction. A controlled negative pressure of 0.7–0.8 kg can be developed with the Malmström or similar vacuum extractor.

The advantages of the vacuum extractor are as follows: Uterine propulsion is combined with synchronous ventouse traction. Hazardous forceps operations are often obviated, and the incidence of cesarean section may be reduced. The volume of the presenting part is not increased; compression of the head is avoided; and tentorial tears and cerebral hemorrhage in the infant are less common. Birth canal lacerations are infrequent, and cervical incision is rarely necessary. Neither particular skill nor anesthesia is required. The patient is usually cooperative. The vacuum extractor may be applied early (cervix > 4–5 cm in multiparas; > 7–8 cm in primiparas) at any station; occasional "high" extraction is feasible. Labor is frequently accelerated and shortened, especially when complicated by uterine inertia and cervical dystocia. "Autorotation" is encouraged and may correct minor degrees of malposition.

The disadvantages are as follows: The vacuum extractor can never completely replace forceps: rotation is difficult, and axis traction cannot be exerted. Scalp suffusion ecchymosis usually occurs, lacerations and cephalhematomas occur frequently, and intracranial injury occurs occasionally. If extraction takes more than 35 minutes, fetal subgaleal hematoma or severe scalp damage is likely. The extractor is rarely applicable in acute fetal distress: very rapid production of a vacuum sufficient for hurried extraction may seriously damage the fetus. The ventouse is not well suited for major cephalic deflexion or malposition problems and cannot be used for uncorrected face or breech presentations. This equipment is expensive.

VERSION

Version is a maneuver or operation by which the fetus is turned within the uterus from an unfavorable position or presentation to one more favorable for delivery. It has been used to convert a transverse lie to a breech (podalic version) or vertex (cephalic version) presentation. Version "by the head" or "by the breech" refers to the polarity after turning.

Version may be accomplished by maternal postural change or by external or internal manipulation. Cesarean section has virtually supplanted version today, because it is far safer for both mother and infant.

External version should be attempted only by physicians trained in this procedure.

Indications for Version

Postural or external version is used to convert transverse lies and breech presentations to vertex.

Because the perinatal mortality rate (including premature, term, and neonatal deaths) following breech delivery is at least 15% as compared with 3% for vertex deliveries, postural and, especially, external version have great theoretic advantages. However, spontaneous version often occurs during the last trimester. External version is successful on the first attempt in about 70% of cases after the 32nd week of pregnancy. With external version, about 1% of fetuses die from placental and cord accidents. The risk to the mother is negligible if no anesthesia is used.

External version with anesthesia is successful in 90% of cases, and the incidence of breech presentations may be reduced from 3–4% to 1.5–2%. However, the incidence of fetal death attributable to the procedure usually rises to 2% or more, and maternal death (due to uterine rupture) occasionally occurs. The author is opposed to external version under anesthesia.

Contraindications to External Version

Low engagement of the presenting part, threatened rupture of the lower uterine segment by a tight uterus, marked fetopelvic disproportion, previous cesarean section or an extensive myomectomy scar, first deliveries in multiple pregnancy, and large pelvic tumors complicating pregnancy are contraindications.

Methods of Accomplishing Version

A. Postural Version: This may be done before or during early labor without anesthesia. The mother is placed in the knee-chest position or on one side with her head and thorax lower than her pelvis. The uterus is thereby raised out of the true pelvis, and more room is thus made available for the fetus to shift. If the patient is cautiously returned to the supine position and rolled towels are applied to the sides of the abdomen and held by a binder, the fetus may be retained in the better presentation thus achieved. Unfortunately, postural version is rarely successful in completely correcting an unsatisfactory fetal lie.

B. External Version: The uterus must be relaxed. The polarity of the fetus can be changed (usually from breech to vertex presentation) by manipulation through the abdominal and uterine walls.

With the patient in the deep Trendelenburg position and without using excessive force, try to bring the fetus around by pushing the breech upward while deflecting the vertex in the other direction. This helps to

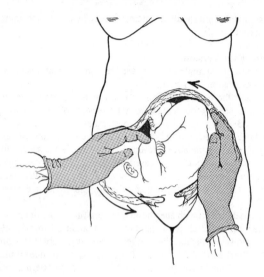

Figure 15–13. External cephalic version.

maintain flexion of the fetal head. The fetus may turn in a somersault movement.

If the fetal heart tones indicate distress, terminate attempts at version; if they do not improve, return the fetus to its original presentation. A short cord or tightening of coils or loops of cord may obstruct fetal circulation during attempted version.

C. Internal Version: This is accomplished during the second stage of labor and is warranted only for the delivery of a second twin in abnormal presentation or with fetal distress. It should be reserved for cases in which the head of the second twin cannot be caused to engage immediately and cesarean section is not feasible. Deep anesthesia is required. One presentation may be substituted for another by inserting the entire hand into the uterus and grasping one or both fetal extremities. Internal version is usually podalic, ie, by manipulation of the feet.

Make a generous mediolateral episiotomy. Grasp the fetus by both feet. Using the abdominal hand to guide the turning, bring the feet down with internal rotation until the knees are delivered at the introitus. At this point, version has been completed. Unless the need for delivery is urgent, the patient should be allowed to resume labor to permit accommodation of the fetus by the lower birth canal.

Complications & Prognosis

Internal version and breech extraction are associated with a 5–25% fetal-neonatal mortality rate. Hemorrhage and asphyxia are the usual causes of death. Neural damage, fractures, dislocations, and epiphyseal separation may complicate the course of many of the survivors.

The maternal mortality rate in internal version is 1–2%. Rupture of the uterus, hemorrhage, and shock are the most common causes of death. Women who survive often sustain severe lacerations of the birth canal and excessive blood loss.

Cesarean section should be substituted for internal version.

BREECH PRESENTATION

A breech presentation is one in which the caudal pole of the fetus presents over the pelvic inlet or lower, within the birth canal. There are 3 types—frank, complete, and incomplete (Fig 15–14).

Fetal polarity is largely determined by the adaptation, attitude, and size of the fetus in relation to the volume and shape of the amniotic sac as well as the placental site. Relatively more primiparas than multiparas deliver infants by the breech. Breech presentation is common until about the 32nd week of pregnancy, when the frequency declines. Only about 3% of term infants are breech births. The perinatal mortality and morbidity and maternal morbidity rates in breech delivery are much higher than with vertex (occipital) presentations. Breech presentation is therefore considered to be unfavorable and a cause of dystocia.

The following factors are probable or possible causes of breech presentation:

(1) Accommodation of the large pole of the infant to the more commodious portion of the uterus. In most cases of breech presentation, the placenta occupies the cornual region of the uterus. In such instances, the breech seems to seek more commodious space (the lower portion of the uterine cavity); the head must then occupy the smaller upper portion.

(2) Position of the legs of the fetus. Flexion of the thighs on the abdomen and extension of the lower legs, as in frank breech presentation, discourages spontaneous or external version.

(3) The size of the fetus in relation to available intrauterine space. Fetuses born by the breech at term are generally smaller than those delivered by the vertex.

(4) Fetal or maternal abnormality. Large congenital goiter, hydrocephalus, and uterus subseptus are frequently associated with breech presentation.

(5) Increased tone and firm contractions of the uterus. An original breech usually changes to a vertex presentation only once. In the last trimester, spontaneous version may be impeded when considerable early

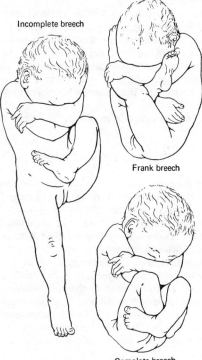

Incomplete breech

Frank breech

Complete breech

Figure 15–14. Types of breech presentation.

uterine activity occurs well before term. As a consequence, the uterine (and abdominal) wall may be tight and the amount of amniotic fluid relatively small.

In breech presentations, the presenting part does not fit or fill the pelvis as well as the vertex would. Delayed engagement and premature rupture of the membranes may occur, and these may cause intrapartal and postpartal infection.

There is no significant difference in the length of the first stage of labor in breech and vertex presentations, nor does the position of the breech affect the length of most labors. Nevertheless, the percentage of abnormal labors is at least 3–5 times higher in breech presentations.

Breech Types

A. Frank (Single) Breech: The legs are extended over the abdomen and thorax so that the feet lie beside the face.

B. Complete (Double) Breech: The so-called fetal position is maintained with the legs flexed and crossed.

C. Incomplete Breech: One or both lower legs and feet (or one or both knees) may prolapse into the vagina. Footling or knee (single or double) presentations are subdivisions of incomplete breech.

Breech Positions

Breech presentations are determined by the relationship between the fetal sacrum and the side of the mother's pelvis toward which it is directed. The point of the sacrum and the genital crease are used for orientation. Six positions are possible (see p 151).

Diagnosis

A. Abdominal Palpation and Auscultation: (See Leopold's maneuvers, Fig 6–5). On abdominal examination, the upper pole of the fetus is globular, firm, and ballottable (if the mother is not excessively obese and the uterus is not contractile, tender, or distorted by tumor). The fetal back is identifiable on one side and the small parts on the opposite side. The lower fetal pole is invariably less distinct, especially if engagement has occurred.

The fetal heart tones will be heard near the midline, slightly above and to one side of the umbilicus—usually higher in the abdomen than in vertex presentations.

B. Vaginal Examination: Vaginal examination may permit palpation of the presenting part, particularly when the cervix is slightly dilated and the membranes are ruptured. Specific identification of frank, complete, or incomplete breech presentation may also be possible.

When the breech presents, insert a finger through the cervix to feel a soft, smooth, irregularly-rounded surface (the genitalia) with a dimpled depression (the anus) nearby. If the finger is gently inserted into the anus, it will be stained by meconium. The genital cleft or crease separates the pudendum from the sacrum (the point of reference for position) and the symphysis. It may be possible to palpate 2 rounded, bony landmarks (tuberosities of the ischium) lateral to the anus for further orientation. One or both feet are usually felt opposite the sacrum in complete or incomplete breech.

C. X-Ray or Ultrasonographic Examination: In problem cases, ultrasonography or roentgenography may provide the diagnosis in breech presentation.

Fetometry in breech presentation is simple with ultrasonography but difficult with x-ray stereoscopy.

Differential Diagnosis

Vaginal examination is essential. Do not depend upon rectal examination for more than an estimation of the station of the presenting breech.

(1) A face presentation may be confused with a breech. If breech presentation is suspected, palpate the mother's abdomen carefully to identify the head in the uterine fundus. On vaginal examination, note that the genital crease is midway between the ischial tuberosities and perpendicular to a line joining them. In a face presentation, the mouth parallels the malar ridges, and the saddle of the nose and the alae of the nostrils are characteristic.

(2) Fetal anomalies such as anencephaly presenting by the vertex may be confused with a breech or face presentation. Virtually no landmarks are felt through the cervix in anencephaly because the calvaria are missing. The soft, irregular vault may be particularly perplexing. Fetal inactivity, polyhydramnios, and postdatism are signs of anencephaly.

(3) A high shoulder presentation may be mistaken for a breech. Vaginal examination generally reveals the parallel ridges of the rib cage, the closed angle of the axilla at the shoulder, and the palpable characteristics of the face.

(4) A hand or a foot (or both) may accompany an unengaged breech or vertex. Differentiating between a hand and a foot is easy, since the great toe parallels the others but the thumb is at an angle to the fingers. In addition, a line drawn across the tips of the fingers forms a curve, whereas a line across the tips of the toes is straight; the foot has a raised heel and the hand does not; and the thumb is readily supinated across the palm, but the great toe cannot be drawn over the sole.

Complications

Lacerations of the birth canal, hemorrhage, shock, and infection commonly follow breech delivery, particularly when surgical procedures such as complete breech extraction are required. Fetal complications include asphyxia and birth trauma.

Prolapse of the cord occurs in about 5% of breech presentations (10 times the incidence in vertex presentations). Shoulder dystocia, single or double nuchal arm (also called nuchal hitch), and dystocia of the aftercoming head (extension, hyperrotation) may be especially serious in breech presentations.

Fractures of the skull, clavicle, and humerus; dislocation of the hip; epiphyseal separation; nerve damage due to hemorrhage; and spinal and nerve plexus traction injury occur much more often with breech than with vertex delivery. The optimal size for a breech infant is 2500–3800 g (5 lb 8 oz–8 lb 6 oz). Notably smaller or larger infants are exposed to a much greater risk of injury during vaginal delivery; thus, in such cases, cesarean section is recommended.

Choice of Vaginal Versus Cesarean Delivery

Elderly primigravidas, patients with obstetric indications for cesarean section, and those with diabetes mellitus or previous obstetric difficulties should be delivered by cesarean section. Fetuses weighing over 3800 g should be delivered by cesarean section if possible. Vaginal delivery of footling breech presentation is too hazardous, and cesarean section is recommended. Cord prolapse occurs in 5–15% of these cases but in only 0.5% of frank breech or vertex presentations. Other indications for cesarean section are listed on p 433.

Factors *favorable* for vaginal delivery include a history of successful vaginal delivery of a previous breech presentation of weight greater than 3800 g (8 lb 6 oz); or vaginal delivery of a vertex presentation of weight greater than 4000 g (8 lb 13 oz).

Infants of moderate size at term (2500–3800 g [5 lb 8 oz–8 lb 6 oz]) who present as frank breeches can be safely delivered vaginally if the mother's pelvic capacity is adequate and labor is good. Pelvimetry by ultrasonography (preferred) or x-ray is necessary to rule out congenital anomaly, to confirm the infant's presentation and position, and to exclude hyperextension of the head. Cautious oxytocin stimulation is reasonable, but all patients who may deliver breech infants vaginally should have electronic fetal monitoring.

The disadvantage of a slight increase in perinatal morbidity due to shoulder dystocia or hypoxia in breech presentations delivered vaginally must be weighed against the more serious problem of increased maternal mortality and morbidity rates if all breeches are delivered by cesarean section.

Obstetric Management of Breech Delivery

Avoid artificial rupture of the membranes, but examine the patient vaginally immediately after spontaneous rupture and at the onset of labor to rule out prolapse of the cord and to confirm the presentation and position.

A trial of labor is not possible with breech presentation. Therefore, it must be decided early in labor whether vaginal delivery is likely or whether cesarean section will be necessary.

If labor is permitted, conservative management is indicated during the first stage. During the second stage, interfere as little and as late as possible.

A. Spontaneous Breech Delivery: Completely spontaneous (unassisted) breech delivery of a normal, living infant at term is uncommon, although premature infants are often born unattended in this way. Because of the many hazards involved, some aid to the infant should be provided.

B. Assisted Breech Delivery: No matter how the remainder of the breech delivery is to be managed, a short loop of cord must be loosened

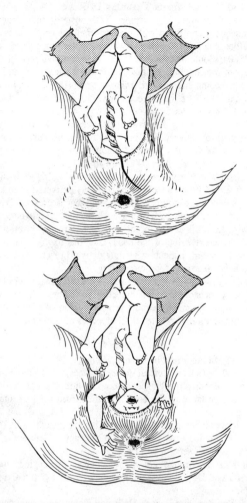

Figure 15–15. Bracht's method of assisted delivery. (Redrawn and reproduced, with permission, from Greenhill JP, Friedman EA: *Biological Principles and Modern Practice of Obstetrics.* Saunders, 1974.)

and drawn down as soon as the umbilicus comes into view. This avoids later umbilical traction and injury and cord compression.

Bracht's method of assisted breech delivery is recommended (Fig 15–15). When the scapulas are visible, gently lift the infant's back toward the mother's abdomen. (Do not overextend the back, or spinal injury may result.) The arms usually emerge spontaneously. Apply suprapubic pressure to force the head into the pelvis. The chin, mouth, nose, and brow emerge from the vagina spontaneously. The advantages of Bracht's method are that it involves no intravaginal manipulation, no traction on the infant's body or neck, and no forced rotation of the infant's thorax. The method is contraindicated with abnormal rotation of the fetus (back caudad), unusual position of the arms, abnormalities of the maternal pelvis and soft parts, or weak uterine contractions and cannot be successful unless the mother cooperates. Bracht's method should be abandoned in favor of extraction if the infant makes vigorous attempts to breathe before it is fully delivered.

C. Partial Breech Extraction: Nitrous oxide or trilene inhalation analgesia is permissible during the second stage, but regional anesthesia must be withheld (if possible) until the breech is crowning. Then make a long mediolateral episiotomy incision, preferably under pudendal block anesthesia. Do not give spinal anesthesia until a multipara is dilated 8 cm or a primigravida is fully dilated with the breech on the perineum.

Slowly draw the thighs downward (not outward); grasp the pelvis with the thumbs over the sacrum (not higher, or renal or adrenal injury may result); and apply traction and slight lateral rotation. When the scapulas are visible, complete the rotation of the infant laterally to bring the bisacromial diameter of the shoulders into the anteroposterior diameter of the mother's pelvis.

Gentle groin traction is then applied as follows: Hook one finger into the angle of the leg flexed on the abdomen of the frank breech if slight traction is needed. Apply slight force downward and slightly backward (as with traction forceps) during uterine contractions or combined with pressure over the fundus to dislodge an impacted breech, then rotate the infant slightly so that the back will be upward when delivered.

To deliver the first arm and shoulder, insert one or 2 fingers into the posterior vagina and sweep the posterior arm and shoulder out of the birth canal; then depress the trunk in the lateral position against the perineum while applying traction to the thighs. The anterior shoulder and arm will usually come beneath the symphysis for spontaneous delivery. Pressure applied medially over the angle of the exposed scapula may bring down the arm, or the arm may be swept out over the chest with the forefinger. The forefinger should be applied parallel to the humerus, as a splint—not at a right angle, as a hook—in order to avoid fracturing the humerus.

Note: Never use more than one finger for fear of dislocating the hip.

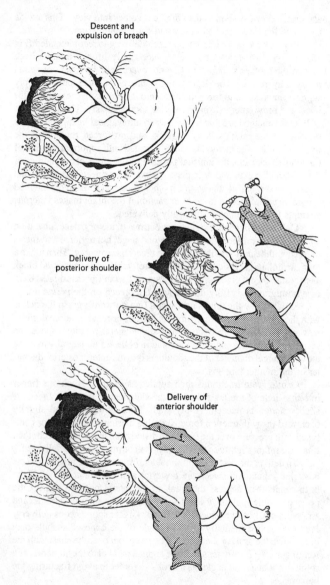

Figure 15–16. Breech delivery.

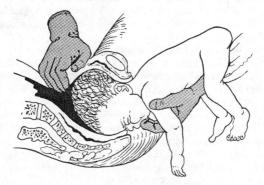

Figure 15–17. Wigand maneuver for delivery of head. Fingers of left hand inserted into infant's mouth or over mandible; right hand exerting pressure on head from above.

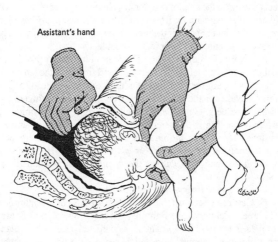

Figure 15–18. Mauriceau-Smellie-Veit maneuver for delivery of head. Fingers of left hand inserted into infant's mouth or over mandible; fingers of right hand curved over shoulders. Assistant exerts suprapubic pressure on head.

The anterior groin is usually the more accessible. It is dangerous to hook fingers into both groins. Use a metal hook for traction only if the fetus is dead. Do not attempt to apply forceps or a vacuum extractor to the breech; they will not hold.

D. Complete Breech Extraction: Pinard's maneuver to flex the extended legs in a frank breech is best done when the breech is not deeply engaged. Introduce a hand into the vagina (the right hand if the fetal back is to the mother's right; the left if the back is to the left), and displace the breech out of the pelvis. Identify the anterior thigh of the fetus. Pass the fingers up along the inner aspect of the infant's thigh to the knee. Abduct the thigh, causing the leg to flex at the knee, and ensure adequate flexion by pressing the index finger into the popliteal space and triggering the second finger over the tibia and fibula. Grasp the foot and apply downward traction in the axis of the vagina. Try to grasp the second foot in a similar manner if this is not too difficult.

E. Delivery of the Aftercoming Head: The head may be delivered in several ways.

1. Assisted delivery–

a. Wigand's method–Hold the infant astride the left arm, insert 2 fingers of the left hand into the infant's mouth (or over the mandible) to direct the head to the anteroposterior or oblique diameter of the pelvis for delivery (also maintaining flexion of the head), and apply strong pressure with the right hand over the mother's symphysis to deliver the head. This avoids traction on the infant's shoulders.

b. Mauriceau's method–Rotate the head to the OA position, support the infant on the left arm, insert the first 2 fingers of the left hand into the infant's mouth (or over the mandible) to flex the head, and place the right hand over the infant's back with one or more fingers curved over the shoulders. Guide delivery with the right hand, using no traction, until the chin is delivered. An assistant then applies suprapubic pressure. Then elevate the infant's body and guide delivery without using traction on the shoulders or excessive force. Hold the jaw to flex the head, and then deliver the occiput from beneath the symphysis.

2. Forceps delivery–See Fig 15–19.

F. Cesarean Section: The many very serious complications possible in breech delivery have rightfully led to the liberal use of cesarean section (see below). The infant is jeopardized more often than the mother, ie, cord compression and hypoxia or birth trauma may be critical. At least two-thirds of all breech presentations should be delivered by cesarean section. Indications include the following:

1. Primigravida or infertility patients where there is a high premium on the infant.

2. Immature fetus (1500–2500 g) presenting by the breech, because of possible central nervous system injury.

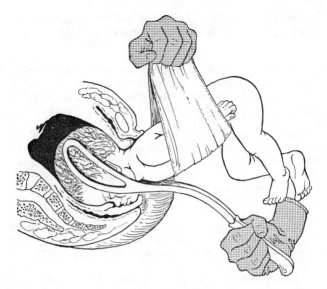

Figure 15–19. Application of Piper forceps and towel-sling support in breech delivery (Savage).

3. Single or double footling breech presentation, because of possible prolapse of the cord.

4. Prior uterine surgery, eg, cesarean section, myomectomy; rupture of the uterus may occur.

5. Pelvic tumor greater than 5 cm in diameter, eg, myoma or ovarian tumor; labor may be obstructed.

6. Obstetric or medical complications, eg, preeclampsia, diabetes mellitus, that may compromise both mother and fetus.

Management of Special Problems

Hydrocephalus is commonly associated with breech presentation. If it is diagnosed before labor, withdrawal of cerebrospinal fluid by transabdominal encephalocentesis can reduce the size of the head sufficiently that vaginal delivery may occur without incident. If this is not feasible, deliver the breech and shoulders and then engage the head. Rotate the back anteriorly. With a right-angled retractor beneath the mother's urethra and bladder, carefully insert a long No. 16 or No. 18 needle obliquely through the infant's foramen magnum and quickly aspirate cerebrospinal fluid. Then apply pressure on the head from above to drain cerebrospinal fluid. Deliver the head when it decompresses. (The fetus is congenitally abnormal and may not survive.)

Prognosis

Even in the absence of a primary indication for cesarean section, each patient with a breech presentation must be considered high-risk. If labor is permitted, it should take place in a well-staffed maternity unit and be closely supervised and monitored by a capable obstetric team. Delivery should be by an experienced obstetrician.

If the mother is a primigravida, if the fetus is large, or if the presentation is complete breech, the prognosis is improved if the mechanism of labor is normal, especially if rapid dilatation and effacement of the cervix occur. In most hospitals, the gross fetal-neonatal mortality rate in breech presentations delivered vaginally is 10–20%. For this reason, cesarean section is more liberally employed.

Although the maternal mortality rate is about the same with breech and with vertex presentations, the maternal morbidity rate is increased in proportion to the degree of operative intervention necessary and is thus higher with breech presentations.

Breech presentation recurs in subsequent pregnancies in about 20% of cases.

CESAREAN SECTION

Cesarean section is delivery, after 28 weeks' gestation, of the fetus and placenta through an incision in the uterine wall. (The term does not include transabdominal recovery of a fetus lying free in the abdominal cavity after laceration or rupture of the uterus.) The surgical approach is usually abdominal, although vaginal cesarean section is also possible. There are 5 types of abdominal cesarean section: (1) classic (Sänger), (2) low cervical (laparotrachelotomy of Krönig and DeLee), (3) peritoneal exclusion (Hirst), (4) extraperitoneal (Physick), and (5) cesarean section followed by hysterectomy.

Cesarean section performed on valid indications will often preserve the life and health of the mother and infant. However, no major operative procedure is without hazard, and cesarean delivery should not be done without good reason.

The incidence of this operation now varies from 10 to 25%, being highest in communities where deformed or contracted pelves are prevalent or where the mode of delivery is decided on the basis of the dictum "once a cesarean, always a cesarean." Repeat cesarean sections account for at least 40% of all cesarean sections in the USA.

Indications

The indications for cesarean section may be permanent or temporary. Some indications are clear and absolute; others are relative. In some cases, fine judgment is needed to determine whether cesarean section or vaginal delivery would be better. Combinations of factors each of which separately would be insufficient to justify cesarean section constitute a weak motive for the operation.

A. Maternal Indications:

1. Fetopelvic disproportion, usually after a trial of labor in vertex presentations, is the most common indication for abdominal cesarean section.

2. Potentially weak uterine scar after myomectomy, unification operation, or prior cesarean section. Partial or complete dehiscence of the site of previous cesarean section uterine incision occurs in 1–3% of cases.

3. Placenta previa covering 30% or more of the cervix.

4. Premature separation of the placenta with marked antepartal bleeding.

5. Primary uterine inertia or desultory or prolonged labor despite stimulation.

6. Ruptured uterus (an abdominal emergency).

7. Pelvic tumors that obstruct the birth canal or weaken the uterine wall.

8. Abnormal presentation (breech when mother is primiparous or infant is large; transverse or shoulder presentation; face or brow presentation with chin posterior).

9. Fulminating preeclampsia-eclampsia.

10. Serious maternal problems such as previous vesicovaginal fistula or carcinoma of the cervix.

B. Fetal Indications: The fetal indications for cesarean section are only occasionally imperative.

1. Fetal distress is recorded in 1–2% of maternity hospital admissions. The problem is generally hypoxia due to short cord, compression of the cord, premature separation of the placenta, or placenta previa.

2. Small (1500–2500 g) or large (> 3800 g) fetuses or those in footling breech or transverse presentation.

3. Maternal diabetes mellitus–Cesarean section is now used to terminate pregnancy in over 50% of cases involving diabetic women. Early delivery helps reduce the high incidence of intrapartal and postnatal death in infants of class B–H diabetic mothers (see p 366).

4. Maternal isoimmunization–Cesarean section is done in an effort to prevent possible fetal death in utero or irreparable damage to the infant from icterus gravis or hydrops fetalis in Rh and ABO isoimmunization of the mother when induction of labor is unsuccessful.

5. Prolapse of the cord in early labor, especially in primigravidas.

6. High social premium on the infant, eg, elderly primigravida with complications, numerous advanced pregnancies without living children, breech presentation in primipara.

7. Maternal herpes labialis or vaginalis.

Types

A. Classic: Classic cesarean section may be chosen in placenta previa (to avoid the vascular lower uterine segment and the placenta itself; see Chapter 11) and in obstetric emergencies such as premature separation of the placenta and prolapsed cord when speed of delivery is essential. A vertical incision is made through the visceral peritoneum and extended through the contractile portion of the uterine corpus. This operation should be used in less than 5% of cesarean sections.

The advantages of the classic operation are that it is the simplest cesarean section to perform and can be done under local infiltration anesthesia and that rapid entry of the uterus and extraction of the fetus are possible. The disadvantages are that bleeding from the thick, vascular uterine wall is marked; good peritonealization of the uterine scar is impossible; bowel adhesions to the uterine scar may cause intestinal obstruction; healing of the myometrium is often faulty; sinus formation and leakage of infected uterine fluid into the peritoneal cavity is common; and in 1–2% of cases, the scar ruptures in subsequent pregnancies.

B. Low Cervical: The low segment operation is the best general-purpose cesarean section. The visceral peritoneum over the uterus is incised at the bladder reflection, and an upper and a lower peritoneal flap are developed. The bladder is separated from its loose attachment to the anterior uterine wall and displaced downward. A vertical or transverse incision is made through the thin lower segment of the uterus several centimeters inferior to the initial entry through the visceral peritoneum. After delivery of the fetus, the uterine wall is closed in layers and the peritoneal flaps secured. Thus, the bladder covers the uterine incision. This type of operation is chosen in over 80% of cases in modern hospitals. A much higher percentage is warranted.

The advantages of a low cervical segment operation are as follows: The danger of drainage of infected uterine fluid into the peritoneal cavity after delivery is minimized. The likelihood of secondary intraperitoneal drainage and peritonitis is reduced because the bladder wall and a peritoneal flap cover the uterine scar. Less blood is lost because the lower uterine segment is thinner and less vascular than the fundus. Omental and bowel adhesion to the uterine scar is prevented. Delivery is reasonably safe even if it must be delayed for 24 hours after rupture of the membranes, which increases the likelihood of potential or subclinical intrauterine infection. Less packing-off of bowel and manipulation of the intestines are necessary, and the postoperative course is smoother than after classic cesarean section.

The disadvantages are that the operation is slightly more difficult and takes longer than the classic operation (especially in repeat cesarean sections), and maternal and fetal blood loss may be marked. A low segment incision may extend to lacerate large vessels laterally (with a transverse incision) or may tear downward into the bladder and cervix (when the incision is vertical). A placenta previa or low-lying placenta attached to the anterior uterine wall may be torn at entry. The incidence of placenta previa occurring over the lower segment scar in subsequent pregnancies is 10% (3 times the normal rate of low implantation).

C. Extraperitoneal: Because peritonitis is unlikely, extraperitoneal cesarean section may be used in neglected frankly infected problem cases, although low cervical cesarean section combined with use of broad-spectrum antibiotics and blood replacement gives almost as good results. A paravesical (Latzko or Norton) or retrovesical (Waters) incision is made into the uterus, avoiding the peritoneal cavity and bladder. The operation is best done after several hours of labor, so that definite planes of cleavage can be identified. This type of cesarean section is difficult and hazardous for an inexperienced operator to perform.

D. Peritoneal Exclusion: Prior to incision of the uterus, the parietal and visceral peritoneal surfaces are sutured together in an attempt to prevent contamination of the peritoneal cavity with infected material from the uterus. If suppuration occurs, drainage will usually be extraperitoneal. In spite of its theoretic advantages, peritoneal exclusion has not reduced maternal morbidity or mortality rates appreciably.

E. Cesarean Hysterectomy: Subtotal cesarean hysterectomy (removing only the uterus) and total hysterectomy (usually removing the cervix also) are often done after classic or low segment cesarean section. In certain unusual cases such as those involving fetal death with intrapartal infection, the uterus containing the fetus may be excised unopened and the infant then delivered through an incision in the uterine wall. The operation may be done for urgent reasons, eg, rupture of the uterus or placenta accreta, or electively, eg, in the treatment of large myomas and as a means of sterilization.

Total cesarean hysterectomy is gradually supplanting the subtotal procedure because it eliminates the possibility of future infection or carcinoma of the cervix.

The complications of cesarean hysterectomy are hemorrhage, shock, and urinary tract injury.

Elective total cesarean hysterectomy carries a lower maternal mortality and morbidity rate than the urgently indicated operation.

F. Vaginal Cesarean Section: Vaginal cesarean section may be performed for early termination of pregnancy in cases of fetal death or anomaly before term and complete dilation of the cervix. The operation is actually an anterior vaginal hysterotomy. Vaginal cesarean section is almost never done in the USA today.

Healing of the Incision

Theoretically, a uterine incision heals by regeneration of the muscle fibers with little or no fibroblastic response. Unfortunately, about half of the incisions studied have healed imperfectly and contained varying amounts of inelastic, weak scar tissue. The length and site of the incision, the accuracy of apposition of the wound edges in suturing, and whether exudation and infection occur all determine the quality of healing.

There is no accurate method of appraising the integrity or tensile strength of the uterine wall before or during labor. One-third to one-half of all disruptions of uterine scars occur before labor, and the rest occur during labor. Following delivery, manual exploration or, later, hysterography may disclose a definite defect, but serious damage may have already occurred.

About 1–2% of classic and 0.5–1% of low segment incisions rupture in subsequent pregnancies. The classic operation scar generally disrupts suddenly, violently, and often totally. The fetus almost always succumbs to asphyxia, and the mother may die of hemorrhage. The low segment scar usually ruptures subtly, silently, and often incompletely. In many cases a "window" is formed in the thin, scarred lower uterine segment, but usually the visceral peritoneum remains intact and bleeding is not extensive. Few infants and fewer mothers die. The rupture is discovered either at repeat cesarean section or subsequent laparotomy; after delivery at uterine exploration; or on a lateral hysterogram taken several months after delivery.

Morbidity & Mortality Rates

A. Maternal: Maternal morbidity and mortality rates vary depending upon the reason for the operation, the duration of labor and the time between rupture of the membranes and surgery, the number of vaginal and rectal examinations, the effectiveness of antibiotic therapy, and the type of cesarean section chosen.

In many large hospitals in the USA, the mortality rate (from all causes) following cesarean section is 0.1–0.2%; it may be 5 times as high as this elsewhere.

Many maternal deaths occur as a result of deficient preoperative preparation, faulty surgical technique, complications of anesthesia, errors in blood typing, inadequate blood replacement, and mismanagement of infection.

B. Perinatal: Perinatal morbidity and mortality rates vary depending upon the status of the fetus prior to delivery, the difficulties encountered in the birth process, postdelivery complications, and the quality of pediatric care.

Despite great improvements during the past decade, the perinatal mortality rate (including premature infants) following repeat, elective cesarean section is 2% in many hospitals. This is about twice as high as for vaginal delivery in the same institutions. Even in many well-staffed hospitals, the perinatal mortality rate in all types of cesarean sections (including both first and repeat operations) is 3–5%.

A well-timed and properly executed cesarean section increases the fetal salvage rate, especially when the surgery is done for an obstetric emergency. Miscalculation of the duration of pregnancy, leading to the delivery of a premature or immature infant, is the most important single factor in perinatal death following cesarean delivery.

Cesarean section, like other obstetric operations, prolonged labor, and preeclampsia-eclampsia, reduces the fetal oxygen supply and thus contributes to fetal morbidity and death. However, the very complications of pregnancy and labor that make surgical delivery mandatory are themselves among the major causes of perinatal morbidity and death.

The causes of perinatal death (in order of frequency) are (1) prematurity due to miscalculation of gestational age, (2) respiratory disorders (hypoxia, atelectasis, respiratory distress syndrome [hyaline membrane disease]), (3) unknown causes (even after clinical and postmortem studies), (4) fetal trauma (cerebral and other hemorrhage, neural injury, shock), (5) infection (bacteremia, pneumonia, omphalitis), and (6) congenital anomalies incompatible with life.

Postcesarean Obstetrics

If the problem for which the original cesarean section was done is still present (contracted pelvis, previously repaired vesicovaginal fistula) and the fetus is of average term size or larger, do a repeat (low segment) cesarean section. Because of the risk of rupture of classic incision scars, repeat elective cesarean section should be done at term or at the onset of labor during the last trimester.

If the indication for the first cesarean section no longer exists (eg, placenta previa, prolapsed cord), a choice must be made between a trial of labor, with vaginal delivery intended if symptoms of uterine rupture do not appear, and repeat cesarean section. The proponents of a trial of labor and vaginal delivery after low cervical cesarean section argue that many instances of disastrous uterine rupture occur before labor and that vaginal delivery may be safer for the mother than the complications which may occur following repeated cesarean section. Few women die of rupture of a low segment uterine scar if labor is carefully observed; maternal morbidity following repeat cesarean section is 5–10 times greater than that following vaginal delivery; and fetal morbidity and mortality rates are lower following vaginal delivery than following elective cesarean section.

Labor should not be induced after a previous cesarean section. Low forceps extraction should be employed to avoid increased intrauterine pressure during the second stage of labor, and the interior of the uterus should be palpated for defects after recovery of the placenta.

If labor is permitted after a previous cesarean section, the physician must remain in the hospital to observe the patient's progress and any indications of uterine rupture. An operating room must be ready and a full surgical team, including an anesthesiologist, in constant attendance. Blood for transfusion must be on hand. If these requirements cannot be met, elective repeat cesarean section is the only alternative. If signs of uterine dehiscence appear, a cesarean section must be done at once.

Elective Appendectomy

Elective appendectomy is generally a desirable and safe procedure at cesarean section unless the appendix is inaccessible or the patient's condition (hemorrhage, preeclampsia-eclampsia, infection) contraindicates the procedure. The operative time will be increased slightly, but significant complications attributable to appendectomy are rare. Not only may appendicitis be averted by this brief additional procedure, but carcinoid and other bowel problems may be reduced. The patient's consent must be obtained, and adequate anesthesia is necessary.

Induced Abortion & Sterilization | 16

INDUCED ABORTION

Induced (elective or therapeutic) abortion is the artificial termination of a previable pregnancy.

The United States Supreme Court legalized elective abortion in January, 1973, by ruling that the termination of an unwanted pregnancy is a matter for the woman and her physician to decide. The Court held that the state's need to preserve and protect the health of a pregnant woman begins to intrude on her right of privacy during the second trimester. The Court appeared to favor abortion when there is a substantial risk that the child would be born with a grave physical or mental defect and when pregnancy results from legally established statutory or forcible rape or incest. The Court further stated that at some time in the last trimester (generally conceded to be after the 23rd week) the fetus becomes viable, ie, capable of extrauterine life. A state "may then go so far as to proscribe abortion—except when it is necessary to preserve the life and health of the mother."

Consent by parents or guardians of minors (in many instances under age 15 years) may be required for abortion in some states. A married minor is free to make her own decision.

There are numerous medical and surgical indications for therapeutic abortion. The assumption that interruption of a pregnancy will improve a seriously ill patient's prognosis for life is only occasionally justified. Before contemplating therapeutic abortion, the physician must be reasonably certain that pregnancy is a threat to the mother's life or health and that the risks of therapeutic abortion will be less than those of continued pregnancy, labor, and delivery. Considering the success of modern therapy, therapeutic abortion is probably imperative only about once in 500 pregnancies even in specialty practice. Most abortions are now done for social indications.

In some instances, if elective abortion is warranted, sterilization may be indicated also. Thirty to 50% of women who are aborted become pregnant again, often before resolution of the problem for which the abortion was done.

If elective or therapeutic abortion is recommended, the advantages, disadvantages, and alternatives should be explained, whereupon the couple must decide. Neither the patient nor her husband should be urged to agree to an abortion, and both should be assured of the physician's continued sympathetic care whatever their decision.

The Roman Catholic Church denounces even therapeutic abortion unconditionally. The Jewish position is somewhat varied, depending on the interpretation by individual rabbis. Nevertheless, it is generally accepted that abortion may be performed only for the preservation of the mother's life or physical health. The Protestant view is much more liberal, with several denominations even recommending that abortion be made available on request.

Medical & Surgical Indications

A. Neuropsychiatric Disorders: Authorities disagree on the importance of emotional illness as an indication for abortion.

B. Renal Disease: Bilateral renal insufficiency and chronic resistant pyelonephritis may be indications for therapeutic abortion. Chronic nephritis is not aggravated by pregnancy in the absence of severe secondary infections or preeclampsia-eclampsia.

C. Heart Disease: (See Classification of Heart Disease, p 328.) Therapeutic abortion is not warranted on medical grounds in patients with class I or class II disability. In class III cases, in patients with atrial fibrillation or coronary occlusion, and in those in whom valvotomy has been unsuccessful, therapeutic abortion may be considered.

Hypertensive cardiovascular disease rarely jeopardizes the pregnant patient directly.

D. Pulmonary Disease: Marked impairment of pulmonary ventilation, with the functional equivalent of less than one lung (vital capacity < 1400 mL in the average-sized person), may justify abortion. Pulmonary tuberculosis is no longer a valid indication for interruption of pregnancy.

E. Metabolic Disorders: Diabetes mellitus is not an indication for therapeutic abortion unless progressive loss of vision or progressive Kimmelstiel-Wilson syndrome occurs as a complication.

F. Hematologic Disorders: Thromboembolic disorders, severe hemoglobinopathies, gammaglobulinopathies, and clotting defects may be indications for therapeutic abortion.

G. Gastrointestinal Disorders: Severe ulcerative colitis may be worsened by pregnancy. When perforations, hemorrhage, or nutritional deficiency becomes critical, abortion may be necessary.

H. Cancer: Invasive cervical cancer and stage II breast carcinoma may be indications for therapeutic abortion. Fulminating Hodgkin's disease early in pregnancy justifies abortion to facilitate radiation therapy, but leukemia or bowel or thyroid carcinoma does not.

I. Obstetric Complications:

1. Rubella–The risk of serious damage to the fetus resulting from maternal rubella before weeks 12–14 of pregnancy may justify therapeutic abortion. Rubella after the 14th week rarely damages the fetus.

2. Influenza and viral hepatitis occasionally affect the fetus, and abortion may be warranted.

3. Isoimmunization–If a woman is severely sensitized to the Rh factor, has a husband known to be Rh-positive, and has delivered several infants with severe Rh hemolytic disease, especially of the hydrops fetalis type, there is a a high probability of the disease in all subsequent children. The degree of jeopardy is uncertain, however.

J. Surgical Complications: Abortion may be justified if continued pregnancy and delivery will compromise a good surgical result, eg, correction of uterine prolapse, urinary diversion procedure, or kidney transplant.

K. Congenital Disorders: Marfan's syndrome or osteogenesis imperfecta may justify abortion.

L. Immunologic Disorders: Hypoimmune diseases, rheumatoid arthritis, lupus erythematosus, or polyarteritis nodosa may justify abortion.

M. Paternal and Fetal Indications: Paternal and fetal indications for therapeutic abortion are usually genetic problems.

Studies on amniotic fluid or its cellular contents may reveal many genetic disorders of the fetus as early as the 12th week. If elective abortion of an abnormal fetus is chosen, subsequent pregnancies may produce normal children.

Social Indications

Social indications for interruption of pregnancy usually are related to preservation of mental health. Rape, incest, poverty, or excessive family size may warrant elective abortion.

Methods

A. Dilatation and Curettage (D&C): Most elective or therapeutic abortions before the eighth week of pregnancy are performed by dilatation and surgical curettage (Figs 16–1 and 16–2). Paracervical, spinal, or general anesthesia may be used. If all goes well, a 1- or 2-day period of inactivity usually gives adequate time for recovery.

B. Suction Curettage: (Fig 16–3.) Suction curettage, preferably after the sixth or seventh week of pregnancy, has supplanted mechanical curettage in many hospitals for the termination of early pregnancy. The advantages and disadvantages are as follows:

1. Advantages–

a. Less dilatation of the cervix is necessary than for surgical D&C; thus, the likelihood of cervical tears and incompetent cervix is lessened.

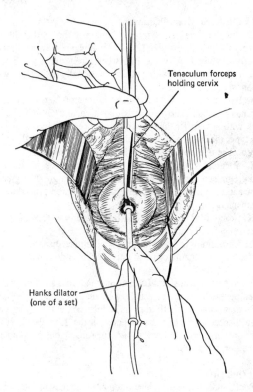

Figure 16–1. Cervical dilatation.

b. The negative pressure is powerful enough that the tip of the instrument need not come into contact with the entire surface of the uterine cavity (even the uterine "dead space" is denuded).

c. Separation of the placenta occurs at its surface contact; thus, the basalis and muscularis layers of endometrium are protected. Therefore, traumatic amenorrhea and intrauterine adhesion (Asherman's syndrome) is less likely.

d. Suction aspiration is much more rapid (3 minutes average) and expeditious than surgical D&C.

e. Less anesthesia and analgesia are required (basal analgesia and paracervical block may suffice).

f. When the uterine cavity is quickly evacuated, the uterus con-

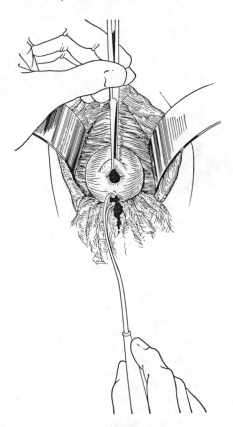

Figure 16–2. Curettage.

tracts rapidly, minimizing blood loss. Measurement of blood loss is possible.

g. The short operating time and minimal use and exchange of instruments reduce the danger of infection.

h. Blunt suction tubes are less traumatic than curets.

2. Disadvantages–

a. The suction tube is not delicate enough that minor changes in architecture of the uterus (partial septa, polyps) can be distinguished.

b. In pregnancy of more than 10 weeks' duration, the suction tube can be blocked by fetal-placental fragments.

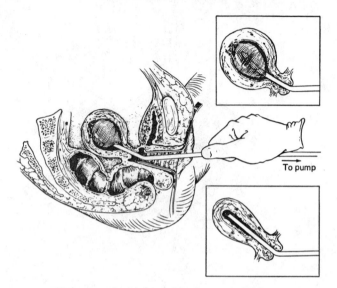

Figure 16–3. Suction method for therapeutic abortion.

c. Distortion and fragmentation of the tissues occurs with suction.

d. If there is a tight fit at the cervix and prolonged suction is applied, excessive blood loss may occur.

C. Menstrual Regulation: Menstrual regulation is also called menstrual or endometrial extraction, menstrual induction, interception, or postconceptive fertility regulation. These are all alternative terms for very early abortion by suction curettage. Suction aspiration of the endometrial cavity is usually performed at a time when the presence of an early pregnancy cannot be diagnosed accurately. In many cases, menstrual regulation is performed on a patient who believes herself to be pregnant, who has missed her menstrual period by 14 days or less (arbitrary), and who has previously had reasonably regular periods. The patient must sign a surgical consent form.

Aspiration generally is performed with a 4- to 5-mm flexible plastic (Karman) cannula attached to a source of low-pressure suction, eg, a 50-mL hand-held syringe. Paracervical block can be used if necessary.

Actually, about 40% of patients who request menstrual regulation fear that they are pregnant but in fact are not. It is unwise—even though the risk is minimal—to perform menstrual regulation when one can use accurate methods of pregnancy testing such as radioimmunoassay. Radioimmunoassay for the β subunit of hCG is a more accurate test for pregnancy than radioimmunoassay for hCG. With the former test, pregnancy can be diagnosed before the first missed period. Such tests are much less expensive than menstrual regulation. If the pregnancy test is positive, menstrual regulation (now properly regarded as early elective abortion) can be done. If the test is negative, reassurance, contraceptive advice, and further observation are all that is required.

Menstrual regulation is contraindicated in women with acute cervicitis or possible salpingitis or in those who are more than 21 days pregnant.

D. Dilatation and Evacuation (D&E): Dilatation of the cervix followed by evacuation of pregnancies of 8–20 weeks' duration is safe if done carefully and skillfully. A laminaria (laminaria tent; see below) inserted into the cervix 6–8 hours before D&E will soften the cervix and allow easier dilatation, or prostaglandin E_2 (PGE$_2$) in a gel applied to the cervix 12–24 hours before D&E may soften the cervix. Slow dilatation of the cervix to approximately 5 cm in diameter to avoid laceration should allow morcellation and removal of the fetus. A large, blunt curet facilitates separation and removal of the placenta. Total evacuation of the uterus must be assured.

Second-trimester D&E is less traumatic medically for the patient than intrauterine instillation procedures. However, long-term consequences such as cervical incontinence have not been adequately assessed.

E. Prostaglandins as Abortifacients: The prostaglandins, 20-carbon, long-chain hydroxy fatty acids present in many tissues of humans and other animals, possess, among other biologic properties, the ability to produce strong uterine contractions.

1. PGE$_2$–Intravaginal PGE$_2$ gel or suppositories effectively induce labor for elective abortion and after intrauterine fetal death. Often, intravenous oxytocin must also be given for more rapid evacuation of the uterus. However, molar pregnancies cannot be evacuated adequately with prostaglandin products; suction or surgical curettage may also be required.

2. PGF$_{2\alpha}$–Prostaglandin $F_{2\alpha}$ (PGF$_{2\alpha}$) is now commercially available (Prostin-F$_{2\alpha}$) as an abortifacient and to induce labor. Intravenous infusion of PGF$_{2\alpha}$ at a rate of 40–50 mg/min generally induces abortion in 12–19 hours, slightly shorter than after injection of hypertonic saline solution. Nausea, vomiting, and diarrhea do occur. Unfortunately, the morbidity rate after prostaglandin induction of labor is increased over that with hypertonic saline solution, and the fetus may be born alive.

F. Intra-amniotic Injection of Solutions: Therapeutic abortion after the 14th week and evacuation of the uterus following fetal death can be accomplished medically within 12–14 hours, almost without exception, by aseptic transabdominal aspiration of amniotic fluid and immediate very slow replacement by a similar amount of sterile aqueous 20% sodium chloride or 50% urea in 5% dextrose and water. Local anesthesia is used, and a No. 14 or 16, 4- to 6-inch needle with obturator is inserted slowly into the uterine cavity. Ideally, 100–200 mL of fluid is withdrawn. In second-trimester pregnancy and missed abortion, only small amounts of amniotic fluid may be available. In such instances, at least 60–90 mL of solution should be injected if possible. A laminaria inserted into the cervical canal 6–8 hours prior to intra-amniotic injection, or PGE_2 in a gel applied to the cervix 12–24 hours before the injection, will facilitate and shorten labor and evacuation in most cases. If uterine contractions are poor, oxytocin stimulation may be necessary. The fetus is always dead at delivery. Saline should not be used for patients with preeclampsia-eclampsia or other disorders in which sodium restriction is desirable. Labor generally requires only 2–3 hours; its cause is uncertain. Whether labor is the result of progestogen block or reduced progestogen production by the placenta is debated.

The coagulation system is altered temporarily by injection of hypertonic saline or urea solution. The plasma fibrinogen concentration is reduced, and the mean platelet count is also decreased. The concentrations of fibrinogen and fibrin degradation products are increased significantly in many patients. However, abnormal bleeding due to coagulopathy is rare with the concentration of substances ordinarily employed.

G. Induction of Labor With Oxytocic Agents: The use of oxytocin without intrauterine hypertonic solutions or other measures invites a high failure rate, a prolonged interval to abortion, or a live-born fetus.

H. Bags, Bougies, and Catheters: These instruments are associated with trauma, infection, and unpredictability. A live-born fetus may be delivered. They should not be used.

I. Hysterectomy: Abdominal hysterectomy is feasible up to 23 weeks of gestation. This method may be used for patients with large myomas or when sterilization is warranted.

Vaginal hysterectomy can be performed up to 12 weeks of gestation without uterine evacuation, and even later if the uterus is emptied first. This technique should be used only by those skilled in vaginal surgery.

J. Hysterotomy: Abdominal or vaginal hysterotomy has the disadvantage of delivering a live fetus if the pregnancy is advanced, and the operation carries a higher complication rate than evacuation followed by tubal ligation. Hysterotomy may also compromise future pregnancies.

K. Laminaria Tent: A small stem segment of sterilized, dehydrated *Laminaria digitata,* or sea tangle, can aid in dilating the cervix. When dry, the laminaria is very hygroscopic, capable of expanding to 2–3 times its original diameter. The laminaria must remain in the cervix for at least 6–8 hours to accomplish dilatation. Marine bacteria are relatively nonpathogenic for humans, but it is now possible to sterilize the laminaria by exposure to gamma radiation and then ethylene oxide.

The laminaria is useful in conditions where the cervix is closed or stenotic, eg, in early elective or therapeutic abortion, for drainage of hematometra, and to obtain endometrial biopsies, especially in postmenopausal patients.

Complications

Induced abortion is a potentially dangerous operation even in healthy women. Perforation of the uterus, pelvic infection, hemorrhage, and embolism are the most common complications. The mortality rate for legal abortions in the USA is about 3 per 100,000. The greater the duration of pregnancy, the greater the threat to the mother's life. A 5% morbidity rate (fever, pelvic infection) is common in the first trimester; the morbidity rate is over 15–20% in legal abortions during the second trimester.

However, in seriously ill pregnant patients whose physical or emotional disease may justify abortion, the mortality rate is 1–2%—at least twice the mortality rate for therapeutic abortions in healthy women. The postoperative morbidity rate is proportionate.

Protracted feelings of guilt and remorse may result from induced abortion, particularly when religious and social conflicts complicate the decision to abort and the patient feels responsible for the loss of the fetus. The reported incidence of debilitating remorse or regrets following an induced abortion has been less than 5%.

Anesthesia for Induced Abortion

The safest anesthesia for abortion by suction curettage or D&C is paracervical block. Unfortunately, some patients are uncooperative or tense when local anesthesia is used. For this reason, thiopental, nitrous oxide, and oxygen are widely used in combination for elective abortion. Regional anesthesia usually is chosen for hysterectomy or hysterotomy.

Evaluation of the Patient Requesting Induced Abortion (Unwanted Pregnancy)

Patients give varied reasons for requesting abortion. Since in some cases the request is made at the urging of the woman's parents, in-laws, spouse, or peers, every effort should be made to ascertain that the patient herself desires abortion for her own reasons. In addition, one should be certain that the patient knows she is free to choose among other methods of solving the problem of unplanned pregnancy, such as adoption or single parenthood. Help from social agencies should be made available as necessary. A complete social history, medical history, and physical examination are required. Particular attention must be given to uterine size and position, gynecologic problems, medical diseases, and psychiatric disorders. The importance of accurate calculation of the duration of pregnancy cannot be overstated. Routine laboratory tests should include pregnancy tests (if in doubt), urinalysis, hematocrit, Rh typing, serologic test for syphilis, culture for gonococci, and Papanicolaou smear.

Follow-Up of Patients After Induced Abortion

Rho (D) immune globulin (RhoGAM) should be administered within 72 hours after abortion if the patient is Rh-negative unless it is known that the father is Rh-negative or that the patient will not have future pregnancies. For first-trimester abortion, the recommended dose of Rho (D) immune globulin given to Rh-negative women to protect against sensitization is 50 μg intramuscularly; for second-trimester abortion, the recommended dose is 1 vial (300 μg). If an unusually large amount of fetal blood has entered the maternal circulation, the dose should be increased.

The patient should take her temperature daily and avoid intercourse and the use of tampons or douches for at least 1 week. She should report fever or unusual bleeding at once. She should also be informed that emotional depression, similar to that following term pregnancy and delivery, may occur after induced abortion. Follow-up care should include careful pelvic examination to rule out endometritis, parametritis, salpingitis, failure of involution, or continued pregnancy. Finally, effective contraception should be made available according to the patient's needs and desires.

Legal Aspects of Induced Abortion

The patient must be informed regarding the nature of the procedure, its risks—including possible infertility or even continuation of pregnancy—advantages, disadvantages, and alternatives. The rights of the spouse, parents, or guardian must also be considered. The necessary permissions must be obtained.

State or provincial laws must be obeyed, with special reference to residence, duration of pregnancy, indications for abortion, consent, and consultations required.

STERILIZATION

Sterilization is the permanent prevention of pregnancy. Elective or compulsory sterilization may be done for men and women who wish to avoid parenthood or are considered unfit to bear, father, or rear children because of incapacitating, often hereditary, disease. Reasons for sterilization include hereditary disease, lack of the ability or determination to practice contraception, unacceptably high risks associated with pregnancy, and the desire to have no more children. Elective sterilization is rapidly becoming an acceptable means of limiting family size in all parts of the world. Voluntary sterilization is legal in all states in the USA.

Compulsory sterilization of mental incompetents may be approved by a state board of eugenics in most states in the USA and by similar agencies in many other countries, in response to written application by the subject's family. The board rarely initiates the action, and it is subject to appeal in the courts.

Indications

Most intractable disorders (eg, severe inoperable congenital heart disease), if they constitute an indication for interruption of pregnancy, are threats to future pregnancies as well. If therapeutic abortion is necessary, sterilization may also be indicated. Sterilization is also indicated when pregnancy is hazardous but contraceptive methods are apt to be unsuccessful or harmful.

A. Neuropsychiatric: Severe mental retardation, advanced schizophrenia, severe epilepsy.

B. Medical: Familial blood dyscrasias, marked cardiovascular or renal disease, severe diabetes mellitus, chronic leukemia, neurofibromatosis.

C. Obstetric: Extreme Rh isoimmunization in a woman whose husband is Rh-positive, uncorrectable uterine abnormality.

D. Surgical: Stage II carcinoma of the breast.

E. Socioeconomic: Frequent pregnancies and inability to rear additional children, patient's desire to have no more children.

Methods of Sterilization in Women

Tubal closure is the most commonly used sterilization procedure, but sterilization may be done by bilateral oophorectomy or salpingectomy, hysterectomy, or bilateral tubal closure.

There are 4 main approaches to the tubes: abdominal (used in 75% of cases), vaginal (used occasionally), transuterine (rarely used), and inguinal (rarely used).

Tubal closure is accomplished by ligation, diversion, or excision. Ligation may be done with segmental resection (Pomeroy, Fig 16–4) or with crushing and ligation (Madlener). Excision may be done by salpingectomy, removal of the infundibular portion of the tube, resection of the isthmic part of the tube (cornual resection), burial of the proximal extremity of the tube beneath the visceral or parietal peritoneum (Irving, Fig 16–5; or Uchida, Fig 16–6), or cauterization-occlusion of the uterotubal ostia through the uterine cavity.

Minilaparotomy, a limited celiotomy procedure for tubal sterilization, can be done safely and rapidly in an outpatient surgical center or during part-day admission to a hospital. Only basic surgical skills and a minimal number of instruments are required. Minilaparotomy is less hazardous than laparoscopy (see below) because it is associated with

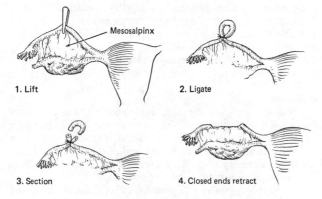

Figure 16–4. Pomeroy method of sterilization.

fewer injuries of the bowel and large blood vessels. Bleeding and infection are rare complications.

Minilaparotomy sterilization requires a small (usually transverse) skin incision with dissection into the peritoneal cavity, often performed under analgesia and local anesthesia. A Vitoon or similar uterine elevator or sound inserted into the uterine cavity prior to surgery can be manipulated by an assistant to elevate the fundus toward the incision in the absence of adhesions. Small angular retractors, or even a Pederson vaginal speculum, should allow inspection of the tubes and ovaries. Local anesthetic is then injected into the mid portion of the tube (when general anesthesia is not employed) for a Pomeroy sterilization, or into the terminal segment of the tubes for a Kroner tubal ligation. Simple closure of the incision in layers, perhaps with a subcuticular catgut suture for reapproximation of the skin edges, completes the operation.

Minilaparotomy is contraindicated when the patient is obese or has an enlarged or immobile uterus or when adnexal disease or endometriosis is suspected. Nonetheless, minilaparotomy is a safer, simpler, and cheaper sterilization procedure than laparoscopy, which requires expensive equipment and endoscopy experience.

Surgical reestablishment of the continuity of one or both tubes is successful in over two-thirds of cases following Pomeroy or Madlener sterilization. Viable pregnancy results in less than one-third of these patients, however.

Recently, the successful use of the laparoscope in the fulguration of a portion of the tubes has made "come-and-go" (1-day) sterilization possible. Occlusion of the oviducts by metal clips or Silastic rubber rings is also possible. This method eliminates the need for thermoenergy to

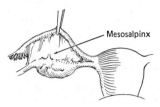

1. Uterine tube lifted and cut.

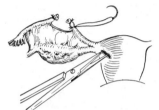

2. Double ligation with gut; one tie left long for traction (special traction suture). Mesosalpinx stripped back.

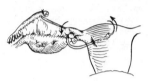

3. Special traction suture inserted in tunnel in anterior uterine wall.

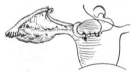

Figure-of-eight fixation suture

4. Implantation of the proximal tubal limb into a tunnel in the anterior uterine wall.

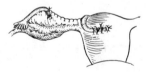

5. Traction suture tied and proximal tube sutured in tunnel.

Figure 16–5. Irving method of sterilization.

ensure tubal closure and has a greater potential for successful future recanalization. With elimination of the need for laparotomy, morbidity and mortality rates have been markedly reduced and costs lessened.

Results of Sterilization in Women

The physician must explain that with tubal interruption alone, no organ is removed; tubal sterilization merely prevents conception. The operation is not "de-sexing" and will not reduce libido, vary the

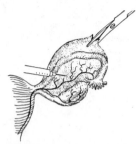

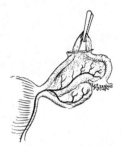

1. Saline with epinephrine injected below serosa, which becomes inflated locally. Muscular tube, and even blood vessels, can be separated from serosa, which is then cut open.

2. Muscular tube emerges through opening or is pulled out to form a U shape.

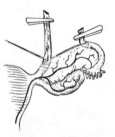

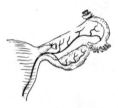

3. Fimbriated end is untouched, while the end leading to the uterus is stripped of serosa. This can usually be done without damaging blood vessels.

4. About 5 cm of muscular tube is cut away; the end is buried automatically in serosa. Fimbriated end and serosa opening are closed and tied together.

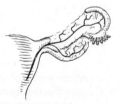

5. Blood supply continues normally between ovary and uterus. Hydrosalpinx or adhesion has not been noted.

Figure 16–6. Uchida method of sterilization.

Table 16–1. Failure rates of minilaparotomy and
laparoscopy sterilization procedures.*

Minilaparotomy Procedure	Failure Rate (%)
Uchida	Nil
Fimbriectomy	Nil
Irving	Nil
Pomeroy	0–0.4
Salpingectomy	0–1.9
Madlener	0.3–2
Simple ligation	20
Laparoscopy Procedure	
Coagulation and excision	0–0.6
Coagulation and division	0.1–2
Coagulation (only)	1–2
Silastic (Falope) rings	0.23
Spring-loaded (Hulka) clips	0.2–0.6

*Data from Department of Medical and Public Affairs, George Washington University Medical Center: *Popul Rep* (May) 1976; Series C, No. 7.

woman's menses, or alter her appearance. There is usually no adverse change in sexual function following tubal sterilization; on the contrary, many women who feared pregnancy before the operation report increased satisfaction in sexual intercourse and are pleased with the operative result. However, 5–10% report less frequent orgasm and regret the procedure.

Only hypophysectomy, bilateral oophorectomy, and ovarian damage by radiation are certain methods of sterilization. Abdominal and tubal pregnancies have occurred (rarely) even after total hysterectomy.

Oophorectomy and sterilization by radiation are usually followed within 4 weeks by vasomotor reactions and a gradual diminution in libido or sexual satisfaction during the next 6 months.

Sterilization in Men

Sterilization of the man by vas ligation (an office procedure) may be far less dangerous than an operation on the woman if she is for any reason an inappropriate candidate for surgery. This alternative should be offered to the couple who must limit childbearing. Impotence does not result. Sterility cannot be assumed until ejaculates are found to be completely free of sperm. Disadvantages of vasectomy include occasional and unlikely spontaneous recanalization (< 1%), the occasional development of a spermatocele, and the possible development of antisperm antibodies. Hematoma formation, epididymitis, and psychologic impotence are occasional complications also. Atrophy of the testes may result from excessive ligation of the vasculature. Vasectomy often is reversible—up to 90% in some reports—but pregnancy results in only 18–60% of cases after reanastomosis.

17 | Emotional Aspects of Pregnancy

Taboos, superstitions, and misinformation regarding menstrual function, sexual practices, and childbirth still cause much needless anxiety and uncertainty among women. Many obstetric and gynecologic illnesses are emotionally induced or aggravated by emotional factors.

Pregnancy and the puerperium are periods of psychologic stress for all women, though some women experience minimal discomfort during this time, and for many it may be the happiest time of life. Conception places the woman in the role of a giver much more than it does the man. Any event that so profoundly affects an individual's present and future life situation may be viewed as a potential threat to emotional adjustment. The clinical manifestations will depend on the degree of stress and the efficiency of the individual's adaptive processes. These in turn relate to the circumstances of her past and present life.

The clinician must attempt to evaluate the patient's response to the pregnancy not only to offer help if it is needed but also because her emotional state often has adverse effects on her physical well-being. Some physicians are highly skilled in dealing with their patients' psychologic problems; many others are not. Some of what is known about the psychodynamics of human gestation will be reviewed here. Prevention and management will be discussed, including the aspects of routine prenatal care that tend to favor a smooth progress through pregnancy and delivery and into a stabilized relationship with the infant and other members of the family. In general, more emphasis should be placed on the parents' roles in rearing children in our complex society than on the actual delivery of the infant.

Aims in Assessment & Management of the Emotional Aspects of Pregnancy

(1) To evaluate the pregnancy and the patient's acceptance of it soon after the last missed menstrual period. If there are contraindications to pregnancy or if the pregnancy is not welcome, abortion should be considered. Serious rejection of the pregnancy may result in mild to severe somatic complaints.

The success of the pregnancy and the outlook for the child and the family may be affected by the motivation for the pregnancy; thus, the motivation should be considered. The ideal motivation for pregnancy, of course, is the need of a mature couple to produce and rear a child as a reflection of their own mutual love and expression of their ability to provide a home in which a child can grow to healthy adulthood. However, some pregnancies are based on "good reasons" and some are motivated by bad ones. For example, the need to become pregnant may be quite different from the need to continue the pregnancy and to have and raise a child. Individuals who feel inadequate as men or women may need to conceive a child in order to demonstrate their biologic validity but may later lose interest in having a child and request an abortion. A woman who feels that having a child will prevent loneliness may be unable to cope with the reality of child rearing. A teenager may feel that, by becoming a mother, she will be in charge of her life and will have a life companion who will always love her and respond to her needs. Pregnancy may also be used as a defense against or compensation for death or some other form of separation from a family member or close friend or as a means of providing continuity and retaining a familiar role and thus avoiding the need for a significant life change.

(2) To inform the patient about the course of pregnancy and labor. Factual information and reassurance help to minimize anxiety and tension.

(3) To assist the parents in accepting the child promptly after delivery. The reproductive instinct often conflicts with personal and social attitudes. Fear and apprehension are commonly associated with the patient's first suspicions that she is pregnant even though she may want the child. A woman having her first child is suddenly faced with the unknown perils of pregnancy, labor, delivery, and parenthood. Paradoxic reactions of happiness and resentment are common.

The principal adverse psychic factors in pregnancy are fear of the unknown, fear of pain during labor and delivery, fear of death, fear of the economic consequences of pregnancy and motherhood, resentment at the imminent loss of personal independence and attractiveness, resentment of the child as a potential competitor for the father's love and affection, and uncertainty about adequacy as a parent.

The Emotional Course of Pregnancy

A. First Trimester: This is the most important phase in the adjustment of the patient, particularly the primigravida. Emotional tension is manifested as symptoms such as headache, nausea, and easy fatigability. In general, patients who accept childbearing as a normal aspect of womanhood will adjust well. Patients who consider menstruation ("the curse"), sexual intercourse, and pregnancy to be woman's "burden" in life are much more likely to suffer the discomforts of psychosomatic illness.

The father is often the "forgotten man" in antepartal care. The physician should welcome him in the office at an early visit, explain the course of pregnancy, and tell him how he can help. Lucid explanations and frank answers to questions will promote a confident, supportive attitude on his part that will be an important source of satisfaction and assistance to the mother. Plans may be made for the father to be present at delivery; the father's presence in the delivery room may afford great support to the mother and may enhance bonding with the infant.

B. Second Trimester: When pregnancy progresses on schedule, the patient will feel fetal movements by about the fourth month. This is an exciting and satisfying experience for almost all women.

During the second trimester, relatives and friends may repeat sadistic rumors and recount harrowing experiences to ''guide'' and warn the patient. The physician must be willing to listen patiently, correct misinformation, and give reassurance as needed.

C. Third Trimester: Tensions mount and anxieties increase as the expected date of confinement approaches. Emphasize the natural and normal nature of pregnancy. The more factual knowledge the patient possesses, the fewer anxieties she will have. Fear of delivery is fear of the unknown; knowledge dispels this fear. Prenatal classes conducted by experienced personnel are often available in the community. Both parents should take a tour of the maternity service of the hospital if possible.

The father's continued display of affection and interest in both the mother and the child is essential. Oversolicitude has an adverse effect, however.

EMOTIONAL ASPECTS OF LABOR & DELIVERY

Emotional adjustment to delivery depends upon prenatal preparation for labor and delivery, the patient's emotional stability, the success of the marriage, the couple's desire for a child, and patient-physician rapport. Adequate emotional preparation for labor and delivery will ease the prelabor period, especially for emotionally immature and apprehensive individuals.

Offer the couple the opportunity to attend parents' classes or preparation for childbirth sessions. Numerous civic and hospital services have organized groups for the presentation and discussion of antenatal and postnatal problems. A doctor or nurse usually acts as moderator. If such meetings are available in the community, the patient and her partner may find them stimulating and informative.

Both parents should visit the hospital before the onset of labor. Maternity service tours will familiarize the couple with the hospital plan and routine. The patient in labor who enters the hospital in the middle of the night without prior knowledge of hospital procedure may receive a fearsome initiation: Under the worst circumstances, she leaves her husband at the hospital desk and is led down a long, dark corridor by an uncommunicative nurse or attendant—often in cap, mask, and gown. She is undressed, put to bed, shaved, and given an enema. Strange individuals do vaginal examinations; "shots" may be administered. During all this, uterine contractions increase in frequency and severity. If the events of the first hours in the hospital are like this, the patient's inherent fear increases, and an emotional milieu is created that must be experienced to be appreciated. As tension mounts, pain is intensified.

The dynamics of pain in labor were outlined as follows by Grantly Dick Read:

(1) Gravida + fear = marked tension. Marked tension + anemia, fatigue, discouragement, panic = severe pain.

(2) Gravida + abnormal pregnancy, poor integration, limited intelligence, previous obstetric disaster = severe pain. But

(3) Gravida + normal pregnancy + confidence + relaxation = little pain + good labor.

Pain in childbirth is minimized by relaxation. The patient must utilize her contractions without working against them. Emotional support is especially necessary during labor. Friendly, attentive nurses and an obstetrician who is frequently in attendance can anticipate the patient's concerns and estimate her emotional status. Personal attention and the use of breathing and relaxation techniques during labor will reduce the patient's discomfort considerably.

The physician should meet the patient at the hospital or see her shortly after admission. The resident physician and nurse should be introduced as a "team" who will assist her during labor and delivery. The physician need not sit continuously for hours with a patient in labor, but the patient must be aware that the physician is actively and successfully supervising her care.

A woman in labor needs companionship and should not be left alone or isolated. If left alone, she may fear that the child will be born suddenly and the call button will not be answered promptly. She should be assured that if she sleeps she will be supervised closely.

The father today is taking a more active part in pregnancy and labor. With proper training, the father can become a valuable member of the obstetric team and need no longer feel like an outsider. Men who have attended prenatal education courses can give their partners great psychologic support and can coach them in helpful exercises and relaxation procedures during labor.

Most of the concerns that led to barring the father from the labor and delivery rooms—increase in incidence of infection, fainting or panic by the father—have not proved to be well founded. Fathers rarely jeopardize the well-being of the patient by disturbing the obstetrician and assistants. In complicated cases or those in which operative obstetrics is likely, it may be advisable to allow the father to be in the labor room but not in the delivery room.

Many physicians feel that conscious experience of childbirth is an important factor in the mother's acceptance of the infant in the postpartal period, and this seems to be true in animal experiments with drugged births. Heavy analgesia and anesthesia seem to be harmful to the mother and child both physiologically and psychologically. "Natural" childbirth, psychoprophylaxis, or regional anesthesia reduces these hazards.

EMOTIONAL ASPECTS OF THE POSTPARTAL PERIOD

If the antepartal period has been well managed and there have been no complications, psychic and physiologic adjustments are comparatively easy following delivery.

The mother should breast-feed her infant (see p 244) unless strong aversions or medical problems (eg, mastitis) interfere. A tremendous emotional lift results from being able to nurse the infant.

Some women do not want to breast-feed because they are employed. Others believe they will not produce enough milk. The fear that nursing will spoil the beauty of the breasts or will interfere with social activities deters others. Most of these objections can be overcome by explanation of the facts. A good start for the child and a quicker recovery for the mother are the goals of breast feeding. If the mother only nurses for several months, this may be sufficient.

When the breasts are full and tender, a temporary emotional depression often occurs ("baby blues"). (See Depressive Reactions, p 461.) The unfamiliar routine of breast feeding may provoke tears and discouragement, and the complete dependency of the infant on the mother may be burdensome at first. This may prove difficult until the mother becomes familiar with the routine of child care and unless she is confident of the assistance of her husband and others. The mother should be forewarned that her infant will seem to become more hungry on about the fourth or fifth day and will want to nurse more often. After 1–2 of these "frequency days," the infant will return to a less frequent feeding schedule. Explanation, demonstration of nursing and child care procedures, and emotional support will help to minimize problems in breast feeding.

A second brief, mild depression may develop about 1 month after delivery, when personal sacrifices and the drudgery of daily routines have taken much of the glamor out of motherhood. The mother may resent both the child and the father. Additional household help, a supportive attitude on the part of the father and the physician, and adequate reassurance usually will prevent serious depression.

The mother may subconsciously consider the child a rival for the father's affections, and the father in turn may resent the transfer of the mother's attention to the infant during the first few months after delivery (the "childbirth triangle"). This may lead to jealousy and discontent unless a good relationship exists between the parents, and they should be cautioned to modify their responses in a constructive way for the good of the family.

If more severe problems exist or are likely to occur, the patient's ability to cope should be assessed by an experienced person (eg, a representative of the Visiting Nurse Association) who can visit the home periodically, at least during the first 2 weeks. If serious problems exist, psychiatric consultation may be required.

Grief & Grieving

Grief reactions may develop after spontaneous abortion, fetal death, or neonatal death. Most women who have a pregnancy loss feel a great sense of guilt for having done "something wrong" to cause the problem. A satisfactory explanation must be given. Moreover, the patient should be encouraged by an empathetic physician or nurse to resolve her grief by "talking it out," perhaps with other women who have had a similar loss.

In personal loss situations, one must distinguish between inadequate grieving and depression, because the treatment and course of each may be different. Unresolved grief with anniversary recognition is not uncommon. When the response is disproportionate or persists long after the event, psychiatric consultation is warranted.

MENTAL ILLNESS ASSOCIATED WITH PREGNANCY

A woman who is physically able to bear a child may not wish to become pregnant at a given time, may not ever wish to have a child, or may not be psychologically adaptable to the stresses involved in pregnancy and parenthood. Many women have no desire for parenthood; others have a basic aversion to pregnancy even though they may claim the contrary.

The fear of pregnancy may be rationalized in many ways, including the following: "It's too soon after marriage" or ". . . after my last baby." "We can't afford it." "My husband is unwilling to accept another obligation." "Our marriage is insecure already." "I'm not well." "I'm absorbed in my career." "I'm afraid of losing my husband's love to the child." These "reasons" for not wanting a child are usually expressions of conscious or unconscious anxiety, conflict, or inadequacy.

Some motivations for pregnancy are discussed on p 455. If a

pregnancy is unwanted or its motivation is poor, the mother, the child, and the family may suffer. Depression, anxiety, and feelings of inadequacy are common in such situations.

Because even the happiest parents cannot escape some concern regarding pregnancy, positive and negative emotions are almost always present. In some cases, the psychic consequences are brief and clinically unimportant; in others, extended and serious. Fortunately, the course of pregnancy is a happy experience for most women.

Mental illness can often be prevented or its severity lessened by a physician alert to patients' unusual signs or symptoms.

During the postpartal period, even women who regarded pregnancy as a joyful time may become tense and disturbed. Breast feeding is often a problem; some women do not want to nurse, and those who do cannot always produce enough milk. "Frequency days" at the end of the first week (see p 458) may add to the mother's responsibilities and tensions. The infant seems to become the central figure in the household and the mother its "servant," providing primary care for a helpless and demanding other person. Responsibilities and obligations are multiplied while personal gratifications are sacrificed. Fatigue is common and may lead to irritability. If the child is in any way abnormal or especially difficult to manage, it may easily seem "too much for one woman to handle." How the mother responds to these challenges is a measure of her emotional stability and maturity.

Psychosis requiring psychiatric intervention occurs in approximately 0.3% of women during pregnancy and the puerperium. About 15% of psychotic breakdowns occur before delivery, 55% during the 2 weeks after delivery (most of these during the first 7 days), and the remainder later in the perinatal period.

Pregnancy itself never causes psychosis, even toxic psychosis. However, some patients may be predisposed to psychotic responses to stress. Gestational psychosis does not exist, and parity is significant to neither the incidence nor the type of emotional illness.

Of the 3 types of psychoses seen postpartum, most are manic-depressive or schizophrenic reactions. Toxic delirium is very uncommon. Rare types of mental illness are alcoholic psychosis, epilepsy associated with psychosis, and psychosis due to general paresis.

A. Manic-Depressive Psychosis: No specific etiologic factor is known, although in many cases there seem to be strong familial predispositions to mental illness. Manic-depressive psychosis is a recurrent disorder of adults.

At least half of psychotic illnesses during or immediately following pregnancy are affective reactions. About 10% of these are major manic or depressive episodes that occur before delivery; the remainder occur during the puerperium. Mania or depression (or both) may occur in one pregnancy and not in others.

1. Manic reactions–These are usually noted 1–2 weeks postpartum and may be preceded by brief periods of depression. Symptoms include agitation, excitement, volubility, inattention, rhyming and punning speech, disorder of dress, and disinterest in food. The patient often becomes dehydrated and exhausted. Manic reactions are brief in duration (1–3 weeks), but the patient can become exhausted early, and vigorous initial therapy is most important.

Refer the patient to a psychiatrist. Electroshock therapy (contraindicated in pelvic infection) or psychotropic drugs or sedatives may be given together with supportive treatment and psychotherapy.

Caution should be used in drug treatment of manic-depressive states during pregnancy. Psychotropic drugs are transmitted across the placenta. Although malformations are possible with heavy or prolonged drug therapy, the fetus is more likely to suffer from accumulation, slower or absent detoxification, enzyme induction, or limited drug excretion.

Neuroleptic drugs produce tremors, hypertonus, poor sucking, sluggish reflexes, and leukopenia in the newborn. Some of these signs may persist for weeks. Neonatal jaundice, enzyme induction, and hyperbilirubinemia from maternal phenothiazines have also been reported. Maternal lithium therapy may cause cyanosis, flaccidity, hypertonia, hypercapnia, or tachycardia in the newborn. These signs are reversible, but they may be serious in a highly vulnerable newborn.

In all cases of psychiatric complications during pregnancy, minimal effective doses of a potent phenothiazine or haloperidol are preferred to lithium if medication is required. Moreover, mania is cyclic and may remit spontaneously. Therefore, all medications should be discontinued as soon as possible. The patient may go to term or complete delivery without the need for additional drugs.

Breast feeding usually is contraindicated when severe psychiatric disorders complicate the puerperium. Nonetheless, nursing mothers should avoid diazepam, lithium, bromides, and reserpine, because these drugs may seriously contaminate the milk (see p 245).

Therapeutic doses of barbiturates, benzodiazepines, and phenothiazines such as trifluoperazine or thioridazine are excreted in breast milk in amounts too small to affect the infant. Antidepressant drugs administered to the mother but safe for the nursing infant include imipramine, desipramine, amitriptyline, and tranylcypromine.

The prognosis for the child is good if it can be separated from the mother until she has recovered.

2. Depressive reactions–Periods of despondency are far more frequent than manic states and are more dangerous for both mother and child. The "baby blues" often deepen and continue into the second week postpartum, and the patient's condition is marked by anxiety, profound fatigue, and anorexia. The amphetamines and antidepressants are of little value. The woman becomes self-accusatory and expresses inappropriate or bizarre thoughts and feelings. Intense depression often follows, and the future seems hopeless. During this critical interval, the mother may kill the child and commit suicide.

The duration of an attack cannot be predicted. Some patients suffer for weeks, others for months. Electroshock therapy usually results in a dramatic improvement, and follow-up psychotherapy is valuable; however, attacks may recur. Both mother and infant do well when they are separated.

B. Schizophrenia: This psychosis of unknown cause occurs with greatest frequency in adolescents or young adults. A sudden onset often follows a seemingly contented pregnancy. Abnormal personality reactions before and during pregnancy are almost always present, however.

The splintering of the personality results from underlying psychic problems and inability to adjust to adult demands. Abnormally shy, quiet, reserved, sensitive, and suspicious women are more prone to develop schizoid personality reactions during pregnancy. They are exceedingly introspective, easily offended, and prone to daydreaming.

The infant is invariably rejected. Hostility toward the husband is obvious to the perceptive physician. The patient often has delusions of immaculate conception or that some man other than the husband is the father of the child.

This disorder progresses from avoidance of social contacts and rationalization of failure to complete abandonment of reason for a small, personal world of unreality. Ideas of reference and influence, delusions and hallucinations, complete distortion of emotional responses, excitement, vulgarity, and confusion of thought content are prominent features of the syndrome. Infanticide occurs occasionally, but suicide is rare.

Hospitalization is required. Electroshock therapy followed by psychotherapy is effective in most cases. Exhaustion or puerperal sepsis are temporary contraindications to shock treatment.

The immediate prognosis for the schizophrenic patient before delivery is fair to good. The prognosis is better if the onset occurs abruptly during the puerperium. Although hereditary tendencies are postulated, the infant is not obviously affected by parental schizophrenia.

C. Toxic Deliria: Exogenous or endogenous toxicosis causes behavioral and mental disorders similar to those seen in acute psychosis. The patient is excitable, confused, incoherent, and restless. The sensorium is clouded, and delusions and hallucinations may lead the patient to believe she is fighting for her life. She may try to flee—injuring herself, her infant, and others in the attempt. The causes are as follows: (1) Drugs, occasionally taken with suicidal intent (eg, alcohol, barbiturates), bromides, opium derivatives, LSD, marihuana, lead; (2) cardiac or renal failure; (3) metabolic aberrations (hypoglycemia, hypothyroidism); (4) trauma (usually cranial); and (5) acute infections (septicemia).

Unless the obstetric patient is eclampsic, has a very long labor, is dehydrated, or receives extremely large doses of analgesics, delirium rarely develops.

Delirium clears with removal of the cause and symptomatic, supportive therapy. Discontinue toxic drugs immediately. Restrict the patient's movements as necessary, but avoid physical restraints. Protect the patient and others from harm. Force fluids and restore electrolytes and blood glucose to normal levels. Prescribe appropriate antibiotics for infection. Rule out other types of mental disease.

The prognosis for both mother and child is good when the toxicosis is mild to moderate and exogenous. The prognosis in endogenous toxicosis depends upon the specific medical circumstances (see Chapter 13).

Emergency Management

The family physician, obstetrician, or gynecologist should not attempt to treat functional psychoses (schizophrenia, mania, etc), because intensive specialized care and institutional management are almost always required. However, the physician must be able to treat acute psychiatric emergencies such as antepartal or postpartal psychosis until consultation can be obtained and the patient transferred.

(1) Diagnose the problem. Observe the patient's behavior and movements, looking especially for muscular weakness and paralysis. Listen for speech impairment, disorientation, and delusional or hallucinatory expressions. Perform an adequate physical examination.

(2) Allay fear. Do not make promises or agree with or humor the patient, but calm her with a reassuring, supportive manner, emphasizing illness (not mental problems or "insanity"). Arrange for a favorite relative or friend to remain with or near the patient. Eliminate shadows and noise and exclude nonessential personnel.

(3) Avoid force. Restrict but do not restrain the patient.

(4) Prevent the patient from harming herself or others. Admit her to a single room on the first floor or to one with barred windows screened on the inside. Remove cords, ties, and sharp or movable heavy objects from the room. Provide special nurses day and night as necessary.

(5) Ensure rest. For excitable patients, consider ataractics (promazine, chlorpromazine), sedatives (paraldehyde, barbiturates), warm tubs, and cold packs.

(6) Provide adequate simple foods and fluids, observing the patient's preferences insofar as possible. Intravenous or gavage feedings may be necessary if the patient is completely resistant to eating or drinking.

PSEUDOCYESIS

Pseudocyesis (false pregnancy) is a fantasy reaction (delusion) noted during the childbearing years in women who have either an intense desire for pregnancy or an extreme fear of it. It occurs once in approximately 5000 general obstetrics cases and is most common in unmarried women and infertile married women. Patients with pseudocyesis are severely psychoneurotic or frankly psychotic. Stubborn, illogical insistence that pregnancy exists is characteristic.

All of the presumptive symptoms of pregnancy may be present: amenorrhea (hypothalamic), nausea and vomiting (psychogenic), breast sensitivity (subjective), abdominal protuberance (obesity, subconscious laxity of posture), quickening (misinterpretation), and waddling gait ("playing the role"). There are no probable signs and no positive evidences of pregnancy. On physical examination, the physician may be deceived by supposed fetal movements that are usually the result of contractions of the intestines or the muscles of the abdominal wall. However, a small uterus usually can be palpated on bimanual examination. In the absence of other disease, the use of certain drugs, or misinterpretation, laboratory tests are negative.

Suicide or a complete psychotic break may occur in patients who are ineptly "convinced against their will" that they are not pregnant or who are ridiculed. Many patients with pseudocyesis are borderline or actual schizophrenics.

The differential diagnosis of pseudocyesis includes intra- and extrauterine pregnancy, missed abortion, pelvic tumor, and psychopathologic states.

Treatment consists of kindly explanation and psychotherapy, usually by a psychiatrist. Hospitalization may be necessary.

The prognosis depends upon the seriousness of the emotional disorder and the success of psychotherapy.

Delivery in the Home or in an Alternative Birthing Center | 18

Selective home delivery is an important phase of maternity care all over the world. Complicated obstetric cases can now be transported to hospitals—or medical personnel and emergency supplies and equipment brought to the patient and her newborn—by improved surface and air transportation. Individualized domiciliary obstetrics will undoubtedly continue to be practiced among the poor, those living in rural areas, and those in whom the rapidity of labor prevents transfer to a hospital and for a large segment of the population during natural catastrophe and war.

In many areas, a scarcity of hospital beds and trained medical personnel requires the integration of home and hospital delivery programs. In some of these situations, good antenatal care, delivery of first infants and subsequent abnormal cases in hospitals, and the availability of experienced doctors and nurses have increased the safety of home delivery; maternal and infant mortality and morbidity rates are often below those reported by hospitals in the same region where obstetric patients both with and without complications are admitted.

Supervision of midwives is the physician's duty in many countries. All physicians must therefore be familiar with the techniques of confinement in the home.

Midwives or nurse practitioners, family practitioners, and consultant specialists have been incorporated successfully into effective obstetric units. These individuals can call upon or refer patients to numerous services for specialty study and care.

The family practitioner should supervise the midwife in obstetric delivery, and both should be under the direction of a specialist when complications develop. Obstetricians cannot hope to manage all deliveries personally; their primary function is to manage problem cases.

Selection of Cases for Home or Alternative Birthing Center Delivery

Home delivery should be done electively only for patients with a history of normal pregnancy and a prognosis of probable uncomplicated delivery; in other words, women for whom minimal medical and surgical intervention is anticipated. Individualized judgments must be made about delivering primigravidas outside an obstetric service.

The site and circumstances of childbirth have become a focus of recent controversy between 2 large groups: couples who seek to make childbirth as natural as possible, thereby enhancing the personally beneficial qualities of the event; and medical personnel who have welcomed advanced technology during labor and delivery to maximize safety. Those who subscribe to the first point of view have seized upon home delivery as their goal despite being accused of seeming to deny almost a century of medical progress. However, their reasons are numerous:

(1) To permit the parturient to be in control of her body and experiences.

(2) To limit or avoid analgesia-anesthesia, thereby heightening the mother's full participation and fulfillment.

(3) To increase mother-father-infant interaction (bonding), permit earlier breast feeding, and strengthen the family unit psychologically.

(4) To deny possibly unnecessary hospital procedures (eg, induction of labor, episiotomy) and to limit risks (eg, iatrogenic or nosocomial infection).

(5) To reduce the expense of childbirth.

The patient's demands notwithstanding, physicians—particularly those who fear a return to poorly supervised, hazardous delivery—have been reluctant to abandon medical security and the emergency facilities available to patients in a hospital.

A better appreciation of the problems, as well as the feasibility of delivery in a less ''medicalized'' and more homelike setting, has led to the limited acceptance of home birth by careful and experienced personnel for low-risk obstetric patients in the USA. A compromise favored by even more lay and medical individuals is delivery in an alternative birthing center.

Most alternative birthing centers are in hospital suites away from the traditional obstetric department but close to the delivery and operating rooms and medical or neonatal intensive care facilities for use when serious problems arise. Birthing rooms have homelike accommodations, including a crib for the newborn. By agreement, medication and instrumentation are limited. Delivery can be accomplished in the mother's bed, with skin-to-skin contact on the mother's abdomen following (usually) spontaneous birth. During labor and delivery, family and friends of the mother's choosing may remain. Early discharge from the center, often during the day of delivery, must meet medical criteria. Many centers arrange for the mother and infant to be seen within 24 hours of dismissal by a nurse midwife or nurse specializing in neonatal care.

Readmission of the mother (because of bleeding or other urgent problems) or transfer of the newborn to the pediatric service for special treatment is readily accomplished.

Contraindications to Home Delivery

Home delivery is contraindicated for patients requiring forceps rotation or extraction and general, spinal, or caudal anesthesia. Other contraindications include high-risk problems such as preeclampsia-eclampsia, multiple pregnancy, breech or transverse presentation, antepartal bleeding, severe isoimmunization, a history of premature or postdate deliveries, grand multiparity, and significant medical and surgical complications in previous pregnancies.

Advantages of Home Delivery

(1) Delivery is often more physiologic within known surroundings. The presence of the patient's husband and family may have a favorable psychic effect on some women.

(2) Rooming-in need not be arranged; the infant may remain with the mother.

(3) Expense is less than in a hospital.

(4) Puerperal sepsis is unlikely (provided strict asepsis is maintained). The residents of a home seem to be partially immune to any pathogenic bacteria that may be present.

(5) Maternity hospital beds are freed for complicated cases.

Disadvantages of Home Delivery

(1) "Normal" cases chosen for home delivery may become complicated despite the greatest care in selection. It is difficult to predict uterine inertia, prolonged second stage of labor, or postpartal hemorrhage.

(2) If emergencies should arise, adequate facilities and personnel are not immediately available.

(3) The specialist called to the home to deal with a complicated delivery rarely knows the patient's antepartal course and prior problems.

Principles to Be Observed in Home Confinement

(1) Expert antepartal evaluation is required to eliminate abnormal cases or those with a doubtful prognosis from the group scheduled for labor and delivery at home.

(2) A physician should check home delivery candidates regularly for the best utilization of time, planning, and consultation. If the patient is to be delivered by a midwife, the physician should see the patient regularly with the midwife.

(3) The midwife's and physician's names and telephone numbers should be posted prominently in the home. Preparations for confinement should be completed by the sixth month of pregnancy, since the patient is likely to be more ambitious before the last trimester and because an unexpected premature delivery may occur.

(4) An obstetric specialist should examine pregnant patients vagi-

nally at about the 36th week (with the midwife and generalist present). The pelvic capacity, presentation, size of the infant, etc, can thus be determined.

(5) If a midwife is scheduled to perform the delivery, the general practitioner should be alerted when the patient goes into labor. The physician must then remain on emergency call until the patient is delivered successfully.

(6) Home facilities may be meager or primitive (eg, poor lighting, few conveniences), and the aseptic field is limited. The precepts of obstetric management are always the same, however, no matter where delivery is accomplished. One can improvise almost everything except water, certain essential instruments, and special medications.

REQUIREMENTS FOR HOME DELIVERY

Bedding
A supply of linen adequate for the patient's needs during labor, delivery, and the first week after delivery will be required: clean sheets, pillow cases, blankets, and bed pads. In addition, the patient should obtain a rubber or plastic sheet to protect the mattress, a 4- to 6-inch stack of unfolded newspapers for padding beneath the patient and for disposal of waste, and light plastic or paper bags and newly ironed ("sterilized") newspapers for storage of sheets and other bedclothing.

Other Supplies
(1) Soap, towels, washcloths, sanitary pads.

(2) A 1-lb roll of absorbent cotton.

(3) A bedpan.

(4) Two sterile basins: one for the physician's hands and another for preparing the patient.

(5) One sterile dipper and 2 kettles: one for sterile hot water and the other for sterile cold water.

(6) An ironing board or piece of wood wide enough to be placed under the mattress for elevation of the patient's hips if delivery in bed is likely.

Labor Room
The mother's own room is usually chosen. It should be clean, light, and attractive. Proximity to a bath and toilet is important. The room should be screened against flies, and measures should be taken to eliminate animal and insect vectors during the lying-in period. Family members with contagious diseases should be excluded.

Delivery Room

It is possible to deliver the patient in her own bed if other prerequisites are at hand.

The kitchen is often selected because the light is usually good and a large table that can even be used for a delivery table is generally available. Water, a tub or sink, and a stove for warmth and sterilization are also customarily available.

Infant's Room

The newborn should have a separate room if possible. It should be warm, well ventilated, sunny, clean, and quiet. Running water in or near the room is desirable. If the mother wishes to keep the child in her room, simpler facilities than these will be sufficient. Only practical furnishings are necessary: a scrupulously clean baby bed, a newly painted baby basket, or a light bassinet or crib. A shelf, stand, or rack for toilet needs; a closet, bureau, or cabinet for clothing; and a table or bathinette for changing and bathing the infant are desirable but not essential. A low armless chair, clothes racks, and hooks should be provided. A covered diaper pail and paper bags for refuse are necessary. Heavy rugs, coarse hangings, and articles difficult to keep clean should be removed.

The Layette

Shirts, nightgowns, quilted pads, a plastic or rubber pad, diapers, baby blankets, and flannelet squares should be provided.

Cotton or synthetic clothing is preferable to wool because the former is easier to launder and cheaper and does not shrink as much and because wool may be too harsh for an infant's skin. Allergies are less common with cotton fabrics.

The infant must have a separate supply of washcloths and bath towels. Terry cloth is preferable, and towels should be at least 1 yard square so that they can be wrapped around the infant after the bath.

Launder all dry goods, and iron and fold the surfaces together while they are still warm. Store in plastic bags, clean pillow cases, or an ironed newspaper.

The Physician's & Nurse's Equipment for Home Delivery

The patient's antepartal record, including pelvic measurements, blood pressure readings, results of serologic tests, Rh titers, x-ray findings, etc, should be available in the home for reference.

The necessities for the average home delivery can be carried in 2 bags.

A. Physician's Bag:

1. Materials–

2 pairs of rubber gloves, sterile if possible (although gloves can be boiled before use at delivery).

2 sterile hand brushes and 1 bar of germicidal soap or detergent.

1 sterile mask, cap, and gown.

1 sterile cord tie and dressing.

1 plastic or rubberized apron.

Labor record and birth certificate.

1 large sterile sheet for draping the patient.

1 small clean sheet for instruments.

Clinistix or Uristix for determining urine glucose and protein.

2. Medications—

Meperidine, 1-mL ampules, for analgesia.

Ergonovine maleate, 0.2-mg tablets, for postpartal bleeding.

Hydroxyzine or other comparable compound (tranquilizer, antihistaminic) in ampules to potentiate analgesia or relieve allergic manifestations.

Phenobarbital, 0.03-g tablets, for sedation.

Magnesium sulfate solution, 2 10-mL ampules (5 g of 50% solution; 500 mg = 4 mEq/mL).

Calcium carbonate, 1 g in 10 mL of solution (10%), for intravenous use in the event of respiratory depression due to magnesium sulfate.

Procaine hydrochloride (1%), 120 mL, for local anesthesia.

Bichloride of mercury or mercuric cyanide tablets, 475 mg. Two such tablets per quart of water yield an antiseptic solution of approximately 1:1000 concentration. *Caution:* This poisonous material must never be given to lay individuals.

Povidone-iodine (Betadine, Isodine, etc) antiseptic surgical scrub; 5 mL will cover about 50 cm². Brush or cleanse thoroughly for 10 minutes; wash with clean water.

Silver nitrate, 1% solution in wax plastules, for ocular instillation.

3. Instruments—Boil instruments and then immerse them in an antiseptic solution before use.

1 scalpel and 1 pair of tissue scissors.

1 smooth and 1 toothed tissue forceps.

3 ring (ovum) forceps.

1 uterine packing forceps.

2 broad vaginal retractors.

1 box of assorted needles, round and cutting.

1 needle holder.

Packs of sutures: chromic and plain 00 and 000 size.

2 10-mL syringes and long needles for local anesthesia.

4 artery forceps.

1 sterile tracheal catheter with DeLee mucus trap.

1 sterile No. 16 soft rubber catheter.

1 pelvimeter.

1 sterile measuring tape.

1 cord clamp or tie.

1 obstetric forceps (Simpson forceps may be the most utilitarian).

4. Emergency materials–

Low-molecular-weight dextran and distilled water diluent; tubing and needles for intravenous administration to treat hypovolemia.

Sterile 6-inch gauze roll for vaginal and uterine packing to control excessive bleeding.

B. Nurse's Bag:

1 large sterile sheet for draping the patient.

1 small clean sheet for instruments, etc.

1 plastic half-sheet to place beneath the patient.

4 sterile towels.

1 package of sterile 4 × 4 inch gauze sponges.

2 sterile hand brushes and 1 bar of germicidal soap or detergent.

1 oral and 1 rectal thermometer.

2 pairs of gloves (sterile, if possible).

1 stethoscope and sphygmomanometer.

1 safety razor and blades.

1 rectal tube with funnel.

1 good flashlight with fresh batteries.

Baby scales.

1 plastic bag for the placenta.

1 clean lifting forceps to remove articles that have been sterilized.

1 sterile 5-mL syringe with short and long No. 22 needles.

Ampules (1 mL each) of oxytocin or ergonovine.

1 plastic or rubberized apron.

Initial Examination at Onset of Labor

(1) Examine the patient externally and rectally.

(2) Administer an enema and clip or shave the perineum.

(3) Assist at a shower or give a vigorous bed bath (with special attention to abdomen, legs, and perineum). Use 1:1000 bichloride of mercury solution as a germicide.

(4) The patient should wear a clean nightgown or slip.

(5) Make the bed with clean sheets (place clean newspapers beneath bed pad).

(6) Remove unnecessary furniture, equipment, and litter.

(7) Provide a good light and an ample stack of clean plastic sheeting or newspapers.

(8) Sterilize diapers and newspapers by baking if facilities and time are available: dampen "like clothes for ironing," then bake like bread (ie, for 45–60 minutes in an oven at 375 °F).

(9) Decide whether delivery should be on a table or in bed, and make the necessary preparations.

Conduct of Labor & Delivery (See Chapter 6.)

Assume that everything but the operative field is contaminated in home delivery. Keep gloved hands, cotton balls, instruments, etc, aseptic.

Keep good records on standard hospital forms. As far as possible, simulate a hospital delivery in professional care and consideration for the patient and her family. Moderate analgesia may be administered and episiotomy may be accomplished in the home just as in the hospital.

If an abnormality develops during labor or after delivery and places the patient or the infant in jeopardy, call for consultation immediately; arrange for ambulance transfer to a hospital if indicated.

Immediate Postpartal Care of the Mother

(1) Make the patient comfortable, keep her warm, and ensure rest and quiet.

(2) Check the fundus every 5 minutes for the first hour; estimate the amount of vaginal bleeding.

(3) Elevate the uterus and massage the fundus lightly every 15 minutes for 1–2 hours. (For subsequent management, see p 160.)

Immediate Care of the Newborn (See also pp 159 and 186.)

A preterm infant or one who appears to be abnormal should be transferred to a hospital at once.

Handle the infant as little as possible. Wrap the infant in a clean towel. Cut and tie the cord, using aseptic technique. Wipe the newborn clean using dry skin technique. *Do not bathe the infant.* Insert 1 drop of 1% aqueous silver nitrate solution into each eye and irrigate with cool boiled water. Dress the newborn in a cotton shirt and diaper. Apply a dressing to the cord. Weigh and wrap the infant in a cotton or wool blanket.

Place the infant in a warmed crib, basket, or box away from fire, animals, and vermin. (A box within a box, with space around for 5 hot water bottles between the sides, is a good arrangement. **Note:** Do not place hot water bottles at the infant's head or in contact with the skin.)

Keep the navel and cord stump dry. The cord separates in 5–10 days. If it appears reddened or becomes odorous, touch with 70% alcohol twice daily and dry the navel by exposure to air.

The Placenta

Examine the placenta grossly. Note whether it is intact or if a portion is missing. Count the vessels in the cord, and place the placenta in a plastic or paper bag for pathologic study or discard.

19 | Gynecologic History & Examination

OUTLINE OF HISTORY & EXAMINATION

Age, Gravidity, & Parity:

Chief Complaint: The patient's main problems in her own words and listed in her order of seriousness.

Present Illness: The character of the patient's health at the onset of illness and the symptoms in sequence. Include facts, dates, and essential details.

Medical & Surgical History: Summary of the patient's childhood and later illnesses in chronologic order together with complications and the treatment prescribed for each. Record operations and injuries with dates and outcome.

Obstetric History: Number of previous pregnancies (with dates), duration of pregnancy, character and duration of labor, complications, weight and sex of infant; stillbirths, abortions, neonatal complications.

Family History: Age and health of parents and siblings. Age, cause, and date of death of principal relatives. Familial or hereditary abnormalities, diseases, bleeding tendencies. Occurrence of cancer, tuberculosis, diabetes mellitus, syphilis, heart disease, high blood pressure, nervous or mental disorders in the family.

Marital or Cohabitation History: Duration of present marriage or living arrangement, age and health of spouse/partner and children, if living, or cause of death and age at time of death; former marriages and nonmarried living arrangements; degree of compatibility. Other marriages and relationships (dates, duration).

Social History: Occupation, hazards. Church, clubs, reaction to other people. Successes, failures, arrests. Health of husbands and children. Success of marriage or nonmarried living arrangement, coitus, contraception. Sleep, exercise, relaxation, hobbies, medications, alcohol, tobacco, drugs. Residence abroad or in the tropics.

System Review

Provide a positive or negative comment for each division in this category, but cover the symptoms relative to the patient's chief complaint in the present illness only.

A. General: Patient's health, allergies, skin disorders. Present weight, average weight, weight prior to present illness. Patient's version of reason for gain or loss.

B. Head and Neck: Pain, tenderness, swelling, restriction of neck, trauma.

    1. Eyes–Vision with and without glasses, double vision, irritation, swelling of lids, prominence of eyes.

    2. Ears–Hearing, pain, "buzzing," discharge.

    3. Nose–Acuity of smell, obstruction to nasal passages, bleeding, discharge.

    4. Mouth–Condition of teeth, gums, tongue; sensitivity of taste; bleeding; chewing difficulties.

    5. Throat–Speech, swallowing, condition of tonsils and pharynx.

C. Cardiovascular: Skin color (pale, ruddy, dusky), precordial or substernal constriction pain, irregular or labored heartbeat, shortness of breath at rest or exercise.

D. Respiratory: Cough, wheezing, sputum, hemoptysis, chest pain with breathing, chills, fever, night sweats.

E. Gastrointestinal: Appetite; thirst; digestive difficulties (nausea, vomiting, pre- or postprandial pain; hematemesis; food intolerance); jaundice; frequency, character, and color of stools.

F. Genitourinary and Menstrual:

    1. Urinary frequency, nocturia, oliguria, dysuria, hematuria, urethral discharge, "sores," swelling, sexually transmitted disease.

    2. Menarche, last menstrual period (LMP), previous menstrual period (PMP), regularity, duration, amount of bleeding, pain, mucous discharge, intermenstrual or postcoital spotting, menopause (date and symptoms).

G. Neuropsychiatric: Skin sensation. Strength, ability to move, walk, work. Ataxia, dizziness, tremor. Headache. "Spells," fits. Acuity of memory. Strange occurrences. Libido.

Physical Examination

    A. General: Appearance, ambulatory or bed patient. Attitude. Color of skin, mucous surfaces. Temperature, pulse, respiration, blood pressure, height, and weight.

    B. Head and Neck: Skull size and shape, hair (amount, color, texture), tumors, tenderness, neck swelling, pulsations, deviation of trachea, tracheal tug, mobility.

        1. Eyes–Prominence of lids or eyes. Size, shape, pupillary reaction to light, character of conjunctiva and sclera, ocular movements, ophthalmoscopic examination (when indicated).

2. **Ears**–Hearing, discharge, cerumen, tophi, tenderness, otoscopic examination (when indicated).
3. **Nose**–Deformity, septal deviation, obstruction, tenderness, discharge, unusual smells, tenderness over sinuses, transillumination of sinuses.
4. **Mouth and throat**–Lips, gums, tongue, dentition, tonsils, oropharynx, postnasal discharge, laryngoscopic examination (when indicated).

C. **Thorax:** Size, shape, symmetry, pulsations, tenderness.

1. **Breasts**–Size, shape, equality, masses, tenderness, scars, nipple discharge.
2. **Lungs**–
   a. Inspection of chest–Breathing (type, rate, depth), equality of inspiration and expiration.
   b. Palpation–Muscle tone, tenderness, tactile fremitus.
   c. Percussion–Resonance, great vessel and cardiac silhouette, excursions of the diaphragm, gastric tympany.
   d. Auscultation–Quality and intensity of breath sounds, rales (especially posttussive), whisper and vocal fremitus, friction rub.
3. **Heart**–Point of maximal impulse at apex, abnormal pulsations, retractions or venous distention in neck or other veins.
   a. Palpation–Record the point of maximal intensity in centimeters to the right and left of the midsternal line, in centimeters in or near the closest inner space. Palpate the precordial area for shocks and thrills.
   b. Percussion–Outline by direct and indirect methods the borders of the heart and great vessels. Orient the left border of the heart with respect to the midclavicular line.
   c. Auscultation–Character of sounds, intensity of tones, rate and rhythm. Location of murmurs, type and intensity of murmur, transmission of murmur, time of murmur. Compare A_2 and P_2. Friction rubs and posttussive rales.

D. **Abdomen:** Note the size, shape, and contour of the abdomen, masses, visible peristaltic waves, prominent veins, herniation.

1. **Palpation**–Thickness of the abdominal wall (panniculus), tenderness, rigidity, masses, hernias; presence or absence of a fluid wave. Palpate organs, liver, spleen, and kidneys, other masses. Costovertebral angle tenderness.
2. **Percussion**–Dullness in the flanks; fluid shift; position of tumors, organs, and bladder.
3. **Auscultation**–Presence of peristaltic tones, "swish" of shifting fluids.

E. **Extremities:** Size, shape, color, and movements of hands; condition of fingers and nails; size and color of arms; size and movement of legs and feet.

F. Peripheral Vascular System: Record blood pressure in both arms, and palpate arteries for thickness and resilience. Note type of radial, femoral, distal pedal, posterior tibial, and popliteal pulses. Observe temperature of extremities, and note presence or absence of cyanosis.

G. Nervous System: Cerebral function, cranial nerves, cerebellar function, motor system, sensory system, and reflexes.

GYNECOLOGIC EXAMINATIONS & PROCEDURES

The gynecologic evaluation of each new patient must include blood pressure determination and examination of the heart, lungs, breasts, abdomen, vagina, rectum, and anus, as well as a combined abdominopelvic evaluation. Particular attention must be devoted to the breasts, abdomen, pelvis; and appropriate laboratory studies must be performed.

An appraisal of other body systems should be done when indicated by the medical history or unusual findings. Do not dismiss a patient following the initial work-up without seeking a disorder of major consequence if signs or symptoms are present. The gynecologic specialist will frequently refer a patient for consultation, eg, to a cardiologist or neurologist, when indicated. The physician who does not specialize may do whatever evaluation is required for complete diagnosis (although it is unlikely, for example, that this would include a complete ophthalmologic examination). If the patient who is seen for gynecologic complaints is already under the care of another physician, the gynecologic examination should be specific and complete with particular reference to the chief complaint.

Breasts (See Figs 19–1, 19–2, and 19–3.)

Examine the breasts in good direct light with the patient first in a relaxed sitting position. Record abnormalities, using a sketch or diagram for clarity. Note the size, shape, symmetry, vascularity, and pendulosity of the breasts. Examine for skin and nipple changes and nipple discharge. A specimen of nipple discharge should be smeared and fixed for cytologic examination.

Palpate one breast at a time. Hold the fingers flat against the breast and carefully feel with the fingertips, using gentle pressure against the firm chest wall. Evaluate the entire breast systematically from the nipple outward. Distinguish tender regions. Observe breast consistency for thickened or firm zones. Identify the cordlike duct structures and any "shotty" or nodular masses, and determine whether masses are fixed to

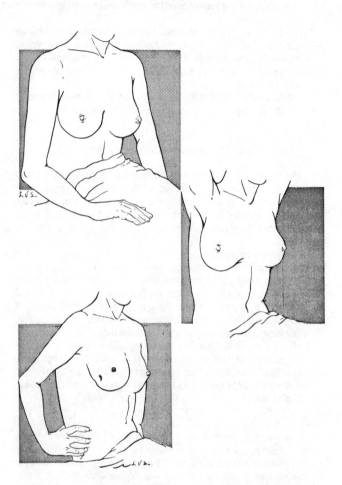

Figure 19–1. Inspection of breasts. Observe breasts with patient sitting, arms at sides and overhead, for presence of asymmetry and nipple or skin retraction. These signs may be accentuated by having the patient raise her arms overhead. Skin retraction or dimpling may be demonstrated by having the patient press her hand on her hip in order to contract the pectoralis muscles. (Reproduced, with permission, from Wilson JL: Chapter 20 in *Current Surgical Diagnosis & Treatment,* 4th ed. Dunphy JE, Way LW [editors]. Lange, 1979.)

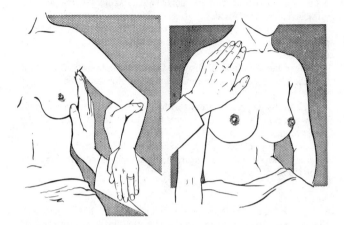

Figure 19–2. Palpation of axillary and supraclavicular regions for enlarged lymph nodes. (Reproduced, with permission, from Giuliano AE: Chapter 20 in *Current Surgical Diagnosis & Treatment,* 6th ed. Way LW [editor]. Lange, 1983.)

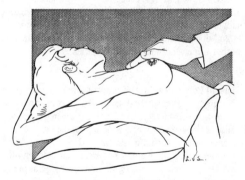

Figure 19–3. Palpation of breasts. Palpation is performed with the patient supine and arm abducted. (Reproduced, with permission, from Giuliano AE: Chapter 20 in *Current Surgical Diagnosis & Treatment,* 6th ed. Way LW [editor]. Lange, 1983.)

the skin or chest wall. Transilluminate the breast in a darkened room to distinguish solid from cystic tumors. Palpate axillary and supra- and infraclavicular lymph nodes.

With the patient's arms raised over her head, observe asymmetry or retraction of the nipple or skin. Use oblique light to confirm surface dimpling.

Have the patient bend forward from the erect position to reveal irregularities or dimpling when the breasts fall forward from the chest wall.

Carefully palpate the breasts with the patient supine. Place a small pillow under her shoulder on the side to be examined to "balance" the breast on the chest wall.

Any unphysiologic mass or discharge should be investigated further because of the possibility of cancer. Mammography is indicated for areas suspicious for cancer.

Abdomen

Drape the patient in the dorsal recumbent position with her knees slightly flexed to improve abdominal relaxation. Inspect for freedom of respiratory movement, prominence or enlargement of internal organs, asymmetry, scars, and significant skin changes (eg, rashes, postirradiation telangiectasia).

Palpate the abdomen gently for evidence of muscle guarding, tenderness, rebound phenomenon, herniation, or masses. Palpate firmly for deep masses or sensitivity, especially over the cecum, colon, and bladder. Identify the liver by percussion and palpate its edge; examine the gallbladder and epigastric region. Check for costovertebral angle tenderness and displacement of the kidneys. Consider splenic enlargement and other upper abdominal abnormalities.

Pelvis

A. General Pelvic (Vaginal) Examination: Place the patient in the lithotomy position, appropriately draped. The physician must be seated to visualize the parts adequately. Use surgically clean gloves, and have a female attendant present as a chaperone and assistant.

1. Inspection of external genitalia–Inflamed, hypertrophied, atrophied, ulcerated, and other abnormal areas can be seen almost at a glance. Separate the labia. Look for vaginal discharge at the introitus. Note abnormalities of the clitoris.

Inspect for skin changes over the perineum, thighs, mons veneris, and perianal region. Note and record the presence of masses and tender areas. Describe discernible external genital lesions.

Observe the urethral meatus for redness, purulent exudation from Skene's ducts, and other abnormalities.

2. Speculum examination (Fig 19–4)–The speculum should be

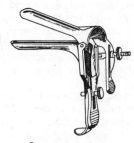
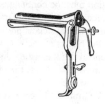

Graves vaginal speculum   Pederson vaginal speculum

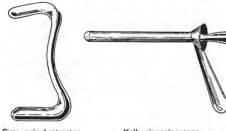

Sims vaginal retractor   Kelly air vaginoscope
                               (cystoscope) for children

Figure 19–4. Vaginal specula and vaginoscope. (These come in various sizes.)

warm. Artificial lubrication of the speculum is rarely necessary because vaginal secretions are normally adequate for this purpose when the speculum is inserted carefully. Warm water may be used if necessary. Cream or jelly lubricants have the disadvantage of interfering with vaginal and cervical cytologic examination, bacterial smears or cultures, and wet preparations for *Trichomonas, Candida,* and *Corynebacterium vaginale.*

The patient should be asked to relax and then bear down as with a bowel movement to reduce muscular resistance as the speculum is introduced. Spread the labia with the gloved fingers of one hand, insert the gloved index finger of the same hand into the vagina, and depress the perineum slightly. Do not insert the speculum directly into the vagina but slightly downward and inward to avoid the urethra. Visualize the vaginal canal while inserting and opening the speculum. If a single-blade speculum is used, merely depress it to view the cervix. To avoid traumatic encounter with a vaginal obstruction, mass, or friable lesion, observation must be continuous as the speculum is advanced. A good light source is required, preferably daylight or a blue-white spotlight, although some physicians prefer a head lamp or head mirror.

As the blades of the bivalve speculum meet the cervix, open the instrument so that the blades slip into the anterior and posterior fornices to fully expose the cervix. Fix the blades in an open position by tightening the screw lock.

3. Vaginal and cervical cytology–Before digital examination, obtain vaginal mucus from the posterior vaginal fornix and from the cervical canal for cytologic examination (see p 575), using the method recommended by the pathologist who will examine the smear, and for culture if indicated.

4. Inspection of the cervix–Examine the cervix carefully. Determine the size, contour, and surface characteristics; significant lacerations; displacement; size and configuration of the external os; distortion and ulceration; type and amount of discharge, blood, or fluid originating in the cervical canal; and the character of the cervical canal (in a patulous cervix).

Touch or gently wipe ulcerations or friable lesions with a cotton-tipped applicator for evidence of contact bleeding. Deliberately move the cervix up and down with moderate force to elicit tenderness on motion. Biopsy of suspicious lesions and topical therapy should be deferred until after bimanual examination to avoid bleeding.

5. Withdrawal of the speculum–Slowly remove the speculum from the vagina while inspecting the vaginal walls. Note the color, the presence or absence of rugae, the apparent thickness of the mucosa, and any abnormalities such as redness, ulceration, or tumors. Be especially alert for zones of contact bleeding.

In cases where cystocele, rectocele, or descensus of the cervix are suspected, open the blades of the speculum widely just within the introitus before complete withdrawal of the instrument, and have the patient "bear down" so that the degree of vaginal relaxation can be determined.

Firmly "strip" Skene's ducts and the distal urethra immediately after removal of the speculum. Observe and make smears and cultures of the discharge expressed.

B. Manual Pelvic (Vaginal) Examination: Digital examination is easiest with the patient in the lithotomy position and the examiner standing with one foot on a step or low stool and the elbow on that knee to brace the examining arm and hand. Ideally, use first one hand and then the other in pelvic examination; masses in the right pelvis will be palpated more easily with the right hand, and vice versa.

Insert the gloved, lubricated index finger gently but deliberately into the vagina. Apply slight backward pressure at the fourchette to aid perineal relaxation, to determine the patient's apprehensiveness and resistance, and to note whether the hymen is intact. After a pause to enhance relaxation, slip the middle finger of the examining hand along the forefinger into the vagina.

1. Palpation of the structures of the introitus–Note tenderness, masses, and thickening. With the thumb external and the palm turned downward, feel for enlargement and sensitivity of Bartholin's glands. Investigate the lower vaginal wall for abnormalities. Feel the urethra for relaxation, local dilatation, masses, and tenderness.

To demonstrate cystocele, rectocele, and descensus of the cervix, turn the hand downward, spread the 2 fingers widely, and ask the patient to strain.

2. Palpation of the cervix–Lightly outline the cervix with the fingers to determine its size, position, contour, consistency, and dilatation. Move the cervix about to stretch the uterosacral and transverse cervical ligaments. This will usually reveal the degree of freedom of the cervix and unusual pelvic tenderness.

3. Palpation of the bladder base–Feel beneath the bladder to determine sensitivity and unusual structures. Slight tenderness and a suggestion of thickening over the normal ureter at or near its insertion into the bladder are normal.

C. Bimanual Examination: The foregoing procedures require only one unaided hand. In bimanual examination, the other hand is used on the abdomen to outline the deeper pelvic structures.

Hold the hand palm down on the abdomen with the fingers together, slightly flexed, and pointed toward the patient's head. Press firmly against the abdominal wall to displace the lower abdominal and pelvic organs toward the fingers in the vagina. The patient should take shallow, rapid breaths with her mouth open to avoid tensing the abdominal wall.

1. Palpation of the uterus–Attempt to depress the fundus of the uterus with the hand on the abdomen while the fingers of the hand in the vagina are resting against the cervix and lower portion of the corpus. Relaxation of the vaginal walls and fornices may permit examination of all or much of the posterior aspect of the uterus and even the fundus via the cul-de-sac. A normally free uterus can usually be brought well downward and forward by the abdominal hand. This makes possible vaginal palpation of both the anterior wall and the fundus of the uterus.

Palpate the uterus to determine its position, size, consistency, contour, and mobility and the patient's discomfort on uterine manipulation. Gently explore the posterior fornix for masses, fullness, fluctuation, and sensitivity. Acute tenderness in this region may temporarily prevent further examination.

2. Palpation of the adnexa–Turn the hand in the vagina so that the palm is upward. Insert the 2 examining fingers slightly posteriorly but high into one of the lateral fornices. Sweep the abdominal examining hand downward over the fingers in the vagina to attempt to trap the ovary and tube between the 2 hands.

The ovary normally lies just lateral to the uterus near its mid portion. If the ovary and tube are not felt initially, check the cul-de-sac, the lateral pelvic wall, or the space anterior to the uterus for a displaced, possibly adherent ovary and tube. If the examining hand is swept laterally from the uterine cornu, it may be possible to follow the uterine tube to the ovary. The ovary is normally slightly tender, which helps to distinguish it from nontender masses such as fecal material within the bowel. Rectovaginal examination may permit the best delineation of the ovary (see below). Observe the position, size, consistency, contour, and mobility of each ovary. Note any unusual tenderness.

Ordinarily the uterine tube is not sensitive, but it is so delicate that a normal tube cannot be palpated. Tenderness, swelling, or a cordlike thickening between the ovary and the uterus indicates tubal disease. Inflammation or tumor may convert the tube into an enlarged mass that may be mistaken for an ovarian tumor.

Salpingitis, endometriosis, or cancer may involve one or both adnexa so extensively that these structures and the uterus become a single mass filling the entire true pelvis. The cul-de-sac may be filled or obliterated, and gynecologic landmarks may disappear.

D. Rectovaginal Examination: Rectovaginal examination should be done routinely even though all of the internal genital structures have been palpated properly on vaginal evaluation. Anal, rectovaginal septal, and even sacral abnormalities may be felt only on rectovaginal examination. This examination is invaluable in children, virgins, and old women, in whom the vaginal introitus is so small that only a single finger can be inserted. Rectovaginal examination is preferred to simple rectal examination because the second finger reaches farther when the first finger is in the vagina.

Rectovaginal examination will permit palpation of the following particularly well: (1) rectocele, (2) an ovary not located by vaginal examination, (3) the posterior uterine wall, (4) cul-de-sac masses, (5) rectovaginal septal masses, (6) sacral nerve trunks, and (7) uterosacral and sacrococcygeal ligaments. Rectovaginal examination may be more informative than 2-finger vaginal examination in patients with vaginal stricture, pelvic masses, acute pelvic tenderness, and other disorders that interfere with vaginal manipulation.

The patient and the examiner are positioned as for bimanual vaginal examination. Lubricate the second finger of the examining hand liberally and apply the finger to the anus. With the patient bearing down slightly to relax the anal sphincter, insert the distal half of the finger into the anal canal. When the examining finger has been inserted a short distance, introduce the forefinger into the vagina. The perineal body will then be between the 2 fingers. Encourage the patient to relax by adopting a gentle, slow, deliberate manner. Finally, reach as high as possible in the pelvis with the tips of both the vaginal and rectal fingers, and palpate bimanually, as with the vaginal examination.

To demonstrate rectocele, bring the rectal finger back to the perineal body, removing the vaginal finger. As this is done, the rectal pouch will be entered, and its protrusion into the vagina may be evident at the introitus. The patient herself may be able to see a rectocele thus demonstrated if she holds a mirror at an appropriate angle.

Laboratory Studies

A. Smears:

1. Bacteria–Obtain specimens for smears for bacteria with surgically clean cotton-tipped applicators. Fluid exudate may be obtained from the urethral meatus, Skene's and Bartholin's ducts, the vaginal walls, the posterior vaginal fornix, and the cervical os. Make a thin spread of the discharge on a clean glass slide and permit it to dry in air. Methylene blue stain (1% aqueous solution) may suffice for a quick rough appraisal of the type and approximate number of bacteria present. For specific etiologic diagnosis (eg, pneumococci and gonococci), use Gram's stain.

2. *Trichomonas vaginalis* –Examine separate preparations from the posterior fornix, the cervical os, and the urethral meatus. Moisten a clean cotton-tipped applicator with normal saline, and swab the site of exudation or dip into the discharge with the applicator. Touch a drop of the exudate to a polished slide and apply a fresh coverslip. Examine microscopically immediately (while still warm) for trichomonads. Hollow-ground glass slides are an unnecessary refinement. If a delay of 5–10 minutes is inevitable, the moistened cotton-tipped applicator carrying a small amount of the fluid to be examined may be transferred to 1–2 mL of warmed Ringer's injection and this fluid examined for trichomonads.

3. *Candida albicans* –The technique is the same as for the demonstration of trichomonads, but use 1–2 drops of potassium hydroxide (10% aqueous solution) on the slide or in the tube to dissolve the epithelial, inflammatory, and red blood cells. The mycelia will be displayed prominently as hyphae and spores. It is unnecessary to warm the slide or solution. The material most likely to show mycelia is the white plaque of "vaginal thrush," which must be rubbed from the mucosa with the cotton applicator.

B. Cultures:

1. Bacteria–Obtain sufficient exudate to saturate a sterile cotton-tipped applicator. Using bacteriologic technique, place the applicator in a sterile, dry test tube and send it immediately to the bacteriology laboratory for culture and identification. Avoid heating and drying the sample. When gonorrhea is suspected, inoculate a sterile chocolate or blood agar plate or Transgrow medium at the time of pelvic examination. Place the applicator in a sterile test tube with the customary flame sterilization, and send all preparations to the bacteriology laboratory for processing without delay.

2. _T vaginalis_–Trichomonads may be cultured aerobically. Trichosel or Difco's hash medium (B-1016T, a modified trypticase medium that does not require addition of serum under sterile conditions) is preferred. However, culturing is rarely necessary in gynecology. If these organisms are not identified in the wet smear, careful inspection of the stained exfoliative vaginal cytologic smear (Papanicolaou) will generally reveal their presence.

3. _C albicans_–In contrast to trichomonads, candidal hyphae and spores are frequently missed in the potassium hydroxide wet smear, especially when the patient does not have curdlike plaques. Therefore, in doubtful cases it is necessary to culture vaginal fluid on Sabouraud's or Nickerson's medium.

C. Urine: Collect a catheterized urine specimen in a sterile test tube, using sterile equipment and technique after thoroughly cleansing the urethral meatus with a mild antiseptic solution.

Other Procedures

A. Sounding the Uterus: Rule out intrauterine pregnancy before sounding the uterus with a sterile, malleable, calibrated Sims or Simpson uterine sound to determine the patency of the cervical canal, the presence of cervical or uterine lesions that will bleed on contact, the size of the uterus, the position of the uterine fundus, and the direction of the uterine canal (before endometrial biopsy).

Carefully wipe the external cervical os with a cotton pledget or gauze sponge saturated with an antiseptic solution. Bend the sound to the estimated curvature of the cervico-uterine axis. The speculum may be surgically clean rather than sterile if one is careful not to touch the speculum blades with the distal 3–4 inches of the sound during its introduction. In the absence of cervical stenosis and extreme flexion of the corpus, gentle sounding of a uterus in an approximately normal position causes only very mild, menstruallike cramps.

It may occasionally be necessary to draw the cervix toward the introitus to make the os accessible or to straighten the canal. For traction, apply a double-toothed Braun or other suitable tenaculum to the anterior cervical lip in either the frontal or sagittal plane. Warn the patient that she may feel sudden, slight discomfort.

Measure and record the length of the cervical canal and the depth of the uterine cavity. Note points of obstruction, distortion, and bleeding. Be careful to avoid perforation of the uterus.

If sounding of the uterus is impossible with the usual instruments, try a fine, soft wire probe. Hegar dilators (No. 5–10) may be used to

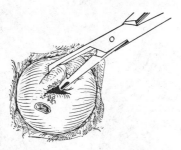

Figure 19–5. Multiple punch biopsy of cervix with Tischler forceps.

dilate a stenotic cervix and for the diagnosis of an abnormally large (incompetent) internal cervical os.

B. Biopsy:

1. General considerations–Infiltrate the site of biopsy with procaine, 0.5–1% aqueous solution, or its equivalent. If the suspicious lesion is 1 cm or less in diameter, it should be totally excised; if it is larger, only a portion should be taken. Include normal-appearing bordering tissue for comparison. One or more fine, nonabsorbable sutures may be required for hemostasis and closure of the defect.

Excisional biopsy of ulcers, tumors, and other lesions over 1 cm in diameter should be done in an operating room where adequate equipment and assistance for anesthesia and hemostasis are available. Wide margins of normal tissue should be taken.

2. Cervix–

a. Punch biopsy–Even multiple biopsy of the cervix may be performed in the office with little or no pain or danger, using the Tischler, Schubert, or similar punch biopsy forceps (Fig 19–5). The Tischler forceps is favored by many because of its simplicity and because its construction allows small or generous "bites" with collecting of the tissue in a small recess at the tip. It is important to use an instrument that will not crush the tissue. Anesthetics are not required, because the cervix is relatively insensitive to pain. The Hyams and other similar electrosurgical instruments should not be used, because they cause physical changes in the specimen that alter the staining characteristics of the tissue.

Steady the cervix with a tenaculum; biopsy the posterior lip first to avoid obscuring other biopsy sites by bleeding. Include samples from the mucosquamous junction. Immediately place tissue fragments in 10% formalin fixative.

Although bleeding from biopsy sites is unpredictable, it is generally minimal and can usually be controlled with light pressure for a few

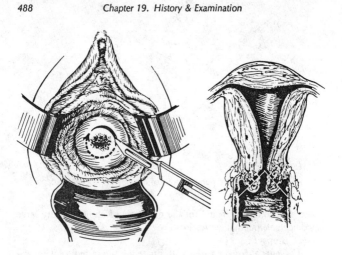

Figure 19–6. Conization of the cervix.

minutes. Control minor ooze with cotton wool or gauze applied with firm pressure. Always ligate individual bleeding points with very fine catgut if possible. Interrupted or figure-of-eight hemostasis sutures may be used also. If these measures do not suffice, touch the bleeding areas with negatol (Negatan), acetone, or 5% silver nitrate solution. Use electrocautery only as a last resort. Cytologic study of repeat biopsy material or examination of the cervix after surgery for residual cancer may be complicated by tissue necrosis and inflammation when traumatic or styptic procedures are used to control bleeding.

b. Scalpel biopsy or cold conization–

Scalpel or "cold conization" of the cervix (Fig 19–6), particularly for investigation of early carcinoma, involves removing a portion of the cervix from the mucosquamous junction to the internal os. For cancer study, the tissue rarely must exceed 0.3 cm in thickness. A suture of nonabsorbable material is usually inserted at the top of the cone to aid the pathologist in orienting the tissue for histologic study.

If the cervix is deeply lacerated, segmental excision of tissue may be required to make up a cone. Each of the fragments must be identified. A diagram should be made, and each fragment should be individually numbered and placed in a separate bottle of fixative to simplify subsequent pathologic study.

Cold knife cone biopsy (and fractional curettage) must be done in surgery. Paracervical or general anesthesia may be required. Suspicious areas that should be biopsied are more readily identified after preliminary application of Schiller's reagent or Lugol's solution. Bleeding is reduced if dilute phenylephrine or other vasoconstrictor drug (eg, epinephrine) in normal saline solution is injected. Except during pregnancy, a uterine sound should be inserted to or just beyond the internal os so that, by directing the tip of the scalpel toward the probe at the internal os, the cervix can be coned without excessive bleeding. Scalpel cervical biopsy requires primary suture closure for control of bleeding. Hemorrhage may necessitate vaginal packing or deeply placed sutures (or both).

3. Endometrium–Sound the uterus (see p 486) to determine bleeding, contour, points of distortion, and other abnormalities. If thorough surgical (therapeutic) curettage is required, it should be done in the operating room and not in the examining room.

Contraindications to endometrial biopsy in the office include possible uterine pregnancy; marked cervicitis; friable, bleeding cervical abnormalities; marked cervical stenosis; and profuse bleeding at the initiation of endometrial curettage.

For endometrial biopsy in the examining room, a Randall, Novak, or Weissman tubular barbed curet is used to obtain strips of endometrium, which become threaded into the instrument. Pass the biopsy curet to the fundus. Stroke it downward against the uterine wall to the cervix in various parts of the uterus to obtain representative bits of endometrium. Finally, secure fragments of the endocervical lining also.

Slight suction from a syringe may be used, but forceful pump or other suction will macerate tissue samples. The tissue obtained by suction can be gently blown into 10% formalin solution by light positive pressure.

C. Colposcopy: The colposcope is a binocular microscope used for direct visualization of the cervix. The most popular magnification in clinical use is $13.5 \times$. This effectively bridges the gap between what can be seen by the naked eye and by the microscope. Some colposcopes are equipped with a camera for the single or serial photographic recording of pathologic conditions.

Colposcopy does not replace other methods of diagnosing abnormalities of the cervix but is instead an additional and important tool. It does not lend itself well to mass screening but is valuable in the next diagnostic step after mass screening. The 2 most important groups of patients who can benefit by its use are (1) patients with abnormal results on Papanicolaou smear and (2) "diethylstilbestrol babies," who may have dysplasia of the vagina or cervix. Colposcopy should be used in follow-up of patients whose mothers received diethylstilbestrol during pregnancy and in pre- and posttreatment assessment of cervical intraepithelial neoplasia (CIN) (see p 562). It may also be used for cancer therapy follow-up, ie, to distinguish radiation changes from recurrent carcinoma and to differentiate acute cervicitis from cancer. However, occult neoplasms in the upper cervical canal, where 10–15% of cervical cancers develop, cannot be detected by colposcopy.

Normally, columnar epithelium covers the ectocervix until adolescence, when it gradually changes to a squamous surface. The transformation zone can be inspected easily with the colposcope and dysplastic surface changes identified, including the following: (1) "white epithelium," eg, sheets of layered metaplastic cells; (2) mosaic structure, eg, sharply outlined cells and cell groups; (3) punctation, eg, vascular tufts between cell clusters; and (4) leukoplakia, eg, abnormal pale cell plaques.

The colposcopist is able to see areas of cellular dysplasia and vascular or tissue abnormalities not visible otherwise, which makes it possible to select areas most propitious for biopsy. Stains and other chemical agents are also used to improve visualization. The colposcope-directed biopsy decreases the number of false-negative results on biopsy and frequently eliminates the need for conization of the cervix, which may have a high morbidity rate.

Colposcopy procedure is as follows:

1. Obtain repeat cytosmears.

2. Cleanse the cervix with 3% acetic acid to remove excess mucus and to blanch the surface. This accentuates abnormal epithelium.

3. Focus the colposcope on the cervix, beginning with low power (usually 13.5 ×). Carefully inspect the squamocolumnar junction (transformation zone). A significantly abnormal area can usually be outlined in its entirety.

4. Take biopsy specimens with a Kevorkian or similar biopsy instrument, and record the sites most suggestive of cancer.

5. Admit for cervical conization and D&C only those patients who have class III–IV Papanicolaou smears and abnormal surface changes extending up the cervical canal beyond the field of vision.

6. Treat benign or malignant disorders appropriately.

To use the colposcope effectively, the physician needs thorough training and the opportunity for extensive experience; this, combined with the high cost of the instrument, leads to the logical decision by many gynecologists not to train themselves in its use but to refer patients needing the service to an expert colposcopist in the community.

D. Culdoscopy: Culdoscopy is visualization of the pelvic structures through the vaginal vault and cul-de-sac, using an optical instrument similar to the cystoscope or laparoscope. It is a hospital procedure and should be attempted only by a physician with adequate experience. Perforation of a viscus, intraperitoneal bleeding, and peritonitis are possible complications. Puncture is incomplete or visualization unsatisfactory in 5–10% of attempts, and diagnostic errors occur in 1–5% of cases. Culdoscopy has been virtually supplanted by laparoscopy (see below), which is more practical and versatile.

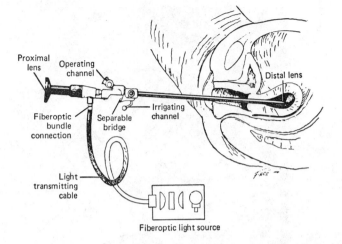

Figure 19–7. Diagrammatic representation of hysteroscope in use. (Reproduced, with permission, from Valle RF, Sciarra JJ: *Minn Med* 1974;57:892.)

E. Hysteroscopy: Hysteroscopy is visual examination of the uterine cavity with a small-bore fiberoptic endoscope (Fig 19–7). Paracervical or light general anesthesia may be required. Intrauterine instillation of 35% dextran, 5% dextrose, or carbon dioxide causes slight distention of the uterus; dextran is preferred because it will not mix with blood and is easily handled.

Hysteroscopy is simple and can be used for the following purposes: (1) removal of a foreign body, eg, "lost" intrauterine device; (2) diagnosis of abnormal uterine bleeding, eg, tumor; (3) biopsy, eg, suspected endometrial carcinoma; (4) lysis of intrauterine synechiae, ie, Asherman's syndrome; and (5) investigation of infertility, eg, canalization of the uterine tubes.

Voluntary sterilization by means of hysteroscopy is not yet acceptably dependable or without complications, but the simplicity of the procedure invites further investigation.

Contraindications to hysteroscopy include pregnancy, acute cervicitis or salpingitis, and hemorrhage.

F. Laparoscopy: Laparoscopy (Fig 19–8) is a transperitoneal endoscopic technique for visualization of the abdominal and pelvic contents. It is an intra-abdominal operation performed through a small subumbilical incision, and it provides excellent visualization of the

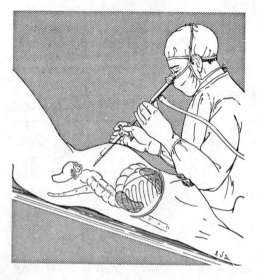

Figure 19–8. Pelvic laparoscopy with patient in Trendelenburg position. (Reproduced, with permission, from Long AE: Chapter 5 in *Current Obstetric & Gynecologic Diagnosis & Treatment,* 4th ed. Benson RC [editor]. Lange, 1982.)

pelvic structures and often permits diagnosis of gynecologic disorders and limited surgery without laparotomy. Fiberoptic illumination, carbon dioxide pneumoperitoneum, and local or light general anesthesia are employed. In addition to the equipment used for observation, a variety of other instruments for biopsy, coagulation, aspiration, and manipulation can be passed through a separate cannula (second puncture technique) or inserted through the same cannula as the laparoscope.

Indications are as follows:

1. Diagnosis–Examples are uterine anomaly; endometriosis; biopsy of ovarian tumors, omentum, spleen, or liver; and differentiation between ectopic pregnancy and salpingitis or between psychogenic and organic pelvic pain.

2. Evaluation–Examples include investigation of infertility, eg, tubal patency test, and assessment of response to treatment in women with ovarian cancer.

3. Therapy–

a. Tubal sterilization by fulguration or application of Silastic rings or metal clips.

b. Lysis of adhesions.

c. Elimination of disorder, eg, fulguration of endometriosis.

d. Removal of foreign body, eg, extruded intrauterine device.

Absolute contraindications to laparoscopy are intestinal obstruction and general peritonitis. Severe cardiac or pulmonary disease is a relative contraindication.

Complications depend upon the problem, the status of the patient, and the expertise of the laparoscopist. Minor problems, eg, abdominal or shoulder pain, are common and rarely serious; other problems such as perforation of a viscus, a thermal burn of the bowel, severe bleeding, or cardiac arrest are rare but often critical. The incidence of major complications (mostly with bipolar instruments) in the USA is less than 5%. The overall mortality rate in sterilization done by laparoscopy is less than 2 per 100,000.

The laparoscope is expensive and easily damaged, and considerable experience is required to achieve facility with the instrument. Nonetheless, in capable hands, laparoscopy is an excellent, direct, well-tolerated surgical method that can often supplant laparotomy or culdotomy for diagnosis or treatment of many intra-abdominal problems. Often, a look is worth 100 sutures.

G. Ultrasonography: See pp 59 and 125.

•   •   •

RAPE

Rape constitutes sexual assault and battery. About 95% of reported rape victims are women. Although forcible coitus is the most common form of rape, fellatio or sodomy also constitutes the offense. In any case, it is no longer necessary to prove that penetration occurred for the assault to be considered a crime.

Statutory rape is defined as intercourse with a female below the legal age of consent (often 18 years) *with* her consent.

Rape represents an expression of anger, power, and sexuality on the part of the rapist. The rapist is usually a hostile, compulsive man who uses sexual intercourse to terrorize and humiliate a woman. He may derive little or no sexual gratification from the act. Rape rarely represents the outcome of a frustrated seduction attempt. The sexual act is a weapon used to degrade and hurt the victim and is the ultimate insult. Women neither secretly want to be raped, nor do they expect, encourage, or enjoy rape.

Rape may be the most underreported major crime; only about one case in 10 is reported to the police. Rape involves severe physical injury in 5–10% of cases and is always a terrifying experience in which most victims fear for their lives. Consequently, all victims suffer some psychologic aftermath. Moreover, some may acquire sexually transmissible disease or may become pregnant.

Because rape is a personal crisis, each patient will react differently. The rape-trauma syndrome comprises 2 principal phases:

(1) Immediate or acute–Shaking, sobbing, and restless activity may last from a few days to a few weeks. The patient may experience anger, guilt, shame, self-blame, and fear of revenge or may repress these emotions. Reactions vary depending on the victim's personality and the circumstances of the attack.

(2) Late or chronic–Problems related to the attack may develop weeks or months later. The life-style and work patterns of the individual may change. Sleep disorders or phobias often develop. Panic may ensue in a situation that is reminiscent of the circumstances surrounding the original attack. Loss of self-worth or esteem rarely leads to suicide, but the patient may resort to the use of alcohol or other drugs.

The rape victim should receive medical assessment and treatment. Short-term crisis intervention and, when indicated, long-term support and counseling should also be provided. Persons close to the patient may also need professional guidance so that they can help the patient.

General Office Procedures

Physicians who are not prepared to care for a patient who has presumably been raped should promptly refer her to a rape control center or to the emergency room of the nearest hospital.

The physician who first sees the alleged rape victim should take the following actions:

(1) Secure written consent from the patient, guardian, or next of kin for gynecologic examination; arrange for photographs (usually by the police photographer) if they are likely to reveal evidence; and release pertinent information and specimens to the authorities.

(2) Notify the police and obtain their permission to examine the patient, or await the arrival of the police physician.

(3) Obtain and record the history in the patient's own words. The sequence of events, ie, the time, place, and circumstances, must be included. Note whether the alleged victim is calm, agitated, or confused (drugs or alcohol may be involved). Record whether the patient came directly to the health care facility or whether she bathed or changed her clothing.

(4) Obtain appropriate tests (see below).

(5) Mark clothing for evidence.

(6) Record findings but do not issue even a tentative diagnosis lest it be erroneous or incomplete.

(7) Treat disease and psychic trauma; prevent pregnancy; counsel the patient, including information about legal rights, eg, filing charges

against the assailant; and explain subsequent therapy and follow-up as well as the prognosis.

Physical Examination

Be empathetic. Begin with a statement such as, "This is a terrible thing that has happened to you. I want to help."

With witnesses present, record the general appearance, demeanor, coherence, and cooperation of the patient. Note torn, stained, or bloody clothing. Identify any lacerations or contusions (these may be more apparent the next day).

Seek, label, and retain foreign matter, eg, sand, leaves, carpet threads, or hair from another person found on the victim. Scrape any material from beneath the fingernails for evidence. Comb the patient's pubic hair with a clean comb and place a few hairs in a designated envelope for possible comparison with those of the assailant.

Search for any signs of vulvar or vaginal trauma, discharge, or bleeding. Illuminate the pudendum with an ultraviolet light (prostatic secretions fluoresce even when dry).

"Rape kits" containing labels, bottles, etc, are now available for physicians. A warm, water-moistened (nonlubricated) speculum or vaginoscope should be used to inspect the vagina and cervix. (If the suspected victim is a child, light general anesthesia may be required.) Prepare cervical and anal cultures for *Neisseria gonorrhoeae* in Transgrow or Thayer-Martin medium. Inject 5 mL of normal saline solution into the vagina, aspirate the fluid from the posterior vaginal fornix, and place the specimens in individual corked test tubes or screw-top vials for police laboratory or authorized hospital laboratory tests for the following: (1) Acid phosphatase. If the reaction is strongly positive, it almost certainly indicates the presence of prostatic fluid ejaculate. (2) Blood group antigen of spermatozoa (to distinguish rape by a second individual following a recent but earlier primary, unforced act of intercourse with a partner whose blood type differs from that of the offender). In cases in which the presence of sperm may not be decisive, this test often is critical. (3) Precipitin tests for human spermatozoa and blood. (4) Spermatozoa. Motile sperm may be seen in a wet-mount preparation. Alcohol-ether-fixed or spray-dried smears may disclose spermatozoa. (Men who have had a vasectomy have sperm-free ejaculate, however.)

Transfer clearly labeled evidence, eg, laboratory specimens, directly to the clinical pathologist in charge or to the responsible laboratory technician, in the presence of witnesses (never via messenger), so that the rules of evidence will not be breached.

Submit marked clothing, photographs, slides, etc, to the police as evidence and obtain a written receipt.

Whether rape has occurred is a legal question, not a medical one.

Hence, the physician must not be bound to a diagnosis verbally or in writing, even at the conclusion of the examination and the report of laboratory tests. Terms such as "alleged victim of rape" or "suspected rape victim" must always be used. The records, which may be subpoenaed, must contain any negative as well as positive evidence to determine the guilt or innocence of the accused.

Treatment

A. General Measures:

1. The physician should assume a sympathetic, concerned attitude—never a skeptical or cynical one.

2. Avoid comments and discussion with others in the presence of the patient.

B. Medical Therapy (With the Patient's Permission):

1. Give analgesics or tranquilizers if indicated.

2. Administer tetanus antitoxin if deep lacerations contain soil or dirt particles.

3. Give prophylactic probenecid, 1 g orally, and 30 minutes later aqueous penicillin G, 4.8 million units intramuscularly, to prevent syphilis and gonorrhea. If the victim is allergic to penicillin, give tetracycline, 30–40 g orally, over a period of 10 days.

4. Prevent pregnancy by using one of the following methods:

a. Administer medroxyprogesterone (Depo-Provera), 100 mg intramuscularly.

b. Give ethinyl estradiol, 0.1 mg, and dl-norgestrel, 1 mg (Ovral or equivalent), 2 tablets orally; repeat in 24 hours. (The effectiveness of this method is still not established.)

c. Insert an IUD (preferably one with a copper addition).

C. Surgical Measures:

1. Suture lacerations and evacuate hematomas.

2. Use menstrual regulation to reduce the likelihood of implantation if pregnancy occurs, or–

3. Perform a D&C for prevention of pregnancy or if pregnancy develops despite hormone or other therapy (see above).

D. Follow-Up: Repeat cultures for gonorrhea 1 week later; perform a nontreponemal serologic test for syphilis 6 weeks later. Perform pregnancy tests if pregnancy is a possibility. Refer the patient for psychiatric assessment and counseling if severe emotional problems persist.

Complications

Strong negative feelings by the woman, eg, humiliation, confusion, and fear of retaliation, may give way to quiet anger, hatred of men, feelings of isolation or worthlessness, distrust, and fear of being raped again. This may lead to deficiencies in expressing affection or relating socially or sexually. A psychotic sequela is rare but may occur, especially in patients with a history of psychosis.

Prognosis

A. For the Patient: The prognosis is excellent if good family support and counseling by trained social workers or rape crisis center (or committee) personnel are provided.

B. For the Rapist: Despite conviction and incarceration or psychotherapy, the rapist often rapes again.

Prevention of Rape

A. At Home: Lock doors and windows, remain in the presence of others, and avoid being "trapped" in an elevator or dark corridor.

B. Away From Home: Take a taxi; avoid hitchhiking; travel on busy, well-lighted streets; walk with someone; run if followed; and lock the car.

C. Resistance: Opinion is divided on whether the rape victim should offer resistance. Many believe that the victim should scream, scratch, kick, bite, etc, when endangered. Some suggest using legal self-defense methods, eg, pushing a lighted cigarette, heavy keys, or a safety pin into the assailant's face or employing karate or judo if the victim is skilled in these methods of self-defense. Other authorities recommend passive compliance to prevent serious injury or death.

D. Weapons: Carrying weapons is not the solution to the problem of rape. A woman who uses a gun, knife, or chemical device to protect herself against rape may face a criminal concealed weapons charge. Moreover, weapons are often ineffective or harmful to innocent persons except in the hands of trained experts. Brandishing a weapon may also have the effect of enraging the attacker, resulting in greater harm to the victim than would have occurred otherwise.

20 | Diseases of the Breast

CARCINOMA OF THE BREAST

Carcinoma of the breast is the most common lethal cancer of women. There were 108,000 new cases of breast cancer and about 35,000 deaths from this disease in the USA in 1980. The peak incidence is at age 40–50, but malignant breast tumors may be diagnosed as early as age 25. At the present rate of incidence, one of every 11 American women will develop breast cancer at some time during her life. The cause is not known.

Perhaps paradoxically, the mortality rate from breast cancer has not changed significantly during the past 20 years, despite a significant increase in the use of estrogens in oral contraceptives and in the management of menopause. During the same period, the overall arrest rate of breast cancer has not improved greatly despite the availability of presumably better diagnostic techniques and methods of treatment.

A familial predisposition to breast cancer is recognized, and cancer tends to occur at an early age in such families. Nulliparas are slightly more prone to breast cancer than multiparas.

The role of nursing in the etiology of breast cancer is unsettled. Chronic mammary dysplasia may predispose to malignancy, but benign tumors, trauma, and inflammation do not.

Risk factors for breast cancer, based largely upon the patient's past and family history, are listed in Table 20–1.

The natural history of untreated breast cancer is variable. Although death claims most of these patients in 3–4 years, survival for over 10 years is not unusual. Such variation is related to the type and grade of the lesion. Treatment is based upon the stage (extent) of the tumor as well as its microscopic appearance. Most breast cancers are very aggressive, and early widespread metastasis is common.

Breast cancer is multicentric in development; more than one malignant focus can be identified in the breast in 40% of patients and in the other breast in about 2% of patients.

Breast cancer occurs in the upper outer quadrant in about 45% of cases; in the central zone in about 25%; in the upper inner quadrant in about 15%; in the lower outer quadrant in 10%; and in the lower inner quadrant in 5%.

Table 20–1. Risk factors in breast cancer.

Major risk factors
    Previous mastectomy for breast cancer
    History of breast cancer in immediate family (mother or sister)
    Lump in breast
    Nipple discharge
    Severe mammary dysplasia, identified by mammography or biopsy
Minor risk factors
    Age over 50
    History of breast cancer in remote family (aunt, grandmother, etc)
    Menarche before age 12
    First child born after age 30
    History of cancer elsewhere, especially uterus, ovary
    Nulliparity
    Recent onset of pain in one breast

The spread of breast cancer is principally by metastasis to the regional lymph nodes: 50–60% of patients who submit to radical mastectomy have positive axillary nodes, and the internal mammary nodes are positive in about 30% of patients who are considered to be operable— especially those with cancer in the central or inner half of the breast or with axillary node metastases.

Hematogenous spread of mammary carcinoma is common also: Dissemination to bone (eg, pelvis, spine, femur, ribs, etc), liver, or lungs is frequent.

Breast cancer is manifested clinically as a firm or hard, nontender, fixed mass or lump with ill-defined margins (because of local invasion). There may be a slight accumulation of fatty tissue above the small, nodular cancer. Occasionally, there will be slight asymmetry of the breasts. Redness, edema, nodularity, or ulcerations may accompany more advanced disease. Enlargement or reduction of breast size and axillary adenopathy may be noted.

Clinical Findings

A. Symptoms and Signs: About 90% of breast abnormalities are discovered by the patient; about 5% are discovered during the course of physical examination performed for other reasons. A painless lump is the initial finding in the great majority of cases of breast cancer. Nipple discharge or ulceration, itching, retraction, or pain is occasionally reported. Enlargement, shrinkage, or firmness of the breast is less common. In rare cases, the first symptom is an axillary mass, swelling of the arm, or bone or back pain from metastases.

Examination of the breast should be methodical, meticulous, and delicate. Breast examination is described on p 477.

It is a curious fact that some patients can identify a lesion 0.5–1 cm in diameter—often too small for an examiner to distinguish. If the examiner cannot confirm the patient's suspicion, the examination should be repeated in 1 month—ideally, in premenopausal women, 1 week after the cessation of a period. Brief tenderness and transient thickening in the breast during the premenstrual phase may suggest a mass lesion. In such cases, reevaluation 1–2 weeks later may be more revealing.

B. Laboratory Findings: A persistently elevated sedimentation rate or elevated serum alkaline phosphatase level may indicate extensive metastases. Hypercalcemia occurs in occasional advanced cases. Otherwise, laboratory studies are not helpful.

C. X-Ray and Ultrasonographic Findings:

1. Mammography–The greatest advance in the diagnosis of breast cancer in the past decade has been the demonstration of occult breast cancer less than 0.5 cm in diameter by mammography or xeromammography. Experienced physicians can detect only about 70% of breast cancers on physical examination; the diagnostic yield of mammography plus physical examination includes approximately 15% of cases that would otherwise be missed. There is a 10–15% rate of false-negative interpretation, and abnormally dense areas may be over-read. Nonetheless, mammography has greatly increased the frequency of breast biopsy and the diagnosis of small, even occult, cancers.

Mammography is indicated (1) to evaluate the opposite breast when a diagnosis of potentially curable breast cancer has been made and at intervals of 1–3 years thereafter; (2) to assess a questionable or ill-defined breast mass or other cancer-suspicious change in the breast (but only if mammographic findings will assist in determining whether or where a biopsy is to be performed); (3) to search for an occult breast cancer in a woman with metastatic disease in the axillary nodes or elsewhere from an unknown primary; (4) to screen at regular intervals a selected group of women who are at high risk for developing breast cancer; (5) to appraise women with large breasts that are difficult to examine; and (6) to reassure women with cancerophobia.

2. Other x-ray findings–Since metastases occur all too often except in very early breast cancer, anterior, posterior, and lateral views of the lumbar spine and pelvis and lateral skull films should be a part of every breast cancer work-up. Prior to definitive surgery, anteroposterior and lateral chest films should be obtained together with bone scans usually utilizing technetium Tc 99m-labeled phosphate or phosphonates. Ultrasonography, CT scan, or radionuclide scanning of the liver or brain is also of value when metastases may have occurred.

3. Ultrasonography–Ultrasonography is more useful in excluding noncancerous masses, eg, cysts, than in identifying probable cancer.

D. Biopsy: Useful methods of biopsy are needle biopsy (aspiration or coring tissue) and directed open biopsy. Breast biopsy is indicated in cases of persistent breast mass, bloody nipple discharge, eczematoid nipple changes, and suspicious or positive results of mammography. About 30% of cases considered strongly suggestive of cancer will be found to be benign on biopsy. In contrast, about 15% of abnormal foci thought to be benign will be diagnosed as malignant on biopsy.

Special Clinical Forms of Breast Cancer

A. Paget's Carcinoma: Clinically, the lesion begins as a pruritic or burning eczematoid ulceration of the nipple that develops as a phase of infiltrating intraductal carcinoma. The nipple may not be grossly involved, and nipple discharge is present only occasionally. Although about 3% of all breast cancers are of the Paget type, this malignancy, derived from the ducts or acini of apocrine glands, may be mistakenly treated as an infection or other dermatologic lesion. Nonetheless, this cancer metastasizes to regional lymph nodes in about 60% of patients who finally come to surgery. Paget's carcinoma must be diagnosed early, and therapy must be as aggressively pursued as with any other breast cancer.

B. Inflammatory Carcinoma: This is the most virulent type of breast cancer. Lactating women may develop this tumor, which begins as a painful, red, rapidly spreading area of induration that soon causes marked enlargement of the entire breast. The skin over the diseased area is erythematous, edematous, tender, and warm (due to rapid local spread of cancer cells), but other signs and symptoms of inflammation do not develop, and dark nipple discharge occurs only rarely. Biopsy is essential, but there will be no discrete localization, and the other breast will be uninvolved. A variety of cellular types may be responsible for inflammatory carcinoma, which obviously involves a deficiency in the patient's immune defenses against cancer. Early dissemination occurs invariably. Radical mastectomy is futile. The patient should not continue to breast feed. Regional irradiation may be palliative, but few patients can be cured by any treatment program.

C. Sarcoma: Sarcoma of the breast is rare, and lack of sharp criteria makes the diagnosis difficult. Because slides are often "overread," the incidence of fibrosarcoma, for example, may be lower than reported. Early diagnosis and wide surgical excision should arrest sarcomas (eg, fibrosarcoma, liposarcoma, rhabdomyosarcoma), although lymphatic or hematogenous spread may occur. Irradiation is important only as palliative therapy.

D. Breast Cancer Occurring During Pregnancy and the Puerperium: Palpation of a cancer-suspicious mass in the breast is more difficult during engorgement associated with pregnancy or lactation. Therefore, most cases of breast cancer are advanced when diagnosed during pregnancy or during the puerperium, and inflammatory carcinoma is most virulent at these times. In fact, at least 60% of obstetric patients with breast cancer already have at least axillary metastases.

Under these circumstances, the 5-year survival rate of such women treated by radical mastectomy is only 5–20%—less than half the overall 5-year survival rate for nonpregnant women of comparable age.

Mammography and biopsy should be accomplished without delay during pregnancy or the puerperium if a breast mass is palpable. If the cancer is small and localized, the prognosis with proper treatment is good; if axillary (or other) nodes contain tumor, the outlook is poor.

Hormone Receptor Sites

The presence or absence of estrogen receptors in the cytoplasm of tumor cells appears to be a primary diagnostic factor and is of paramount importance in managing patients with recurrent metastatic disease. Patients whose primary tumor is estrogen receptor-positive have a more favorable course after mastectomy than those whose tumors are receptor-negative. About 60% of patients with metastatic breast cancer will respond to hormonal manipulation if their tumors contain estrogen receptors, but less than 10% of patients with metastatic, estrogen receptor-negative tumors can be successfully treated with hormonal manipulation. If progesterone receptor sites are also present in the tumor, a favorable response to hormonal treatment is likely in over half of patients. Other substances—eg, tamoxifen citrate, an antiestrogen medication—may also compete for hormone-binding sites.

It is advisable to obtain receptor assays on every breast cancer patient at the time of initial diagnosis. Specimens will require special handling, and the laboratory should be alerted.

Prevention

Because the causes of breast cancer are unclear and probably multiple, prevention is not yet possible. Death can be postponed and serious complications partially or completely avoided by early diagnosis and prompt therapy.

All women over age 20 should be taught how to examine their breasts. Examination should be done monthly in premenopausal women, just after the period. The breasts should be inspected initially while standing before a mirror with the hands at the sides, overhead, and pressed firmly on the hips to contract the pectoralis muscles. Masses, asymmetry of the breasts, and slight dimpling of the skin may become apparent as a result of these movements. Next, the woman should lie supine and carefully palpate each breast with the fingers of the opposite hand. Any mass or other abnormality should be reported to the physician at once.

Differential Diagnosis

The lesions most often to be considered in the differential diagnosis of breast cancer are the following, in order of frequency: mammary dysplasia (cystic disease of the breast), fibroadenoma, intraductal papilloma, duct ectasia, and fat necrosis. The differential diagnosis of a breast lump should be established without delay by biopsy, by aspiration of a cyst, or by observing the patient until disappearance of the lump within a period of a few weeks.

Treatment

Before specific methods of treatment can be determined, 5 basic questions must be answered: (1) Is the patient pre- or postmenopausal? (2) What is the clinical stage (International or American Joint Committee staging)? (3) What type of cancer does the patient have? (4) What is the patient's age and general medical condition? and (5) What problems of acceptance of treatment are presented, if any?

Treatment may be curative or palliative. Curative treatment is advised for clinical stage I and stage II disease; extirpative surgery

Table 20–2. Clinical and histologic staging of breast carcinoma and relation to survival.*

Clinical Staging (American Joint Committee)	Crude 5-Year Survival (%)
Stage I	85
Tumor < 2 cm in diameter	
Nodes, if present, not felt to contain metastases	
Without distant metastases	
Stage II	66
Tumor < 5 cm in diameter	
Nodes, if palpable, not fixed	
Without distant metastases	
Stage III	41
Tumor > 5 cm or—	
Tumor any size with invasion of skin or attached to chest wall	
Nodes in supraclavicular area	
Without distant metastases	
Stage IV	10
With distant metastases	

	Crude Survival (%)	
Histologic Staging	5 Years	10 Years
All patients	63	46
Negative axillary lymph nodes	78	65
Positive axillary lymph nodes	46	25
1–3 positive axillary lymph nodes	62	38
> 4 positive axillary lymph nodes	32	13

*Reproduced, with permission, from Giuliano AE: Chapter 11 in *Current Medical Diagnosis & Treatment 1983.* Krupp MA, Chatton MJ (editors). Lange, 1983.

Table 20–3. Classification of mammary carcinoma according to the cellular growth pattern.*

Type I: Rarely metastasizing (not invasive)
  1. Intraductal or comedocarcinoma without stromal invasion. Paget's disease of the breast may exist if the epithelium of the nipple is involved.
  2. Papillary carcinoma confined to the ducts.
  3. Lobular carcinoma in situ.
Type II: Rarely metastasizing (always invasive)
  1. Well-differentiated adenocarcinoma.
  2. Medullary carcinoma with lymphocytic infiltration.
  3. Pure colloid or mucinous carcinoma.
  4. Papillary carcinoma.
Type III: Moderately metastasizing (always invasive)
  1. Infiltrating adenocarcinoma.
  2. Intraductal carcinoma with stromal invasion.
  3. Infiltrating lobular carcinoma.†
  4. All tumors not classified as types I, II, or IV.
Type IV: High metastasizing (always invasive)
  1. Undifferentiated carcinoma having cells without ductal or tubular arrangement.
  2. All types of tumors indisputably invading blood vessels.

---

*Reproduced, with permission, from Kouchoukos NT et al: *Cancer* 1967;**20**:948.
†Infiltrating lobular carcinoma has been moved from type II to type III because of growing experience with its metastasizing potential.

affords the greatest chance of permanent arrest for these stages. Radiation therapy usually is added in extensive stage II disease. Stage III is a borderline category amenable to only limited salvage, usually by combined surgery and radiation therapy. Stage IV patients are essentially incurable but may benefit greatly from palliative irradiation, chemotherapy, or hormonal therapy as well as supportive counseling and other psychologic methods of management.

   A. Surgical Therapy: In selecting the best operation for any given patient, the question is not which procedure is best for treatment of breast cancer as such, but rather which method is most rational for management of each of the advancing clinical stages of breast cancer. Thus, clinical and histologic staging is all-important (Tables 20–2 and 20–3). An expert panel convened by the National Cancer Institute of the National Institutes of Health in 1979 generally agreed that the treatment standard for women with stage I breast cancer should be modified radical mastectomy and axillary node dissection rather than radical mastectomy. The panel based its opinion largely on 6-year data from the National Surgical Adjuvant Breast Project (NSABP) involving 1680 cancer patients. The more conservative procedure was also preferred for patients with stage II disease (tumor < 5 cm in diameter with positive axillary nodes), usually followed by irradiation. This is admittedly a tentative recommendation, because long-term follow-up will be necessary to establish final procedure. Moreover, the NSABP did not sufficiently consider the multicentricity of breast cancer or variables based on histologic examination of tumors.

The major procedures available for surgical treatment of breast cancer are as follows:

1. Standard radical mastectomy–This extensive, meticulous operation consists of en bloc removal of the breast, pectoral muscles, and axillary lymph nodes in stage I (breast lesion < 2 cm) or stage II (axillary nodes < 2.5 cm in diameter) disease. No other method of treatment is superior to this approach, although lymphatic drainage is compromised, significant edema occurs in 10–30% of patients, and arm weakness may result. If local disease cannot be removed completely, however, the radical operation should not be attempted.

2. Modified radical mastectomy–In this operation, the breast and often the pectoralis minor muscle are removed, with preservation of the pectoralis major. The axillary nodes are usually sampled but may or may not be excised in stage II patients. While this method is not as complete, the cosmetic result is better, ie, there is less disfigurement and less arm edema.

3. Simple mastectomy–This operation is accomplished with or without staging by axillary lymphadenectomy. Generally, irradiation is added in extensive stage II or in stage III cases.

B. Radiation Therapy: It has been amply demonstrated that intensive supervoltage therapy can destroy small primary cancers as well as cancer in the axillary and internal mammary nodes. Thus, in recent years, wide excision of the lesion or simple mastectomy followed by radiation therapy has yielded results almost as good as those of radical or modified radical mastectomy in selected cases.

The advantages of preoperative versus postoperative radiation therapy are still debated.

C. Adjuvant Therapy: The indications listed below are widely accepted criteria for various forms of adjuvant therapy.

1. Radiation therapy–
a. Presence of over 3 positive axillary nodes.
b. Centrally or medially situated breast cancer.
c. Inflammatory carcinoma (probably metastatic).
d. Bone metastases–Pain or pathologic fracture.

2. Chemotherapy–
a. Premenopausal patients with 1–3 positive axillary nodes.
b. Compromising metastatic lesions, eg, spread to liver.

3. Hormone therapy–
a. Antiestrogens in pre- or postmenopausal patients with positive estrogen receptor assays.
b. Estrogen or testosterone in postmenopausal patients.

4. Ablative surgery—

a. Consider ablative surgery for patients with positive estrogen receptor binding assays who later develop metastatic lesions, particularly in bone. If a favorable response is obtained for 1 year by ovariectomy in premenopausal patients, adrenalectomy may be helpful also.

b. Postmenopausal patients with bone pain from metastatic breast cancer may be benefited by ablative surgery, including adrenalectomy or hypophysectomy.

D. Treatment During Pregnancy and the Puerperium: Therapeutic abortion is not medically indicated in patients with localized breast cancer of a favorable microscopic type and positive estrogen or progesterone receptor site determinations. It is not yet known whether early interruption of pregnancy will benefit women with negative receptor site determinations. Interruption of an early pregnancy may palliate patients with advanced breast cancer. Ovariectomy may also have an ameliorating effect, and, if this is confirmed, adrenalectomy may extend the palliation. However, if pregnancy has progressed beyond 20 weeks, it should be allowed to continue to term. In the absence of obstetric contraindications, vaginal delivery will be in the best interests of mother and offspring.

Follow-Up Care

After primary therapy, patients with breast cancer should be followed for life for at least 2 reasons: to detect recurrences and to observe the opposite breast for a second carcinoma. During the first 3 years, the patient is examined every 3–4 months. Thereafter, examination is done every 6 months until 5 years postoperatively and then every 6–12 months. Special attention is given to the remaining breast, because of the increased risk of developing a second primary. The patient should examine her own breast monthly, and a mammogram should be obtained annually.

After the first few days following mastectomy, active motion of the arm and shoulder on the operated side should be encouraged. If a full range of motion is not possible by 10–14 days after the operation, physical therapy may be required. Chronic edema is managed by elevation of the arm and by a snugly fitted elastic sleeve slipped over the arm from hand to shoulder.

After radical mastectomy, the arm on the operated side becomes more than normally susceptible to infection. The patient should be warned to avoid activities likely to cause superficial wounds and infections of the arm; if infection occurs, it must be treated promptly.

The Service Committee of the American Cancer Society sponsors a rehabilitation program for postmastectomy patients called Reach for Recovery and will provide useful literature upon request. Women who have had a mastectomy may be valuable counselors for the patient before and after operation. The patient's morale is improved by a temporary breast prosthesis held in place by a comfortably fitted brassiere before she leaves the hospital. She should also receive information on where to obtain a more permanent device.

Advice regarding future pregnancies should be individualized. Pregnancy is generally unadvisable for patients with axillary metastases who have had definitive treatment for breast cancer; if pregnancy occurs, it should probably be interrupted at least until 5 years have passed without recurrence. Patients with stage I breast cancer who have no evidence of recurrent disease 3–5 years posttreatment are less likely to harbor occult metastases, and pregnancy is correspondingly less hazardous.

Prognosis

Evidence is mounting that breast cancer may be a systemic as well as a neoplastic disease and that the prognosis is therefore closely related to cell-mediated immune defenses against the tumor. Regional lymph nodes seem to play a role in the immune mechanism whether the nodes contain cancer cells or not. There is as yet no way of measuring immunity to cancer, however.

The 5-year survival statistics of patients treated for breast cancer do not accurately reflect the outcome of therapy because of numerous recurrences of breast cancer 5 or even 10 years after treatment. Nonetheless, because few studies of 10- or 20-year survivors are available, it is still customary to refer to 5-year arrest data.

When cancer is confined to the breast, the 5-year clinical cure rate by accepted methods of treatment is 75–90%. When breast cancer involves the axillary nodes, the rate drops to 40–60% at 5 years; after 10 years, the clinical cure rate is only about 25%. The least favorable anatomic site for breast cancer is the median portion of the inner lower quadrant.

Breast cancer is probably somewhat more malignant in younger than in older women.

MAMMARY DYSPLASIA
**(Fibrocystic Disease of the Breast,
Chronic Cystic Mastitis)**

Mammary dysplasia is the most common disorder of the breast. While frequently diagnosed in premenopausal women, it is rare after the menopause. For this reason, it is believed that ovarian hormones, especially estrogen, may be responsible, at least in part. The chief pathologic feature of cystic disease of the breast is the formation and growth of microscopic cysts derived from terminal ducts and acini. The term fibrocystic disease is misleading, provokes anxiety, and probably should be abandoned. Mammary dysplasia, especially when proliferation occurs—eg, papilloma formation or solid hyperplasia—is associated with an increased incidence of breast cancer.

Clinical Findings

Most patients with mammary dysplasia complain of cyclic tenderness and dull heaviness in both breasts. These symptoms increase premenstrually and call attention to sensitive breast irregularities, lumps, or cysts. The cysts usually are palpable and may be 1–2 cm in diameter. They are clear to transillumination. Clearly, mammary dysplasia is not periodic mastalgia due to exaggerated physiologic activity. However, mammary dysplasia may be relatively asymptomatic, and discovery of one or more cysts may occur only accidentally.

Rapid appearance or disappearance of the cysts is common in mammary dysplasia. The multiplicity of lesions, usually involving both breasts, is helpful in differentiating clinical cystic mastitis from carcinoma. However, transition from clinical cystic disease to cancer occurs about twice as often in patients with mammary dysplasia as in controls. If skin retraction is noted, one must assume that cancer is present until it can be ruled out by biopsy.

Prominent cysts and fibrosis in themselves are not a cause for concern, but marked proliferation is.

Pathologists now classify ductile changes according to degree. On a scale of 1 to 5, epithelial alteration progresses from control (stage 1) through 3 stages of hyperplasia with and without atypia to carcinoma in situ (stage 5).

Treatment

When a classic history of cystic disease of the breast is made in a young woman, aspiration of a discrete cyst under local anesthesia is reasonable. The typical aspirate from such cysts is yellow, greenish, or brown turbid fluid. If the fluid is reported as benign on cytologic study, further surgery is not indicated, and frequent follow-up examinations are in order. If malignant or cancer-suspicious cells are reported, biopsy confirmation is required.

In most cases, absolute diagnosis or exclusion of malignant change in mammary dysplasia is impossible by physical examination alone, and biopsy is necessary. Deeply embedded cysts, clusters of cysts, sclerosing adenosis, or dense fibroplasia may constitute a mass that mimics cancer. Definitive surgery in chronic cystic mastitis should be conservative, because the primary objective is to diagnose or exclude malignancy. In general, needle biopsy should be done if the case is classic or the diagnosis has already been established or is almost certain, and directed open biopsy should be done if no fluid is obtained on aspiration or the mass persists or recurs. If malignant disease is diagnosed, the patient must be treated appropriately. In any case, close follow-up is most important.

Analgesic drugs may afford considerable relief for chronic cystic mastitis. Low-dose oral contraceptive therapy is beneficial, although it never cures the disorder. Danazol, a synthetic androgen, may produce dramatic improvement, but the side-effects are often objectionable. Long-term restriction of methylxanthines (eg, coffee, tea, and chocolate) may be helpful. A well-fitted brassiere worn day and night and the avoidance of trauma are most helpful. Diuretics for the reduction of fluid retention often give relief from periodic mastalgia.

Prognosis

Strictly speaking, severe mammary dysplasia is a precancerous disorder, and patients with this problem must be followed carefully for an indefinite time.

The signs and symptoms of chronic cystic mastitis subside after the menopause, but they may persist or recur if excessive, prolonged estrogen therapy is given. All women should examine their breasts regularly, and examination by a physician is indicated whenever a palpable mass is identified.

FIBROADENOMA OF THE BREAST

Fibroadenoma of the breast is a benign, usually unilateral, firm, discrete, and nontender tumor that may develop in women 20–40 years of age. It is rare after the menopause. It occurs more frequently and earlier in black than in white or Oriental women and is usually diagnosed during a general physical examination.

Cancer or mammary dysplasia is more likely than fibroadenoma in women over 30 with a breast mass. However, if aspiration fails to yield fluid, fibroadenoma or cancer may be the correct diagnosis. Needle biopsy or local excision of the tumor and an assessment by a pathologist is in order. If fibroadenoma is identified, further surgery is not necessary.

Cystosarcoma phyllodes (giant mammary myxoma) is a type of breast fibroadenoma with unusually proliferative cellular stroma. It is rarely malignant. The tumor may grow rapidly to large size and may recur if incompletely excised. Hence, a wide margin of excision is essential.

FAT NECROSIS

Fat necrosis of the breast is uncommon but may be the basis for confusion and misdiagnosis of cancer. Trauma is presumed to be the cause, but only about half of patients give a history of injury to the breast. Ecchymosis or local tenderness may not develop. Nonetheless, a sensitive mass, perhaps with slight skin retraction, often develops. Although breast trauma is never a cause of cancer and fat necrosis as a rule resolves without therapy, biopsy in puzzling or poorly documented cases to rule out malignancy is the best policy, especially in older women.

Diseases of the Vulva & Vagina | 21

VAGINAL HERNIAS
(Cystocele, Urethrocele, Rectocele, Enterocele)

Cystocele and rectocele (Figs 21–1 and 21–2) are herniations of the bladder and rectum, respectively, through faults in the vaginal septa; enterocele (Fig 21–3) is a herniation, usually of intestine, through the cul-de-sac or other pelvic floor defect into the vaginal vault. Cystocele is frequently accompanied by a urethrocele or sagging (not sacculation) of the mid and proximal urethra into the vagina. Most vaginal hernias are multiple and are due to childbirth injuries, but tissue weakness due to any of several causes (postmenopausal estrogen deficiency, obesity, and other problems of increased intra-abdominal pressure; neurologic deficits; operative trauma; congenital defects) is often a contributory factor. White women develop cystocele and rectocele more often than Oriental or black women.

At least half of all parous women develop some degree of cystocele or rectocele, usually after the menopause, but only about 10% of the lesions become symptomatic. Significant enterocele occurs in all cases of uterine or vaginal vault prolapse.

Vaginal herniations are rarely observed early, even after a traumatic delivery. The defects become evident only months or years later, perhaps following subsequent apparently normal deliveries. The climacteric and the persistent stress of increased intra-abdominal pressure gradually stretch the supports of the damaged bladder, rectum, or pelvic floor. The protrusion may eventually become so large that it presents at the introitus.

Voiding is incomplete with cystocele because some urine always remains in the pouch below the bladder neck. Residual (stagnant) urine soon becomes contaminated, and urinary tract infection results. Urinary frequency and urgency incontinence are due to overflow voiding. Stress incontinence is not a symptom of cystocele per se. Urethrocele does not itself interfere with urinary function.

Rectocele enlarges slowly with constipation and straining.

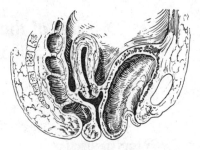

Figure 21–1. Cystocele.

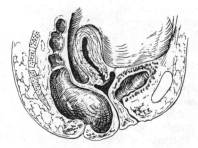

Figure 21–2. Rectocele.

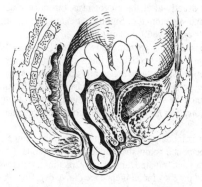

Figure 21–3. Enterocele and prolapsed uterus.

Clinical Findings

A. Symptoms and Signs: Cystocele, rectocele, or enterocele of slight to moderate degree is usually asymptomatic, but many women describe a sensation of bladder and vaginal distention and urinary frequency, especially when erect. Stress incontinence develops when injury involves the bladder neck structures. Urethrocele causes no symptoms. Rectocele and enterocele, which both cause constipation and are worsened by it, are responsible for a "bearing down" sensation and vaginal fullness, particularly when the patient is standing. With a large cystocele or rectocele, the patient may have to reduce the herniation manually in order to urinate or defecate.

Vaginal hernias are apparent on rectovaginal examination. The rectal finger will enter the rectocele pouch to accentuate the posterior vaginal wall defect. With the patient in the lithotomy position, a single-blade vaginal speculum should be inserted. When the patient strains, cystocele will cause the anterior vaginal wall to bulge while the posterior wall is depressed by the speculum; rectocele will cause the posterior wall to bulge while the speculum is retracted upward.

The diagnosis of a small enterocele may be difficult, and some are discovered only at surgery. However, most hernias of this type can be distinguished by seeking the bulge of an enterocele just above that of a rectocele as a bivalve speculum is slowly withdrawn from the vagina of the supine patient. The diagnosis can be confirmed by performing rectovaginal examination and asking the patient to cough; an impulse will be felt against the fingertip held against an enterocele (upper bulge) but not a rectocele (lower bulge).

B. X-Ray Findings: Lateral x-rays with contrast medium in the bladder, large bowel, or small bowel may demonstrate a cystocele, rectocele, or enterocele, respectively.

C. Special Examinations: Cystoscopy and proctoscopy will corroborate a diagnosis of cystocele or rectocele. Passage of a firm catheter will demonstrate a urethrocele or cystocele.

Complications

Urinary tract infection is generally recurrent and often serious.

Damage to the pubococcygeus portion of the levator musculature and the endopelvic fascia, often associated with a large cystocele, weakens and displaces the bladder neck and causes incontinence.

Progressive enlargement of a cystocele, usually with uterine prolapse, may result in acute urinary retention.

Most patients with rectocele also have hemorrhoids.

Rectocele may cause obstipation, fecal impaction, and diverticulosis. Intestinal obstruction occurs rarely in an enterocele containing small amounts of feces.

Differential Diagnosis

Cysts of vestigial (wolffian) origin, semisolid tumors of the vaginal septa, and large inclusion cysts may be mistaken for cystocele or rectocele. A large cystocele may overshadow a urethrocele. The fullness of a large, high rectocele; prolapsed and adherent adnexa; a markedly retroflexed uterus; a soft cervical or uterine myoma; or retained fecal material may be confused with enterocele.

Prevention

Childbirth injury should be avoided. Obesity, chronic cough, and straining should be corrected promptly. Postmenopausal estrogen therapy is of value. Neurologic disorders should be prevented or treated promptly. Gross enlargement of pelvic and vaginal hernias must not be neglected.

Treatment

A. Emergency Measures: The lower bowel and bladder must be emptied if acute retention occurs. In enterocele, if incarceration of the intestines is not relieved by placing the patient in the knee-chest position or by vaginal packing, laparotomy and surgical release will be required.

B. General Measures: Overweight women must be encouraged to lose weight. Pelvic tumors must be removed and ascitic fluid drained and reaccumulation prevented. Cough and constipation should be treated appropriately. Cyclic estrogens in small doses usually are beneficial to postmenopausal women.

C. Specific Measures: Pessaries, especially doughnut, ball, and crescentic (Gehrung) supports, afford temporary symptomatic relief but are never curative. Surgical correction of cystocele, urethrocele, or rectocele by colporrhaphy may be required. Enterocele should be repaired surgically by cul-de-sac herniorrhaphy.

D. Treatment of Complications: Bladder drainage and antibacterial therapy are required for urinary retention and infection. Fecal impaction may be relieved by oil instillation, digital evacuation, enemas, and laxatives.

Prognosis

A recurrence rate of at least 15% is reported after vaginal hernia repair.

VULVOVAGINITIS & LEUKORRHEA

Leukorrhea is a usually whitish vaginal discharge that may occur at any age and affects almost all women at some time. It is not a disease but an abnormal sign. It is usually due to infection of the vagina or cervix;

other causes include uterine tumors, estrogenic or psychic stimulation, trauma, foreign bodies, excessive douching (especially with irritating medications), and estrogen depletion. The presence of some vaginal mucus is normal; when soiling of the clothing or distressing local symptoms occur, the discharge must be considered abnormal.

Protozoa, notably *Trichomonas vaginalis,* and candidal infections are frequent causes of leukorrhea. Candidal infections are especially common in diabetic patients and during pregnancy. *Gardnerella vaginalis (Corynebacterium vaginale, Haemophilus vaginalis)* infections, *Chlamydia trachomatis* infections, and gonorrhea and other venereal infections are causes of leukorrhea; *Mycobacterium tuberculosis* is rarely responsible; helminths, especially *Oxyuris,* occasionally cause leukorrhea in children.

When estrogen and progesterone levels are normal, the genital tract resists infection. During childhood and the menopause, these hormones are absent or present in low concentrations, and the thin vulvar and vaginal surfaces are more susceptible to bacterial invasion.

Elevated estrogen levels, as occur during pregnancy, cause the production of cervical mucus in large amounts. Excess mucus production also occurs normally in the newborn; as a result of sexual or other emotional stimulation; during anovulatory menstrual cycles; with feminizing tumors of the ovary; and after excessive estrogen administration.

Estrogen depletion after the menopause causes atrophy of the genital tract, decreased mucus production, and a more alkaline vaginal fluid. This encourages local infection because lactobacilli are supplanted by a mixed flora or one in which cocci predominate.

The most common sites of origin of genital discharge (in order of frequency) are the cervix, vagina, vulva, and uterine corpus.

T vaginalis infection is a diffuse vaginitis usually characterized by a thin, yellow-green, occasionally frothy leukorrhea with a fetid odor. Numerous red points (''strawberry patches''), which rarely bleed, are scattered over the vaginal surface and cervical portio. The cervix, urethra, and bladder may be involved secondarily.

T vaginalis vaginitis is almost always a sexually transmitted infection. Vaginal, oral, and enteric trichomonads are distinctly different morphologically, and the gastrointestinal tract is not the site of origin of genital trichomoniasis. The vaginal organism can often be traced to the male partner, who may harbor the flagellate beneath the prepuce or in the urethra or prostate.

Candida albicans and related yeast pathogens are natural inhabitants of the bowel and are also found on the perineal skin. Vaginal contamination from these sources is common. The thin vaginal discharge due to candidal infection may have no odor. White curdlike collections of exudate are often present, and some are lightly attached to the cervical and vaginal mucosa. When these are removed, slight oozing frequently occurs.

Chlamydial infections cause vaginitis and cervicitis as well as nongonococcal urethritis, salpingitis, neonatal infections, and lymphogranuloma venereum. The infection usually begins as a mucopurulent, often odorous or pruritic discharge. Giemsa staining of the discharge may reveal intracellular organisms, but cultures are usually required for diagnosis.

G vaginalis (C vaginale, H vaginalis) is normally found in the respiratory tract. It is found in the vaginal flora of about 30% of normal women. Genital transmission is by sexual intercourse. A "fishy" odor, often intensified by potassium hydroxide solution, is often evident.

Gonorrheal vulvovaginitis in children is usually due to hand-to-body contact by an infected adult. It may be due to sexual abuse. In adolescents and adults, gonorrhea is sexually transmitted almost without exception.

Herpesvirus type 2 infection is a common cause of painful papulovesicular ulcerative vulvovaginal (and cervical) lesions, usually in young adults. It is sexually transmitted.

Metazoal vaginal infestations occur as a result of fecal soiling of the introitus.

Cervicitis may be present even when the appearance of the ectocervix is not remarkable. Chronic cervicitis is usually accompanied by a thick, viscid mucopurulent discharge with an acrid (or no) odor.

Clinical Findings

A. Symptoms and Signs: Vaginal discharge, with or without itching, may be associated with formication when urine contaminates the inflamed introitus. The patient may complain of pudendal irritation, proctitis, vaginismus, or dyspareunia.

B. Laboratory Findings: Blood findings usually do not suggest infection. Papanicolaou smears are indicated to rule out cancer. Specific tests should be performed for infections or infestations.

A fresh wet preparation of vaginal fluid should be inspected for motile *T vaginalis. G vaginalis* probably will be present if there is a heavy clouding of the spread, especially when epithelial cells appear dusted with bacteria ("clue cells"). *Gardnerella vaginalis,* formerly called *Corynebacterium vaginale* and *Haemophilus vaginalis,* is a small, nonmotile, nonencapsulated pleomorphic rod that stains variably with Gram's stain. To aid visualization of candidal hyphae and spores, add 10% potassium hydroxide to the preparation to lake blood cells. Add 1 drop of Lugol's solution to color the organisms. Intracellular gramnegative diplococci *(Neisseria gonorrhoeae)* and other predominant bacteria and helminths may be identified in a Gram-stained smear. Scrapings of ulcerative areas spread on a slide, fixed, and stained—

preferably with hematoxylin and eosin—may reveal multinucleated giant cells containing viral aggregations. Vaginal specimens should be smeared for acid-fast staining and cultured if *M tuberculosis* is thought to be present.

If possible, vaginal fluid should be cultured anaerobically and aerobically to identify bacterial pathogens. Thioglycolate medium is useful for culture of *Haemophilus* and *Chlamydia. Candida* can be demonstrated by inoculation of Nickerson's or a similar medium.

Serologic tests are used to distinguish leukorrhea due to syphilis; lymphogranuloma venereum is diagnosed by use of a complement fixation test.

Complications

T vaginalis vaginitis is often followed by chronic bacterial cervicitis, a major factor in infertility.

G vaginalis vaginitis may be atypical and even more troublesome when other pathogens are also present.

Candidal vaginal infections may lead to dermatitis of the thighs and pudendum.

Gonococcal vulvar or vaginal infections in infants may be accompanied by gonorrheal ophthalmia and blindness. In adults, bartholinitis, skenitis, cervicitis, salpingitis, and peritonitis may occur.

Urethritis, salpingitis, or chronic granulomatous ulcerations due to lymphogranuloma venereum may progress to cancer; or rectal strictures may be caused by chlamydiae. Lymphogranuloma venereum causes suppurative inguinal buboes.

Genital herpesvirus infection is a postulated cause of carcinoma of the cervix. If open herpetic lesions are present, vaginal delivery may result in neonatal infection and death.

Tuberculosis of the genital tract, usually secondary to pulmonary or gastrointestinal tuberculosis, may extend to the urinary organs or the peritoneal cavity and its contents.

Benign genital tumors may bleed and become infected; malignant tumors may spread locally and metastasize.

Prevention

The sexual partner should use a condom if infection or reinfection is likely. Sexual promiscuity and borrowing of douche tips, underclothing, or other possibly contaminated articles should be avoided.

Long-term antibiotic treatment, especially with tetracyclines, may permit overgrowth of *Candida* in the vagina and bowel.

Treatment

A. Specific Measures: Treat infection or infestation with specific drugs (listed below). If sensitivity develops, discontinue the drug and substitute another as soon as practicable. Treatment should continue during menstruation; choose a route of administration (eg, vaginal suppositories, oral tablets) that need not be discontinued because of bleeding.

1. T vaginalis vaginitis–Either of the following may be used:

a. Metronidazole, 2 g orally as a single dose. Treat the partner similarly during the same interval. (*Caution:* This drug has a disulfiramlike effect [intolerance to alcohol]. It may also encourage the growth of *Candida*. Rapid disappearance of leukorrhea due in part to trichomoniasis may mask the fact that concurrent gonorrhea has not been cured.) Metronidazole should not be given to nursing mothers or to women in the first trimester of pregnancy because of the possible risk to the fetus. During the second and third trimesters, metronidazole probably should be restricted to symptomatic patients in whom topical measures have proved inadequate. Patients must be informed of the side-effects of the drug: nausea and vomiting, dark urine, alcohol intolerance, and possible dizziness and ataxia.

b. Vagisec Plus suppositories (polyoxyethylene nonyl phenol, aminacrine, and sodium edetate), one inserted twice daily for 2 weeks. This treatment is less effective than metronidazole.

2. C albicans vaginitis–Both of the following have been approved by the FDA for use during pregnancy:

a. Miconazole nitrate (Monistat), 2% aqueous cream, one applicatorful daily at bedtime for 7 days.

b. Clotrimazole (Gyne-Lotrimin), 2 tablets vaginally nightly for 3 nights, then 1 tablet for 1 night.

3. G vaginalis vaginitis–Treat the sexual partner also. Give metronidazole, 2 g orally as a single dose, or ampicillin, 500 mg orally 4 times daily for 7 days. These are the most effective agents.

4. Chlamydial vaginitis–Chlamydiae can be eradicated from the urethra, vagina, and cervix by tetracyclines or erythromycin, 500 mg orally 4 times daily for 1 week.

5. Herpesvirus–No specific therapy exists. Symptomatic relief can be expected from occasional application of local anesthetic creams and acidic douches.

6. Atrophic (senile) vaginitis–

a. Dienestrol vaginal cream, one-third applicatorful every third day for 3 weeks. Omit medication for 1 week, then resume cyclic therapy.

b. Diethylstilbestrol, one 0.5-mg vaginal suppository every third day for 3 weeks. Omit medication for 1 week (to avoid uterine bleeding); then resume cyclic therapy indefinitely unless contraindicated.

6. Gonorrheal vaginitis–See p 521.

B. General Measures: Use menstrual tampons to reduce vulvar soiling, pruritus, and odor. Coitus should be avoided until a cure has been achieved. Relapses are often reinfections. Re-treat both partners.

Antipruritic medications are disappointing unless an allergy is present. Specific and local therapy will usually control itching promptly.

C. Local Nonspecific Measures: Occasional acetic acid douches (4 tablespoons of white [distilled] vinegar per liter of water) may be beneficial in the treatment of leukorrhea. (*Caution:* Never use alkaline [soda] douches. They are unphysiologic and often harmful because they raise the pH and inhibit the growth of the normal vaginal flora.)

Douches are not essential to cleanliness or perineal hygiene. Douching is an ineffective contraceptive measure. Too frequent douches of any kind tend to increase mucus secretion. Irritating medications cause further mucus production.

In severe, resistant, or recurrent trichomonal or candidal vaginitis, treat the cervix (even when it is apparently normal) by chemical or light thermal cauterization. Examine the urinary tract and Skene's and Bartholin's ducts, and treat these areas if they appear to be reservoirs of infection.

D. Surgical Measures: Cryosurgery, conization of the cervix, incision of Skene's glands, or bartholinectomy may be required. Cervical, uterine, or tubal disease (eg, tumors or infections) may necessitate laparotomy, irradiation, or other appropriate measures.

Prognosis

Leukorrhea, especially when due to *C albicans,* is difficult to cure in pregnant, debilitated, or diabetic women. Repeated or even continuous treatment for 3–4 months may be required until the patient is delivered or the diabetes is controlled. The ultimate prognosis is good, however, if a specific diagnosis is made promptly and proper, extended, intensive therapy given.

Although nonpregnant patients have no serious sequelae from *G vaginalis* vaginitis, chorioamnionitis, septicemia, and death of the fetus or newborn may occur when a pregnant woman is infected with *G vaginalis*.

DERMATITIS OF THE FEMALE GENITALIA

Eczema

Eczema is a nonspecific term for a common pruritic, moist dermatitis characterized by excoriation and crusting, with later lichenification. Eczema is often a contact dermatitis caused by irritants in soap, bath oils, or deodorant medications; dyes in clothing; or allergy to wool or silk. Sensitivity tests and exclusion of other dermatitides aid in diagnosis.

Treatment depends upon elimination of the antigen or irritant. Apply Burow's solution followed by steroid creams twice daily.

Psoriasis

The cause of psoriasis is not known. Pruritic, reddened, slightly elevated, flattened lesions (without the typical silvery scale seen on elbows and knees) are seen in body folds. The elbows and knees are frequently affected by scaly lesions. Psoriasis is a chronic disorder that is often familial. Exacerbations often occur in the winter.

Treatment includes improved hygiene and soothing medications such as 0.5% hydrocortisone cream applied periodically.

Lichen Rubor Planus

The cause of this condition is unknown. Pruritus accompanies the purplish, raised papules, which have no tendency to ulcerate. Rare vesicles or bullae may develop, and, occasionally, atrophy or hyperpigmentation occurs with healing. The disease may follow nervous stress, and the lesions are usually characteristic. The buccal and vulvovaginal surfaces are often involved together with the skin.

There is no specific treatment. Give phenobarbital or tranquilizers as necessary for symptomatic relief. Apply steroid cream topically.

NONVENEREAL VIRAL INFECTIONS OF THE FEMALE GENITAL TRACT

Herpes Zoster

Herpes zoster virus, morphologically identical to the varicella virus, is the causative agent. Severe, persistent burning and aching pain occur together with small, unusually unilateral blisters. Zonal vesicular or bullous ulcerative lesions develop along the distribution of one or more sensory nerves, often on the sacrum or buttocks. Eventual suppuration and scarring are characteristic.

Treatment is nonspecific. Palliative therapy includes Burow's compresses and liberal doses of analgesics for pain.

One attack usually confers immunity.

Molluscum Contagiosum

An autoinoculable virus with an incubation period of 1–4 weeks is responsible. Asymptomatic pink to gray, discrete, umbilicated, epithelial skin tumors less than 1 cm in diameter develop on the vulva. The histologic picture, with numerous inclusion bodies in the cell cytoplasm, is diagnostic.

Each lesion may be treated by desiccation, freezing, or curettage and chemical cauterization of the base.

SEXUALLY TRANSMITTED DISEASES
(Venereal Diseases)

The term sexually transmitted diseases is now preferred to the term venereal diseases, which has a pejorative implication, to denote disorders spread principally by sexual contact. These diseases are caused by organisms peculiarly adapted to growth in the genital tract.

The list of diseases traditionally thought of as venereal infections has been extended recently to include lymphogranuloma venereum, cytomegalovirus disease, herpes simplex type 2, and even hepatitis B.

1. GONORRHEA

Gonorrhea is the most prevalent reportable communicable disease in the USA, with an estimated 2.5 million or more infectious cases annually. It is most commonly transmitted during sexual activity and has its greatest incidence in the 15- to 29-year-old age group.

Gonorrhea is caused by *Neisseria gonorrhoeae*, a gram-negative diplococcus typically found inside polymorphonuclear cells. The organism may be recovered from the urethra, cervix, anal canal, or pharynx. It is best isolated by culture in a selective medium such as Thayer-Martin or Transgrow. *N gonorrhoeae* is killed rapidly by drying, sunlight, heat, and most disinfectants.

The columnar and transitional epithelium of the genitourinary tract is the principal site of invasion. Gonococci may enter the upper reproductive tract, causing salpingitis with attendant complications. It has been estimated that at least 20% of women with gonorrhea develop pelvic infection if untreated.

Clinical Findings

A. Symptoms and Signs: The incubation period is usually 2–8 days. Early symptoms, when they occur, are localized to the lower genitourinary tract and include vaginal discharge, urinary frequency or dysuria, and rectal discomfort. Pharyngitis may occur after oral intercourse; acute proctitis, after rectal intercourse.

Pelvic examination should be complete. The vulva, vagina, cervix, and urethra may be inflamed and may itch or burn. If the patient is symptomatic or may have been exposed to gonorrhea, specimens of discharge from the cervix, urethra, and anus should be taken for culture.

Unilateral swelling in the inferior lateral portion of the introitus suggests infection of Bartholin's duct and gland. In early gonococcal infections, pus containing gonococci may be gently expressed from the duct. Enlargement, tenderness, and fluctuation signify abscess formation; *N gonorrhoeae* is infrequently recovered at this stage. Spontaneous evacuation of pus often occurs if drainage by incision is not done. The infection may result in asymptomatic cyst formation.

An infant delivered through an infected birth canal may develop ophthalmia neonatorum.

Gonococcal invasion of nonkeratinized membranes in young girls, which is rare, produces severe vulvovaginitis. Typical signs are a purulent vaginal discharge with dysuria and red and swollen genital mucous membranes. The infection is commonly introduced by adults, and in such cases the physician must consider the possibility of child molesting and take appropriate steps to protect the child.

B. Laboratory Findings: A presumptive diagnosis of gonorrhea can be based on finding gram-negative intracellular diplococci on a stained smear, but confirmation requires positive identification of gonococci grown on selective media. Oxidase-positive gram-negative diplococci grown on selective media such as Thayer-Martin or Transgrow are usually *N gonorrhoeae*. Carbohydrate fermentation tests may be performed, but they are time-consuming and expensive and occasionally yield other species of *Neisseria*. Cultures therefore are reported as "presumptive of *N gonorrhoeae*."

Complications

The major complication in females is salpingitis and its sequelae. *N gonorrhoeae* can be recovered from the cervix in about half of women with salpingitis. Bacteremia due to the gonococci (disseminated gonococcal infection) may involve the tendons, joints, endocardium, or meninges. For unknown reasons, these infections are more common during pregnancy.

If other sexually transmitted diseases acquired from the same exposure or from more than one infected source go undetected and untreated, they can cause problems.

Differential Diagnosis

Vaginitis and urethritis due to other causes may be associated with dysuria, frequency, or vaginal discharge. Once the adnexa are involved, the entities listed in the section on differential diagnosis of salpingitis (see p 629) must be considered.

Vaginitis may be caused by any of the following: trichomoniasis, nonspecific cervicitis, candidiasis, cervical polyps and neoplasms, aging changes, or *G vaginalis* or chlamydial infection. Gram staining may be helpful in distinguishing the cause.

Any of the above may cause urethritis, which may also be associated with bacterial cystitis, coital trauma, chemical irritation, urethral diverticula, or herpes simplex infection.

Vulvovaginitis in children is usually associated with self-insertion of seemingly innocuous foreign bodies, with secondary infection by perineal flora.

Cervicitis (see p 553) or bartholinitis (see p 543) may be due to other causes.

Prevention

Prevention is based on education, mechanical or chemical prophylaxis, and early diagnosis and treatment. Gonorrhea is a reportable disease that can only be controlled by detecting and treating asymptomatic carriers and their sexual consorts. Intensive search for sexual contacts by public health agencies must rely on physician reporting. Contacts are sometimes given full treatment for gonorrhea on epidemiologic grounds, without individual diagnosis, to reduce the reservoir of infection. All high-risk populations should be screened for gonorrhea. Effective drugs taken in therapeutic doses within 24 hours of exposure can abort an infection. Preexposure prophylaxis with penicillin is no longer widely effective; in fact, penicillin prophylaxis contributes to the selection of penicillinase-producing gonococci. Reexamination is mandatory to rule out reinfection or failure of therapy. The use of condoms can reduce the risk of infection with most sexually transmitted diseases.

Ophthalmia neonatorum is prevented by the instillation of an adequate prophylactic agent (1% silver nitrate solution or 1% tetracycline ointment or erythromycin ointment) into each conjunctival sac immediately after birth.

Treatment

Note: Any patient with gonorrhea must be suspected of having syphilis also and managed accordingly. A serologic test for syphilis should be performed before treatment.

A. Antibiotics: One of the following antibiotic regimens should be given:

1. Uncomplicated infections–

a. Aqueous procaine penicillin G, 4.8 million units intramuscularly in 2 injection sites, combined with probenecid, 1 g orally. This is the regimen of choice and is also effective as treatment for concomitant syphilis.

b. Ampicillin, 3.5 g orally, combined with probenecid, 1 g orally.

c. Tetracycline, 1.5 g orally, followed by 0.5 g 4 times daily for 4 days (total dose, 9.5 g). This drug may also eliminate chlamydiae.

d. Spectinomycin, 2 g intramuscularly, is the drug of choice if treatment with penicillin, ampicillin, or tetracycline fails. It is relatively ineffective against pharyngeal infections and is not effective against syphilis. Spectinomycin may be given as primary therapy for patients who are allergic to penicillin and cannot tolerate oral tetracycline.

2. Salpingitis–See p 630.

3. Disseminated gonococcal infection–Crystalline penicillin G, 15 million units intravenously daily for 3 days. Alternatives are tetracycline or erythromycin.

B. Local Treatment: Local therapy should consist of hot sitz bas, application of hot moist compresses, and avoidance of coitus. Incision and drainage of Bartholin's ducts may be necessary. Prompt, aggressive treatment is the best way to prevent complications, notably salpingitis.

C. Follow-Up Treatment: Test-of-cure procedures are recommended at approximately 7–14 days after treatment. Specimens for culture should be obtained from the endocervix, urethra, and anus. If the cultures are positive for *N gonorrhoeae,* uncomplicated gonorrhea in females should be re-treated with spectinomycin, 2 g intramuscularly, or oral tetracycline, 0.5 g orally 4 times daily for 10 days (total dose, 10 g). The patient should not be considered cured until 2 consecutive sets of cultures have revealed no gonococci. A serologic test for syphilis should be repeated 2 weeks and 2 months after treatment.

Prognosis

The prognosis with prompt, effective treatment and proper follow-up is excellent. The steady rise in drug-resistant gonococci is responsible for an increasing number of cases that require re-treatment. With recurrent infections or relapses, infertility may result.

2. SYPHILIS

Syphilis is caused by *Treponema pallidum,* a spirochete. Treponemes will pass through intact mucous membranes or abraded skin. Transmission is most often by direct (usually sexual) contact with an infectious lesion, but the organism can survive for days in fluids and can therefore be transmitted in blood from infected persons. Syphilis can be transferred via the placenta from mother to fetus after the tenth week of pregnancy (congenital syphilis). A primary lesion (chancre) develops 10–90 days after the treponemes enter, persists for 1–5 weeks, and then heals spontaneously. Serologic tests for syphilis are usually nonreactive when the chancre first appears but become reactive 1–4 weeks later. Two weeks to 6 months after the primary lesion disappears, the generalized cutaneous eruption of secondary syphilis may appear. The skin lesions heal spontaneously in 2–6 weeks. Serologic tests are almost always positive during the secondary phase. Latent syphilis may follow the secondary stage; it may last a lifetime, or tertiary syphilis may develop. Tertiary syphilis occurs in one-third of untreated cases, usually 4–20 years or more after the primary lesion disappears. The complications are fatal in almost 25% of cases, but 25% of patients with tertiary syphilis never show any ill effects.

Clinical Findings

A. Symptoms and Signs:

1. Primary syphilis–The chancre, an indurated, firm, painless papule or ulcer with raised borders, develops at the portal of entry 10–90 days (average, 21 days) after exposure. Genital lesions are not usually seen in women unless they occur on the external genitalia; however, careful examination may reveal a typical cervical or vaginal lesion. Primary lesions may occur in all body locations, and darkfield examination is required for all suspect lesions. Groin lymph nodes may be enlarged, firm, and painless. Serologic tests should be done every week for 6 weeks.

2. Secondary syphilis–About 2 weeks to 6 months (average, 6 weeks) after the disappearance of the primary lesion, a rash develops. The typical lesions are maculopapular, follicular, or pustular. "Moth-eaten" alopecia in the occipital area of the scalp is characteristic. The lateral third of the eyebrows may be lost. Moist papules occur in the anogenital area and the mouth—this eruption, known as condyloma latum, is diagnostic of the disease. *T pallidum* may be recovered from the lesions, and serologic tests are positive. Lymphadenopathy is an important finding; occasionally, splenomegaly is noted. Needle aspiration of enlarged lymph nodes produces fluid that is usually positive for syphilis by darkfield examination.

3. Latent syphilis–By definition, latent syphilis has no clinical signs or symptoms. The only positive finding is reactive serum and, sometimes, spinal fluid. In early latency (the first 4 years after infection), infectious lesions may recur. After this, the disease is rarely communicable except from mother to fetus.

4. Tertiary syphilis–Neurologic, vascular, and other lesions characteristic of tertiary syphilis may be reviewed in standard textbooks.

5. Syphilis during pregnancy–At least two-thirds of pregnant women with syphilis are 20–30 years of age. Pregnancy appears to decrease the severity of syphilis in many pregnant women. The chancre is often unnoticed, insignificant, and asymptomatic; and the nonpruritic rash may be transitory. Occasionally, the primary and secondary phases may be florid and complicated by secondary infection. Pregnancy will neither alter relapses after inadequate treatment nor modify latent or tertiary syphilis.

The effect of syphilis on pregnancy and the fetus depends largely upon whether the maternal infection occurs before pregnancy, at conception, or later. As the years pass from the time the mother contracted syphilis, the likelihood of a fetus showing serologic or other evidence of syphilis diminishes despite lack of treatment. Untreated syphilis contracted more than a few months to several years prior to pregnancy usually causes midtrimester abortion or fetal death. Abortion early in pregnancy is uncommon. When infection occurs at the time of conception or early in pregnancy and is not treated, the fetus, deformed by congenital syphilis, is often delivered prematurely. Syphilis contracted in the second half of pregnancy may or may not result in a syphilitic infant.

6. Congenital syphilis–The newborn with congenital syphilis may be undergrown, with wrinkled facies because of reduced subcutaneous fat. The skin may have a brownish (café au lait) tint. The most common lesion of early congenital syphilis in the newborn is a bullous rash, so-called syphilitic pemphigus. Large blebs may appear over the palms and soles and occasionally in other areas. Seropurulent fluid from the lesions swarms with treponemes.

Mucositis identical with that of secondary syphilis in older subjects may be noted in the mouth and upper respiratory passages of the newborn. The nasal discharge ("syphilitic snuffles") is very infectious because it contains large numbers of *T pallidum*.

The newborn may have lymphadenitis and an enlarged liver and spleen. The bones usually show signs of osteochondritis and an irregular epiphyseal juncture (Guérin's line) on x-ray. Abnormalities of the eyes, central nervous system structures, and other organs may be apparent at birth, or defects may develop later in untreated cases.

Any infant with the stigmas of syphilis should be placed in isolation until a definite diagnosis can be made and treatment given.

Newborns with congenital syphilis may appear healthy at birth but often develop symptoms weeks or months later. If the mother's serologic test is positive at delivery, the infant's will also be positive. At intervals of 3 weeks over a period of 4 months, examine the infant for stigmas of syphilis and obtain blood for serial quantitative serologic tests for syphilis. A rising titer indicates congenital syphilis and the need for treatment.

B. Laboratory Findings:

1. Microscopic examination–*T pallidum* can usually be identified by darkfield examination of specimens from cutaneous lesions, but the period during which treponemes can be recovered is very brief; in most cases, diagnosis depends on the history and serologic tests. An immunofluorescence technique for demonstrating *T pallidum* in dried smears of fluid from early syphilitic lesions is now available.

2. Serologic tests–Serologic tests become positive several weeks after the primary lesion appears.

a. Nontreponemal antigen tests–Commonly employed nontreponemal antigen tests are of 2 types: flocculation (VDRL, Hinton) and complement fixation (Kolmer, Wassermann). The flocculation tests are rapid, inexpensive, and easy to perform and are therefore used primarily for routine (often automated) screening for syphilis.

The VDRL test (the nontreponemal test in widest use) usually becomes positive 4–6 weeks after infection, or 1–3 weeks after the appearance of the primary lesion; it is almost invariably positive in the secondary stage. The VDRL titer is usually high in secondary syphilis and tends to be lower or even nil in late forms of syphilis, although this is highly variable. A falling titer in treated early syphilis or a falling or stable titer in latent or late syphilis suggests satisfactory response to treatment. These serologic tests are not highly specific and must be closely correlated with other clinical and laboratory findings. "False-positive" serologic reactions are frequently encountered in nonvenereal treponematoses and a wide variety of nontreponemal states including collagen diseases, infectious mononucleosis, malaria, many febrile diseases, leprosy, vaccination, drug addiction, old age, and possibly pregnancy. False-positive reactions are usually of low titer and transient and may be distinguished from true positives by specific treponemal antibody tests.

The rapid plasma reagin (RPR) test is a simple, rapid, and reliable substitute for the traditional VDRL test and gives comparable results. It is suitable for automated screening tests.

b. Treponemal antibody tests–The fluorescent treponemal antibody absorption (FTA-ABS) test is the most widely employed treponemal test. It measures antibodies capable of reacting with killed *T pallidum* after absorption of the patient's serum with extracts of nonpathogenic treponemes. This test shows excellent specificity and sensitivity. It is the first to become positive in early syphilis, and it usually remains positive for many years after effective treatment of early syphilis. It cannot be used to monitor the efficacy of treatment. The FTA-ABS test has now generally replaced the *T pallidum* immobilization (TPI) test, which assays the ability of a patient's serum to immobilize live virulent spirochetes.

A treponemal passive hemagglutination (TPHA) test is comparable in specificity and sensitivity to the FTA-ABS test but becomes positive somewhat later in infection.

Pregnant women should have a routine nontreponemal serologic test for syphilis at the first antenatal visit. Those suspected to be at increased risk for syphilis should be retested late in pregnancy and again on admission to the hospital. Seroreactive patients should be evaluated promptly. Evaluation includes the history (including prior therapy), a physical examination, a quantitative nontreponemal test, and a confirmatory treponemal test. If the FTA-ABS test is nonreactive and there is no clinical evidence of syphilis, treatment may be withheld. Both the quantitative nontreponemal test and the FTA-ABS test should be repeated in 4 weeks. If the diagnosis of syphilis cannot be excluded with reasonable certainty, the patient should be treated as outlined below.

Patients for whom there is documentation of adequate treatment for syphilis in the past need not be re-treated unless there is clinical or serologic evidence of reinfection (eg, 4-fold rise in titer of a quantitative nontreponemal test).

A positive serologic test is not proof of syphilis, nor is a negative test an absolute refutation of the diagnosis. False-positive non-treponemal serologic tests occur in up to 10% of clinic patients; the causes are listed above. False-positive treponemal antibody tests occur rarely in systemic lupus erythematosus and some disorders associated with abnormal hemoglobins.

Differential Diagnosis

Primary syphilis must be differentiated from chancroid, granuloma inguinale, lymphogranuloma venereum, herpes genitalis, carcinoma, scabies, trauma, lichen planus, psoriasis, drug eruption, aphthosis, mycotic infections, Reiter's syndrome, and Bowen's disease.

Secondary syphilis must be differentiated from pityriasis rosea, psoriasis, lichen planus, tinea versicolor, drug eruption, "id" eruptions, perlèche, parasitic infections, iritis, neuroretinitis, condyloma acuminatum, acute exanthems, infectious mononucleosis, alopecia of other origin, and sarcoidosis.

Prevention & Control

At present, the incidence of syphilis (and other sexually transmitted diseases) is rising in most parts of the world. With the exceptions of congenital syphilis and the rare occupational exposure of medical personnel, syphilis is acquired through sexual exposure. An infected person may remain contagious for 3–5 years during "early" syphilis. "Late" syphilis, of more than 5 years' duration, is usually not contagious. Because the cutaneous lesions of syphilis are highly infectious and the disease may be spread by direct contact, aseptic technique should be used in caring for syphilitic patients.

Control measures depend on (1) teaching young people about the disease and its consequences; (2) prompt and adequate treatment of all discovered cases; (3) follow-up on sources of infection and contacts so they can be treated; (4) sex hygiene; and (5) prophylaxis at the time of exposure. Both mechanical prophylaxis (condoms) and chemoprophylaxis (eg, penicillin after exposure) have great limitations. Washing the genitalia after exposure may afford some protection to males. Several venereal diseases can be transmitted simultaneously. Therefore, it is important to consider the possibility of syphilis when any sexually transmitted disease has been found.

Patients with infectious syphilis must abstain from sexual activity until rendered noninfectious by antibiotic therapy. All cases of syphilis must be reported to the appropriate public health agency for assistance in identifying and investigating all contacts.

Treatment

A. Penicillin Regimens:

1. Primary syphilis–Give benzathine penicillin G, 1.2 million units in each buttock, for a total dose of 2.4 million units once. Sometimes a dose of the same size is given twice more at weekly intervals, especially when a typical lesion was not observed by the physician. Other regimens of penicillin are less desirable.

2. Secondary syphilis–Treatment is as for primary syphilis unless central nervous system disease is present, in which case treatment is as for neurosyphilis (see below). Isolation of the patient is important.

3. Latent syphilis–Give benzathine penicillin G, 2.4 million units intramuscularly 3 times at 7-day intervals. If the cerebrospinal fluid is not examined or if there is evidence of cerebrospinal fluid involvement, treat as for neurosyphilis.

4. Late syphilis–

a. Neurosyphilis–There is no simple established treatment schedule for neurosyphilis. The minimum acceptable therapy is as given for latent syphilis, but acute or treatment-resistant neurosyphilis is often treated with larger doses of short-acting penicillin (eg, aqueous penicillin G, 20 million units intravenously daily for 10–14 days).

It is most important to prevent neurosyphilis by prompt diagnosis, adequate treatment, and follow-up of early syphilis. Involvement of the central nervous system must be considered in all cases except those that are treated early and effectively and followed. Lumbar puncture should be performed on all patients with syphilis in the secondary or later stages. In the presence of definite cerebrospinal fluid or neurologic abnormalities, treat for neurosyphilis. The pretreatment clinical and laboratory evaluation should include detailed neurologic, ocular, psychiatric, and cerebrospinal fluid examinations.

All patients must have spinal fluid examinations at 3-month intervals for the first year and every 6 months for the second year following completion of antisyphilis therapy. The adequacy of response may be gauged by clinical improvement and effective and persistent reversal of cerebrospinal fluid changes. A second course of penicillin therapy may be given if necessary.

b. Cardiovascular syphilis–After treatment of cardiac problems, give benzathine penicillin G as for latent syphilis.

c. Benign late syphilis (cutaneous, osseous, and visceral gumma)–Treatment is as for latent syphilis.

5. Syphilis in pregnancy–For pregnant patients with syphilis, the preferred treatment is with penicillin in dosage schedules appropriate for the stage of syphilis (see above). Penicillin prevents congenital syphilis in 90% of cases, even when treatment is given late in pregnancy.

For patients definitely known to be allergic to penicillin, the drug of second choice is erythromycin (base, stearate, or ethylsuccinate) in dosage schedules appropriate for the stage of syphilis. Such treatment is safe for the mother and the child, but the efficacy is not clearly established. Therefore, the documentation of penicillin allergy is particularly important before a decision is made not to use the first-choice drug. Erythromycin estolate and tetracycline are not recommended because of potential adverse effects on the mother and fetus.

The infant should be evaluated immediately and at 6–8 weeks of age (see above).

If the patient is in labor and has untreated syphilis, give an initial 3 million units of aqueous procaine penicillin G intramuscularly and 2 million units every other day for a total of 6 million units. Treat the infant for congenital syphilis.

6. Congenital syphilis–Adequate treatment of the mother before the 16th–18th week of pregnancy prevents congenital syphilis. Treatment thereafter may arrest syphilitic infection in the fetus, but some stigmas may remain. If the cerebrospinal fluid is normal, give benzathine penicillin G, 50,000 units/kg intramuscularly as a single dose. If the diagnosis of congenital neurosyphilis cannot be excluded, the infant should receive aqueous penicillin G, 50,000 units/kg/d in 2 divided doses intravenously or intramuscularly for 10 days; or aqueous procaine penicillin G, 50,000 units/kg/d intramuscularly for a minimum of 10 days.

B. Alternative Antibiotics for Adults: Oral tetracyclines and erythromycins are effective in the treatment of syphilis for patients who are sensitive to penicillin. Tetracycline, 30–40 g, or erythromycin, 30–40 g, is given over a period of 10–15 days in early syphilis; twice as much is recommended for syphilis of more than 1 year's duration. Since experience with these antibiotics in the treatment of syphilis is limited, careful follow-up is necessary. For alternative antibiotics to be used during pregnancy, see above.

3. CHANCROID
(Soft Chancre)

Chancroid, an acute, localized, sexually transmitted disease characterized by a painful genital ulcer, is caused by the short, gram-negative, nonmotile bacillus *Haemophilus ducreyi*. Exposure is usually via coitus, but accidentally acquired infections of the hands have occurred. The incubation period is usually 3–5 days, but if the organism enters an open wound, it may appear within 24 hours.

Clinical Findings
A. Symptoms and Signs: The initial lesion is a vesicopustule on the pudendum, vagina, or cervix. Later, it degenerates into a saucer-

shaped ragged ulcer circumscribed by an inflammatory wheal. The lesion is typically very tender and produces a heavy, foul, highly contagious discharge. A cluster of ulcers may develop.

Painful inguinal adenitis occurs in over half of cases. The buboes may become necrotic and drain spontaneously.

B. Laboratory Findings: Gram staining of material from lesions may show gram-negative rods in strands. Swabs from lesions are best cultured on chocolate agar with 1% Isovitalex and vancomycin, 3 μg/mL, to yield *H ducreyi*. The chancroid skin test may become positive and remain positive for life. Mixed infection with sexually transmitted organisms (including syphilis and herpes) is very common, as is infection of the ulcer with fusiforms, spirochetes, and other organisms.

Differential Diagnosis

Syphilis, granuloma inguinale, and lymphogranuloma venereum should be ruled out.

Prevention

Chancroid is a reportable disease. Routine antibiotic prophylaxis is not warranted. Condoms give good protection. Soap and water liberally used are more effective than common antiseptics. Education is essential.

Treatment

A. Local Treatment: The early lesions should be cleansed with mild soap solution.

B. Antibiotic Treatment: Give trimethoprim, 160 mg, and sulfamethoxazole, 800 mg, orally every 12 hours for 2 weeks. Sulfonamides have the advantage of not interfering with the diagnosis of syphilis.

The tetracyclines are effective in doses of 500 mg orally 4 times a day for 2 weeks or until healing is complete.

Prognosis

Untreated or poorly managed cases of chancroid may persist, and secondary infection may develop. Chancroid usually responds to treatment and tends to be self-limited. In rare cases, it becomes widely destructive, with multiple serpiginous or even phagedenic ulceration.

4. GRANULOMA INGUINALE

Granuloma inguinale, a chronic, relapsing ulcerative granulomatous disease that usually develops in the perineum and inguinal regions, is caused by *Calymmatobacterium granulomatis*. Mononuclear leukocytes containing intracytoplasmic cysts filled with bacteria (Donovan bodies) are pathognomonic. Transmission is via coitus. The incubation period is 8–12 weeks.

Clinical Findings

A. Symptoms and Signs: Granuloma inguinale most often involves the skin and subcutaneous tissues of the vulva and inguinal regions. A malodorous discharge is characteristic. The infection often begins as a papule that then ulcerates, developing a beefy-red granular zone with clean, sharp edges. The ulcer heals very slowly, and satellite ulcers may unite to form a large lesion. There are usually no local or systemic symptoms. Lymphatic permeation is rare, but lymphadenitis may result when the cutaneous lesion becomes superimposed on lymphatic channels. Inguinal swelling is common, with late formation of abscesses (buboes). Chronic cervical lesions may occur. They produce an inflammatory exudate containing many lymphocytes, giant cells, and histiocytes. Granuloma inguinale may mimic carcinoma of the cervix and must be distinguished from this as well as other neoplastic diseases.

The chronic ulcerative process may involve the urethra and the anal area, causing marked discomfort. Introital contraction may make coitus difficult or impossible; walking or sitting may become painful. Other sexually transmitted diseases may coexist. Granuloma inguinale spreads to other areas in about 7% of patients.

There are various types of lesions:

Vegetative or exuberant lesions are covered by soft, red, velvety hypertrophic granulation tissue.

Ulcerative lesions are described above. Secondary infection with spirochete-fusiform organisms is common and makes the lesion fetid and painful.

Chronic cicatricial lesions are characterized by a keloidlike scar.

B. Laboratory Findings: Gram-negative bipolar rods (Donovan bodies) within mononuclear leukocytes may be seen on a direct smear of a specimen taken from beneath the surface of an ulcer. These are seen best in Wright-stained smears. When smears are negative, a biopsy specimen will usually show granulation tissue infiltrated by plasma cells and scattered large macrophages containing Donovan bodies. Pseudoepitheliomatous hyperplasia often is seen at the margin of the ulcer.

The diagnosis is made if histologic sections or smears stained with Wright's, Giemsa's, or silver stain show large mononuclear cells containing one or more intracytoplasmic cysts filled with Donovan bodies—small round or rod-shaped particles that stain deeply.

Prevention

Use of condoms and washing the genitalia with soap and water immediately after intercourse are the best methods of prevention. Treatment immediately after exposure may abort the infection.

Treatment

A. Antibiotics: Tetracycline is the drug of choice. The recommended dose is 500 mg orally 4 times daily for 2 weeks. Occasionally, doses of 40–60 g may be required in resistant cases. Penicillin is not effective.

Streptomycin is effective but more toxic. The dose is 1 g intramuscularly 2–3 times daily for 7–10 days for a total of 21 g. As with tetracycline, 40–60 g may be necessary to ensure a cure. The disease will recur in 10% of cases.

B. Surgery and X-Ray: In chronically resistant cases, surgical debridement may be of value. Radiotherapy combined with administration of antibiotics is also effective in such cases.

C. General Measures: Because *C granulomatis* is probably present in the moist secretions from the lesions, care must be taken in handling dressings and contaminated articles.

The patient's underclothing should be laundered thoroughly by hand with iodine-containing soaps to prevent cross-contamination.

5. *GARDNERELLA VAGINALIS* VAGINITIS
(*Corynebacterium Vaginale* Vaginitis, *Haemophilus Vaginalis* Vaginitis)
(See Vulvovaginitis & Leukorrhea, p 514.)

6. LYMPHOGRANULOMA VENEREUM

Lymphogranuloma venereum is an acute and chronic disease caused by *Chlamydia trachomatis* types L_1–L_3. These chlamydiae are related to the agents of psittacosis and trachoma. Lymphogranuloma venereum is a sexually transmitted disease, but it is also transmitted by contact with exudate from active lesions, eg, in soiled dressings or clothing. The disease remains contagious until the lesions stop draining. *C trachomatis* disseminates through the lymphatics or bloodstream to create a chronic localized inflammatory disease. The incubation period is 5–21 days.

Clinical Findings

A. Symptoms and Signs:

1. Early–Initially, a vesicopustular eruption may go undetected; with inguinal (and vulvar) ulceration, lymphedema, and secondary bilateral invasion, the condition becomes excruciating. Sitting or walking may cause pain. During the inguinal bubo phase, which usually appears within 10–30 days after exposure, the groin is exquisitely tender. The buboes are red to purplish-blue, hard cutaneous indurations that may occur bilaterally. Anorectal lymphedema occurs early; defecation is painful, and the stool may be blood-streaked.

2. Late–Late manifestations are chronic cicatrizing inflammation of the rectal and perirectal tissue. Rectal stricture makes defecation difficult or impossible, and rectovaginal and perianal fistulas may develop. Vaginal narrowing and distortion may cause severe dyspareunia. Systemic invasion may occur, causing fever, headache, arthralgia, chills, abdominal cramps, skin rashes, conjunctivitis, and iritis.

B. Laboratory Findings: The diagnosis can be proved only by isolating *C trachomatis* from appropriate specimens and confirming the immunotype. These procedures are seldom available, so less specific tests are employed.

A complement fixation test utilizing a heat-stable antigen that is group-specific for all *Chlamydia* species is available. This test is positive at a titer of $\geq 1{:}16$ in more than 80% of cases of lymphogranuloma venereum. If acute or convalescent sera are available, then a rise in titer is particularly helpful in making the diagnosis.

Specific immunofluorescence tests for antibody can be performed. The Frei test (intradermal skin test) is obsolete. The nontreponemal serologic test for syphilis (VDRL) may be falsely positive.

Serum globulin levels are greatly elevated and the albumin/globulin ratio is usually reversed in chronic lymphogranuloma venereum. There may be slight leukocytosis with a shift to the left. Stained smears of pus, buboes, or biopsy material may be examined, but particles are rarely recognized. On histologic study of a biopsy specimen fixed with formalin or Bouin's solution, the lesion is seen to be a granulomatous tubercle with central fibrinoid necrosis (not caseation) surrounded by plasma cells (microabscesses). Lymph node tissue has a similar appearance.

Differential Diagnosis

As with any disseminated disease, the systemic symptoms of lymphogranuloma venereum may resemble meningitis, arthritis, pleurisy, or peritonitis. The cutaneous lesions must be differentiated from those of granuloma inguinale, tuberculosis, early syphilis, and chancroid. If lesions are present in the colon, proctoscopic examination and mucosal biopsy are needed to rule out carcinoma, schistosomiasis, and granuloma inguinale.

Complications

Perianal scarring and rectal strictures—late complications—can involve the entire sigmoid colon, but the urogenital diaphragm is rarely involved. Vulvar elephantiasis produces marked distortion of the external genitalia.

Prevention

The disease is reportable. Use of condoms or refraining from coitus minimizes the risk of infection, but it must be remembered that exudate from active lesions is infectious and can transmit the disease nonsexually. Case-finding and early treatment of infected persons are essential.

Treatment

A. Antibiotics: Tetracyclines should be given orally in daily doses of 2 g for 10–15 days according to tolerance. If disease persists, the course of therapy should be repeated. Sulfonamide drugs are only suppressive.

B. Local and Surgical Treatment: Place the patient at bed rest, apply warm compresses to buboes, and give analgesics. Anal strictures should be dilated manually at weekly intervals. Severe stricture may require diversionary colostomy. If the disease is arrested, complete vulvectomy may be done for cosmetic reasons. Abscesses should be aspirated, not incised, using aseptic technique.

C. Nursing Care: Aseptic technique (gowning, hand washing, gloving) is indicated. Because *C trachomatis* is present in exudates, contaminated dressings must be burned.

Prognosis

Prompt early treatment will cure the disorder and prevent late complications. Nevertheless, the longer treatment is delayed, the more difficult it is to eradicate the infection and to prevent gross distortion and ultimate marked disability. Late vulvar or rectal carcinoma is not uncommon in lymphogranuloma venereum.

7. HEPATITIS B
(Long Incubation Hepatitis, "Serum" Hepatitis, HBV)

Hepatitis B is a viral infection of the liver usually transmitted by inoculation of infected blood or blood products. However, the surface antigen (HBsAg) has been found in most body secretions, and it is known that the disease can be spread by oral or sexual contact. Hepatitis B virus (HBV) is highly prevalent in homosexuals and intravenous drug abusers. Other groups at high risk include patients and staff at hemodialysis centers, physicians, dentists, nurses, and personnel working in clinical and pathology laboratories. Approximately 5–10% of infected individuals become carriers, providing a substantial reservoir of infection. Forty to 70% of infants born to HBsAg-positive mothers will develop antigens to hepatitis B in the bloodstream. Fecal-oral transmission of virus B has also been documented. The incubation period of hepatitis B is 6 weeks to 6 months. Clinical features of hepatitis A and B are similar; however, the onset in hepatitis B tends to be more insidious.

The symptoms, general management, and outcome of hepatitis B are the same as those of hepatitis A (see p 352). Hepatitis B hyperimmune globulin may protect against hepatitis B if given in large doses within 7 days of exposure and again at 30 days. At present, this preparation is recommended for individuals exposed to HBsAg-contaminated material via the mucous membranes or through breaks in the skin. Persons who have had sexual contact with patients with acute HBsAg-positive disease should also receive hepatitis B hyperimmune globulin. Hepatitis B hyperimmune globulin is also indicated for newborn infants of HBsAg-positive mothers; give 0.5 mL very soon after birth and at ages 3 and 6 months. Hepatitis B hyperimmune globulin does not seem to be indicated in the prevention of transfusion-associated hepatitis.

A newly available vaccine for the prevention of hepatitis B has been extensively tested and found safe.

8. CYTOMEGALOVIRUS DISEASE
(See p 374.)

9. CONDYLOMATA ACUMINATA
(Genital Warts, Anal Condylomas)

These pink, elongated, pointed, soft, moist pruritic excrescences are often seen in the vagina, cervix, or anal canal or over the perineal and perianal regions. The causative agent, a papovavirus, is transmitted by coitus. The lesions become especially exuberant during pregnancy or during long-term immunosuppressive treatment. They may aggregate into a large mass that may even block the introitus during late delivery. Secondary infection is common. Condylomas usually regress markedly during the puerperium and may even disappear.

Podophyllum resin and fluorouracil are often effective in treating condylomata acuminata in nonpregnant individuals but are noxious to the fetus and therefore contraindicated during pregnancy. Pregnant women with condylomata acuminata should be treated by use of a laser beam, cryotherapy, fulguration, or excision of the lesions. Contraceptive creams appear to have both preventive and ameliorating effects. Local cleanliness and the frequent use of a talc dusting powder are beneficial.

Laryngeal papillomas are caused by a similar and perhaps identical virus, suggesting that infants may be infected by the genital wart virus of their mothers. While laryngeal papillomas are rare, they may obstruct the larynx and have to be removed repeatedly by surgical means.

10. NONGONOCOCCAL URETHRITIS (NGU)

Nongonococcal urethritis (NGU), a sexually transmitted disease, is an occasional problem in obstetric and gynecologic practice. NGU not caused by *Chlamydia trachomatis* immunotypes D–K is usually caused by *Ureaplasma urealyticum* (formerly called T strains of mycoplasmas).

NGU is more likely to be symptomatic in men, but women can be reservoirs for the offending organisms. Chlamydiae are often recovered from the cervix, and there may be overt cervicitis, salpingitis, or pelvic inflammatory disease. In pregnant women, carriage of *U urealyticum* in the cervix has been associated with chorioamnionitis and low-birth-weight infants. Both chlamydiae and *U urealyticum* can be transmitted to the newborn during its passage through the birth canal. Chlamydiae cause neonatal inclusion conjunctivitis, which is now far more common than gonococcal ophthalmia neonatorum though not as serious, and chlamydial pneumonitis, which appears in the first 2–6 months of life.

The diagnosis depends upon culture of the organism or, occasionally, on the demonstration of specific antibody titers in serum or ocular or genital secretions. Neonatal pneumonitis produces high titers of antichlamydial IgM antibody.

Both sex partners must receive antibiotic therapy. For chlamydial infections, give tetracycline HCl, 0.5 g 2–4 times daily for 2 weeks, or erythromycin, 0.5 g 2–3 times daily for 2 weeks. Pregnant women should be treated with erythromycin. Neonatal inclusion conjunctivitis can be managed by topical tetracycline in the conjunctival sac, but systemic erythromycin, 40 mg/kg/d, may be preferred if active chlamydial pneumonitis is suspected. Nongonococcal urethritis associated with *Ureaplasma* may be treated with trimethoprim-sulfamethoxazole, 2 tablets twice daily for 2 weeks.

11. HERPES GENITALIS

Herpes simplex virus type 2 infection of the lower genital tract is a sexually transmitted disease of increasing frequency and seriousness. It has been estimated that there are 500,000 cases of primary herpes simplex genitalis annually in the USA. The incidence varies greatly but may be one in 750 in obstetric or gynecologic clinic patients. This is many times the incidence among private patients and probably exceeds that of syphilis and gonorrhea in some social groups.

Patients complain of fever, malaise, anorexia, local genital pain, leukorrhea, dysuria, and even vaginal bleeding. Typical genital lesions are multiple shallow ulcerations, vesicles, and erythematous papules. Painful bilateral inguinal adenopathy is usually present. Scrapings and biopsies may show the characteristic homogeneous "ground glass"

appearance of cellular nuclei with numerous small intranuclear vacuoles, small scattered basophilic particles, acidophilic inclusion bodies,
and giant cells; these are best seen on hematoxylin and eosin stained
preparations. A scraping taken from the base of a vesicular or pustular
lesion of herpes and stained as a Papanicolaou smear will show the
characteristic giant cells of herpes genitalis in about two-thirds of cases.
However, these may be confused with malignant cells even by a
pathologist. Virus is easily recoverable from acute lesions if facilities for
tissue culture are available. Herpesvirus is very sensitive to drying and
cold, so specimens should be sent directly to the virus laboratory without
freezing. Approximately 85% of patients develop antibodies to type 2
virus within 21 days of primary infection.

Healing of the primary lesions is usually complete in 1–3 weeks.
Most women develop recurrent herpes after resolution of the primary
lesions, and recurrent episodes are the major cause of morbidity of
congenital herpes. Recurrent lesions are not as painful as the primary
ones and last only about 10 days. Affected individuals probably harbor
the virus indefinitely.

Acyclovir, 5% ointment (Zovirax), applied topically may give
some relief in primary genital herpes infections. It is of no benefit in
recurring herpes.

For recurrent lesions, local analgesic ointments (eg, 2% lidocaine)
may alleviate the pain, especially during vesiculation and ulceration.
Treatment for less than 2 weeks is suggested in order to avoid sensitization. Topical or systemic corticosteroids are not helpful in vulvovaginal
herpes. Ethyl ether is of no value.

The use of neutral red or proflavine and ultraviolet light to inactivate the virus has been disappointing. Moreover, this therapy may be
oncogenic.

Genital herpes is especially susceptible to secondary infection by C
albicans. Miconazole nitrate vaginal suppositories may be used prophylactically or therapeutically for this associated problem. Gonorrhea
and syphilis may coexist and must be ruled out.

Herpesvirus type 2 is associated with later cervical dysplasia and
may be a carcinogenic agent. Necrotizing cervicitis due to herpesvirus
may even resemble stage 2 squamous cell carcinoma. Herpesvirus infection during pregnancy is responsible for a higher incidence of spontaneous abortion, stillbirth, and neonatal death.

Genital herpes during pregnancy is especially hazardous for the
fetus. The overall risk to the offspring after 32 weeks of pregnancy is
about 10%. An infant delivered through an infected birth canal with
active lesions has approximately a 50% chance of developing
disseminated herpesvirus infection; if this occurs, the mortality rate is
about 50%. The risk is lessened if elective cesarean section can be
undertaken less than 4 hours after rupture of the membranes, but cesa-

rean section is no guarantee that the infant will not be infected. A mature fetus who contracts herpesvirus infection will usually have elevated serum IgM levels. The fetus or newborn with disseminated herpesvirus infection will probably die. Only supportive therapy is available. Strict isolation of the mother and fetus is mandatory.

Women who have contracted genital herpes must be educated about the disease—especially the fact that it is communicable when active lesions are present—and have long-term follow-up for possible cervical tumors.

The general rules for prevention of dissemination are as follows: (1) Precautions are unnecessary in the absence of active lesions. (2) Small lesions situated away from the oral or vaginal orifices may be covered with adhesive or paper tape during coitus. (3) In the presence of active lesions, whether or not the partner contracts the disease depends upon previous exposure to herpes. A nonimmune partner usually will be infected. If a regular partner has had genital herpes or has not been infected after prolonged exposure, no precautions will be necessary. If a casual partner has a history of genital herpes, a contraceptive cream or foam should be used, followed by genital cleansing with soap and water. If a partner has no history of genital herpes, a condom should be used.

PARASITIC INFECTIONS & OTHER INFESTATIONS OF THE FEMALE GENITAL TRACT

Trichomoniasis

See p 515.

Pediculosis Pubis

The crab louse, *Pthirus pubis,* is transmitted by sexual contact or from shared infected bedding or clothing. The louse eggs are laid at the base of pubic, axillary, or scalp hair shafts. When the eggs hatch, the lice must attach to the host's skin to survive; intense itching results. Minute pale-brown insects and their ova may be seen attached to the hair shafts near the skin.

Treat by applying 1% gamma benzene hexachloride (Kwell) cream, lotion, or shampoo according to the directions on the package insert (not recommended for pregnant or lactating women); or apply pyrethrins (Rid, Pyrinate 200) to the infested and adjacent hairy area and wash off after 10 minutes. Re-treat in 1 week if necessary. Treat all contacts, and sterilize infected bedding and clothing.

Scabies

Sarcoptes scabei causes intractable itching and excoriation of the surface in the vicinity of minute skin burrows where the parasites have deposited ova. The mite is usually transmitted directly from an infested person. An entire family may be affected.

Treat by applying 1% gamma benzene hexachloride (Kwell) cream or lotion (not recommended for pregnant or lactating women, infants, or children under 10 years of age) from the neck down overnight and washing off thoroughly after 8 hours, or use 10% crotamiton (Eurax) cream or lotion applied from the neck down nightly for 2 nights and washed off thoroughly after the second application. Contacts must also be treated to prevent recurrence, and all potentially infested clothing and bedding must be washed in hot water or dry-cleaned.

Enterobiasis (Pinworm, Seatworm)

Enterobius vermicularis, a short, spindle-shaped roundworm often called the pinworm, commonly infects children. Nocturnal perianal itching is described by the patient, and perianal excoriation can be observed. The most reliable diagnostic technique consists of applying a short strip of sealing cellulose pressure-sensitive tape (eg, Scotch Tape) to the perianal skin, spreading the tape on a slide, and examining the slide for adult worms or ova. Three such preparations made on consecutive mornings before bathing or defecation will establish the diagnosis in about 90% of cases.

Patients with enterobiasis must wash their hands and scrub their nails after defecation and again before meals. Their underclothes must be boiled.

Apply 1% ammoniated mercury ointment to the perianal region twice daily for relief of itching. Pinworms succumb to systemic treatment with pyrantel pamoate, mebendazole, or pyrvinium pamoate. Mebendazole should not be used during pregnancy.

MYCOTIC INFECTIONS
OF THE FEMALE GENITAL TRACT

Fungal Dermatitis

Tinea cruris is a superficial fungal infection of the genitocrural area. It is more common in men than in women and is usually caused by *Trichophyton mentagrophytes* or *Trichophyton rubrum.* This chronic pruritic skin disorder begins with superficial reddened, dry, scaly, confluent annular lesions on the inner upper thighs. Scratching causes lichenification. The diagnosis depends upon microscopic examination (as for *Candida*); culture on Sabouraud's medium is final proof. Treatment with tolnaftate, 1% haloprogin, 2% miconazole, or 1% clotrimazole is effective. Local measures to keep the involved area dry and prevent chafing are beneficial.

Deep Cellulitis Caused by Fungi

Blastomycosis is a deep mycosis that usually affects internal organs but may also involve the skin. Actinomycosis is a similar disease formerly thought to be a mycosis but now known to be caused by filamentous bacteria that superficially resemble fungi. Involvement of the vulvar skin in these diseases is very rare in the USA. The diagnosis is usually made by a process of exclusion of the granulomatous sexually transmitted diseases, tuberculosis, and other causes of chronic infection by laboratory means. Actinomycosis in some women is associated with an intrauterine contraceptive device. In such cases, the bacterial filaments are seen in discharge or diseased tissue as compact masses called sulfur granules. Anaerobic culture is required to distinguish *Actinomyces* from *Nocardia,* because specific treatment differs radically.

Treatment of blastomycosis with amphotericin B or hydroxystilbamidine is not very satisfactory. Actinomycosis can usually be treated successfully with penicillin G, 10–20 million units intramuscularly daily for 4–6 weeks.

Candidiasis

See p 515.

TOXIC SHOCK SYNDROME

This is characterized by abrupt onset of high fever, vomiting, and watery diarrhea. Sore throat, myalgias, and headache are often complaints. Hypotensive shock with renal and cardiac failure are ominous manifestations in severe cases. A diffuse macular erythematous rash and nonpurulent conjunctivitis are common, and desquamation, especially of palms and soles, is typical as the victim recovers. Reported fatality rates range from 3.2 to 15%.

Although toxic shock syndrome has occurred in children 8–17 years old and in males, the great majority of cases (90% or more) have been reported in women of child-bearing age. Of these, 95% or more have begun within 5 days of the onset of a menstrual period in women who have used tampons. If a woman recovers from the syndrome, she should forgo use of tampons. Outbreaks have also developed in surgical patients.

Staphylococcus aureus has been isolated from various sites including nasopharynx, vagina, rectum, or wounds, but blood cultures are negative. It is probable that the cause is a toxin produced by some strains of staphylococci. The toxin has not been definitely identified.

Important aspects of treatment include rapid rehydration, antistaphylococcal drugs, and management of renal or cardiac insufficiency.

SUPPURATIVE INFECTIONS
OF THE FEMALE GENITAL TRACT

Impetigo

Impetigo is a contagious and autoinoculable infection of the skin caused by staphylococci or streptococci or both. The infected material may be transmitted to the skin by dirty fingernails. In children, the source of infection is often another infected child.

Itching is the only symptom. The lesions consist of macules, vesicles, pustules, and honey-colored gummy crusts (streptococcal) that when removed leave denuded red areas. The face and other exposed parts are most often involved.

Impetigo neonatorum is a highly contagious, potentially serious form of staphylococcal impetigo occurring in infants. It requires prompt systemic treatment and protection of other infants (isolation, exclusion from the nursery of personnel with pyoderma, etc). The lesions are bullous and massive and accompanied by systemic toxicity. Death may occur.

The patient must be segregated and the blebs incised surgically, the ulcerative areas exposed, and specimens taken for culture; the crusts should be removed aseptically. Neomycin or bacitracin cream should be applied twice a day for 1 week.

Furunculosis

Furunculosis (boils) is a staphylococcal infection that appears as perifollicular abscesses. Throbbing pain and regional tenderness are present. Pustular areas require incision and drainage. Specimens from the opened lesions should be cultured.

The patient must be segregated and topical moist heat applied periodically. Prescribe systemic antibiotics (eg, a cephalosporin) when indicated.

Erysipelas

Erysipelas, an acute inflammation of the skin and subcutaneous tissue caused by beta-hemolytic streptococci, appears as a reddened, slightly raised, and confluent induration. It occurs classically on the cheek. Vulvar erysipelas is extremely rare and usually follows trauma to the vulva or vulvar surgery. Fever, vulvar burning and aching, and acute local tenderness are typical. The onset is usually rapid. Culture the drainage for beta-hemolytic streptococci.

The patient must be isolated. Place the patient at bed rest with the head of the bed elevated, apply hot packs, and give aspirin for pain and fever. Intensive treatment with systemic antibiotics such as procaine penicillin G, 1–2 million units intramuscularly and the dose repeated in 12 hours, is indicated.

Hidradenitis

Hidradenitis is a refractory infection of the apocrine sweat glands, usually caused by staphylococci or streptococci. It is analogous to cystic acne. Symptoms are soreness and local swelling, with edema, cellulitis, and suppuration, often of the groin. Involvement of apocrine glands establishes the diagnosis.

Treatment consists of hot, wet packs, drainage, and specific antibiotics chosen on the basis of organism sensitivity tests. Excision may be necessary; the wound must be allowed to heal by second intention.

Tuberculosis (Usually Vulvovaginal Lupus Vulgaris)

Pudendal tuberculosis is manifested by chronic, minimally painful, exudative "sores" that are tender, reddish, raised, moderately firm, and nodular, with central "apple jelly"-like contents. Ulcerative, undermined, necrotic, discharging lesions develop later. There is some tendency toward healing, with heavy scarring. Induration and sinus formation are common in the scrofulous type of infection. Cancer and sexually transmitted disease must be ruled out and tuberculosis sought elsewhere in the body. *M tuberculosis* should be identified by acid-fast smear, culture, or guinea pig inoculation.

Wet compresses of Burow's solution are helpful. Antituberculosis chemotherapy should be given.

BARTHOLIN DUCT ABSCESS & CYST

A soft swelling within the labia minora at the juncture of its mid and lower thirds usually indicates occlusion of Bartholin's duct. This is almost invariably the result of pyogenic infection, often with *N gonorrhoeae*. Secondary infection, usually with streptococci, staphylococci, or *Escherichia coli,* causes recurrent discomfort and enlargement of the duct. One duct is affected much more commonly than both ducts. Bartholin duct cysts are frequently seen in clinic patients but are not common in private practice.

Bartholin's duct is susceptible to infectious occlusion because of its narrowness, not because of its transitional cell lining. Infectious organisms pocketed within the passage form an abscess; the inflammation finally resolves, but permanent occlusion of the distal tract causes retention of mucus produced by the gland, and a cyst develops. The gland is almost never as seriously involved as the duct.

Enlargement of Bartholin's duct or gland in the postmenopausal patient should arouse a suspicion of cancer, and biopsy is indicated.

Clinical Findings

Acute symptoms are ordinarily due to infection, which results in pain, tenderness, and dyspareunia. The surrounding tisues become inflamed and edematous. One or both labia are swollen, and the introitus is distorted. A fluctuant mass can usually be palpated.

Unless there is an extensive inflammatory process, few systemic symptoms or signs of infection are likely. Smears and cultures of the ostium of Bartholin's duct and the cervical canal are required for specific bacteriologic diagnosis, eg, gonorrhea.

Differential Diagnosis

Bartholin duct cyst must be differentiated from inclusion cysts (after vulvar laceration or episiotomy), large sebaceous cysts, hidradenoma, congenital anomalies, primary cancer, and secondary cancer metastatic to the vulvovaginal area.

Treatment

Primary treatment consists of drainage of the infected cyst or abscess, preferably by marsupialization (Fig 21–4). Marsupialization, or permanent fistula formation, is simple and effective. The procedure is feasible under local anesthesia. Fine, interrupted catgut sutures usually are employed.

Simple incision and drainage may provide temporary relief. However, the opening tends to become obstructed, and recurrent cystic dilatation and infection may result. Appropriate antibiotics should be given if considerable surrounding inflammation develops. Bed rest, local dry or moist heat (or both), and analgesics should be used as indicated.

Prognosis

Recurrent infection resulting in cystic dilatation of the duct is the rule unless a permanent opening for drainage is established.

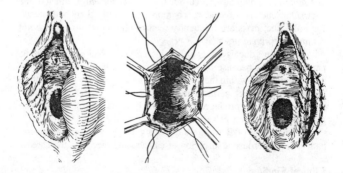

Figure 21–4. Marsupialization of Bartholin's cyst.

CANCER OF THE VULVA

Cancer of the vulva is the fourth most common female genital cancer (following cancer of the endometrium, the cervix, and the ovary) and accounts for about 5% of gynecologic cancers. About 85–90% of these tumors are epidermoid cancers. Less common tumors are extramammary Paget's disease, carcinoma of Bartholin's gland, basal cell carcinoma, melanoma, sarcoma, and metastatic cancers from other sites.

More than 50% of patients with vulvar cancer are over age 50; the average age is 65 years. However, it may occur at any age.

The cause of cancer of the vulva is not known. The disease is so common among the poor of all races that a causal relationship with poor personal hygiene and lack of medical care seems likely. Many vulvar cancers develop from or are associated with so-called premalignant conditions, eg, Paget's disease of the vulva. Predisposing and contributing causes, often so-called white lesions, include the following:

A. Leukoplakic Vulvitis: This is a hypertrophic-atrophic disorder of the genital skin and, to a lesser degree, the mucosal surface of the introitus. Several stages of leukoplakic vulvitis may be noted in different areas in the same patient. Cancer is infrequently associated with the early (hypertrophic) stage; often preceded and accompanied by the intermediate (leukokraurotic) phase; and only occasionally associated with the late kraurotic stage.

B. Chronic Granulomatous Disorders: Patients with long-standing lymphogranuloma venereum, granuloma inguinale, or syphilis have a much higher incidence of cancer of the vulva than others.

C. Chronic Irritation: Persistent scratching or excoriation of the vulva over a period of months or years as a result of pruritus vulvae may play a part in the development of vulvar cancer.

D. Paget's Disease of the Skin: Paget's disease is a forerunner of cancer. It arises from apocrine glands, particularly those in supernumerary breast tissue, which may be found in the labia majora. Although Paget's disease of the breast is much more common than its vulvar counterpart, the types are morphologically similar, and both affect patients in the same age group (50 years and over).

Paget's disease of the vulva is characterized by a red, moist, granular, nonsensitive area, usually in the labium majus. Numerous Paget's cells within a disordered epidermis are a diagnostic feature. These large, rounded, vacuolated cells do not have prickle projections and never become keratinized. Their cytoplasm contains mucopolysaccharide, and their prominent, dark nuclei often include several nucleoli. Malignant change may occur centrally or peripherally.

E. Pigmented Moles: Pigmented moles subjected to prolonged chafing by clothing or perineal pads may develop into malignant melanoma.

F. Irradiation: Radiation treatment of nonspecific pruritus vulvae or pelvic cancer has been postulated to cause vulvar cancer, but this has not been proved.

G. Intraepithelial Carcinoma: Bowen's disease of the vulvar skin, or carcinoma in situ, may ultimately develop into invasive epidermoid cancer. The frequency with which carcinoma in situ progresses to invasive vulvar cancer has not been established. Bowen's disease may appear as a bright red, velvety, slightly raised area, with an irregular margin in the labial skin. Unless infection or excoriation occurs, the skin is unbroken before invasive cancer develops. Biopsy is required for diagnosis.

Because of its origin and external location, vulvar cancer more closely resembles skin cancer than genital cancer. Cancers of the vulva are diagnosed most often (in order of frequency) in the labia majora, the prepuce of the clitoris, the labia minora, Bartholin's gland, and the vestibule of the vagina.

Most vulvar cancers begin as surface growths that ulcerate and extend downward and laterally. Only rarely do they progress from a deep site toward the surface. They grow slowly and, although metastases are unpredictable, the malignant cells probably remain in the regional lymph nodes for some time before they disseminate further. They then metastasize via the lymphatic drainage channels of the vulva to the superficial and deep inguinal and femoral nodes and the external iliac and obturator nodes.

Because the vulva is a bilateral, joined structure, the lymphatics anastomose and cross, and tumor cells spread from one side to the other by embolic transfer or by permeation of the lymphatic channels. The more anaplastic the tumor, the more likely it is to metastasize.

A classic early invasive epidermoid cancer of the vulva is a small, reddened, crusted, slightly exudative, nontender lesion with some peripheral thickening. Patients with chronic variable infections have fissured or exuberant areas that may not be typical of carcinoma but may include epidermoid cancer.

Histologically, typical grade I epidermoid carcinomas of the vulva are composed of well-differentiated spinal or prickle cells, many of which form keratotic pearls. Occasionally mitoses are seen. Malignant cells invade the subepithelial tissues, and leukocytes and lymphocytes infiltrate the stroma and tissues adjacent to the tumor. Less well differentiated tumors (grades II and III) also occur.

Malignant melanomas are usually single, hyperpigmented, raised, nontender, ulcerated lesions that bleed easily. Early spread via the venous system is common, and local recurrences frequently develop.

Basal cell carcinomas are ulcerated lesions composed of small, rounded, basophilic malignant cells derived from the innermost layers of the epidermis. The cells are arranged in irregular groups that often penetrate the underlying connective tissue. Occasional mitoses are observed, but there is no keratinization. Unlike keratinizing epidermoid carcinoma, basal cell carcinoma metastasizes late and infrequently; like malignant melanoma, it frequently recurs locally.

Adenocarcinoma arising in Bartholin's gland, most often seen in postmenopausal women, is at first indistinguishable from the gland itself. Gross enlargement and induration occur relatively late.

Clinical Findings

A. Symptoms and Signs: Nodular ulcerative lesions, especially those occurring in postmenopausal women and containing granulomatous or leukoplakic changes, are particularly suggestive of vulvar cancer.

Pruritus vulvae is the most common symptom of ulcerative vulvar cancer. Nodulation ("a lump") may be present for months or years before the patient consults a physician. Ulceration ("a sore"), odorous discharge, and bleeding usually occur late, but in postgranulomatous cases, these signs are often present early. Lymphadenopathy is always suggestive of carcinomatous metastases. Pain is a late symptom that depends upon the size and location of the tumor and the presence or absence of infection.

B. Recommended Diagnostic Procedures:

1. The admission work-up must include a complete blood count and differential count; hematocrit; blood urea nitrogen, creatinine, SGOT, lactate dehydrogenase, and electrolyte determinations; urinalysis; and chest x-ray and intravenous urography. An ECG will identify patients at potential high risk from anesthesia or operative procedures.

2. Any vulvar lesion that may be cancerous should be biopsied. Toluidine blue dye, a vital stain, may help to identify these sites for biopsy. Colposcopy may demonstrate a need for multiple biopsies. The diagnosis can only be made by histologic examination of biopsy specimens.

3. A skeletal survey should be performed if fixation is noted or other symptoms suggest possible bony metastasis.

4. Lymphangiography is indicated if the cancer is stage II–IV (Table 21–1).

5. Colposcopy, proctoscopy, or barium enema is required if symptoms suggest involvement of pelvic organs by the tumor or damage to pelvic organs during the course of therapy.

6. A liver scan is required if the diagnosis is malignant melanoma.

C. Staging: See Table 21–1.

Table 21—1. Staging of carcinoma of the vulva.*

Cases should be classified as carcinoma of the vulva when the primary site of the growth is in the vulva. Tumors present in the vulva as secondary growths from either a genital or extragenital site should be excluded from registration, as should cases of malignant melanoma. (See also Cancer of the Vagina.)

FIGO Nomenclature

Stage 0   Carcinoma in situ.

Stage I   Tumor confined to vulva—2 cm or less in diameter. Nodes are not palpable or are palpable in either groin, not enlarged, mobile (not clinically suspicious of cancer).

Stage II   Tumor confined to the vulva—more than 2 cm in diameter. Nodes are not palpable or are palpable in either groin, not enlarged, mobile (not clinically suspicious of cancer).

Stage III   Tumor of any size with (1) adjacent spread to the urethra and any or all of the vagina, the perineum, and the anus, and/or (2) nodes palpable in either or both groins (enlarged, firm, and mobile, not fixed but clinically suspicious of cancer).

Stage IV   Tumor of any size (1) infiltrating the bladder mucosa or the rectal mucosa or both, including the upper part of the urethral mucosa, and/or (2) fixed to the bone or other distant metastases. Fixed or ulcerated nodes in either or both groins.

TNM Nomenclature

1.1 Primary Tumor (T)

     TIS, T1, T2, T3, T4

         See corresponding FIGO stages.

1.2 Nodal Involvement (N)

     NX   Not possible to assess the regional nodes.

     NO   No involvement of regional nodes.

     N1   Evidence of regional node involvement.

     N3   Fixed or ulcerated nodes.

     N4   Juxtaregional node involvement.

1.3 Distant Metastasis (M)

     MX   Not assessed.

     MO   No (known) distant metastasis.

     M1   Distant metastasis present.

         Specify _____

*American Joint Committee for Cancer Staging and End-Results Reporting; Task Force on Gynecologic Sites: Staging System for Cancer at Gynecologic Sites, 1979.

Complications

A. Without Treatment: Untreated vulvar cancer pursues a slow, inexorable course marked by foul odor, bleeding, and soiling; vesicovaginal and rectovaginal fistulas; and breakdown and drainage of inguinal glands containing cancer metastases followed by lymphedema, pain, and thrombophlebitis. The patient usually dies of debility, inanition, or hemorrhage.

B. With Treatment:

1. Recurrence–Early recurrences may be local or remote; most appear within 1–3 years. Incomplete excision and unrecognized wide dispersion of cancer are the causes. Late recurrences (after 3 years) are almost invariably vulvar and tend to remain localized.

Wide excision prevents recurrences; lymphadenectomy, which must include the inguinal, superficial, and deep femoral nodes, is required.

2. Lymphedema of the legs is due to incompetent lymphatic and venous return; it may be caused by postoperative infection and scarring or by recurrence of cancer.

3. Hernia–Femoral and inguinal hernias result from weakened tissues, severance of Poupart's ligament, and incomplete repair of the musculofascial layers of the abdominal wall after lymphadenectomy.

4. Marked vaginal stenosis is not common. If pregnancy occurs after vulvectomy, cesarean section is only rarely required because of contracture of the introitus.

5. Prolapse of the cervix and uterus and urinary stress incontinence may occur as a consequence of wide, deep excision. To prevent these problems, an attempt should be made to reconstruct the levator fascia and perineal body. These parts of the pelvic floor are important for adequate support of the viscera.

Differential Diagnosis

Benign ulcerative or granulomatous lesions, eg, lymphogranuloma venereum, must be distinguished from various common cancers of the vulva or vagina.

A few vulvar carcinomas are secondary to breast, kidney, ovarian, bladder, or bowel tumors, and these primary tumors must also be diagnosed and treated.

Prevention

Early diagnosis and treatment of irritative factors that predispose to vulvar carcinoma will prevent many cases. Periodic gynecologic examination and excision biopsy of suspicious lesions allows early diagnosis and successful treatment. Simple vulvectomy is indicated for extensive lesions. Prominent or enlarging pigmented moles of the vulva should be removed before they become malignant.

Treatment

A. Surgical Measures: The primary treatment of vulvar cancer is wide excision of the tumor and extirpation of potential routes of dissemination. Surgery should always be done unless it is refused or contraindicated. The physician should be encouraging but firm and should make every reasonable effort to convince the patient and her family that the benefits of treatment are worth the substantial risks involved. A patient should not be denied a palliative vulvectomy because she is "a questionable operative risk." Expeditious, well-planned surgery, perhaps under local anesthesia, is usually well tolerated even by very old women. Relief from the offensive odor, discharge, bleeding, and pain makes surgery worthwhile. With modern surgical techniques, anesthesia, and appropriate supportive therapy, at least 80% of patients are operable.

Anemia and metabolic or cardiovascular disease should be treated intensively before surgery. Preoperative wide-spectrum antibiotic therapy for several days may be beneficial if local infection is likely.

The operation involves (1) extraperitoneal resection of the superficial and deep inguinal and femoral lymph nodes and (2) wide, deep excision of the entire vulva. Low-grade cancer does not justify less radical surgery. It is desirable to complete the entire procedure in one operative session if feasible. Large tumors are necrotic and infected with aerobic and anaerobic organisms, and prophylactic antibiotic therapy beginning on the evening before and for 24 hours after surgery may be desirable. Although an attempt must be made to isolate a large necrotic tumor during the operation, it may be difficult to accomplish vulvectomy without contaminating the operative wound. For this reason, groin dissection with or without extraperitoneal pelvic lymphadenectomy should be performed before vulvectomy. Postoperative suction drainage is also worthwhile because of the wide dissection, often in debilitated patients.

The extent of surgery should not be compromised in order to achieve primary closure, because in about 30% of cases closures will partially reopen anyway. Healing by second intention and use of Thiersch or full-thickness skin grafts may be necessary.

Basal cell carcinoma metastasizes so rarely and so late that most cases can be treated by wide, deep excision without lymphadenectomy. Radical vulvectomy without lymphadenectomy is probably sufficient for cancer that develops in chronic granulomas, because metastases are not likely to occur through lymphatics that have been occluded by infection.

In general, the operation should not be confined to one side; bilateral involvement is common because malignant and premalignant tissue usually exists in several sites and the lymphatic channels anastomose and cross.

When glands appear to be involved in the cancer process, a gland biopsy should not be done; the entire gland and all others in that area should be removed.

B. Irradiation: Radiotherapy is not often curative but is of great value in the treatment of recurrences, especially of basal cell carcinoma. It is also valuable in many instances of known incomplete surgery and for palliation of inoperable cancer. Unless metastases are discovered in the lymph glands, supplementary x-ray therapy does not improve the results of surgery sufficiently to justify the skin and other tissue damage that it may cause.

C. Chemotherapy: Recurrent or metastatic malignant melanoma may respond to anticancer drugs.

Prognosis

An approximate 5-year survival rate of 60% should be expected after complete surgical treatment of invasive epidermoid cancer. The primary factors determining survival are tumor size and nodal metastases. With tumors less than 2 cm in diameter, the incidence of nodal metastases is 10–15%. With nodal metastases, the 5-year survival rate varies from 15 to 30%. Only rarely do patients survive for 5 years after radical treatment of malignant melanoma.

The operative mortality rate is about 5%. Death may be due to cardiovascular complications, primary or secondary hemorrhage, infection, or venous thrombosis.

CANCER OF THE VAGINA

Primary cancer of the vagina represents about 1–2% of gynecologic cancers. It usually develops about 10 years after the menopause but may occur in children. Females 10–30 years of age whose mothers received diethylstilbestrol (or an analog) during early pregnancy may develop clear cell adenocarcinoma of the vagina or cervix. The upper third of the vagina is the most common site, but this tumor is multicentric and often involves both the vagina and the cervix.

About 75% of primary vaginal cancers are epidermoid cancers; the

Table 21–2. Staging of carcinoma of the vagina.*

Preinvasive carcinoma		
Stage	0	Carcinoma in situ, intraepithelial carcinoma.
Invasive carcinoma		
Stage	I	Carcinoma limited to the vaginal wall.
Stage	II	Carcinoma has involved the subvaginal tissue but has not extended to the pelvic wall.
Stage	III	Carcinoma has extended to the pelvic wall.
Stage	IV	Carcinoma has extended beyond the true pelvis or involved the mucosa of the bladder or rectum. Bullous edema as such does not permit allotment of a case to stage IV.
Stage	IVA	Spread of carcinoma to adjacent organs.
Stage	IVB	Spread to distant organs.

*American Joint Committee for Cancer Staging and End-Results Reporting; Task Force on Gynecologic Sites: Staging System for Cancer at Gynecologic Sites, 1979.

remainder, in decreasing order of frequency, are adenocarcinomas, sarcomas, and melanomas. Sarcomas are often botryoid in children and old women. Loose connective tissue and a rich vascular and lymphatic circulation favor rapid growth and early dissemination of the cancer. Tumors of the lower vagina metastasize like vulvar cancers; those in the upper vagina, like cervical cancers.

Painless bleeding is the initial manifestation in about 50% of cases and leukorrhea in about 25%. Less common complaints are a vaginal mass, pruritus, and constipation. Pain, weight loss, and swelling are late manifestations.

There are no typical gross characteristics. Most vaginal tumors are ulcerative and firm. A few are papillary or nodular. Careful physical examination and biopsy are required for diagnosis, although the appearance of the vaginal cytologic smear may be suggestive.

Primary vaginal cancer must be distinguished from extensions of vulvar or cervical cancer and from cancer metastases from the urinary tract, gastrointestinal tract, or ovary.

Treatment by irradiation is preferred in most cases. Radical surgery is usually chosen for vaginal cancers near the introitus, for sarcomas, and for definitely localized cancers involving the bowel, urethra, or bladder.

The prognosis depends upon the type, location, and extent of the tumor and the adequacy of treatment. With adequate treatment, the 5-year survival rate in stage I and II carcinoma in situ is about 70–75%. Melanomas are very malignant, and few respond to treatment. Survival data are not available for sarcoma of the vagina, but the prognosis is usually poor.

Diseases of the Cervix | 22

CERVICITIS

Cervicitis, the most common of all gynecologic disorders, affects over 50% of women at some time during adult life. It is usually characterized by eversion due to outward growth of endocervical cells. Chronic cervical infection is the most frequent cause of persistent leukorrhea and is a major etiologic factor in infertility, dyspareunia, and abortion. It may even be a stimulus (eg, herpesvirus infection) to the development of cervical carcinoma.

Over 60% of parous women have cervicitis. Cervicitis of variable duration occurs following virtually every delivery because the forcefully dilated cervix inevitably sustains many small lacerations, which become infected. Spontaneous and induced abortion and traumatic instrumentation are likewise often followed by cervicitis.

Other factors in the pathogenesis of cervicitis are poor hygiene (anal-vaginal contamination), diminished resistance to infection in estrogen depletion or vitamin deficiency, and irritation caused by tailed intrauterine contraceptive devices.

Acute and chronic cervicitis may be caused by gonorrhea that affects the cervix early in the disease. Although specific antibiotics usually destroy the gonococci, secondary invading organisms may persist for months or years as a cause of cervical infection.

The cervix is the reservoir for chlamydiae, microorganisms that cause inclusion conjunctivitis. Because genital tract symptoms are minimal, the primary infection may go unheeded.

Viruses may also infect the cervix. Herpesvirus—almost always type 2—produces an extensive transient superficial vesicular ulceration. Condylomata acuminata of the cervix, vagina, or vulva (see p 536) are caused by the same virus that produces the common skin wart (verruca vulgaris).

Cervicitis begins as a surface infection, but the endocervix becomes involved within hours. In 1–2 days, even the remote depths of the cervix are inflamed, and hypertrophy and hyperplasia of the glandular cells follow. Irritation due to infection results in hyperfunction of the glandular epithelium, producing copious leukorrhea. Because the infected glands evacuate poorly, they become dilated, and the fibromuscular supporting framework shields the inflammatory process.

When the columnar endocervical cells and the squamous portio cells are in functional equilibrium in adult life, their juncture is just within the external os. If the balance is disturbed by infection or hormonal aberrations, eversion or redness about the external os results as columnar cells extend beyond the os. With the reestablishment of equilibrium by hormone regulation or elimination of infection, the vaginal and endocervical pH becomes normal, and columnar cells regress toward the os. Complete obliteration of evidence of eversion or ectropion may not be possible, however; once columnar cells become established exteriorly, a zone or patch of reddish mucosa often persists, and glands in the portio continue to function, a few becoming cystic (nabothian cysts) when their drainage is obstructed.

"Erosion" is not a proper term for cervical redness except in cases of limited denudation of the mucosquamous junction that occurs early in virulent infection or after cauterization. In such acute processes, the squamous epithelium is lost for a very brief time and is replaced by either substituted tall columnar cells or squamous elements.

Cervical secretions depend upon hormonal, psychogenic, and irritative stimulation. A major role of the cervix in reproductive physiology is production of a thin, clear, acellular mucus in average amounts at ovulation. The mucus plug screens out pathogenic bacteria and permits the collection and transport of sperms to the uterine cavity. Reproduction is hindered by infected, thick, tenacious mucus or the absence of mucus. Heavy bacterial contamination causes loss of sodium chloride and water from the cervical mucus, and this results in increased viscosity and a decreased pH. Leukocytes and bacteria in the mucus are inimical to sperms, and few active sperms can be found in such mucus (negative Sims-Huhner test; see p 729).

Clinical Findings

A. Symptoms and Signs: In the absence of infection, the cervical mucus is thin, clear, and acellular at the time of ovulation or after moderate estrogen stimulation. In the late secretory phase, the mucus is mucopurulent and may be tenacious.

1. Leukorrhea–The most common presenting complaints referable to cervicitis are viscous, often odorous leukorrhea (see p 514); vulval burning; and pruritus.

2. Infertility–This is also a common presenting complaint referable to cervicitis. Thick, viscid, acid, pus-laden cervical mucus is noxious to sperms and prevents fertilization.

3. Backache–Lymphangitis of the uterosacral structures causes pain that is usually referred to the sacrum.

4. Lower abdominal pain, dyspareunia, dysmenorrhea–Pelvic congestion and parametritis often cause these symptoms.

5. Dysuria, frequency, urgency–Urinary distress may be due to posterior ureteritis and trigonitis secondary to cervicitis.

6. Metrorrhagia–Hyperemia of the infected cervix produces a freely bleeding surface. Such cervical ooze accounts for intermenstrual (often postcoital) spotting.

7. Abortion–Cervicitis is frequently followed by deciduitis and placentitis that lead to abortion early in pregnancy.

8. Cervical dystocia–Cervical fibrosis and stenosis may follow chronic cervical infection. Delayed or incomplete dilatation of the cervix may result.

9. Other symptoms and signs–Speculum exposure of the cervix in good light will often reveal a thick mucoid discharge exuding from the canal. Lacerations, eversion, and hypertrophy of the cervix may be apparent, together with occluded superficial cervical glands (nabothian cysts). Patulousness of the deeply lacerated external os exposes the endocervical canal, which may bleed when wiped with a cotton applicator. The portio and the upper vagina usually appear normal.

B. Laboratory Findings: In acute cervicitis, smears of the discharge reveal a thin purulent spread containing myriads of polymorphonuclear leukocytes. A Gram-stained smear may show intracellular gram-negative diplococci in gonorrhea. Staphylococci, streptococci, and *Escherichia coli* may also be found. The dried smear never shows the normal "fern" formation with clinical cervicitis.

Urine specimens obtained by catheterization of patients with cervicitis usually contain only occasional white cells, rare or absent erythrocytes, and no casts. Culture of the urine is generally negative in urethritis and trigonitis secondary to cervicitis.

The white blood count and differential count are rarely abnormal.

C. X-Ray Findings: Hysterograms may disclose hypertrophic rugous folds within the endocervical canal or even partial stenosis.

D. Colposcopy: Inflammatory changes will be seen.

Complications

Leukorrhea, cervical stenosis, and infertility are sequelae of chronic cervicitis. Chronic infection of the urinary tract may follow persistent cervicitis. Salpingitis is common with gonorrhea, chlamydial infection, and acute postabortal cervicitis.

It is postulated that carcinoma of the cervix may be caused by herpesvirus infections.

Differential Diagnosis

Leukorrhea and metrorrhagia also occur in early carcinoma of the cervix. Vaginal and cervical cytologic smears and scrapings and biopsies of the reddened areas are required for a definitive diagnosis. Sexually transmitted infections (eg, granuloma inguinale) and tuberculous involvement of the cervix must also be considerd.

When cervical discharge is present, rectovaginal examination should be done to detect pelvic tenderness, induration, and mass formation above the cervix.

Prevention

Prophylactic measures include (1) avoidance of traumatic delivery and instrumentation; (2) meticulous postpartal repair of cervical lacerations over 1.5 cm deep; (3) persistent, methodical treatment of cervical infections following pregnancy and delivery until the cervix is healed; (4) periodic gynecologic examination, including vaginal smears and cultures, and prompt treatment of cervical infection; (5) wider use of total (rather than subtotal) hysterectomy; (6) avoidance of sexual contact with infected individuals, or condom protection during coitus; and (7) good hygiene.

Treatment

Treatment depends upon the age of the patient and her desire for pregnancy, the severity of cervical involvement, the presence of complicating factors (eg, salpingitis), and previous treatment.

A. Acute Cervicitis: Acute gonococcal cervicitis must be treated promptly (see p 523). When acute cervicitis is associated with a specific vaginitis, treatment must be directed against the organism involved (see p 517). Instrumentation and vigorous topical therapy should be avoided during the acute phase and before the menses, when upward spread of the infection may occur.

B. Chronic Cervicitis:

1. Medical treatment–Medical treatment should be used initially for patients during and after the childbearing period. If the patient is unimproved after 2–3 months, minor surgical therapy is indicated.

a. A retroposed uterus should be repositioned and a pessary inserted to reduce chronic passive congestion.

b. Chemical cauterization of the ecto- and endocervix with 5–10% silver nitrate solution or 2–5% sodium hydroxide solution is effective when done during the midcycle.

c. Aqueous vaginal creams of low pH are helpful. Aci-Jel, one application after an acetic acid douche every night for 3 weeks during the intermenstrual period, may be used concomitantly with endocrine or antibiotic therapy at midcycle. The criterion of cure is a microscopically clear mucus with the consistency of saliva at ovulation.

2. Surgical treatment–Before treating cervicitis by surgery, one must consider the results desired; the likelihood of postoperative bleeding, infection, stricture formation, and infertility; and the implications for vaginal delivery in future pregnancies. Dilatation of the cervix and puncture of nabothian cysts may be done in the office at any time during the cycle. Any other type of surgery for cervicitis must not be done within 7 days of a menstrual period, because of the danger of salpingitis.

a. Severe chronic cervicitis or a cervical canal widely exposed by lacerations may be treated by cryotherapy or minor surgery. Minor surgical procedures include light electrocauterization with low-frequency current and a nasal tip or small Post electrode, or mild electrocoagulation with a high-frequency monopolar electrode. These procedures may be used to treat chronic cervicitis during or after the childbearing years.

With electrocoagulation (and electrosurgery), both incision and coagulation are possible, and the penetration of heat and destruction of diseased gland tissue are uniform and controllable. Cauterization or coagulation should be done radially (Fig 22–1). The latter is preferred. Complications (salpingitis and cervical stenosis) are more frequent following cauterization. Only portions of the canal and portio should be treated at any one visit, preferably during the first half of the cycle. In general, undertreatment is best. Several treatments 1 week apart may be required. Anesthesia is usually unnecessary for minor surgical treatment.

Immediately after cauterization, daily acetic acid douches or sulfonamide cream or suppositories locally for 3–4 days may be prescribed to suppress infection. Following extensive coagulation, the cervix should be gently dilated occasionally over the following 2 months to ensure patency of the canal.

b. Conization of the cervix (see p 488) may be indicated during the childbearing years, but lesser measures are usually successful.

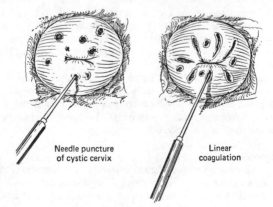

Needle puncture
of cystic cervix

Linear
coagulation

Figure 22–1. Cauterization (coagulation) of the cervix (after Ball).

c. Cryosurgery destroys tissue by a freeze-thaw sequence rather than by heat. The refrigerant (carbon dioxide, Freon, nitrous oxide, or nitrogen—all in liquid state) is passed through a hollow probe placed in the cervical canal and against the external os. The procedure can be done in the office. There is little or no pain, and anesthesia is usually not required. Serious scarring of the cervix or cervical stenosis rarely occurs, and excessive postoperative bleeding is exceptional. The disadvantages include copious serous discharge (a minor problem) and a prolonged healing period (3–6 weeks) following extensive cryosurgery. Sepsis occasionally develops. Expensive and somewhat cumbersome equipment is required.

C. Treatment of Complications:

1. Cervical hemorrhage–This may follow electrotherapy or trachelorrhaphy. The bleeding vessels must be sutured and ligated. Point coagulation of bleeding areas is often successful. Styptics such as negatol (Negatan) applied topically with snug vaginal packing are often helpful.

2. Salpingitis–Administer procaine penicillin G, 1.2 million units intramuscularly daily for 3–5 days, or tetracycline, 500 mg orally 4 times daily for 1 week.

3. Leukorrhea–Discharge is usually due to persistent infection. Re-treat, if necessary, after taking specimens for culture.

4. Cervical stenosis–Gentle passage of graduated sounds through the cervical canal at weekly intervals during the intermenstrual period for 2–3 months following treatment should prevent and correct stenosis.

5. Infertility–Absence of cervical mucus, which is necessary for sperm migration, often causes infertility and may be due to too extensive destruction (coagulation, cauterization) or removal (conization, trachelorrhaphy, amputation of the cervix) of the endocervical glandular cells. Conjugated estrogens (Premarin or equivalent), 0.3 mg orally daily for 3–4 days before and on the day of ovulation, may stimulate the remaining endocervical cells to produce more mucus. Artificial insemination may be required.

6. Cancer–(See p 561.) Tissue obtained at conization (see p 488) or amputation of the cervix must be examined by a pathologist. Later, vaginal and cervical cytologic smears, biopsies, or even repeat conization may be required if cancer is suspected. Treatment depends upon the type and stage of the cancer.

Prognosis

With a conservative, systematic, and persistent treatment program, cervicitis can almost always be cured. Mild chronic cervicitis usually responds to local therapy in 4–8 weeks; more severe chronic cervicitis may require 2–3 months of treatment.

CERVICAL POLYPS

Polyps are small, pedunculated, often sessile or tessellated tumors. The cause of polyp formation is not known, but local inflammation is a possible cause. Cervical polyps are common and may occur at any time after the menarche; the great majority are seen during the reproductive years, and an occasional one may form after the menopause. Most originate from the endocervix; a few arise from the portio. They eventually cause discharge or abnormal bleeding.

Endocervical polyps are usually red, flame-shaped, fragile growths rarely over 2 cm in length. They protrude from the os, are delicate, and bleed easily. They are supported by a connective tissue framework containing blood vessels centrally and mucous glands peripherally, and their surface is covered by tall, columnar mucus-producing cells typical of those within the endocervical canal.

Ectocervical polyps are pale, flesh-colored, and rounded or elongated, often with a broad pedicle. They arise from the portio and are less likely to bleed than endocervical polyps. They are more fibrous than endocervical polyps, have fewer, if any, mucous glands, and are covered by stratified squamous epithelium.

Inflammation, often with necrosis at the tip (or more extensively), is typical of both endocervical and ectocervical polyps. Metaplastic change is common, but carcinomatous change is rare. Endometrial cancer may involve polyps secondarily; sarcoma rarely develops within a polyp.

Botryoid sarcoma, an extremely malignant embryonal tumor of the cervix or vaginal wall, resembles small pink or yellow grapes and contains striated muscle and other mesenchymal elements.

Polypoid structures are vascular and often become infected, and they are subject to displacement or torsion. Discharge commonly results, and bleeding, often metrorrhagia of the postcoital type, follows.

Because polyps are a potential focus of cancer, they must routinely be examined for malignant characteristics on removal.

Clinical Findings

A. Symptoms and Signs: Leukorrhea is the most common sign. Abnormal vaginal bleeding is often reported, including postmenopausal bleeding in older women. Infertility may be traceable to cervical polyps and cervicitis.

B. Laboratory Findings: Vaginal cytologic smears show signs of infection and often abnormal cells of Papanicolaou class II–III (Table 22–2). Blood and urine studies are not helpful.

C. X-Ray Findings: Hysterosalpingography, using a blunt-tipped cannula, may disclose an occult endocervical polyp in the canal.

D. Special Examinations: Sounding the cervix may reveal a polyp within the canal not yet visible at the os. Surgical D&C (see p 441) may be required to outline and remove a polyp high in the canal.

Complications

All polyps are infected, some by virulent pathogens. Rarely, acute salpingitis may be initiated or exacerbated by polypectomy. A broad-spectrum antibiotic should be administered at the first sign or symptom of spreading infection.

It is unwise to remove a large polyp and then do a hysterectomy several days thereafter, because pelvic sepsis may complicate the latter

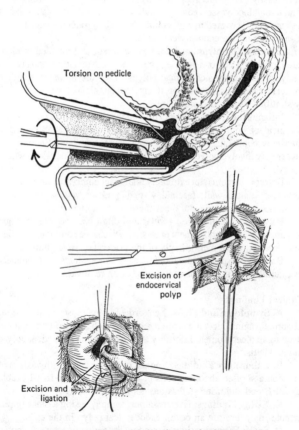

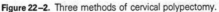

Figure 22–2. Three methods of cervical polypectomy.

procedure. An interval of several weeks between polypectomy and hysterectomy is recommended.

Differential Diagnosis

Masses projecting from the cervix may be polypoid but not polyps. Adenocarcinoma or sarcoma of the endometrium may present at the external os or even beyond. Discharge and bleeding usually occur.

Small submucous pedunculated myomas or endometrial polyps arising low in the uterus often result in dilatation of the cervix, so that they present just within the os and appear to be cervical polyps.

The products of conception, usually decidua, may push through the cervix and resemble a polypoid tissue mass, but other signs and symptoms of recent pregnancy are usually present.

Prevention

Cervicitis should be treated early and thoroughly. Periodic vaginal examination may disclose asymptomatic cervical polyps.

Treatment

A. Specific Measures: Remove the polyp by avulsion, scalpel excision (Fig 22–2), or high-frequency electrosurgery (all office procedures). Submit all tissue to a pathologist for histologic examination.

If the cervix is soft, patulous, or definitely dilated and the polyp is large, surgical D&C (see p 441) should be done, especially if the pedicle is not readily visible. Exploration of the cervical and uterine cavities with the polyp forceps and curet may disclose multiple polyps or other important lesions.

B. Local Measures: Warm acetic acid douches after polypectomy will usually control an inflammatory reaction. Prophylactic antibiotic therapy is not usually necessary.

Prognosis

Simple removal is usually curative.

CANCER OF THE CERVIX

Cancer of the cervix is the third most common malignant disease in women (breast and colon cancer occur more frequently). Cervical cancer accounts for two-thirds of all malignant disease of the female reproductive tract. It has been estimated that about 2% of all women over age 40 will develop cancer of the cervix. The average age at diagnosis of patients with cervical cancer is 45, but the disease can occur even in the second decade of life and occasionally during pregnancy.

Squamous cell carcinoma accounts for about 87% of cases and

adenocarcinoma or mixed adenosquamous carcinoma for about 13% of malignant epithelial cancers of the cervix. Sarcomas occur occasionally.

The cause of cervical cancer is not known, but certain predisposing factors are recognized. Sexual activity seems to be positively correlated with the disease, and intercourse at a relatively early age or with multiple partners is a highly significant factor. Conversely, celibacy and nulliparity reduce the statistical risk. Cancer of the cervix is rare among Jewish women, perhaps because of hereditary immunity or because Jewish males are circumcised in infancy and genital hygiene is better.

Numerous females whose mothers received even small amounts of diethylstilbestrol or other nonsteroidal synthetic estrogens during the first trimester of pregnancy have developed cervical anomalies, adenosis, or a particularly aggressive so-called clear cell carcinoma.

Pathology

A. Cervical Intraepithelial Neoplasia (CIN): CIN forms a continuum beginning with mild dysplasia and ending with invasive carcinoma. CIN almost always arises within the transformation zone—that area of the ectocervix near the external os where everting columnar epithelium from the endocervical canal has been "transformed" by metaplasia into squamous epithelium. Hormonal changes and local disease processes are responsible.

The degree (grade) of CIN is determined by the extent to which the neoplastic cells involve the full thickness of the cervical epithelium. The designation is mild dysplasia (CIN grade 1) if the neoplastic cells are confined to the lower third of the epithelium; moderate dysplasia (CIN grade 2) if they occupy up to two-thirds of the thickness of the epithelium; severe dysplasia (CIN grade 3) if undifferentiated neoplastic cells extend almost to the surface; and carcinoma in situ (CIS, but still CIN grade 3) if the full thickness of the epithelium is composed of undifferentiated neoplastic cells. While controversy continues over the definition of the early stages of disease and the natural history of each, it is agreed that CIN may follow 3 courses: regression, persistence, or progression to cancerous invasion. The risk of progression increases with increasing anaplasia. Spontaneous regression rarely occurs once CIS is established, and invasive cancer often occurs in 5–10 years. Thus, the cancer must be eradicated as soon as it is diagnosed.

The peak age at which carcinoma in situ appears is 30–40 years, but CIN grade 1 occurs most often in the teens, when sexual activity often begins.

In most cases, CIN changes occurring in the transformation zone over the portio of the cervix, where initial columnar epithelium is replaced by metaplastic squamous cells, can be detected by colposcopy (see p 489). Occasionally, CIN may begin within the endocervical canal, probably from islands of so-called reserve epithelial cells.

The prognosis is good except in extensive, severe cervical dysplasia, which may represent underdiagnosed carcinoma.

B. Epidermoid Carcinoma: Basal cell hyperplasia and CIN usually precede carcinoma in situ (CIS), which often becomes invasive cancer. At least 90% of squamous cell carcinomas of the cervix develop in the intraepithelial layers at or near the squamocolumnar junction.

Epidermoid cancers of the cervix are graded according to the predominant cell type or degree of differentiation (Broders' index). Grade 1 carcinoma is highly differentiated; grade 2, moderately well differentiated; and grade 3, completely undifferentiated.

The histologic criteria for grading squamous cell carcinoma are as follows:

In grade 1, there are many epithelial pearls, marked keratinization, easily identifiable intercellular bridges, fewer than 2 mitoses per high-power field, and minimal variation in the size and shape of tumor cells.

In grade 2, there are infrequent epithelial pearls, moderate keratinization, occasional intercellular bridges, 2–4 mitoses per high-power field, and moderate variation in size and shape of tumor cells.

In grade 3, there are no epithelial pearls; slight keratinization; no intercellular bridges; more than 4 mitoses per high-power field; often marked variation in size and shape of tumor cells; occasional small, elongated, closely packed tumor cells; and numerous giant cells.

Malignancy roughly parallels the grade: the undifferentiated variety metastasizes earlier but also responds better initially to radiation therapy.

C. Adenocarcinoma: Adenocarcinoma of the cervix arises from the glandular elements of the cervix. It is composed of tall, columnar secretory cells arranged in an adenomatous pattern with scant supporting stroma. A much less common adenocarcinoma, derived from mesonephric (wolffian) duct remnants within the cervix, is characterized by small, cuboidal, irregular cells and a less well defined glandular pattern. Adenocarcinoma of the cervix is not usually diagnosed until it is advanced and ulcerative.

During pregnancy, hypertrophic and hyperplastic squamous and glandular elements are obvious on biopsy. Intraepithelial as well as invasive carcinoma may also be present, however. Gestational changes should not be permitted to confuse the diagnosis.

Adenocarcinoma is graded as well differentiated, moderately well differentiated, and poorly differentiated. However, precise classification is not possible even after examination of numerous isolated fragments, because tissue variability is marked.

D. Invasive Carcinoma: Ulceration always implies necrosis of the epithelium. A carcinomatous process usually has a firm, somewhat raised edge; the base of the ulcer is indurated, irregular, and granular. If extensive necrosis is present, it is imperative that biopsy be done at the margin of the ulcer to compare abnormal with normal tissue.

Clinical Findings

A. Symptoms and Signs: There are no signs or symptoms of noninvasive cancer of the cervix.

Metrorrhagia is the most common sign of invasive malignant cervical ulceration, but hypermenorrhea may be reported, especially in advanced cervical cancer. Leukorrhea, usually sanguineous or purulent, odorous, and nonpruritic, may be present in invasive cervical cancer. Bladder and rectal dysfunction or fistulas are late symptoms. Pain is present only when obstruction occurs or when local pelvic nerve involvement develops. Anemia, anorexia, and weight loss are signs of advanced malignant disease.

Table 22—1. International classification of cancer of the cervix.*

Preinvasive carcinoma	
Stage 0	Carcinoma in situ, intraepithelial carcinoma.
Invasive carcinoma	
Stage I	Carcinoma strictly confined to the cervix (extension to the corpus should be disregarded).
IA	Microinvasive carcinoma (early stromal invasion).
IB	All other cases of stage I. (Occult cancer should be labeled "occ.")
Stage II	Carcinoma extends beyond the cervix but has not extended onto the pelvic wall. The carcinoma involves the vagina, but not the lower third.
IIA	No obvious parametrial involvement.
IIB	Obvious parametrial involvement.
Stage III	Carcinoma has extended to the pelvic wall. On rectal examination, there is no cancer-free space between the tumor and the pelvic wall. The tumor involves the lower third of the vagina. All cases with hydronephrosis or nonfunctioning kidney.
IIIA	No extension onto the pelvic wall.
IIIB	Extension onto the pelvic wall and/or hydronephrosis or nonfunctioning kidney.
Stage IV	Carcinoma extended beyond the true pelvis or clinically involving the mucosa of the bladder or rectum. Do not allow a case of bullous edema as such to be allotted to stage IV.
IVA	Spread of growth to adjacent organs (ie, rectum or bladder with positive biopsy from these organs).
IVB	Spread of growth to distant organs.

*American Joint Committee for Cancer Staging and End-Results Reporting; Task Force on Gynecologic Sites: Staging System for Cancer at Gynecologic Sites, 1979. *Note:* The interpretation of the physical and microscopic findings is to some extent subjective, and the personal opinion of the examiner unavoidably influences the staging of various cases. This is especially true with stages II and III. Therefore, when the results of therapy for carcinoma of the cervix are being reported, all cases examined should be reported so that the reader can determine what series of cases in his or her own experience the data are applicable to. In reporting the results of therapy for stage II carcinoma at a given institution, the statistics for stage III should be included so that the reader may compare the reported results with a more surely comparable series of cases at another institution.

B. Staging: The deeper the malignant cells invade beyond the basement membrane, the wider the extent of primary cancer within the cervix and the more likely that secondary or metastatic cancer has occurred. It is customary to stage cancers of the cervix and lymph node metastases as shown in Table 22–1 and Fig 22–3. Stage IA cervical cancer (microinvasion) is superficial invasion with minimal (< 3 mm) local spread only; otherwise, it is morphologically identical to frank epidermoid carcinoma. The diagnosis can be made only by systematic examination of serial sections from a cone biopsy specimen.

Microinvasion must be distinguished from occult cancer in which there are confluent, definite invasive foci of carcinoma.

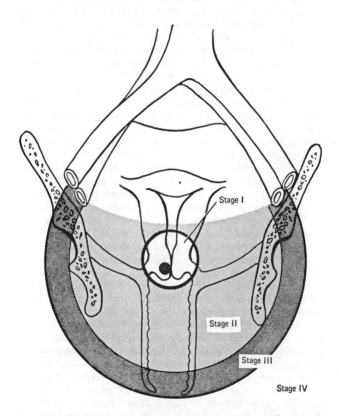

Figure 22–3. Staging of metastases of cervical cancer (corresponding to international classification; see Table 22–1).

The lymph nodes most often involved in the spread of carcinoma of the cervix are, in order of frequency, the obturator, hypogastric, common iliac, external iliac, aortic, sacral, and inguinal.

Although the bladder and rectum and the nerves within the pelvis are often invaded in advanced cervical cancer, metastases to distant organs such as lungs, liver, brain, and bone tend to occur late. They may not be identified clinically but are frequently recognized at autopsy.

C. Laboratory Findings: Blood counts are significant only when infection or anemia has developed as the result of hemorrhage or gross metastases to bone, or following intensive radiation therapy.

Carcinoma cells exfoliate from the surface of noninvasive tumors even more freely than from invasive lesions. Endometrial, tubal, ovarian, or other intraperitoneal cancers may shed cells that find their way down the genital tract. In an area of invasive cancer, infection causes cytolysis. Cytologic study and colposcopy and biopsy of suspicious areas facilitate early diagnosis and cure of cancer of the cervix. A positive cytologic smear calls for further investigation (see section on cervical intraepithelial neoplasia, above). Fewer than 2% of cytologic smears are falsely positive, but approximately 6% are falsely negative. Because inflammatory elements are present in greater numbers in invasive cancer and because in situ lesions shed malignant cells more readily, reports of cytologic studies are more frequently falsely negative in invasive lesions. Clinical signs and symptoms that suggest cancer require investigation despite a negative cytologic examination.

1. Schiller test–Aqueous solutions of iodine stain the surface of the normal cervix brown because normal cervical epithelial cells contain glycogen. Zones of cancer within the epithelium over the cervix do not contain glycogen and thus remain unstained when painted with Lugol's or Schiller's iodine solution, as do scars, erosion, eversion, cystic mucous glands, and zones of nonmalignant leukoplakia.

2. Vaginal cytologic (Papanicolaou) smear–See p 575.

D. X-Ray Findings: When invasive cervical cancer has been diagnosed, chest x-rays, intravenous urograms, a skeletal survey, and a barium enema study should be performed in an attempt to identify extensions or metastases. Pelvic lymphangiography may show involvement of the pelvic or periaortic lymph nodes.

E. Special Examinations: For any stage of invasive cancer of the cervix, the following studies and procedures are recommended: hemogram to detect anemia or infection; liver function tests and blood urea nitrogen determination to diagnose liver metastases or liver disease that might compromise chemotherapy; cystoscopy to detect extension of cancer to the bladder or associated bladder pathology; and sigmoidoscopy (for patients over age 50 years or those with bowel symptoms) to detect extension of cervical cancer and prevent colon complications due to irradiation. Ultrasonography is also useful to detect metastases.

Carcinoma in situ is not visible except by colposcopy. Upon colposcopic examination, preinvasive cervical carcinoma usually is seen as an area of coarse mosaicism and punctation. There is no ulceration, and no irregularity or mass can be seen or felt. Once sanguineous vaginal discharge or abnormal bleeding occurs, penetration of the cancer into the substance of the cervix is certain. Occasionally, a small patch of leukoplakia that represents preinvasive carcinoma may be found, or a thickened area in an eversion of the cervix may show such changes. Biopsy or cold conization of the cervix is required.

Biopsy should be avoided initially unless a definitely ulcerative or suspicious lesion is found. Four-quadrant biopsy of the cervix (Fig 19–5) or actual conization of the cervix and D&C may be required to identify or exclude invasive cancer when repeated, confirmed reports of suspicious or probable exfoliated carcinoma cells are made by the pathologist.

Complications

Metastases to regional lymph nodes occur with increasing frequency from stage I (about 15%) to stage IV (at least 60%).

Extension occurs in all directions. Most commonly, the tumor grows laterally in the base of the broad ligaments on one or both sides. The ureters are often obstructed lateral to the cervix. Hydroureter and hydronephrosis impair kidney function. Almost two-thirds of patients with carcinoma of the cervix die of uremia when ureteral obstruction is bilateral. Perivascular, perineural, and lymphatic channels facilitate cancer spread.

Cervical carcinoma may invade the uterus by direct surface extension up the cervical canal; downward extension often involves the vagina.

Invasion of the rectum is by posterior extension from the cervix along the uterosacral ligaments.

Anterior extension is followed by invasion of the bladder in stages III and IV.

Pain and swelling in the leg, particularly the upper thigh, may indicate lymphatic occlusion or obstruction of the venous return by carcinoma.

Pain in the back and in the distribution of the lumbosacral plexus indicates chronic infection or neurologic involvement by extending cancer.

Pelvic infections may complicate cervical carcinoma. Obstruction of the cervical canal may require drainage of a pyometra and chemotherapy to reduce infection.

Death due to hemorrhage occurs in about 10–20% of cases of extensive invasive carcinoma of the cervix. Protracted bleeding will cause anemia.

Vaginal fistulas involving the gastrointestinal and urinary tracts are particularly discouraging. Incontinence of urine and feces are major complications, particularly in debilitated individuals.

Metastasis to the liver is common, but spread to lung or brain is rare.

Differential Diagnosis

Eversion and redness around the cervical os caused by infection, irritation, or hormonal imbalance is smooth, soft, and minimally irregular, unlike carcinoma; is not exudative; and does not bleed easily.

The hard chancre of primary syphilis is a shallow, oval or circular ulceration with a glistening surface and a firm edge and base. It begins as a tiny papule 1–2 mm in diameter and gradually enlarges to 1 cm or more. There is minimal serous discharge, and bleeding is uncommon. *Treponema pallidum* may be identified by darkfield examination of the thin exudate. Serologic tests for syphilis are positive.

The characteristics of chancroid (soft chancre), granuloma inguinale, and lymphogranuloma venereum are described in Chapter 21. Cervical tuberculosis is discussed on p 574.

Abortion of a cervical pregnancy results in a nontender, deep, freely bleeding cavity, usually within the cervical canal. The cervix is soft and patulous, and hemorrhage is severe. Biopsy of the tissue lining the cavity will usually disclose trophoblastic debris but no cancer cells.

Metastatic choriocarcinoma or other secondary cancer must be considered in the diagnosis, as must rare conditions such as actinomycosis, amebiasis, and schistosomiasis.

Prevention

Although the causes of cervical cancer are still unknown, predisposing factors are recognized. Complete chastity is associated with almost total freedom from cervical cancer. Theoretically, then, cancer of the cervix (and penis), particularly before middle age, may be considered to be a carcinogen-induced neoplasm involving intercourse. The incidence of cervical cancer should therefore be reduced by (1) improved personal hygiene, including prevention and prompt treatment of vaginitis and cervicitis, male circumcision in infancy, and precoital washing of the penis or habitual use of condoms; (2) avoidance of intercourse at an early age; limitation of the number of consorts; use of condoms; (3) regular periodic cytologic screening of all women, especially parous women in low socioeconomic groups and those who have had numerous sexual partners; and (4) prompt treatment of suspicious cervical lesions.

Treatment of Cervical Dysplasia

A. Mild or Moderate Dysplasia: Many CIN grade 1 or 2 lesions regress (approximately 60% and 30%, respectively) or persist (approximately 25% and 5%, respectively), and only a minority progress to CIN grade 3 (approximately 15% and 20%, respectively). Therefore, it is reasonable to follow such patients with serial cytologic studies every 6 months. Cryosurgery and electrocoagulation are the methods most often used to treat CIN of grades 1 and 2.

B. Moderate to Severe Dysplasia (CIN Grade 3): CIN grade 3 lesions require cryotherapy or laser or coagulation therapy. If extension up the cervical canal is not found, cold conization is required initially.

C. Severe Dysplasia (CIS): The most effective method of treatment of CIS, and the one usually recommended for women over age 40, is total abdominal hysterectomy with a wide vaginal cuff. Whether to remove the ovaries is a decision that must be based upon the patient's age and the status of the ovaries.

Cervical conization may be considered for patients who desire pregnancy or who are reliable and can be carefully supervised. In either case, cervical smears every 6 months are recommended.

Treatment of Cervical Cancer

A. Emergency Measures: Vaginal hemorrhage originates from gross ulceration and cavitation in stage II–IV cervical carcinoma. Ligation of bleeding points and suturing are impractical. Styptics such as negatol (Negatan), 10% silver nitrate solution, or acetone are effective, although later slough may result in further bleeding. Vaginal packing or irradiation (if tolerance permits) is helpful. Ligation of the uterine or hypogastric arteries may be lifesaving when other measures fail.

B. General Measures: The patient should be admitted to the hospital for thorough study and rest before therapy is begun. Vaginal, urinary, and pelvic infections should be eradicated before surgery or irradiation. Anemia must be corrected and nutrition improved. Debilitated patients should be kept in the hospital for supportive therapy during radiation treatment, and discharged patients should be readmitted if radiation is poorly tolerated.

Pain may be controlled with analgesics such as aspirin compound with codeine, 8 or 15 mg, 1 tablet 4 times daily as necessary. Give diphenoxylate (Lomotil), 2.5 mg, or paregoric, 4–8 mL, 4 times daily as necessary for diarrhea. For urinary frequency and dysuria, give bladder sedative mixture, 4 mL every 4 hours as necessary.

C. Local Measures: During radiation therapy, plain warm water douches may be permitted when necessary for comfort and hygiene.

D. Treatment According to Stage:

1. Stage IA (microinvasive carcinoma) (depth of invasion < 3 mm)–Total extrafascial abdominal hysterectomy with a wide vaginal cuff is current therapy. Patients with invasion greater than 3 mm have a small but definite likelihood of lymph node metastasis. Therefore, we believe they should be treated as for stage IB (see below).

2. Stage IB–External supervoltage radiation and intracavitary and forniceal radium therapy or radical hysterectomy and pelvic lymphadenectomy are probably equally effective in the treatment of stage IB carcinoma. The latter often is favored in young, otherwise healthy, slender patients. The ovaries need not be removed unless they are abnormal or the woman is perimenopausal. Older patients, obese patients, and those who have serious medical problems are best treated by irradiation.

3. Stages IIA and IIB–With rare exceptions, stage II cervical cancer should be treated by irradiation. In some centers, pretreatment laparotomy for biopsy of para-aortic lymph nodes may be done in stage IIB patients. If the nodes are cancer-positive (about 15%), para-aortic extended-field radiation therapy should increase survival, although complications may be more frequent and severe. (Even when cancer-containing nodes are found beyond the pelvis, the original staging must remain the same.)

4. Stages IIIA and IIIB–Radiation therapy is used for all stage III cases. Pretreatment para-aortic lymph node sampling is important, however, because the nodes will be positive in 30–50% of patients, and extended-field therapy may be beneficial in such cases.

5. Stage IV–Supervoltage external radiation therapy to the whole pelvis is best for almost all stage IV patients. If the cancer has extended anteriorly or posteriorly without spread elsewhere, anterior or posterior exenteration may be chosen as primary therapy.

Treatment must be individualized for cervical stump cancers, bulky or "barrel-shaped" cancerous cervices, and laterally recurrent lesions.

Chemotherapy using cisplatin may be appropriate if the patient fails to respond to conventional therapy. Neurosurgery for relief of pain may be considered in selected cases.

E. Radiation Therapy: Irradiation is generally considered to be the best treatment for invasive carcinoma of the cervix. X-ray, ^{60}Co, radium, a cyclotron, a linear accelerator, or other sources of radiation may be used. All stages of cancer may be treated by this method, and there are fewer medical contraindications to irradiation than to radical surgery. Optimal results have been achieved with use of externally applied supervoltage radiation combined with intracavitary and paracervical vaginal radium.

The objectives are destruction of primary and secondary carcinoma within the pelvis and preservation of tissues not involved in the cancer. The amount of radiation required to destroy cancer varies from patient to patient. A safe cancericidal dose for cervical carcinoma is about 7000 R to point A and about 5000 R to point B (see p 572) administered over a period of 4–5 weeks.

Although it is impossible to administer adequate homogeneous radiation to destroy cancer throughout the pelvis without damaging vital structures such as the bowel, bladder, ureters, and blood vessels, the cervix can be treated intensively because it has a high tolerance to radiation. The structures immediately lateral and posterior to the cervix are damaged more easily and so must be protected from exposure to high doses. The cervix and vagina can tolerate 24,000 R, but the bladder and ureter will be seriously injured by doses higher than 7000 R and the bowel by doses higher than 4000–4500 R. Major blood vessels have approximately the same tolerance to radiation as the intestine. Therefore, dosage is determined by the radiosensitivity of both cancer cells and noncancerous tissue. In practice, the experienced oncologist or radiologist applies as much radiation as possible to the cancer within a reasonable time, with particular concern for the neighboring organs.

Physicians who prefer to begin therapy with external radiation do so because they feel that the spread of cancer beyond the cervix is generally what kills the patient and that the primary objectives of therapy are containment and destruction of cancer within the lymphatics beyond the primary lesion. External radiation therapy will often eradicate cervical infection, control hemorrhage, and reduce the size of the tumor; and it is far less uncomfortable for the patient early in treatment than surgery for the insertion of a radium source.

Physicians who prefer to begin therapy with radium or its equivalent do so because they believe that the cancer within the cervix should be treated as soon as possible to prevent metastases. Statistical evidence for the superiority of one method over the other is equivocal.

When vaginal contractures, a cervical stump, or the patient's condition precludes radium therapy, external radiation may be used alone. Radium alone is often used when the cancer is small and medical or surgical problems contraindicate protracted external radiation therapy.

1. Methods of radium application–Numerous methods have been developed for the application of radium in the treatment of cervical cancer. There are essentially 2 schools of thought regarding the relationship between radiation dosage and time—the Stockholm method and the Paris method. The Manchester method combines the Stockholm technique and the Paris applicators to allow more flexibility.

a. Paris method–This method involves low doses of intracavitary radiation from radium in an intrauterine tandem over a period of 8–10 days. A radium applicator is placed in each fornix; these are held by a bent spring to distend the fornices. An applicator is pressed against the cervix at the external os. Vaginal packing is used to retain the radium.

b. Stockholm method–This method delivers relatively high doses of intracavitary radiation over a short period of time. It uses (1) an intrauterine tandem containing linear radium sources (radium is not placed in the cervical canal), (2) metal boxes containing radium needles placed in each fornix, and (3) a box applicator applied to the cervix. Snug vaginal packing is required.

c. **Manchester method**–The Manchester method, one of the most logical and popular methods, uses a combination of the Stockholm technique and the Paris applicators to allow some degree of flexibility in the radium applications. This method emphasizes the importance of calculating the radiation dosage as delivered to 2 precise points in the pelvis. Point A is defined as lying 2 cm lateral to the central canal of the cervix and 2 cm above the lateral fornix in the axis of the uterus (approximately the point where the uterine artery crosses the ureter). Point B lies 5 cm lateral to the central canal of the cervix and 2 cm above the lateral fornix (at the pelvic side wall). Point B represents a lymph node focus adjacent to the iliac vessels; this point is a pelvic focus for metastatic cancer from the cervix.

Rubber applicators for carrying radium tubes in tandem are available in 3 lengths for the deep, average, and shallow uterus. Paracervical rubber ovoids for radium application are designed so that the distance of the radium from points A and B can be varied by changing the amount of radium used, the thickness of the 3 graduated ovoids, and rubber spacers. The dosage depends upon the amount of radium inserted and the distribution employed. By using both intrauterine and paracervical radium applicators, a cross-fire is established. This is far more effective than a radium tandem placed in the cervix alone or radium placed only in the vagina.

The optimal predetermined dosage from radium alone to point A is 7000 R. This dosage is delivered in 2 sessions of 2–3 days each, the first preceding external radiation therapy and the second following it. Treatment is more effective if external radiation therapy is also used. An external radiation dose of 3000 R is given through 2 anterior and 2 posterior ports to the parametrium (point B) within 4 weeks.

2. Treatment of cervical cancer during pregnancy–

a. First trimester–Deliver 6000 R of external radiation to the pelvis through each of 4 ports. Concurrently, give 2 courses of intra- and paracervical radium, and await spontaneous abortion.

b. Second trimester–Deliver intra- and contracervical radium. In 7–10 days, perform an abdominal (classic) hysterectomy. Two weeks after surgery, begin 6000 R of external radiation, and then give a further course of intra- and contracervical radiation during the last week of external radiation.

c. Third trimester–Perform classic cesarean section when the infant is viable. In 7–10 days, begin 6000 R of external radiation, and then give 2 courses of intra- and paracervical radium 1 week apart, the first during the last 7–10 days of external radiation.

F. Surgical Measures: (See also Treatment According to Stage, above.) Total hysterectomy with removal of a wide vaginal cuff is the surgical treatment of choice for women over age 40 with in situ carcinoma of the cervix. Deep conization of the cervix may be acceptable for younger women who wish to have more children, but this is a calculated risk even when the woman understands the need for vaginal cytologic smears every 6 months for an indefinite time.

Radical total hysterectomy (Clark-Wertheim or Okabayashi) together with pelvic lymphadenectomy is performed for treatment of stage I and stage II cervical carcinoma by surgeons skilled in the technique required for this exacting procedure. The 5-year survival rate with operation is as good as that for radiation therapy in selected cases. Obesity, advanced age, and serious medical problems that are likely to complicate surgery or convalescence greatly reduce the number of candidates for elective cancer surgery. In general, the hazards of the operation exceed those of radiation therapy.

Nevertheless, the Wertheim operation and pelvic lymphadenectomy are often used as definitive treatment of cervical cancer if (1) the patient is pregnant, (2) large uterine or adnexal tumors are present, (3) the patient has chronic salpingitis, (4) there are small or large bowel adhesions in the pelvis or to the abdominal wall, (5) the patient is under age 35 and wishes to keep her ovaries, or (6) she refuses or abandons radiation therapy but is a good surgical risk.

Cancer will recur or persist within the cervix or vaginal vault in a small proportion of patients with cervical cancer treated initially with radium and external radiation. Radical hysterectomy and lymph node resection may be indicated for low-risk patients in this group because of the serious hazards of repeated irradiation.

When recurrence or extension of cervical cancer involves the bladder or bowel, exenteration may be justified, provided that the patient is a good surgical risk. Exenteration should be attempted only when metastases to the pelvic glands have not occurred (uncommon) and when the patient is fully aware of the problems of a permanent colostomy and urinary diversion.

Complications of Therapy

The mortality rate due to irradiation is about 1% and that due to surgery about 2%; the morbidity rates are approximately 2% and 5%, respectively.

Radiation therapy may cause early troublesome side-effects, including nausea and vomiting, weight loss, dysuria, and urinary frequency. Side-effects such as tissue fibrosis, hemorrhagic cystitis, small or large bowel stenosis, or fistulas may develop later.

One of the most troublesome complications of radical abdominal hysterectomy is ureteric fistula. However, the incidence of this complication has lately been reduced to 3–5% by improvements in operative technique. Other serious problems include hemorrhage, wound infection or dehiscence, pulmonary embolism, atonic bladder with urinary retention, and cystic lymphangioma.

Prognosis

The earlier the stage at which cancer is found, the better the prognosis. Preinvasive cancer commonly is diagnosed in women under age 30 years, but most patients with invasive carcinoma are 40–50 years old at the time of diagnosis. Thus, it appears to take 5–10 years for carcinoma to penetrate the basement membrane and become invasive. Untreated patients usually die 3–5 years after invasion occurs.

Reported survival rates according to the stage at which the cancer is discovered vary widely. A composite of 5-year survival rates at major cancer centers worldwide where radiotherapy is the primary method of treatment is as follows: stage I, 86–89%; stage II, 43–70%; stage III, 27–43%; and stage IV, 0–12%.

• • •

CERVICAL TUBERCULOSIS*

Tuberculosis of the cervix is almost never primary but is secondary to tuberculosis of the upper genital tract, which is uncommon in the USA. Less than 2% of patients with tuberculosis of the uterine tubes and endometrium develop cervical tuberculosis. In cervical tuberculosis, foul-smelling discharge and contact bleeding from an ulcerative or granulomatous area occur. On biopsy, the tuberculous lesion is characterized by tubercles undergoing central caseation. Cultures and acid-fast stained smears of the discharge are required to demonstrate *Mycobacterium tuberculosis*.

Cervical tuberculosis is treated by extended chemotherapy. The reader should consult other texts for the details of treatment.

CERVICAL STENOSIS

Cervical stenosis of congenital, inflammatory, or surgical origin may be either partially or completely occlusive. Most cervical stenosis follows treatment of chronic cervicitis by cauterization or coagulation of the cervix. Obstruction to menstrual drainage inevitably results in hematometra, which is characterized by amenorrhea or cryptomenorrhea, abdominal discomfort, and a soft, slightly tender midpelvic mass.

Dilation of the cervical canal several weeks after cauterization, coagulation, or chemical treatment of the cervix will prevent or correct stenosis. Dilation of the cervix, usually with the patient under general

*See also p 543.

anesthesia, is required in the treatment of hematometra. A tubular drain within the cervix may be required for 1 or 2 weeks, especially if infection complicates hematometra.

CERVICAL PREGNANCY
(See Chapter 11.)

EXFOLIATIVE CYTOLOGIC STUDY; PAPANICOLAOU (PAP) SMEAR

Early cancer that cannot be detected by other techniques may be diagnosed upon examination of exfoliated cells from the secretions, exudates, transudates, or scrapings of various internal organs and tissues. Exfoliative cytologic examination of specimens from the lower genital tract has been so valuable in the detection of early cancer of the uterus and uterine cervix that it should be performed annually for all women over age 15.

Exfoliated cells may also be obtained from the oral mucosa, trachea and bronchi, stomach, rectum and colon, urinary tract, serous sac fluids, cyst fluids, synovial fluids, cerebrospinal fluid, glandular excretions, and exudates. Methods for obtaining, collecting, and preserving such specimens may vary slightly according to the pathologist's preference. The smears should be stained and interpreted only by properly trained, experienced pathologists or cytologists.

Papanicolaou smears should be performed, usually yearly, according to the following recommendations:

A. Premenopausal Women:

1. Teenage daughters of women who received diethylstilbestrol (or an analog) during that pregnancy.

2. Sexually active women age 18 or younger.

3. Women whose initial smear is satisfactory and without significant atypia should have a second smear within 1 year to rule out a false-negative smear.

a. The American College of Obstetricians and Gynecologists recommends yearly smears for premenopausal patients with negative smears.

b. The Walton Report (Canada), favored by the American Cancer Society, recommends that premenopausal women with negative smears have smears at 3-year intervals until age 35 and then at 5-year intervals until age 60. The Walton Report recommends yearly smears for the high-risk subgroup (early onset of sexual activity with or without multiple partners). This includes women seen in family planning clinics, student health clinics, youth clinics, venereal disease clinics, prenatal clinics, and penal institutions.

Materials Needed:

One cervical spatula, cut tongue depressor, or cotton swab.

One glass slide (one end frosted). Identify by writing the patient's name on the frosted end with a lead pencil.

One speculum (warm but without lubricant).

One bottle of fixative (97% ethanol) or spray-on fixative, eg, Pro-Fixx or Aqua-Net.

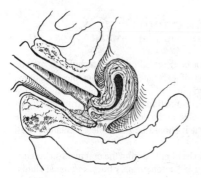
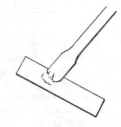

1. Obtain vaginal pool material from the posterior fornix.

2. Place adequate drop 1 inch from end of slide, smear, fix, and dry.

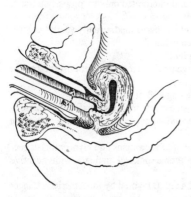
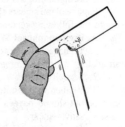

3. Obtain cervical scraping from complete squamocolumnar junction by rotating spatula 360° around external os, high up in the endocervical canal.

4. Place the material 1 inch from end of slide, smear, fix, and dry.

Figure 22–4. Preparation of a Papanicolaou cytosmear.

B. Postmenopausal Women:

1. The American College of Obstetricians and Gynecologists recommends yearly smears.

2. The Walton Report indicates that women over age 60 who have had repeated negative smears may be dropped from a screening program and assumed to be no longer at risk for the development of cervical squamous carcinoma.

3. Postmenopausal patients with bleeding must have endometrial sampling.

C. Hysterectomized Women: For women who have had a hysterectomy for previous benign disease, if an initial smear following surgery is negative, a smear every 3 years is sufficient (American College of Obstetricians and Gynecologists).

Vaginal Aspiration & Cervical Scrapings

A. Vaginal Cytologic Smears: Material from the vagina can be obtained by aspiration or with a cotton swab, spatula, or cut tongue depressor (Fig 22–4).

B. Cervical Scrapings: After vaginal fluid is obtained, a vaginal speculum (moistened in warm water) is inserted and the cervix is inspected. No lubricant should be used. With use of a cotton swab, spatula, or cut tongue depressor, the second specimen is taken from the region of the squamocolumnar junction. Since most cancers of the cervix develop in this area, over 90% of them will be detected by these scrapings. (Specimens should always be taken from any clinically abnormal area of the cervix.) Although vaginal smears detect only 50% of cervical cancers, they are more likely to show malignant cells from the endometrium, uterine tubes, ovaries, and peritoneum. In addition, they may reveal infections and can be used for hormonal evaluation.

Laboratory Reports

The cytology report from the pathology laboratory usually describes the cell specimens as (1) normal, repeat in 1 year; (2) abnormal, repeat immediately or in not more than 3 months (if still abnormal, do colposcopy, biopsy); or (3) positive, take biopsy. The degree of inflammation, the presence of atypical cells and pathogens, and hormonal evaluation are commonly included in the report.

Vaginal cytology for cancer is reported as shown in Table 22–2.

Abnormal and positive smears must be adequately followed up. Perhaps the most important caution relates to "suspicious" smears. Repeat smears should be taken at once to pinpoint possible problems, since trichomonad infection, atrophic changes, or other clinical conditions unrelated to cancer may be the reason for the abnormal or atypical cells. After infection has resolved, dysplastic cells (CIN) may be identified.

Table 22–2. Vaginal cytology for cancer.

American Cancer Society	Papanicolaou Class	Results
Normal	I	Negative for malignant cells.
Suspicious	II	Negative for malignant cells but contains atypical benign elements (including those with radiation changes).
	III	Markedly atypical cells suspicious of cancer.
Positive	IV	Probably malignant cells.
	V	Cells cytologically conclusive of cancer.*

*Note: Cytology reports are unacceptable if only the class (I–V) is given; a description of the smear and comments (similar to a histologic diagnosis) are mandatory. Vaginal cytologic findings alone *never* justify an unequivocal diagnosis of cancer; examination of tissue (biopsy, curettings, etc) is required for confirmation before definitive therapy.

Occult asymptomatic lesions should be suspected if abnormal cytology (> class III) is reported. In the absence of a definite lesion, colposcopy, directed biopsy of suspect areas, and curettage of the endocervix should be done. A visible abnormality, especially an ulcerative area, must be biopsied.

General Rules in Obtaining Specimens

(1) The fixative should be ready for use. Cells dry rapidly once they are smeared, so they must be fixed immediately after the smear is made.

(2) Cotton swabs, if used, must not be contaminated by epithelium from the manufacturer's, examiner's, or patient's skin. They should be prepared just before use by picking up a small amount of nonabsorbent cotton with the tip of an applicator stick and rolling it against the coat sleeve or a clean towel.

(3) The speculum must be introduced with no lubricant. For the patient's comfort, it should be warm. If necessary, water may be used to moisten the speculum and assist introduction.

(4) Specimens should be obtained when the first opportunity arises. Bleeding and douching within the previous 24 hours are not contraindications to specimen collection. These conditions do yield a higher percentage of unsatisfactory specimens, however, and repeat studies may become necessary. To prevent anxiety, the patient should be advised of this possibility.

(5) Prompt light spraying of the smear with a cytologic fixative, eg, Pro-Fixx, will eliminate the need for ether-alcohol fixation. Inexpensive hair spray is equally effective.

Diseases of the Uterus | 23

CONGENITAL UTERINE ANOMALIES

Clinically significant anomalies of the uterus and cervix (absence, duplication, or distortion) occur in about one in 1000 females. Gross developmental deficiencies are of special obstetric and gynecologic concern. Whether or not normal function is possible depends upon the degree of the anomaly and the ultimate size of the uterus.

Congenital absence of the uterus and cervix occurs in ovarian dysgenesis (ovarian agenesis of Turner) as a result of chromosomal aberration; the cause of other uterine abnormalities is not known. Associated abnormalities involving the urinary tract are common.

Chromosomal sex determines the basic character of the internal genitalia. Paired X chromosomes (XX) are apparently required for a normal uterus and cervix. An XO combination occurs in ovarian dysgenesis. Other genital abnormalities may occur with irregular chromosomal division and mosaicism.

The uterine tubes, the uterus, and the upper two-thirds of the vagina are of müllerian duct origin (see p 4). The lower portions of the müllerian ducts normally fuse in the midline to develop a single uterus, cervix, and vagina. A variety of congenital anomalies result from incomplete fusion or abnormal resorption of portions of the müllerian system.

Classification

The rarest and most extreme anomaly is the development of 2 separate adjacent genital tracts, one a mirror image of the other (uterus didelphys bicollis; Fig 23–1). There are usually 2 independent uteri and 2 cervices but only one uterine tube inserting into each fundus laterally. Each organ is capable of menstruation and may support a pregnancy.

A more common type of anomaly is partial fusion of the müllerian ducts with persistence of the mesial walls to include 2 cervices (uterus duplex bicornis bicollis; Fig 23–2). Failure of fusion at a higher level results in 2 uterine corpora with only one cervix (uterus bicornis unicollis; Fig 23–3).

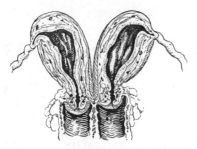

Figure 23–1. Uterus didelphys bicollis.

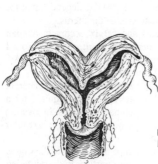

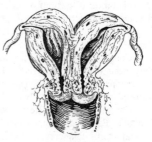

Figure 23–2. Uterus duplex bicornis bicollis.

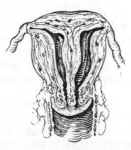

Figure 23–3. Uterus bicornis unicollis.

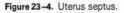

Figure 23–4. Uterus septus.

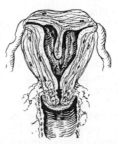

Figure 23–5. Uterus subseptus.

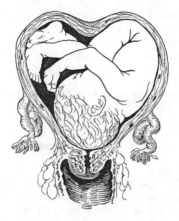

Figure 23–6. Gravid uterus arcuatus.

A complete, usually firm septum may separate the uterus into 2 isolated compartments (uterus septus; Fig 23–4). The division may be only partial (uterus subseptus; Fig 23–5), or the septum may be only a ridge and the uterine exterior and interior will be heart-shaped (uterus arcuatus; Fig 23–6).

Rarely, one müllerian duct may fail to develop (uterus unicornis). If the uterus is not too small, it usually functions normally.

A small, rudimentary uterus may be identified in congenital absence of the vagina (Rokitansky-Küster-Hauser syndrome).

Clinical Findings

A. Symptoms and Signs:

1. Nonpregnant women–Amenorrhea occurs with absence of the uterus, occlusions of the cervix, and imperforate hymen; oligomenorrhea with uterine hypoplasia; and dysmenorrhea with uterine maldevelopment.

2. Pregnant women–Abortion, premature labor, and delivery will occur if the fetus overdistends the maldeveloped uterus. Malpresentation and lack of engagement may occur if the contour of the uterine cavity is abnormal. Dystocia may be caused by inadequate, poorly coordinated forces of contraction or by soft tissue obstruction (as with congenital cervical stenosis or in a uterus bicornis bicollis). Postpartal hemorrhage may be due to uterine atony or lacerations of the uterus or birth canal.

B. X-Ray Findings: Hysterosalpingography, often augmented by pneumoperitoneum, is the most effective diagnostic procedure for detection and delineation of uterine anomalies in nonpregnant women.

C. Special Examinations: Hysteroscopy may disclose intrauterine abnormalities. Laparoscopy may be justified for the diagnosis of müllerian dysplasia, but the uterus and adnexa should be examined for abnormal development whenever laparotomy is done for other reasons.

Complications

Hematometra or infection may occur in an obstructed horn of a double uterus. Perforation of a congenitally deformed uterus during instrumentation and uterine rupture during pregnancy or labor are serious complications. Obstructive uropathy and fistula formation are complications of hysterectomy or irradiation therapy.

Differential Diagnosis

Tumors of the uterus and adnexa may suggest a bicornuate uterus. Malposition of the corpus with adherence of the tubes and ovaries may be mistaken for an abnormally formed uterus. Unilateral tubal occlusion must be considered when a presumptive diagnosis of uterus unicornis is made.

Treatment

Consider operation for septal excision and unification of the uterus in patients in whom repeated late abortion is related to a uterocervical anomaly. Remove a diminutive horn of a double uterus when abnormal bleeding, tumor formation, or obstruction develops on the deformed side.

Prognosis

The prognosis depends upon the extent of the abnormality. Pregnancy and the delivery of a normal infant are not usually prevented by minor degrees of anomalous development. Fetal salvage is reasonably good after unification operations, even with vaginal delivery.

Familial repetition of anomalies of the female generative tract is rare.

MALPOSITIONS OF THE UTERUS
("Tipped Uterus")

Significant displacement of the uterus may cause signs or symptoms such as pelvic pain, backache, menstrual aberrations, and infertility. Displacement may be lateral, anterior, or posterior. Virtually all women with symptoms that may be due to displacement are premenopausal. Almost all postpartum patients have a temporarily retroposed uterus.

The uterus is not a fixed organ, and the position may vary transiently as a result of pelvic inclination or prolonged sitting, standing, or lying. The body of the uterus is directed forward in about 80% of women; in the remaining 20%, it is retroposed. However, fewer than 5% of women with retroposed uteri will have a bona fide complaint referable to posterior version of the uterus. Normally, the cervix is directed posteriorly in the vaginal vault in nulliparas. After parturition, the cervix is often in the vaginal axis, an attitude caused by slight retrodisplacement of the corpus. The cervix and uterus often are aligned following relaxation of the pelvic floor. Laxity of the transverse cervical and round ligaments accounts for a posterior deviation in uterine position. Moderate uterine prolapse is usually associated with a retroposed uterus. Retroversion and retroflexion are more or less synonymous terms. Retroversion implies that the axis of the body of the uterus is directed to the hollow of the sacrum, but the cervix remains in its normal axis. If angulation of the corpus on the cervix is extreme, the condition is called retroflexion. Retrocession implies that both cervix and uterus have gravitated backward toward the sacrum. Acute anteversion probably does not cause either obstruction to uterine discharge or circulatory alteration. Free dextroversion or levoversion is of little clinical importance unless tumors, shortened supports, or other disorders are present. Adherent lateral deviation of the uterus indicates primary pelvic disease, eg, salpingitis. Enlargement of the uterus, whether by pregnancy or tumor, may alter its relative position. Pelvic infections or endometriosis may obliterate the cul-de-sac; a pyo- or hydrosalpinx may drag the corpus backward and downward by its weight, whereupon adhesions add restriction to cause immobility (Figs 23–7 to 23–10).

The patient's complaints uncommonly arise solely as the result of free retroposition. Nevertheless, dysmenorrhea and menometrorrhagia may be due to utero-ovarian congestion; backache is frequently caused by similar turgescence or taut uterosacral ligaments. Prolapse of the ovaries accounts for dyspareunia with uterine retroposition. Infertility occasionally results from anterior displacement of the cervix, because the ejaculate in the seminal pool in the posterior fornix does not bathe the cervix.

Constipation due to displacement of the bowel or pressure by the uterine fundus on the rectum is unlikely. Bladder dysfunction secondary to malposition of the uterus rarely occurs.

During early pregnancy, a retroposed uterus may become incarcerated, often because of adhesions, and cause acute urinary retention. In addition, because adherence prevents normal fetal growth and development, abortion may result.

Clinical Findings

A. Symptoms and Signs: Pelvic pain, backache, abnormal menstrual bleeding, and infertility are commonly but uncritically related

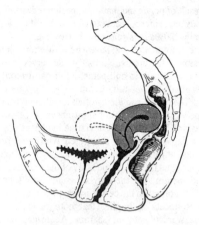

Figure 23–7. Retroflexion in an anteverted uterus.

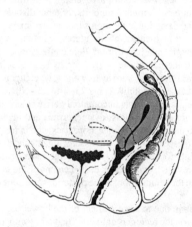

Figure 23–8. Retrocession of uterus.

to malposition of the uterus. A combined abdominal and retrovaginal examination should be done to determine uterine position, and the degree of misalignment of the uterus and cervix as well as adherence and tumefaction should be estimated.

B. X-Ray Findings: Hysterography will reveal malposition of the uterus, especially when both anteroposterior and lateral films are ob-

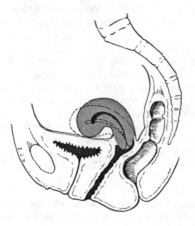

Figure 23–9. Anteflexion of uterus.

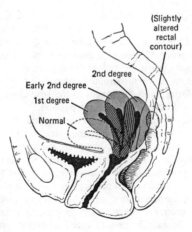

Figure 23–10. Degrees of retroversion of uterus without retroflexion.

tained. Pneumoperitoneum or contrast media placed within the rectum and bladder will enhance hysterography, especially when malposition is related to pelvic tumors.

C. Special Examinations: In the nonpregnant patient, gently insert a sterile curved uterine sound into the uterine cavity after applying a topical antiseptic to the external cervical os and distal canal. The direction of the instrument will indicate the position of the corpus.

Differential Diagnosis

A fundal fibroid or ovarian tumor resting in the cul-de-sac may be mistaken for a retroposed fundus, and vice versa.

Adherent retroposition of the uterus may cause the same symptoms as uterine malposition. Basically, however, the disorder may be salpingitis, endometriosis, or a tumor.

Uterine retroposition can but does not usually cause backache, which is most often due to orthopedic disorders. Abnormal posture, fatigue, myositis, arthritis, and herniation of an intervertebral disk should be considered as possible causes of backache.

Prevention

Avoidance of the causes of pelvic infection and early, specific therapy when infection occurs will reduce the incidence of adherent malposition of the uterus.

Treatment

Retroposition of the uterus is now regarded as clinically important when replacement and support by a vaginal pessary relieve the symptoms. **Note:** Knee-chest exercises alone are of questionable value.

A. Emergency Measures: Elevate an incarcerated, nonadherent uterus, especially when the patient develops acute urinary retention during pregnancy or when abortion threatens. Rectovaginal manipulation of the corpus, with the patient in the knee-chest position, may facilitate the restoration of uterine anteposition.

B. Specific Local Measures: In nonpregnant patients, neither an asymptomatic retroposition nor a normally involuting retroposed puerperal uterus requires treatment. For gynecologic patients with pelvic pain or abnormal bleeding and for recently delivered women with subinvolution and persistent lochia or bleeding, reposition the uterus and insert a properly fitted vaginal pessary (see below). Unless discomfort develops, leave the pessary in place for 6–8 weeks and record the result. If anteversion and relief follow pessary support, no further therapy will be necessary. Reinsert the pessary after 2 months if symptoms recur.

Bimanual replacement of the retrodisplaced uterus (Fig 23–11) is performed as follows: With the patient in the lithotomy position, insert one or 2 gloved fingers into the vagina, elevate the fundus, and press against the cervix. With the other hand, bring the corpus forward. Fit a vaginal pessary of the Hodge type to support the uterus in anteposition.

If this procedure is not successful, insert a pessary of the Hodge type into the posterior vaginal fornix (Fig 23–12). Have the patient sit up and then assume the knee-chest position. Apply pressure on the lateral

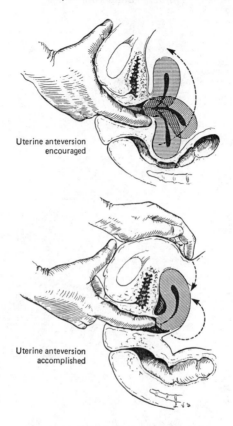

Uterine anteversion
encouraged

Uterine anteversion
accomplished

Figure 23–11. Bimanual replacement of uterus.

bars of the pessary and displace the cervix backward while the patient coughs; the nonadherent uterus will usually fall forward. Have the patient slip slowly into the prone and then into the lithotomy position. Seat the pessary to maintain the uterus in forward position.

C. Surgical Measures:

1. Suspend the uterus as a primary procedure when repeated replacement of the corpus by the use of a pessary has alleviated symptoms and signs or when adherence of the uterus and prolapse of the adnexa are probable causes of disability.

2. Suspend the uterus as a secondary procedure and concluding

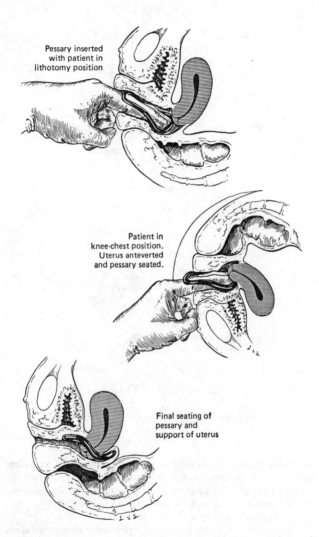

Pessary inserted
with patient in
lithotomy position

Patient in
knee-chest position.
Uterus anteverted
and pessary seated.

Final seating of
pessary and
support of uterus

Figure 23–12. Insertion of Hodge pessary if bimanual replacement of uterus is not successful.

step in surgery done to eliminate specific pelvic disease such as chronic recurrent salpingitis or progressive pelvic endometriosis.

D. Treatment of Complications: Occasional warm acetic acid douches may relieve irritation and prevent discharge caused by a vaginal pessary. (Even a well-fitted one may cause irritation.)

Prognosis

The prognosis is good if correction of the uterine malposition follows an accurate diagnosis of symptomatic displacement but poor if uterine suspension is done without a convincing indication.

UTERINE PROLAPSE
(Descensus Uteri)

Uterine prolapse (pelvic floor hernia, pudendal hernia) is abnormal protrusion of the uterus through the pelvic floor aperture or genital hiatus.

Uterine prolapse occurs most commonly in postmenopausal, multiparous white women as a gradually progressive and delayed result of childbirth trauma, congenital anomaly, musculofascial weakness (which may account for uncommon prolapse in nulliparous women), pelvic tumor, or sacral nerve disorders, especially injury to S1–4 (as in spina bifida), diabetic neuropathy, caudal anesthesia or other accidents, and sacral tumors. It is usually associated with enterocele, cystocele, and rectocele. Ascites and internal genital tumors accelerate the development of prolapse. Other predisposing factors are obesity, asthma, chronic bronchitis, and bronchiectasis. Corrective surgery for uterine prolapse accounts for about 15% of major gynecologic operations.

The principal components of the basinlike pelvic floor are the pelvic bones (including the coccyx), the levator musculature, and the endopelvic fascia. Normally, the pelvic floor supports and contains the pelvic viscera and withstands increased intra-abdominal pressure during straining, lifting, or coughing when the individual is erect. A potential weak zone of the pelvic floor is the central anterior portion where the slotlike pelvic aperture permits the urethra, vagina, and rectum to penetrate the pelvic floor. The puborectalis and pubococcygeus muscles and iliococcygeus portions of the levator muscle group lateral to the pelvic aperture act as a sphincter mechanism for the conduits. Injury to the levator musculature, the endopelvic fascia, or cardinal and uterosacral ligaments may occur during delivery of a very large infant, with a long or tumultuous labor, or as a result of a badly executed forceps delivery or breech extraction.

Both retroposition and prolapse of the uterus develop as a result of relaxation of uterine supports. When the corpus is in the vaginal axis, the

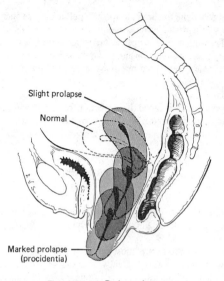

Slight prolapse

Normal

Marked prolapse
(procidentia)

Figure 23–13. Prolapsed uterus.

uterus exerts a pistonlike action with each episode of increased intra-abdominal pressure.

The degree of uterine prolapse (Fig 23–13) parallels the extent of separation or attenuation of its supporting structures. In slight intravaginal or incomplete prolapse, the uterus descends only partway down the vagina; in moderate prolapse, the uterus descends so deeply that the cervix presents at the introitus; in marked or complete prolapse (procidentia), the entire cervix and uterus protrude beyond the introitus and the vagina is inverted.

Anterior and posterior vaginal relaxation, as well as incompetency of the perineum, often accompany prolapse of the uterus. Large cystocele is more common than rectocele in prolapse because the bladder is easily carried downward.

For unknown reasons, the cervix often becomes elongated in prolapse. Before the menopause, the prolapsed uterus hypertrophies and is engorged and flabby. After the menopause, the uterus atrophies. In procidentia, the vaginal mucosa thickens and cornifies to resemble skin.

Clinical Findings

Most patients with uterine prolapse have a history of at least one traumatic or operative delivery. Nevertheless, the symptoms are often minor even with a considerable degree of prolapse. A sense of heaviness or "dragging" in the low back, pelvis, or inguinal regions, often ascribed to enteroptosis, is related to traction on the uterine and cervical ligaments by the inadequately supported uterus. A firm, mobile mass is palpable in the lower vagina.

In premenopausal women with prolapse, leukorrhea or menometrorrhagia frequently develops because of uterine engorgement. Such women may be infertile. However, once pregnancy is well established, it usually continues to term. After the menopause, excessive vaginal mucus and bleeding may be due to trophic ulceration and infection of the prolapsed cervix.

Compression, distortion, or herniation of the bladder by the displaced uterus and cervix may be responsible for residual urine, which leads to urinary tract infection, frequency and urgency, and overflow voiding. Retention occurs, but incontinence is rare. Constipation and painful defecation occur with prolapse as a result of pressure and rectocele. Voiding and defecation may be easy and complete when the patient manually reduces the prolapse. Cramping and obstipation may follow intestinal constriction within a large enterocele.

Pelvic examination with the patient supine or standing (first with the patient at rest and then straining) will demonstrate downward displacement of a prolapsing uterus. Traction on a tenaculum applied to the cervix, particularly when the patient is standing, will disclose the maximal degree of descensus.

Herniation of the bladder, rectum, or cul-de-sac is also diagnosed by vaginal examination. A prolapsed uterus is invariably accompanied by an enterocele, the dimensions of which depend upon the size of the pelvic floor defect and degree of uterine descent. The tubes and ovaries are drawn downward by the prolapsing uterus. Uterine or adnexal tumors and ascites associated with uterine prolapse should be noted.

Rectovaginal examination may reveal a rectocele. An enterocele may be behind and perhaps below the cervix but in front of a rectocele. A metal sound or firm catheter within the bladder may be used to determine the extent of concomitant cystocele.

Complications

Leukorrhea, abnormal uterine bleeding, and abortion may result from infection or disordered uterine or ovarian circulation in prolapse. Chronic decubitus ulceration may develop in procidentia, but whether the ulcers predispose to cancer is uncertain. Urinary tract infection is common in patients with prolapse and cystocele. Partial ureteral obstruction with hydronephrosis may occur in patients with procidentia. Hemorrhoids result from straining to overcome constipation. Small bowel obstruction may occur within a deep enterocele.

Differential Diagnosis

Prolapse of the uterus must be distinguished from hypertrophic cervical elongations or tumors of the cervix or uterus, cystocele, rectocele, uterine inversion, fecal impaction, or a large bladder stone. Myomas or polyps may coexist with prolapse of the uterus, causing unusual symptoms.

Despite the variety of possibilities, the history and physical findings in uterine prolapse are so characteristic that the proper diagnosis is usually not a problem.

Prevention

A program of postpartum exercises (Kegel) to strengthen the levator musculature, avoidance of obstetric trauma, and avoidance of obesity will prevent or minimize prolapse. Prolonged cyclic estrogen therapy for postmenopausal women will often conserve the strength and tone of the pelvic floor constituents.

Treatment

A. General Measures: Palliative therapy with bed rest and a well-fitted pessary (eg, soft or firm doughnut-type, Gellhorn, or Menge) may give relief if surgery is refused or is contraindicated. Ulcerated areas should be biopsied; surgical D&C are indicated to investigate bleeding and rule out cancer. Prescribe acetic acid douches, medicated tampons, or chemotherapy for ulceration. Give estrogens in suppository or vaginal cream form to elderly patients. Treat urinary tract infection, diabetes mellitus, or cardiovascular complications appropriately. Prescribe laxatives or enemas for constipation. Obese patients should lose weight. Girdles and garments that increase intra-abdominal pressure and other factors (physical, occupational, etc) that have a similar effect should be avoided or modified.

B. Surgical Measures: Selection of the surgical approach depends upon the patient's age and desire for menstruation, pregnancy, or coitus and upon the extent of prolapse. Uterine suspension or ventrofixation is not effective in the treatment of prolapse, since attachments give way and the cervix continues to elongate.

In young women, restore the pelvic floor. The Manchester-Fothergill operation is preferred if conservation of the uterus is important. Otherwise, vaginal hysterectomy with correction of hernia defects may be elected.

In postmenopausal women who are sexually active, vaginal hysterectomy and repair are logical. In elderly patients, colpocleisis or colpectomy is often chosen.

C. Treatment of Complications: Infection of the operative area or of the urinary tract may require antibiotic therapy. Prescribe a pessary or reoperate for recurrence.

Prognosis

Prolapse of the uterus may remain unchanged for months or years, but it will never regress and will ultimately progress unless corrected surgically. The age of the patient is less important than her medical status and the surgical prognosis. Nevertheless, the likelihood of cure of prolapse after proper preparation and well-chosen, properly performed surgery is excellent.

• • •

VAGINAL PESSARIES

The vaginal pessary is a prosthesis that is now made of rubber or plastic material, often with a metal band or spring frame. A great many types have been devised, but fewer than a dozen are helpful.

Pessaries are principally used to support the prolapsed uterus or cervical stump (ie, in pelvic floor hernias). They are effective because they reduce vaginal relaxation and increase the tautness of the pelvic floor structures. Little or no leverage is involved. The retrodisplaced uterus remains forward after it is repositioned and a pessary inserted, because the tension produced on the uterosacral ligaments draws the cervix backward. In most cases, adequate anterior support and a reasonably good perineal body are required; otherwise, the pessary may slip from behind the symphysis and extrude from the vagina.

Indications

A. Obstetric Use: Indications include (1) to avert threatened abortion presumed to be due to marked uterine retroposition and chronic passive congestion, (2) to promote healing of trophic cervical ulceration associated with prolapse during pregnancy, (3) to relieve acute urinary retention due to retroposition of the uterus in mid pregnancy, (4) to protect against midtrimester abortion in suspected cervical incompetence, and (5) to prevent or relieve postpartum subinvolution or retroversion.

B. Gynecologic Use: Indications include (1) to treat poor-risk patients or those who refuse surgery for uterine prolapse or other gynecologic hernias, (2) to aid preoperative healing of cervical stasis ulcerations associated with uterine prolapse, (3) to reduce cystocele or rectocele, (4) to alleviate hypermenorrhea, dysmenorrhea, or dyspareunia related to free uterine retroposition and adnexal prolapse, (5) to determine whether hysteropexy will relieve backache due to retroversion, (6) to correct urinary stress incontinence by exerting pressure beneath the urethra or improving the posterior urethrovesical angle, (7) to aid conception in the management of infertility (in some cases, the cervix may be displaced anteriorly, away from the posterior fornix seminal pool; in others, angulation of tubes or chronic passive congestion may be secondary to retroposition), and (8) to facilitate hysteropexy by holding the uterus in position for surgery.

Contraindications

Pessaries are contraindicated in patients with acute genital tract infections and in those with adherent retroposition of the uterus.

Gehrung

Gellhorn

Lucite ring

Ball

Hodge

Doughnut

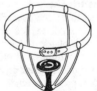

Napier cup and stem
with waistband

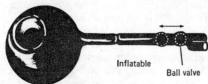

Inflatable

Ball valve

Figure 23–14. Types of pessaries.

Types of Pessaries (See Figs 23–14 and 23–15.)

The Hodge pessary (Smith-Hodge, or Smith and other variations) is an elongated curved ovoid. This type of pessary supports the uterus after it has been repositioned.

The Gellhorn and Menge pessaries are used for correction of marked prolapse when the perineal body is reasonably adequate.

The Gehrung pessary rests in the vagina with the cervix cradled between the long arms; this arches the anterior vaginal wall to reduce a cystocele.

A ring pessary, either of hard vulcanite or plastic composition or of the soft "doughnut" type, distends the vagina, elevates the cervix, and reduces cystocele and rectocele.

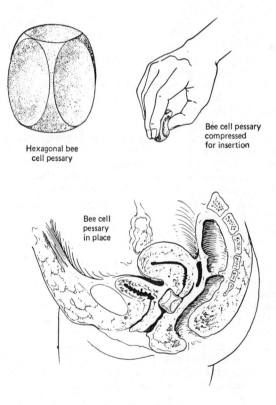

Hexagonal bee
cell pessary

Bee cell pessary
compressed
for insertion

Bee cell
pessary
in place

Figure 23–15. Bee cell pessary.

A hollow plastic ball or sponge rubber (bee cell) pessary functions much like a ring pessary and is used for similar purposes. A moderately intact perineum is necessary for retention.

A uterine supporter (Napier pessary) is a cup-stem arrangement supported by a belt. This device elevates a prolapsed cervix or uterus in cases when the perineum is incompetent.

The inflatable pessary (Milex) functions much like a doughnut pessary. The ball valve controls inflation. When the ball is in the "down" position, air fills the pessary. When it is in the "up" position, the air is sealed in and inflation is maintained.

Fitting of Pessaries

Fitting requires a trial of various shapes and sizes of pessaries. Pessaries that are too large will cause irritation and ulceration. Those too small may not remain in place and may extrude. The forefinger should pass easily between the sides of the frame and the vaginal wall at any point; otherwise, the pessary is too large. A solid vulcanite pessary can be molded in hot water and reshaped for a better "fit."

The pessary should be lubricated and inserted with its widest dimension in the oblique diameter of the vagina; this will avoid painful distention at the introitus. With a finger of the opposite hand, depress the perineum to widen the introitus.

The Hodge pessary should be rotated slightly after it is in the vagina. Using the forefinger of one hand, slip the posterior bar behind the cervix. Bring the anterior bar upward so that the pessary will be wholly within the vagina (ie, no portion of it will be visible).

The patient should be shown how to withdraw the pessary if it becomes displaced, is uncomfortable, or requires cleaning. (Bee cell and inflatable pessaries should be removed nightly to clean them and to preserve the vaginal mucosa.) The patient should be cautioned that a contraceptive vaginal diaphragm cannot be used while a vaginal pessary is in place. Frequent low-pressure acetic acid douches are helpful while vaginal pessaries are being worn.

Firm pessaries should be removed once every 4–6 weeks, when a pessary of slightly different size and shape can be substituted. During pregnancy—and as a preoperative trial in gynecologic patients—a pessary should be worn for 2–3 months. In many cases, if uterine retroposition is corrected with a pessary, the uterus will remain forward after it is removed.

Vaginal pessaries are never curative, but they may be used for months or years for palliation. Their use should be properly supervised.

A neglected pessary may cause fistulas or favor genital infections, but it is doubtful that a modern pessary can cause cancer.

•   •   •

MYOMA

Myoma is the most common tumor of the female genital tract. It is a discrete, rounded, firm, pale pink, benign myometrial tumor composed of smooth muscle and connective tissue. It causes at least 10% of gynecologic problems and is slightly more common in women who have not borne children and among women of dark racial groups. The cause of myoma formation is not known.

Minute myomas may be present in the newborn, but they do not develop until after puberty. Estrogen is a stimulant to the enlargement of myomas. After the menopause, their growth is stimulated by greater than physiologic doses of estrogens. The dependence of myomas on hormonal stimulation and vascular nutrition is well demonstrated in pregnancy; these tumors generally increase in size after the first trimester and subside after delivery.

Classification

Myomas develop from immature smooth muscle cells sheathing myometrial arterioles; they include but are not derived from connective tissue. Because they resemble fibromas, myomas are also called fibroids, fibroid tumors, and fibromyomas.

Uterine myomas are classified by anatomic location (Fig 23–16). Intramural myomas cause the uterus to contract so that the tumor moves toward the cavity (submucous) or toward the peritoneal surface (subserous). A myoma becomes intraligamentous when it extrudes retroperitoneally between the leaves of the broad ligament. Adherence to the bowel or other intra-abdominal structures is rare. A myoma eventually becomes parasitic when its blood supply is derived from the new attachment. It then separates from the uterus or retains only a few adhesive bands to the parent organ.

Two to 3% of uterine myomas are cervical in origin.

Pathology

The uterus may contain many myomas in various stages of development and degeneration. As many as several hundred have been found; only about 2% are solitary. Some grow to massive size; the largest recorded weighed over 45 kg (100 lb). Each tumor is limited by a pseudocapsule—a potential cleavage plane useful for surgical enucleation. Vascular channels enter at the periphery and arborize within the tumor.

On cut section, a typical developing myoma reveals a pattern of whorls of smooth muscle and fibrous connective tissue in varying proportions. The myelocytes are remarkably uniform in size, and the nuclear cytoplasm gives a characteristic benign appearance. Young myomas are well vascularized; older ones are not. Telangiectasia or lymphectasia is occasionally seen.

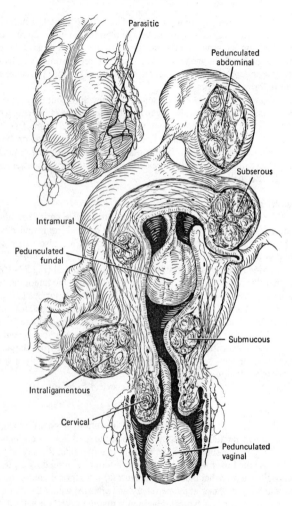

Figure 23–16. Myomas of the uterus.

Benign degeneration is of the following types: atrophic, hyaline, cystic, calcific (calcareous), septic, carneous or red, and myxomatous or fatty. Malignant change is generative, not degenerative. Leiomyosarcoma develops in about 0.1–0.5% of patients with myoma. (The incidence is uncertain because not all myomas are studied microscopically.)

Clinical Findings

A. Symptoms and Signs: Symptoms depend upon the situation, size, and state of preservation of the tumor and whether the patient is pregnant.

1. Site of tumor–Intramural, subserous, or intraligamentous tumors may distort or obstruct other organs, causing pain or bleeding. Submucous tumors remain asymptomatic until they become large enough to displace neighboring viscera. They may cause dysmenorrhea, leukorrhea, hypermenorrhea, or metrorrhagia (especially if pedunculated and protruding through the cervix). Torsion of a sessile submucous tumor may cause acute recurrent pain. Cervical tumors cause vaginal discharge, vaginal bleeding, dyspareunia, and infertility. Large cervical tumors may fill the true pelvis, displacing other pelvic structures and thereby occluding the cervical canal and impeding labor. Parasitic tumors cause intestinal obstruction if they are large or involve the omentum or bowel.

2. Condition of patient–In nonpregnant women, myomas may or may not cause problems. About 25%, however, cause abnormal uterine bleeding. Some patients complain of pelvic fullness or heaviness. Backache and neurologic complaints are rarely reported.

Before or after pregnancy, myomas may cause pelvic pressure and distention (due to excessive size and weight of the tumor); urinary frequency (due to displacement of neighboring organs); menometrorrhagia (due to thinning of the endometrium); constipation (due to pressure on contiguous structures); dysmenorrhea (due to increased uterine contractility); retention cysts (due to reduced ovarian circulation); and infertility (due to obstruction of the genital tract).

In pregnant women, myomas may cause the following additional problems: abortion (due to atrophic circulatory changes in the endometrium); malpresentation or abortion (due to distortion of the uterine cavity); failure of engagement (due to displacement of the uterus); premature labor (due to increased uterine irritability); pain (due to torsion or to degeneration of the tumor); dystocia (due to obstruction of the birth canal); and desultory labor and postpartum hemorrhage (due to reduction of uterine contractility).

B. Laboratory Findings: Anemia may be present as a result of abnormal uterine bleeding and infection. Polycythemia (occasionally) and leukocytosis may be present with myoma and endometritis or carneous, septic degeneration. With degeneration, the white blood cell count may be elevated to about 20,000/μL, and the sedimentation rate may be increased.

C. X-Ray Findings: A plain film of the pelvis may show phlyctenular opacities if calcific degeneration has occurred. Hysterography (contraindicated during pregnancy) and angiography may reveal a cervical or submucous tumor. A pelvic pneumogram may demonstrate enlargement and asymmetry of the uterine contour, but such a tumor can be palpated readily unless the patient is very obese or uncooperative.

D. Special Examinations: In nonpregnant women, vaginal examination under anesthesia and surgical dilatation and curettage may be necessary to delineate myomas. The tumor may be outlined by the curet as a protrusion from the uterine wall. Ultrasonography will identify a pelvic tumor.

Laparoscopy may allow visualization of subserous fundal or parasitic fibroids. Hysteroscopy may become a feasible approach to the diagnosis of intracavitary masses.

Differential Diagnosis

Uterine enlargement or irregularity may be due to any of the following in addition to myoma: pregnancy; adenomyosis; benign hypertrophy; subinvolution; congenital anomaly; adherent adnexa, omentum, or bowel; and sarcoma or carcinoma. Even when the diagnosis of myoma has been made, other neoplastic diseases, cervicitis, cervical stenosis, endometrial polyp, and other gynecologic disorders must be considered.

Prevention

Give minimal-dose oral contraceptives to patients with myomas.

Excessive doses of estrogens should not be given to postmenopausal women with uterine fibroids.

Treatment

Selection of the most appropriate method of treatment depends upon the size and location of the tumors, their state of preservation, the patient's symptoms, her age and parity, whether she is pregnant, her desire for future pregnancies, and her general health.

A. Emergency Measures: Blood transfusions may be necessary to correct anemia. Surgery is indicated for acute torsion of a pedunculated myoma or intestinal obstruction caused by a pedunculated or parasitic fibroid. Myomectomy is contraindicated during pregnancy, however, except for a torsive fibroid, since it may cause abortion.

B. Surgical Measures:

1. Indications and contraindications–

a. Nonpregnant women–Asymptomatic patients with small myomas require only periodic observation and reassurance. Several years after the menopause, myomas are rarely palpable even though they may have been at one time as large as a uterus at 14 weeks of pregnancy. Intramural and subserous myomas rarely require surgery unless they are larger than a uterus at 14 weeks of pregnancy or are multiple or distorting. Cervical myomas larger than 3–4 cm in diameter should be removed surgically.

b. Pregnant women–The mere presence of myomas that were not clinically of much significance prior to pregnancy is not an indication for cesarean hysterectomy in the absence of compelling reasons for abdominal delivery or for removal of the uterus. Uterine surgery will jeopardize the fetus. If a myomatous uterus is no larger than during a 6-month pregnancy by the 16th week of gestation, an uncomplicated course is probable. If a fibroid mass—especially a cervical myoma—is the size of a uterus at 5–6 months of pregnancy by the second month, abortion will probably occur. If myoma occurs during pregnancy, cesarean hysterectomy sometimes is a sensible solution to the problem for a woman who wants no more children. On the other hand, although rather small myomas may increase appreciably in size during pregnancy, they usually regress just as dramatically after delivery, and one must not overlook the hazards (blood loss, urinary tract damage) associated with removal of a huge puerperal uterus. Surgery should usually be deferred until 5–6 months after delivery, when involution of the uterus and regression of the tumor will be complete.

2. Preoperative counseling–Before hysterectomy or oophorectomy, counsel the patient and her husband about the effects of the operation on menstruation, menopause, and libido.

3. Surgical procedures–Preserve the uterus during the childbearing years, if possible.

a. Myomectomy–Myomectomy (contraindicated during pregnancy) permits excision of multiple myomas and restoration of normal uterine size, contours, and function. It is the treatment of choice during the childbearing years. Place a rubber (catheter) tourniquet snugly around the uterus beneath the round ligaments and tubes to control bleeding. Employ transcervical drainage after entry into the uterine cavity.

b. Hysterectomy or oophorectomy–Total hysterectomy is necessary when myomectomy is so extensive as to leave the uterus grossly distorted and incompetent. Abdominal hysterectomy is indicated for removal of large tumors (especially intraligamentous fibroids), exploration of the abdomen, and coincidental appendectomy and treatment of endometriosis or chronic salpingitis. Subtotal abdominal hysterectomy is required when salpingitis or endometriosis makes removal of the cervix extremely difficult. In premenopausal patients, if the ovaries are diseased or if their blood supply has been destroyed, oophorectomy is necessary; otherwise, the ovaries should be preserved. Vaginal hysterectomy may be employed if the myoma is no larger than a uterus at 14 weeks of pregnancy and if the uterus is mobile and descends appreciably. However, morcellation may be difficult. Associated cystocele, rectocele, and enterocele may then be corrected also.

c. Excision of pedunculated myoma–A pedunculated submucous myoma protruding into the vagina may sometimes be removed vaginally with a looped wire snare.

Prognosis

Surgical therapy is curative. Pregnancy is possible after multiple myomectomy. Cesarean section may be necessary if the uterine cavity has been entered widely or if the uterine wall has been weakened. Menopause will not occur prematurely following a well-executed hysterectomy if normal ovaries are left with a good blood supply.

ADENOMATOUS (ATYPICAL) HYPERPLASIA

Adenomatous hyperplasia, in contrast with the cystic variety, may be a forerunner of cancer. The epithelial components tend to be prominent because of pseudostratification, basophilic cytoplasm and dense nuclei, satellite glands around the primary lumen, and (perhaps) increased mitotic activity. The stromal component is reduced.

Adenomatous hyperplasia occasionally is very difficult to distinguish from low-grade adenocarcinoma, because mitoses are present in both and there may be minimal anaplasia of epithelial cells. In such instances, the final diagnosis and treatment may depend upon an experienced consultant.

CARCINOMA OF THE ENDOMETRIUM
(Corpus or Fundal Cancer)

Adenocarcinoma of the endometrium is the most common cancer of the female genital organs and accounts for more than 90% of endometrial cancers. Almost 5% of women between 20–50 years of age will develop adenocarcinoma if they live to old age; about 10% of women with hypermenorrhea just prior to the menopause will have the disease. It is most prevalent in women between 60–70 years of age; only occasionally is it diagnosed in patients under 35 years of age. The incidence is 3 times as high in nulliparous as in parous women.

The cause of endometrial cancer is unknown, but abnormal estrogen balance has been linked with the development of endometrial adenocarcinoma for the following reasons: (1) The number of cancer patients who have received continuous estrogen therapy, including oral contraceptives, is high. (2) Many cancer patients had abnormal uterine bleeding (endometrial hyperplasia) requiring D&C early in life. (3) The association of feminizing ovarian tumors and endometrial cancer is high. (4) Women who have had ovariectomy in early adult life have a low incidence of endometrial cancer.

Inasmuch as the occurrence of cancer may be influenced by variations in the endometrial cycle or its functions, postmenopausal estrogen therapy should be cyclic, with progestrogen added for the last 7–10 days.

Obesity, diabetes mellitus, hypertension, and polycystic ovary disease are commonly associated with endometrial cancer, perhaps because of abnormal estrogen metabolism. Endometrial polyps and uterine myomas do not increase the likelihood of adenocarcinoma of the endometrium.

Classification & Staging

Primary cancers of the endometrium are of the following types:

(1) Adenocarcinoma, the most common type, is obviously derived from endometrial elements.

(2) Adenosquamous carcinoma is an uncommon pleomorphic variant that is characterized by malignant adenomatous and squamous cells. It is a very aggressive cancer that metastasizes early.

(3) Squamous cell carcinoma is a rare lesion arising from squamous rests, perhaps from the isthmic portion of the uterus near the endocervical canal. Initially, it usually extends by surface spread.

(4) Adenoacanthoma is a variant of adenocarcinoma in which benign-appearing squamous cells (derived presumably by metaplasia) are admixed with adenocarcinoma. This suggests a favorable differentiation and therefore a good prognosis.

(5) Carcinosarcoma is a rare double cancer displaying malignant adenocarcinomatous elements and sarcomatous changes, usually poorly differentiated. The prognosis is poor.

(6) Endometrial sarcoma may originate from the endometrial stroma (chondrosarcoma, leiomyosarcoma, myxosarcoma, etc).

In addition to frank adenocarcinoma, forms of endometrial hyperplasia should be mentioned as possible precursors:

(1) Cystic glandular hyperplasia (Swiss cheese endometrial hyperplasia) is often associated with benign uterine bleeding, generally ascribed to anovulation. When ovulatory cycles resume, cystic glandular hyperplasia is replaced by proliferative secretory endometrium. However, long-term cystic glandular hyperplasia is problematic.

(2) Adenomatous hyperplasia is a complicated variant of endometrial hyperplasia with a more complex pattern of cells lining the cystic spaces. It is still benign and undoubtedly reversible by use of endogenous or exogenous cyclic estrogen-progesterone.

Table 23—1. Clinical staging of carcinoma of the endometrium.*

Stage 0	Carcinoma in situ. Histologic findings suggestive of malignant growth. (Cases of stage 0 should not be included in any therapeutic statistics.)
Stage I	Carcinoma is confined to the corpus.
Stage IA	Length of uterine cavity is ≤8 cm.
IB	Length of uterine cavity is >8 cm. Stage I cases should be graded by histologic type as follows:
G1	Highly differentiated adenomatous carcinoma.
G2	Differentiated adenomatous carcinoma with partly solid areas.
G3	Predominantly solid or entirely undifferentiated carcinoma.
Stage II	Carcinoma has involved the corpus and the cervix.
Stage III	Carcinoma has extended outside the uterus but not outside the true pelvis.
Stage IV	Carcinoma has extended outside the true pelvis or has obviously involved the mucosa of the bladder or rectum. Bullous edema as such does not permit a case to be allotted to stage IV.

*Approved by the International Federation of Obstetricians and Gynecologists. Adopted by ACOG, 1976.

Note: On occasion, it may be difficult to decide whether the cancer involves the endocervix only or both the corpus and the endocervix. If a clear differentiation is not possible upon examination of a specimen obtained by fractional curettage, adenocarcinoma should be classified as carcinoma of the corpus and epidermoid carcinoma as carcinoma of the cervix.

(3) Atypical adenomatous hyperplasia is even more anaplastic in appearance than adenomatous hyperplasia. Irregularities of cell groupings and pseudostratification of epithelial cells lining the acinar spaces are notable. Nuclear abnormalities are relatively uncommon. Although this type of hyperplasia may be reversible, it is considered by many to be progressive in most cases and probably precancerous.

(4) Adenocarcinoma in situ carries all the cellular stigmas of cancer, but the process is limited, without invasion. Although these in situ foci may be sloughed, the changes may not all be reversible.

Clinical staging of carcinoma of the endometrium is shown in Table 23–1. The overall impression or grade—and especially the stage or progress of the cancer—bears a good relationship to the patient's survival. However, staging of an adenocarcinoma of the uterus is not always satisfactory, because specimens from different portions of the lining of the cavity vary in appearance. A well-differentiated adenocarcinoma, formerly called an "adenoma malignum," is merely a grade 1 lesion. Others show intermediate degrees of differentiation, and extremely bizarre, unclassifiable types are also seen. Two-thirds of all adenocarcinomas are graded as 1 or 2 on a scale of 1 to 4.

Pathology

Early malignant lesions originating in the endometrium are gener-

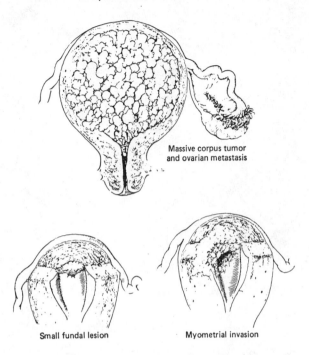

Massive corpus tumor
and ovarian metastasis

Small fundal lesion   Myometrial invasion

Figure 23–17. Adenocarcinoma of the endometrium.

ally minute, in situ changes confined to the functionalis layer, but the cancer finally involves most, if not all, of the endometrial surface. Fortunately, invasion of the myometrium and metastasis occur relatively late (Fig 23–17). When invasion of the uterine wall does occur, the lymphatics are involved first and the venous and arterial channels later. On rare occasions, adenomyosis of the uterus becomes the primary focus for the development of endometrial cancer, either adenocarcinoma or sarcoma.

Endometrial carcinoma may spread in any of the following ways: (1) within the endometrium as a surface growth into the cervical canal, (2) into the myometrium to the peritoneum and parametrium, (3) via the tube to the ovaries, (4) to the uterine and cervical lymphatics, (5) to the uterine arteries and veins, or (6) to the pelvic and abdominal viscera by penetration through the serosa.

As the cancer progresses, the uterus usually becomes larger, more globular, and irregularly softened. The cervix may soften, and the os

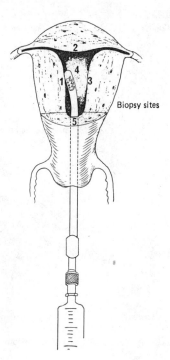

Figure 23–18. Technique of endometrial biopsy.

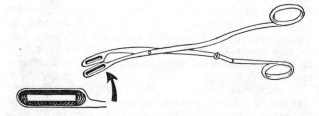

Figure 23–19. Overstreet endometrial polyp forceps.

may appear slightly patulous. Many cases of adenocarcinoma in post-menopausal women are not diagnosed, because the cervix is stenotic and closed while the cancer continues to develop within the fundus. The cancer may spread to the cervix, and pyometra or hematometra is commonly associated with this type of carcinoma. The iliac, obturator, and sacral lymph nodes are seeded when endometrial cancer involves the endocervix (as they are with primary cervical carcinoma).

Obstruction of the cervix and the damming of blood and mucus-containing malignant cells within the uterine cavity permit a reflux of fluid-containing cancer cells into the uterine tubes; neoplastic cells finally escape from the fimbriated ends of the tubes to be implanted laterally and posteriorly to the uterus, just as with retrograde menstruation and the development of endometriosis. However, lymphatic spread is more common than transtubal progression.

Vaginal metastases occur in 10–15% of patients following hysterectomy; most of these are in the vaginal vault or along the urethra 1–2 cm from the urethral meatus. Vaginal metastases may be blood-borne, disseminated through the lymphatics, or implanted at operation. Spread also occurs via uterosacral ligaments and presacral lymphatics to the iliac and periaortic nodes. Hematogenous metastases in the liver, lungs, and bones are not common.

Clinical Findings

A. Symptoms and Signs: Cancer of the corpus is the cause of about half of cases of menopausal menometrorrhagia and postmenopausal bleeding. Abnormal uterine bleeding is the initial symptom in about 80% of cases of adenocarcinoma of the endometrium. Pain occurs late in the disease or when intrauterine infection occurs. A watery, serous or sanguineous, malodorous vaginal discharge, often yellow or brown, is occasionally described instead of (or in addition to) spotting. When obstruction of a senile cervix prevents drainage of discharge, a slow, progressive, painless enlargement of the uterus occurs followed by mucometria or hematometra. The uterine wall becomes extraordinarily thin, and if drainage is not established, the uterus will rupture.

B. Laboratory Findings: The sedimentation rate may be elevated in advanced cancer or when pyometra is present. Cytologic examination of vaginal smears may show endometrial carcinoma cells whether or not symptoms are present. Aspirated material from the cervical canal and uterus should also be examined, as well as the tissue removed from the endometrial cavity during biopsy (Figs 23–18 and 23–19). Use of Isaacs' (or similar) aspiration cannula will increase the diagnostic success to above 95% in cases in which cytology is accurately assessed.

Upon D&C (see p 441), about 90% of endometrial cancers are found to be adenocarcinomas. Squamous cell cancers may be identified on rare occasions. The remainder of uterine cancers are sarcomas. The approximate percentages of various grades of adenocarcinoma of the endometrium are as follows: grade 1 (best differentiation), 60%; grade 2, 25%; and grade 3, 15%.

C. X-Ray Findings: Hysterosalpingography is helpful in the diagnosis of cancer of the endometrium. The contrast media should be injected with minimal pressure—sufficient to fill the uterus without distending the tubes—to avoid transtubal spread of the cancer.

Complications

Mucometria, hematometra, and pyometra may be followed by salpingitis before but rarely after the menopause, and this may be followed by peritonitis. Rupture of the uterus or transtubal spread of the fluid to the peritoneal cavity may occur. Perforation of the uterus may complicate curettage, particularly when the fundus is soft and ill-defined. Bleeding through such a perforation into the abdominal cavity or parauterine spaces is uncommon but may lead to infection or spread of cancer at the site of penetration. Metastatic spread to the vaginal vault or lower vagina, ovaries, tubes, and peritoneal cavity, as well as distant organs, is a serious complication.

Staging Work-Up Recommendations

In contrast with cervical cancer, which spreads rapidly, uterine cancer usually remains localized a long time before metastases occur. For this reason, uterine cancer staging is not done extensively. Nonetheless, the following procedures are recommended:

(1) Fractional curettage is performed to determine possible cervical involvement by cancer.

(2) The patient is anesthetized and then examined to identify parametria and adnexa (or other) spread. Vaginal metastases must also be sought, particularly along the urethra and in the vaginal vault. Anesthesia is important because many uterine cancer patients are obese.

(3) Cystoscopy and sigmoidoscopy should be performed to determine possible bladder or bowel cancer seeding.

(4) Intravenous urography is performed to identify deviation or obstruction of the ureters by tumor.

(5) Laparotomy and definitive surgery may be done singly or with irradiation. At operation, the lateral pelvic, sacral, and para-aortic nodes should be explored carefully (and sampled when indicated).

Differential Diagnosis

Although cystic glandular hyperplasia of the endometrium as such is not a precursor of cancer, adenomatous (atypical) hyperplasia may be, particularly when it is bizarre or of long standing or when premenopausal ovulatory failure and abnormal uterine bleeding have recurred. Because the differentiation of papillary adenocarcinoma of the endometrium and adenomatous or atypical hyperplasia may be extremely difficult, repeat endometrial biopsy or curettage in 4–6 months usually is indicated to prove the persistence and seriousness of the disorder. Special stains are not helpful in making the diagnosis.

Adenocarcinoma may extend to the endometrium from the tubes or the cervix to involve the uterine cavity secondarily. Ovarian, bladder, bowel, and breast cancers also spread to the endometrium.

Adenocarcinoma of the cervix is composed of taller, larger cells that have a greater tendency to form large acinar patterns (in contrast with endometrial cancer elements). Sections containing adenocarcinomatous tissue from the cervix usually also contain more stroma than tissue derived from endometrial cancer.

Adenocarcinoma cells arising in wolffian duct remnants in the lateral aspect of the uterus or cervix are less well differentiated and contain curious frayed or irregular elements.

Carcinosarcoma is diagnosed by the presence of sarcomatous and adenocarcinomatous elements. Sarcoma of the endometrium is usually of the stromal or spindle cell variety. Polypoid intracavitary growths are typical.

Prevention

Endometrial biopsy or aspiration sampling should be done on all peri- or postmenopausal patients before hormone therapy is started.

Routine screening of all women by periodic vaginal cytologic smears—or, even better, by endometrial biopsy—will disclose many incipient as well as clinical cases of endometrial cancer. D&C should be done promptly on patients who report abnormal menstrual bleeding or postmenopausal uterine bleeding.

In women who have recently received estrogens and are bleeding, discontinue the hormone. Repeat cytologic smears and perform an endometrial biopsy 1 month later, even if the earlier cytologic or tissue preparations were not suggestive of cancer.

Pelvic examination of postmenopausal women every 9–12 months is necessary for the recognition and correction of cervical stenosis and other gynecologic problems.

Treatment

A. Emergency Measures: An infected, fluid-distended uterus must be drained without delay to avoid progression of infection. Perforation of the stenotic, occluded cervix usually requires an anesthetic and a small cruciate incision with a bistoury blade. Insert a small mushroom catheter or rubber drain; suture it securely within the cervix, and leave it in place for 2–5 days. Send specimens for culture and bacteriologic sensitivity tests. Surgical curettage or aspiration biopsy should be done when infection has subsided, about 1 week after drainage of the uterus.

B. Supportive Measures: Patients with endometrial cancer are often in an age group in which other diseases are prevalent. Debilitated patients should be restored to reasonable health before definitive cancer therapy is instituted.

C. Principles of Treatment:

1. Despite the general assumption that endometrial carcinoma is well-contained for long periods, approximately 10% of patients with stage I or stage II disease will have pelvic lymph node involvement. The lymph nodes will be involved in 25–30% of stage II patients. Lymphatic spread of adenocarcinoma of the endometrium is likely when the tumor has invaded halfway or more through the myometrium. Moreover, the more undifferentiated the cancer, the greater the likelihood of early metastatic spread. Hence, early diagnosis and treatment are very important in all but indolent tumors.

2. If the cervix is involved in endometrial cancer, the situation is more serious. The mode of spread is likely to be that of cervical cancer, and more extensive treatment will be required.

3. Vaginal spread, while rare, indicates disseminated disease. Approximately 5–10% of patients will have vault or vaginal seeding, but pre- or postoperative irradiation should reduce the incidence of vaginal recurrence to less than 5%.

4. Distant metastases to the ovaries, the cul-de-sac and other peritoneal surfaces, the omentum, the lungs, and the liver are late manifestations of endometrial cancer. In contrast, sarcomas are largely blood-borne, and early dissemination to the liver and lungs often occurs.

D. Treatment Methods: See Table 23–2.

1. Surgery–Extrafascial total abdominal hysterectomy and bilateral salpingo-oophorectomy are mandatory in patients with uterine cancer who can withstand surgery. The additional advantage of radical hysterectomy with pelvic lymphadenectomy is slight, and the complications are too great for most patients. However, if the cervix is involved, if gross spread is unlikely, and if the woman is a good operative risk, radical surgery, including lymph node dissection, may be warranted.

Patients with stage I, grade 1 endometrial carcinoma with less than 50% myometrial invasion can be treated by surgery alone.

2. Radiotherapy–Radiation therapy, usually a combination of intrauterine and supervoltage external pelvic radiation, is recommended for patients who are poor candidates for surgery. However, adjunctive radiation therapy has become popular in combination with surgery for the arrest of possible cancer foci in the pelvis. Combined treatment methods include the following:

a. Preoperative external pelvic irradiation that includes the primary tumor site and the pelvic nodes. A tumoricidal dose of 5000 R to the pelvic axis and 5000 R to the pelvic side walls may be administered. Generally, surgery is scheduled 4–5 weeks later.

Table 23—2. Endometrial carcinoma treatment protocol.

Pretreatment evaluation
1. Fractional D&C in nonenlarged uterus.
2. Chest x-ray.
3. Intravenous urogram.   } May be omitted in patients
4. X-ray following barium enema.   } with stage IA, grade 1 disease
5. SMA-12 or comparable blood chemistry panel and complete blood count.
6. CT scan if a palpable pelvic mass is present.

Treatment

Stage 1A and IB, grades 1 and 2:
1. Surgery: Laparotomy, abdominal washings, and palpation of pelvic and para-aortic nodes. Excision of suspicious nodes. Aortic node biopsy if deep invasion of myometrium has occurred. Total abdominal hysterectomy with adnexectomy is indicated.
2. Radiotherapy: Indications for radiotherapy in grade 2 disease are as follows:
   a. Invasion of more than half of myometrium.
   b. Lymph node involvement.
   c. Large volume of tumor; vascular or lymphatic invasion.

Stage IA and IB, grade 3:
1. Surgery: As above, but aortic node biopsy is not required.
2. Radiotherapy: Radiotherapy is indicated in all cases of grade 3 disease.

Stage II:
1. Gynecologic and radiotherapy oncology consultation before beginning therapy.
2. Consider need for preoperative radium tandem, ovoids, or external radiotherapy.

Stage III and IV: Gynecologic and radiotherapy oncology consultation.

b. Preoperative internal irradiation using capsules of radium or cesium is aimed at the central focus of endometrial carcinoma because little radiation extends to the vagina or pelvic side walls. Patients with stage I, grade 2–3 carcinoma or those with bulky lesions or extension toward the cervix should receive preoperative internal irradiation.

Some uterine sarcomas, eg, endometrial stromal cell sarcoma or mixed mesodermal sarcomas, may respond also to preoperative pelvic irradiation.

c. Postoperative vaginal radium therapy may be elected to prevent vaginal spread of endometrial cancer.

d. Postoperative external pelvic irradiation may be given to patients with anaplastic tumors and to those found to have deep myometrial penetration or a more advanced stage than anticipated.

3. Chemotherapy–Patients with advanced or recurrent adenocarcinoma may respond to palliation by progestogen administration, because many adenocarcinomas of the endometrium are estrogen-dependent. Favored preparations are megestrol acetate (Megace), 80 mg orally 3 times daily, or medroxyprogesterone acetate (Depo-Provera),

400 mg intramuscularly twice weekly. Fluid retention may be a problem if the patient has impaired cardiovascular or renal function. Doxorubicin is the most promising anticancer drug for patients with advanced or recurrent endometrial carcinoma.

Prognosis

The prognosis varies with the stage and grade of carcinoma. At least 80% of endometrial carcinomas are clinically stage I. The following are composite (all modalities combined) approximate 5-year survival rates: stage I, 70–75%; stage II, 45–50%; stage III, 25%; and stage IV, 5%. However, the prognosis is less favorable if the grade of the tumor is high or there is involvement of the cervix or deep (> 50%) invasion of the cervix. Moreover, medical problems such as diabetes mellitus and cardiovascular complications cause about half of deaths in patients undergoing treatment for uterine cancer.

SARCOMA

Sarcomas are heterogeneous, highly malignant tumors of mesodermal origin and constitute almost 2% of all uterine cancers. The corpus of the uterus is affected more frequently than the cervix.

The cause is not known, but women who have received radiation treatment for benign uterine tumors or bleeding have a much higher incidence of uterine sarcoma than a comparison group. Parity or gravidity is not a causative factor. Sarcoma of the uterus occurs most frequently in postmenopausal women, but even infants may be afflicted.

Classification & Staging

Primary sarcomas are classified as follows:

(1) Leiomyosarcomas are homogeneous, pink or grayish, soft, and porklike, with minimal fibrous structure; there is no capsule or limiting membrane. The tumor invades the myometrium with spread of tumor tissue within tissue spaces and along blood vessels. Sarcoma soon penetrates these channels and metastasizes rapidly to lungs and liver. "Recurrent fibroids" (low-grade leiomyosarcomas) may be pathologically benign, but they are clinically malignant. They may develop in the cervix after subtotal hysterectomy.

(2) Mixed mesenchymal tumors contain embryonic striated muscle, osteoid elements, fat, and edematous polymorphous tissue. They develop in the wall of the uterus but may be found in the cervix and resemble pale grapes as they protrude through the os (sarcoma botryoides). Elderly women are affected almost as often as children.

(3) Endometrial stromal cell sarcomas display pale, smooth, firm, polypoid coxcomblike extensions that protrude into the uterine cavity and invade the myometrium.

Table 23–3. Clinical staging of sarcoma.

Stage I	Sarcoma is confined to the corpus.
IA	Length of uterine cavity is ≤ 8 cm.
IB	Length of uterine cavity is > 8 cm.
Stage II	Sarcoma has involved the corpus and the cervix.
Stage III	Sarcoma has extended outside the uterus but not outside the true pelvis.
Stage IV	Sarcoma has extended outside the true pelvis or has obviously involved the mucosa of the bladder or rectum. A bullous edema as such does not permit a case to be allotted to stage IV.

(4) Malignant mixed müllerian tumors have such a wide variety of histologic patterns that diagnosis and classification are difficult. Biologic behavior of tumors may be easier to predict if pure stromal sarcomas (see below) are distinguished from mixed mesodermal tumors. Homologous mixed mesodermal tumors are composed of carcinomatous elements as well as elements of myosarcoma, stromal sarcoma, fibrosarcoma, or mixtures of these varieties of sarcoma. Heterologous mixed mesodermal tumors exhibit carcinoma plus mesenchymal structures not normally seen in the uterus, with or without areas of homologous sarcoma.

(5) Carcinosarcoma grossly resembles endometrial stromal cell sarcoma. Epithelial carcinoma cells in an adenomatous pattern are combined with round sarcoma cells.

(6) Angiosarcomas arise from blood vessels and are delicate and highly vascular, invading the myometrium without restriction.

(7) Reticulum cell sarcoma is a loose, poorly organized and vascularized connective tissue tumor.

Secondary sarcomas may be leiomyosarcomas (occurring in about 0.1–0.5% of myomas) or, rarely, endometrial stromal cell sarcomas (occurring in areas of adenomyosis within the uterine wall).

Clinical staging of sarcoma is shown in Table 23–3.

Pathology

About 25% of sarcomas originate in myomas. About 55% are derived from smooth muscle (leiomyosarcoma) by heteroplasia; 40% are mixed mesenchymal or mesodermal tumors probably derived from endometrial stroma cells; less than 5% are carcinosarcoma; and the remaining 5% develop from such structures as blood vessels (angiosarcoma) or from connective tissue (reticulum cell sarcoma).

Sarcoma cannot be diagnosed by histologic examination of immature, undifferentiated forms of the tumor. Great variation in cell size, hyperchromatism, and 10 or more mitoses per 10× field indicate high-grade malignant growth.

Sarcomas begin as localized silent tumors, but they become diffuse and symptomatic upon extension into and beyond the myometrium. Development is gradual; pain, obstruction, and inflammation do not occur until the tumor is moderately advanced. Extension into the uterine cavity or formation of polypoid growths causes leukorrhea and abnormal bleeding. Metastases occur early via the bloodstream, but lymphatic spread may ensue.

Clinical Findings

A. Symptoms and Signs: A rapidly enlarging uterus or myoma may suggest sarcoma in a young girl or postmenopausal woman. Protrusion of polyps through the cervix is ominous. Common complaints are abnormal uterine bleeding, abdominal enlargement, leukorrhea, urinary frequency, and pelvic discomfort. Late manifestations are loss of weight, pain, orthopnea, jaundice, and edema of the legs.

B. Laboratory Findings: Anemia, increased sedimentation rate, and eosinophilia are reported in well-established sarcoma.

C. X-Ray Findings: Radiopaque coin-shaped densities in the lung fields indicate pulmonary metastases.

D. Special Examinations: Vaginal cytologic examination may disclose malignant cells of endometrial sarcoma and mixed mesenchymal tumors but rarely leiomyosarcoma or other sarcomas. Biopsy of polyps and D&C confirm the diagnosis.

Complications

Relentless local extension and blood-borne distant metastases occur despite therapy in most cases.

Differential Diagnosis

Rapidly growing myomas (particularly submucous fibroids) are usually benign during the period of menstrual activity; postmenopausally, they may be stimulated to resume growth by large doses of estrogen.

Metastatic carcinoma should be considered in the differential diagnosis. Epithelial cells are present only in the uncommon carcinosarcoma.

Diagnosis of sarcoma depends upon thorough pathologic study, including numerous sections and special stains. The presence of "giant cells" and hyperchromatism may indicate degeneration rather than malignant growth.

Treatment

Treatment consists of extracapsular total hysterectomy and bilateral salpingo-oophorectomy. Even more radical primary or secondary surgery may be justified in well-differentiated sarcomas as contrasted with poorly differentiated tumors. Radiation therapy may retard tumor growth and relieve distressing symptoms but may not significantly increase life expectancy. Chemotherapy (eg, with alkylating agents) is only palliative.

Prognosis

Low-grade sarcomas (eg, stromatosis; see below) have a better prognosis than those of more malignant morphology or extent of growth. Well-encapsulated sarcomas incidentally discovered within fibroid tumors metastasize infrequently, and cure is likely. Without treatment, invasive sarcoma of the uterus is fatal within 18 months in 75% of patients. After therapy, approximately 18% survive 5 years.

ADENOMYOSIS

Adenomyosis is a proliferative process wherein benign endometrium, including glands and stroma, has passed into the wall of the uterus beyond the basalis; it usually involves the posterior regions but sometimes penetrates the anterior or cornual regions.

The condition has also been called "adenomyoma," which implies an isolated, distinct regional abnormality. However, a scattered, diffuse type also occurs. Neither type has a sharp limitation or pseudocapsule. "Endometriosis interna" is erroneously used as a synonym; the origin, symptoms, and treatment of the 2 are different.

The cause of adenomyosis is not known. It is unlikely that it could develop primarily from wolffian rests within the uterine wall. Adenomyosis occurs infrequently in nulliparous women; multiparous women are affected 4 times as frequently as primiparous women. Rapid reduction in size of a markedly distended uterus may "fold" the endometrium into the uterine wall at delivery; however, this does not explain adenomyosis when it occurs in nulliparous women. Adenomyosis is found in at least 15% of hysterectomy specimens. It causes difficulty in approximately 70% of proved cases; about 30% of cases are asymptomatic and discovered incidentally. Adenomyosis is generally symptomatic in women between the ages of 45 and 50; it is exceptional after the menopause.

Pathology

The uterus is enlarged (often symmetrically), irregularly firm, and vascular. Incision reveals a coarse, stippled, or granular trabeculation with small yellow or brown cystic spaces containing fluid or blood. Cut surfaces appear convex and bulging, exuding serum. The endometrial-myometrial juncture is often irregular, with the endometrium dipping down into the myometrium. The abnormal zone contains and is surrounded by coarse and whorled strands of muscular tissue.

Adenomyosis is confirmed when both of the following are present: (1) penetration of the myometrium by the endometrium of more than 2 low-power (50×) fields; and (2) associated muscle hypertrophy and hyperplasia.

A grossly yellow specimen suggests stromal adenomyosis (stromatosis). This probably is a low-grade stromal cell sarcoma. There is more stroma than glandular elements, plugs of which are found within tissue spaces and in vessels.

Pain and abnormal uterine bleeding may be caused by increased vascularity of the uterus before and during the menses or by poor vascular control secondary to weakening of myometrial contractility by ectopic endometrium. Intramyometrial bleeding probably does not occur regularly during menstruation, but blood or hemosiderin deep in the myometrium is occasionally seen later in the cycle. Ectopic glands usually resemble those in the basalis; they respond to progesterone in only 20% of patients.

Extension of adenomyosis from the uterine cornu to the tube (salpingitis isthmica nodosa) occurs in 15–20% of patients. It rarely causes infertility, because both tubes are not usually blocked.

Clinical Findings

A. Symptoms and Signs: Adenomyosis is diagnosed and later confirmed at surgery in 65% of patients who are 40–50 years old and complain of abnormal uterine bleeding, increasingly severe dysmenorrhea, and an enlarging, firm, tender uterus.

B. X-Ray Findings: Contrast hysterography may be diagnostic, but the medium must penetrate the glands.

C. Special Examinations: Pelvic examination should be done just prior to or during the early phase of menstruation. Areas of adenomyosis are softened and tender (Halban's sign) as a result of the vasodilating effect of estrogen.

Complications

There are no acute phenomena. Chronic, severe anemia may result from persistent hypermenorrhea. Stromal adenomyosis is rare and originates as an indolent sarcoma in an area of adenomyosis. Equally rare is the development of adenocarcinoma in an area of ectopic endometrium.

Differential Diagnosis

A. Submucous Myoma: Myomas are present in 50–60% of cases of adenomyosis, but the 2 disorders have different symptoms. Myomas may cause excessive and progressive metrorrhagia and pain. The uterus is firm and nontender even during menstruation. The vasodilating effect of the estrogens late in the menstrual cycle causes softening and tenderness (Halban's sign). Discomfort occurs if the myoma is pedunculated and in the process of extrusion. D&C are diagnostic.

B. Endometrial Cancer: This is also diagnosed by D&C.

C. Pelvic Congestion Syndrome (Taylor's Syndrome): The diagnosis of pelvic congestion syndrome should be considered in emotional or hysterical patients with chronic complaints of continuous pelvic pain and menometrorrhagia. The uterus is enlarged, symmetric, and minimally softened; the cervix is cyanotic and somewhat patulous.

D. Pelvic Endometriosis: Pre- and comenstrual dysmenorrhea, adherent adnexal masses, and "shotty" cul-de-sac nodulations are typical. This disorder is associated with adenomyosis in about 15% of patients.

Treatment

Maximal benefit is obtained by surgery. Hysterectomy is best because en bloc excision is required in the absence of a capsule or distinct margin. In premenopausal women, the ovaries should not be removed unless they are diseased. Other accompanying abnormalities such as vaginal relaxation should be corrected.

Radiation therapy will eliminate ovarian function, arrest progress of adenomyosis, and stop pain and bleeding. While therapeutically effective, irradiation should be used rarely in women under 40 because it induces menopause.

Hormone therapy is not effective.

Prognosis

After corrective surgery of classic adenomyosis, the prognosis is excellent. Unless the uterus and areas of possible extension of stromal adenomyosis are widely excised, regional recurrence is likely. Distant metastases are rare.

ENDOMETRIOSIS

Endometriosis is the extrauterine occurrence of endometrium; it most often involves the visceral peritoneal surfaces and may cause pelvic pain, infertility, and abnormal uterine bleeding. Most patients (75%) with endometriosis are 30–40 years of age. The disorder is more common in women who marry late and in nulliparous women. In gynecologic inpatients, the ratio of white to black patients with endometriosis is 2:1. Endometriosis is discovered in at least 5% of obstetric and gynecologic patients.

Endometriosis may originate as a result of partial occlusion of the cervix so that menstrual flow passes through the tubes into the abdominal cavity, where it may implant; in peritoneal (coelomic) metaplastic changes; by vascular and lymphatic dissemination; from embryonic rests; or by surgical implantation.

Staging

The staging of endometriosis is shown in Table 23–4. Aberrant endometrium is found in many different locations: in the ovaries, in the tubes, and over the posterior surface of the uterus; over the anterior surface of the rectum; and even on the appendix. The sigmoid colon and rectum are often involved and show a firm, crescentic or annular, constricting tumefaction. Endometriosis may also distort and obstruct the ureters or invade the bladder. Endometriosis has been reported to occur in the cervix, vulva, umbilicus, and pelvic lymph nodes and in

Table 23–4. Clinical staging of endometriosis.*

Stage I	Broad ligaments: No implants > 5 mm in diameter.
	Tubes: Avascular adhesions; fimbria free.
	Ovaries: Avascular adhesions; no fixation.
	Cul-de-sac: No implants > 5 mm in diameter.
	Bowel: Normal.
	Appendix: Normal.
Stage IIA	Broad ligaments: No implants > 5 mm in diameter.
	Tubes: Avascular adhesions; fimbria free.
	Ovaries: Endometrial cyst ≤ 5 cm in diameter, stage IIA1; > 5 cm, stage IIA2; ruptured, stage IIA3.
	Cul-de-sac: No implants > 5 mm in diameter.
	Bowel: Normal.
	Appendix: Normal.
Stage IIB	Broad ligaments: Covered by adherent ovary.
	Tubes: Adhesions not removable by endoscopy; fimbria free.
	Ovaries: Fixed to the broad ligament; implants > 5 mm in diameter.
	Cul-de-sac: Multiple implants; no adherent bowel or fixed uterus.
	Bowel: Normal.
	Appendix: Normal.
Stage III	Broad ligaments: May be covered by adherent tube or ovary.
	Tubes: Fimbria covered by adhesions.
	Ovaries: Adherent with or without implants or endometriomas.
	Cul-de-sac: Multiple implants; no adherent bowel or fixed uterus.
	Bowel: Normal.
	Appendix: Normal.
	Bladder: Normal.
Stage IV†	Uterus: May be fixed and adherent posteriorly.
	Cul-de-sac: Covered by adherent bowel or fixed retrodisplaced uterus.
	Bowel: Adherent to the cul-de-sac, uterosacral ligaments, or corpus.
	Appendix: May be involved.
	Bladder: Implants.

*Based on laparoscopic findings. (Kistner, 1977.)
†Stage IV is usually combined with Stages I, II, and III.

operative abdominal and vaginal scars following uterine surgery. Rare distant foci, eg, in the axilla or lung, probably are benign metastases.

Pathology

Minute (never large), rounded, raised, cystic "blueberry spots" of endometriosis are scattered over the pelvic structures. Discolored "powder-burn" points and minute stellar scars are characteristic. Dense fibrinoplastic distorting adhesions restrict the organs involved. The uterus may be immobilized in retroversion; the cul-de-sac is obliterated. The tarry endometriotic cysts in the ovary may be microscopic or large (up to about 10 cm in diameter). They contain chocolate-colored, thick, syrupy material, the residue of old hemorrhage (chocolate cysts of the ovary).

The endometrial implants are identical to uterine endometrium: tubular or simple branched epithelial glands or lymphoidlike stroma (or both). The histologic characteristics of ectopic endometrium depend upon the type and amount of circulating ovarian hormone and the response of the ectopic endometrium to these hormones. During pregnancy, endometriotic foci react by developing typical decidua.

Malignant change, eg, adenocarcinoma or stromal cell sarcoma (stromal endometriosis or stromatosis), is rare in endometriosis.

Ectopic endometrium, like uterine endometrium, responds to steroid sex hormones. The response is conditioned by the presence of either adenomatous or stromal tissue, or both; the site and viability of the ectopic endometrium; the phase of the ectopic endometrium at the time of examination; and the extent of endometrial involvement and degree of reaction by underlying tissue. Endometriosis is unresponsive when pressure within the cyst reduces the function of the endometrial cells; when menstrual bleeding grossly disrupts the cystic epithelial lining; or when scarring or thrombosis diminishes the circulation to the lesion. Stromal endometriosis does not react to cyclic hormonal variations.

Most extrauterine foci may be considered miniature uteri because they bleed at menstruation. The greatest response is to estrogen and progesterone in ovulatory cycles. When blood cannot escape, especially from buried lesions, it distends and infiltrates the surrounding tissues. Slow, partial absorption and phagocytosis of blood products follow. Chemical irritation causes the bowel and omentum to seal off many endometriotic bleeding points. The lesions gradually enlarge, adhere, and scar.

The discomfort of endometriosis generally ceases during pregnancy. In most cases, remissions occur following delivery of a viable infant. In such cases, necrosis of decidua, dissolution of the endometriosis, and healing may occur. The menopause terminates the activity and progress of endometriosis unless large, repeated doses of estrogen are administered.

Clinical Findings

A definite diagnosis is not possible until after laparotomy and tissue appraisal; symptoms alone, in the absence of pelvic findings, are not sufficient to establish the diagnosis.

A. Symptoms and Signs: Pre- and comenstrual pelvic pain is practically constant, beginning a few days to a week before the menses and increasing in severity until the flow has virtually ceased. Dysmenorrhea is generally most marked where the endometriosis is advanced. Pain is due to local engorgement and regional bleeding and is often of a "grinding" type. It may be referred to the inguinal region or hips or toward the rectum or coccyx, depending upon the location of the endometriosis. However, one-third of patients have no pain, despite typical pelvic findings.

Defecation is painful if the lesions are on the bowel or in a rectovaginal septum. Dyspareunia of the acquired, deep-thrust type occurs in ovarian and cul-de-sac involvement. Infertility may result from peritubal and ovarian endometriosis. Hypermenorrhea and shortening of the menstrual interval (more rarely metrorrhagia) may occur when the ovary is the site of ectopic endometrium. The rectum and bladder often bleed at the time of the menses when these organs are invaded.

In the absence of a history of salpingitis, pelvic examination will reveal an adherent, retroverted uterus; "shotty" nodulation in the cul-de-sac; adnexal induration and ovarian cyst formation; and increased pelvic tenderness just prior to and during menses.

B. X-Ray Findings: X-rays may be helpful in differentiating endometriosis from inflammatory or malignant disease. The colon is involved in about 50% of extensive cases of endometriosis. In such cases, barium enema x-rays may show that the colon is fixed and constricted in one area; thickened regionally by a plaque or concentric stenosing lesion with sharp demarcations; or restricted in motion, with rounded, intraluminal projections (rare).

C. Special Examinations: Laparoscopy, sigmoidoscopy, and cystoscopy may reveal endometriosis, but bleeding will be seen only at the time of menstruation.

Complications

Tubal, bowel, and ureteral obstruction have been reported in patients with endometriosis. Destruction of the ovary may complicate ovarian endometriosis. Rupture of large endometriotic cysts—particularly during pregnancy, when the enlarging uterus disrupts adhesions—may lead to intra-abdominal bleeding and a low-grade chemical peritonitis.

Differential Diagnosis

Endometriosis must be distinguished from infection and cancer.

A. Postabortal or Postgonococcal Salpingitis: Salpingitis is initiated by an acute illness; endometriosis develops gradually. Fever and elevation of the white blood cell count and sedimentation rate are unlikely in endometriosis but common in salpingitis.

B. Pelvic Tuberculosis: Endometriosis must be differentiated from tuberculosis involving the ovaries, tubes, cul-de-sac, or bowel. Pain (particularly crescendo type dysmenorrhea and dyspareunia, varying with the menstrual cycle), painful defecation, and bleeding from the bowel and bladder are not typical of pelvic tuberculosis. Debilitation and anemia occur with tuberculosis.

C. Ovarian Cancer: Pre- and comenstrual pain, dyspareunia, infertility, and abnormal menses do not occur in ovarian cancer with pelvic implants. Ascites often accompanies pelvic carcinoma. Laparoscopy and biopsy are diagnostic.

D. Bowel Cancer: This is an intrinsically silent tumor that rapidly invades the intestinal wall from within; secondarily, it causes adherence and tumor formation. Bloody stools accompany cancer of the colon. Minimal periodic bleeding from the bowel occurs even in severe endometriosis involving the colon. Proctosigmoidoscopy should be performed.

Prevention

Annual examination of all women during the childbearing years is recommended.

Treatment

Treatment depends upon the stage of endometriosis, the patient's age, and her desire for pregnancy. Pregnancy or pseudopregnancy will halt the spread of endometriosis in many cases, although amenorrhea must continue for at least 6 months to be beneficial. Women who wish to have children should be urged to become pregnant without delay. Procedures to investigate infertility, such as hysterosalpingography, may release peritubal adhesions and obliterate kinks and distortions of the oviducts caused by endometriosis.

Women with suspected mild endometriosis should be examined every 6 months until the menopause or until the diagnosis is confirmed or ruled out.

A. General Measures: For pain, give analgesics such as codeine, 0.03 g, and aspirin, 0.6 g, orally every 4–6 hours when necessary during the immediate premenstrual interval.

B. Endocrine Therapy:

1. Danazol–Danazol (Danocrine) is a weak androgen that suppresses the production of FSH and LH and thus suppresses ovulation. It may suppress endometriosis directly via estrogen receptors. When given in doses adequate to suppress endometriosis, ie, 400 mg orally twice daily for 6 months, danazol causes "pseudomenopause." Danazol is very effective against endometriosis, but it aggravates acne and hirsutism and may cause fluid retention.

2. Estrogens–In the past, patients with endometriosis were treated with large doses of diethylstilbestrol (or comparable drug) to induce pseudopregnancy for 6 months. Because more effective agents with fewer side-effects are now available, estrogen therapy has been abandoned.

3. Androgens–Methyltestosterone, 5–10 mg/d sublingually, generally relieves pain and retards the growth of endometriosis. With the smaller dose, ovulation usually continues, and pregnancy often occurs. The patient must be observed for signs of virilization and the drug discontinued if they appear.

4. Gestogens–Norethynodrel with mestranol (Enovid) induces pseudopregnancy. A dose of 10 mg orally daily is given for 2 weeks beginning on the fifth day of the menstrual period and is increased by 10 mg every 2 weeks until the dose reaches 40 mg/d. The drug should be given for 6–9 months for optimal effect. Sodium intake should be restricted to avoid fluid retention.

C. Surgical Measures:

1. Incidental endometriosis–Small foci should be excised or cauterized during surgery for other indications.

2. Moderately extensive endometriosis–If medical treatment is unsuccessful, surgery is indicated.

a. Patients under age 35–Resect the lesions, free adhesions, and suspend the uterus, but avoid sacrificing reproductive ability. About 30% of such patients become pregnant, although 50% must undergo surgery again later when the disease progresses.

b. Patients over age 35–If both ovaries are involved, both ovaries and tubes and the uterus may have to be removed. If only one ovary is affected, its removal may be sufficient.

3. Very extensive endometriosis–Excision of both ovaries, both tubes, and the uterus is almost always required regardless of the woman's age. Danazol or gestogen therapy may improve the pathologic picture so that an easier and less radical operation will be feasible.

D. Radiation Therapy: If surgery is contraindicated or hazardous, castrating doses of external radiation will relieve the symptoms and cause almost complete regression of the lesions. Nevertheless, one must obtain a definite diagnosis of extensive endometriosis, either by biopsy at exploratory laparotomy or from a previous operation, before this is justified.

E. Treatment of Complications: Bowel obstruction or ureteral occlusion due to endometriosis will require laparotomy for confirmation and decision regarding definitive therapy. Danazol may eliminate the problem, but resection and reanastomosis may be required. If the ovaries are removed or the woman is sterilized by irradiation, the stenotic areas usually resolve spontaneously. Signs of intraperitoneal bleeding or peritonitis will require exploratory surgery, even during pregnancy.

Prognosis

With proper medical or surgical treatment, the prognosis is favorable in patients with early and even moderately advanced endometriosis. When bilateral ovariectomy is not permitted in advanced endometriosis, the prognosis is unfavorable. With appropriate treatment, reproductive capacity is usually regained if endometriosis is minimal; in moderately extensive endometriosis, fertility can be restored in about 15% of women. Few women with extensive endometriosis can ever conceive even with the most intensive treatment.

24 | Diseases of the Uterine Tubes

ANOMALIES OF THE UTERINE TUBES

Congenital absence or distortion of the uterine tubes (oviducts, fallopian tubes) is frequently associated with anomalies of the uterus. It may occur as a result of aplasia or dysplasia of the müllerian ducts or regional injury to the tubes during fetal life. Any variation—absence, atresia, shortening, or lengthening—may occur and is usually unilateral. Infertility may result.

SALPINGITIS
(Pelvic Inflammatory Disease [PID])

Inflammation of the uterine tubes may be acute or chronic and unilateral or bilateral. It accounts for 15–20% of gynecologic admissions to large hospitals. It is more common in urban areas, especially where sexually transmitted diseases are prevalent, obstetric care is poor, and tuberculosis is not well controlled.

Almost all cases are due to bacterial infection, usually with gonococci, chlamydiae, streptococci, staphylococci, tubercle bacilli, or mixed flora. Rare types include actinomycetes, schistosomes, and *Oxyuris* infections.

Gonorrheal or chlamydial infections are responsible for 65–75% of cases. The organisms spread across the mucosal surface of the cervix and endometrium to the endosalpinx. Streptococcal salpingitis, especially that caused by anaerobic strains of enterococci, is still a common sequela of obstetric mishaps. Ascending bacterial infections, notably gonorrhea and postabortal or postpartal infections, almost always involve one or both uterine tubes within 1–3 days after the initial infection. Childbirth and postabortal infections cause 5–10% of cases. Infection caused by staphylococci or streptococci reaches the tubes by lymphatic and vascular pathways in the parametrium and mesosalpinx.

Tuberculous salpingitis is now rare in the USA. It occurs via descending hematogenous spread from a pulmonary, intestinal, or urinary tract focus. Tuberculous salpingitis may not be diagnosed until many months or years after recognition of the primary tuberculous lesion. Mixed infections are often responsible for recurrences or treatment failures.

Factors that predispose to salpingitis include transvaginal instrumentation of the cervix and uterus (especially before and during menstruation), operative delivery, intrauterine devices, peritonitis of bowel origin, degenerative cervical or uterine tumors, and hysterosalpingography performed with excess of oily medium.

Women in the childbearing age group are most commonly affected, but the condition is unusual during pregnancy. Salpingitis may occur in prepuberal girls (often tuberculous) or in postmenopausal women (during the treatment of endometrial cancer, with diverticulitis causing left pelvic peritonitis).

Chronic salpingitis (often inappropriately called pelvic inflammatory disease) is one of the principal causes of infertility in women, menstrual disorders, and gynecologic disability.

Pathology

The tubal inflammation may pass through various stages. Acute pyogenic infection may develop into chronic hydrosalpinx or tubo-ovarian abscess. Either of these may result in fixed retroversion of the uterus with bilateral tubo-ovarian masses. The pathologic findings are as follows:

A. Acute Stage:

1. Gonococcal–Both tubes are generally dependent, injected, and edematous. The tube contains a purulent exudate that may drain from the swollen, fimbriated extremity. Peritonitis frequently accompanies fulminant salpingitis, and fibrinous adhesions soon wall off the tubes, uterus, ovaries, and nearby loops of bowel and omentum. Occlusion of the distal extremities of the tubes is the rule. Occasionally, the tube and ovary are so closely involved that a tubo-ovarian abscess is created (Fig 24–1). Early microscopic examination of stained sections shows severe inflammation of the mucosa; deeper structures soon become involved. Plical swelling, turgescence of all layers, and gross exudation into the tubal lumen are typical.

In untreated cases, *Neisseria gonorrhoeae* usually cannot be identified in the uterine tubes after 3–4 days. Secondary invaders, usually a mixed group of cocci, replace the gonococcus. Reinfection of the tubes by *N gonorrhoeae* does not commonly occur, but flare-ups due to other organisms do.

2. Due to other pyogenic infections–*Chlamydia, Bacteroides,* and anaerobic streptococci may infect one or both tubes. The tubes resemble those seen in acute gonococcal salpingitis, but the redness, swelling, and induration are usually more marked in postabortal or

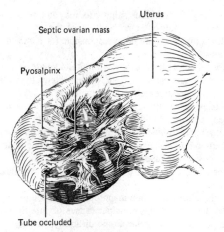

Figure 24–1. Tubo-ovarian abscess.

puerperal salpingitis. Parametritis is often present. Microscopic examination shows infiltration of interstitial tissues and muscle layers of the
tubes with polymorphonuclear leukocytes. Mucosal inflammation and
exudation into the tubal lumen often are only moderate.

Extension of an infectious process from the appendix—to the
uterine tube, for example—is relatively common but is seldom diagnosed correctly before surgery. The infection usually is limited to the
perisalpinx and adjacent structures; the mucosa and tubal lumen are
seldom involved. Pelvic abscesses frequently involve the original focus,
ie, in the appendix, ileum, uterine tube, or ovary.

3. Tuberculous–A seroexudative reaction often occurs in the tube
with the development of tubercles, especially in the deeper layers of the
endosalpinx and the inner muscular layers.

B. Chronic Stage:

1. Gonococcal–The tubes become fluid-filled and ''retort-
shaped''; curved, bulbous, thickened in certain areas and thinned in
others. Both ends are usually closed. The tubes frequently adhere to the
ovary, uterus, or other neighboring structures. Subdiaphragmatic or
subhepatic adhesions, also involving the bowel and omentum, may
indicate prior upper abdominal peritonitis due to salpingitis. As the
infection resolves, the exudate in the tube is reabsorbed; however, up to
180 mL of thin, tawny, serous fluid may remain in the occluded tube
(hydrosalpinx). Adhesions usually persist. If considerable distention of
the tube occurs, the plicae become flattened, and the microscopic pattern

on cross section is referred to as hydrosalpinx simplex. Agglutination of numerous rugous folds, with minimal distention of the tube by fluid, results in hydrosalpinx follicularis. Patchy loss of the endosalpingeal mucosa, scar tissue formation, and persistence of lymphocytes and plasma cells in the mucosa of the tubes are to be expected. Repeated acute infections in the absence of pyosalpinx formation result in a firm, adherent tubal enlargement, the consequence of thickening of the wall of the tube (chronic interstitial salpingitis). Resolution of a tubo-ovarian abscess leaves a tubo-ovarian cyst. With repeated episodes of salpingitis, the heavy infected tubes drag the uterus backward into the cul-de-sac, where it becomes densely fixed in retroposition.

2. Due to other pyogenic infections–The sequence of events is much like that in chronic gonococcal infection.

3. Tuberculous–The tubes are thickened, rigid, rather straight, and occasionally adherent. Curiously, they may be patent. Small raised, pale, firm tubercles may be seen beneath the serosal surface. Caseation and multiple minute cold abscesses within the tube can be observed on stained sections. Granulomatous infiltration, necrosis, and tubercle formation usually occur. Giant cells may be difficult to find.

4. Granulomatous endosalpingitis–This may follow salpingography when excessive oily medium collects in a hydrosalpinx.

Clinical Findings

A. Symptoms and Signs: The symptoms and signs depend upon the infectious agent and the type, extent, and stage of infection.

In the acute phase, lower quadrant pain, the most common complaint, is unilateral or bilateral depending upon whether one or both tubes are involved. In acute salpingitis, the pain is severe, aching, often cramplike but not wholly remitting, and nonradiating. Pain is often described as dyspareunia or dysmenorrhea of the comenstrual and post-menstrual type. Severe sacral backache (referred pain) may be present. Occasionally, associated right upper quadrant pain (gonococcal perihepatitis, Fitz-Hugh–Curtis syndrome) may be noted.

In about 10% of cases of nontuberculous salpingitis, a piercing right upper quadrant pain that radiates toward the back results from accumulation of purulent exudate below the diaphragm. The pain may localize below the right costal margin.

Shaking chills and a high intermittent fever to 104 °F (40 °C) often develop. Menstruation usually exacerbates salpingitis because of the pelvic engorgement with which it is associated. Menstrual disturbances occur. Other findings include profuse, seropurulent leukorrhea; thin, purulent discharge from Skene's and Bartholin's ducts (in gonococcal infections); slight enlargement and tenderness of the uterus (in postabortal salpingitis); and marked bilateral adnexal tenderness without mass formation. Adynamic ileus is usually present in acute salpingitis.

The onset and course of tuberculous salpingitis are insidious; an explosive, dramatic onset is rare.

In the chronic phase of salpingitis, the character of the pain depends upon the extent of the disease. Symptoms and signs include purulent discharge from Skene's ducts, Bartholin's duct cysts, mucopurulent leukorrhea, menometrorrhagia or hypermenorrhea, a tender unilateral or bilateral pelvic mass, severe sacral backache (referred pain), abdominal tenderness and adnexal restriction without abdominal rigidity, dyspareunia, and low-grade fever. Occasionally, several ounces of thin clear or straw-colored fluid from a hydrosalpinx may discharge suddenly via the uterine cornu (hydrops tubae profluens).

B. Laboratory Findings: Stained smears of specimens from the cervix or urethra may reveal *Neisseria gonorrhoeae*, chlamydiae, or other pathogens capable of causing salpingitis. Smears of cervical samples may reveal *Clostridium perfringens (Clostridium welchii)* in certain instances of septic abortion. In postabortal and puerperal infections, cervical or uterine specimens should be inoculated on both blood agar and nutrient broth and grown under both aerobic and anaerobic conditions to identify the pathogen. The organism's sensitivity to antibiotics should also be determined.

In acute salpingitis, the white cell count may be as high as 20–30 thousand/μL, and a marked shift to the left is always present; the red cell count is normal. In tuberculous salpingitis, the white and red cell counts are often within normal limits; monocytes may be increased, and there may be a relative lymphopenia.

C. X-Ray Findings (in Tuberculous Salpingitis):

1. Hysterosalpingography often reveals evidence of tuberculosis. The uterus fills slowly with the contrast medium; the corpus is trumpet-shaped, with a fuzzy or shaggy convex inner outline; and the fundal and lateral shadows bulge.

2. Salpingography may not be possible because of occlusion of the tubes after suppurative salpingitis. In other cases, contrast media may fill the tubes to reveal tuberculous changes. A flat film before injection of radiopaque fluid may reveal calcific tubo-ovarian densities. If the tubes fill at all, they fill by slow, jerky progress of the medium. Uneven, blurred beading, segmentation, or sacculation—even fistula formation—is revealed. These changes are more likely to be seen in the isthmic and ampullar portions of the tubes. The tubes are relatively straight, rigid, and drooping, often with diverticula near the fimbriated extremities. They are usually narrowly patent, and both are usually affected. Contrast filling of the blood and lymph vessels occurs occasionally.

D. Special Examinations:

1. Laparoscopy may reveal distorted, adherent tubes and ovaries.

2. Culture of menstrual discharge for *Mycobacterium tuberculo-*

sis–Collect sanguineous fluid in a contraceptive diaphragm, a menstrual cup (Tassette), or a test tube worn vaginally. Blood may also be aspirated from the posterior vaginal fornix on the first or second day of the period. Inoculate the specimen into Petragnani's or Sabouraud's medium; incubate at 37 °C for 4 weeks. Smear, fix, and stain for acid-fast organisms. (Nonpathogenic acid-fast bacteria are smaller and more readily stained than *M tuberculosis.*)

3. Tine test–If the test is strongly positive, suspect an active tuberculous focus, possibly tubal.

4. Endometrial biopsy may give evidence of associated endometrial tuberculosis.

Complications

Salpingitis rarely remains confined to the tube; the peritoneum, ovary, and distal intestinal and urinary tracts soon become involved.

Complications of gonococcal, streptococcal, or staphylococcal salpingitis include the following:

(1) Torsion of the swollen, deformed adnexa.

(2) Rupture of tubo-ovarian or other abscesses into a neighboring adherent viscus. The initial step in abscess formation may have been ovulation that resulted in an infected corpus luteum. Sometimes tubo-ovarian abscesses drain spontaneously into the bladder or point laterally above the pelvic brim, in which case incision and drainage may be feasible. Rupture into these areas may be considered fortunate, since rupture into the peritoneal cavity may have lethal consequences. Pyosalpinx or pelvic abscess may become localized in the posterior cul-de-sac. Unless surgical drainage is instituted through the vagina, spontaneous rupture into the rectum may occur.

(3) Diffuse generalized peritonitis that may extend beyond the pelvis to the upper abdomen (especially on the right side). This is far more devastating than the acute tubal disease itself. Gonococcal septicemia and endocarditis occur rarely. Metastatic gonococcal abscess formation, especially in the skin and joints, has been reported. Broad ligament cellulitis, pelvic thrombophlebitis, periphlebitis, lymphangitis, and septic pulmonary embolism are critical complications of streptococcal or staphylococcal salpingitis.

(4) Small bowel obstruction.

(5) Infertility. Inability to conceive is common even after mild, short-lived gonococcal, streptococcal, or staphylococcal salpingitis. About 50% of patients with tuberculous salpingitis seek medical assistance with no other complaint than infertility.

Differential Diagnosis

A history of previous salpingitis is helpful in identification of the residua of pelvic infection.

Salpingitis must be differentiated from appendicitis and ectopic pregnancy so that appropriate therapy can be given. (See Table 11–1.)

To differentiate between appendicitis and acute right-sided salpingitis, palpate the patient's abdomen while she lies in different positions. If the point of maximal tenderness is originally over the region of the right ovary and tube while the patient is supine but disappears or diminishes markedly while the patient is in the Trendelenburg position, appendicitis is the more likely diagnosis.

A tetrad of symptoms—menstrual abnormality followed by uterine bleeding, pelvic pain, and pelvic mass—indicates ectopic pregnancy in most cases when the woman is of childbearing age.

Salpingitis isthmica nodosa, or endosalpingiosis, is related to endometriosis and is characterized by areas of nodular thickening of the isthmus of the uterine tube. On section, glandular spaces are observed to be interspersed with an irregularly hypertrophied myosalpinx. Cells suggestive of chronic inflammation may be present. This disorder is bilateral in about one-third of cases, and less than half of cases are due to infection. Few cases are diagnosed preoperatively. The outstanding clinical problem is infertility due to tubal occlusion. Treatment consists of salpingectomy and wedge resection of the cornu.

Prevention

Many cases of salpingitis can be prevented by early diagnosis and treatment of cervical and uterine neoplasms (which may become infected); by avoidance of obstetric and instrumental trauma; by avoidance of cervical contraceptive pessaries and the selective use of intrauterine devices; and by hygienic and anti-infective measures to prevent and control sexually transmitted infections. Use of condoms will reduce the incidence of sexually transmitted diseases that cause salpingitis.

Treatment

A. Specific Measures:

1. Gonococcal, streptococcal, and staphylococcal salpingitis– Penicillin is effective against most gonococci, most strains of streptococci, and many types of staphylococci. A single dose of 4.8 million units of penicillin G intramuscularly, half the dose into each buttock, will cure most uncomplicated cases.

Spectinomycin is an alternative to penicillin for the treatment of gonorrhea, and this is its sole indication. It should be used if the patient is hypersensitive to penicillin or the gonococcus is penicillin-resistant. A single injection of 2 g, half the dose into each buttock, is reported to cure about 90% of patients with gonorrhea. About 10% of gonococci may be resistant to spectinomycin. Pain at the injection site, nausea, or fever may be side-effects.

Kanamycin, often given with penicillin, broadens the chemotherapeutic attack, especially in resistant (retreatment) cases or mixed pyogenic infections. Give 1 g intramuscularly followed by 0.5 g intramuscularly 4 times daily.

Chloramphenicol and the tetracyclines are also effective in the treatment of chlamydial and other nontuberculous salpingitis. Give 500 mg orally and then 250 mg every 6 hours for 1 week. The parenteral dose is about half the oral dose.

2. Tuberculous salpingitis–Several regimens are useful. In general, 2 or 3 of the following drugs are used in various combinations and treatment schedules: isoniazid (INH), *p*-aminosalicylic acid (PAS), streptomycin, ethambutol, cycloserine, and rifampin. Combination therapy is used to minimize toxicity and prevent the emergence of resistant strains. The reader should consult other texts for details of management of genital tuberculosis.

B. General Measures: Complete bed rest in Fowler's position during the acute stage aids in localization of the infection. A hot water bottle or hot pad applied to the hypogastrium relieves lower abdominal pain. Pelvic pain can be relieved with heat applied deep in the pelvis by diathermy (or equivalent), especially when an abdominal and vaginal electrode is used, or warm (1-gallon) vaginal douches. Aspirin, 0.3–0.6 g, and codeine, 30–60 mg, orally every 4 hours as necessary, usually relieve pain adequately, although morphine may be necessary at first in severe acute infections.

C. Surgical Measures:

1. Acute salpingitis–Abdominal surgery is contraindicated. If the peritoneum is opened in error, the tubal inflammatory process should not be disturbed and the abdomen should be closed immediately without drainage. Colpotomy or extraperitoneal drainage of large pelvic abscesses may be required.

2. Chronic salpingitis–Every effort must be made to treat the patient medically to conserve organs and function. Surgery is indicated, however, when conservative management fails, repeated exacerbations occur, and disability develops. Pelvic abscesses should be drained through the vagina or extraperitoneally. Large pelvic masses are less common with antibiotic and other methods of medical treatment.

In general, it is a good rule to be conservative. If conservative management fails, definitive surgery should be performed. If tuboovarian masses are not present and the patient is young, simple bilateral cornual resection and preservation of both tubes and ovaries may be curative without sacrificing ovarian function. If both tubes and ovaries are extensively diseased despite prolonged medical therapy, bilateral salpingo-oophorectomy and hysterectomy, total if possible, are indicated even in a young woman. If the diseased tube can be removed by careful dissection, the ovary should not be removed if it appears to be reasonably normal. If bilateral salpingectomy is required, the uterus and cervix should be removed. The vena cava and the infundibulopelvic vessels should be ligated after repeated septic pulmonary embolization.

If a tubo-ovarian abscess develops or persists after 3–4 months of chemotherapy for tuberculous salpingitis, laparotomy is indicated. Total hysterectomy and adnexectomy, or at least bilateral salpingectomy, is warranted for women over 40 years of age. Avoid injury to the bowel or bladder lest persistent fistulas develop. Antituberculosis chemotherapy should be resumed postoperatively. Isoniazid may have to be given on a long-term basis.

Salpingostomy after severe acute salpingitis has seldom proved satisfactory, even with the most modern techniques.

Prognosis

The earlier and more adequate the treatment, the better the prognosis. While inflammation usually resolves rapidly, tubal obstruction occurs in many cases. Recurrent salpingitis with subsequent infertility usually occurs if an abscess develops within or near the tube.

CARCINOMA OF THE UTERINE TUBES

Primary cancer of the uterine tube (characteristically unilateral) is almost always an adenocarcinoma. It is the least common malignancy of the müllerian system; fewer than 1500 cases have been described in the literature to date. Metastatic carcinoma, usually from the endometrium or ovary, is more common.

Most cases occur in nulliparous postmenopausal women. Symptoms include one or more of the following: pain, brownish vaginal discharge, and unilateral pelvic mass. Salpingitis is probably not a causative factor, since there is a disparity of incidence between tubal cancer and tubal infection.

Carcinoma of the uterine tube usually occurs in the ampullary or fimbriated portion; the right tube is more frequently involved than the left. The tube in the area of carcinoma is rounded at first but later becomes fusiform or even sausage-shaped. The surface is glistening and red or purple; the tube is firm but not hard or nodular.

The tube contains yellow-brown grumous necrotic cancer tissue and dark-brown or straw-colored sanguineous fluid. Minute hemorrhagic points are commonly present. The fimbriated extremity is usually closed. Spread occurs when the malignancy extrudes or grows through the fimbriated end, and the tube, ovary, and uterus are ultimately bound together in an irregularly shaped fixed mass.

In premenopausal women, exclude the following in differential diagnosis: salpingitis, tubal pregnancy, ovarian enlargement and carcinoma, endometrial disease, hydrosalpinx, and a soft pedunculated myoma. Tubal tuberculosis often produces a highly adenomatous picture that may be mistaken for tubal cancer, particularly the papillomatous type.

Treatment

Surgery is required. The success of treatment depends upon the type of tumor and the stage of the disease when the diagnosis is made. Except when the tumor is very small and diagnosed histologically as an incidental finding, the long-term survival rate is extremely poor. When the diagnosis has been confirmed, the treatment of choice is bilateral salpingo-oophorectomy, total hysterectomy, and postoperative irradiation. When there is direct extension to adjacent viscera, ie, the rectosigmoid, every effort should be made to resect the affected structures.

Prognosis

The presently available therapeutic techniques are relatively ineffective, and the prognosis is exceedingly poor. The 5-year survival rate is less than 15%.

25 | Diseases of the Ovaries

OVARIAN CYSTS

A cyst is a sac that contains fluid or semisolid material. Ovarian cysts cause ovarian enlargement and may develop at any time, although they occur most commonly from puberty to the menopause. They range in size from a microscopic cyst to a large pelvic mass and may cause difficulty if pulsion, traction, torsion, infection, malignant change, or rupture occurs.

The following factors must be evaluated in any ovarian enlargement: size, persistence, bilaterality, adherence, hormone production, surface nodulation, papillar formations or neighboring irregularities, and ascites. In postmenopausal women, it is usually impossible to palpate the ovary, and what may appear to be a ''normal or slightly enlarged'' ovary may actually represent an ovarian cyst that may be malignant. In this case, diagnostic evaluation should not be delayed.

Ovarian cysts are usually small and clinically unimportant. Most resolve spontaneously within a few months, and only a few require removal. Cysts that do not resolve in that time may be inflammatory, endometrial, or malignant. Surgery is generally required if a tense ovarian enlargement progresses to more than 6 cm in diameter within 4 months. Abdominal pain, bleeding, or a palpable pelvic mass may require exploratory laparotomy. Treatment must be based upon an estimate of whether the growth is benign or malignant, the consequences of its development, and the risk of its elimination.

Classification

Ovarian cysts may be classified as functional cysts (follicle, granulosa lutein, theca lutein), inflammatory cysts (tubo-ovarian), endometrial cysts (endometriomas), inclusion cysts, and parovarian cysts.

A. Functional Cysts: Follicle and corpus luteum cysts are normal transient physiologic structures. Malignant change does not occur in functional cysts.

1. Follicle (retention) cysts–Follicle cysts are common, frequently bilateral, multiple cysts that appear at the surface of the ovaries as pale blebs filled with a clear fluid. They vary in size from microscopic to 4 cm in diameter (rarely larger). These cysts represent the failure of an incompletely developed follicle to resolve by atresia. They are commonly found after anovulatory cycles, in prolapsed adherent ovaries, or when a thickened, previously inflamed ovarian capsule restricts ovarian function. Symptoms are usually not present unless torsion or rupture with hemorrhage occurs, in which case the symptoms and signs of an acute abdomen may develop. Large or numerous cysts may cause aching pelvic pain, dyspareunia, and occasionally abnormal uterine bleeding. The ovary may be slightly enlarged and tender; the vaginal smear will often show a high estrogen level and a lack of progesterone stimulation.

Salpingitis, endometriosis, lutein cysts, and neoplastic cysts must be considered in the differential diagnosis. Any cyst that becomes larger than 6 cm in diameter or persists longer than 60 days probably is not a follicle cyst.

Most follicle cysts disappear spontaneously within 60 days without any treatment. When symptoms are disturbing, warm douches, pelvic diathermy, and reestablishment of the ovarian hormone cycle may be helpful. Ovulation may be simulated following progesterone in oil, 5 mg as a single intramuscular injection, or medroxyprogesterone (Provera), 10 mg orally daily for 7 days. Ovulation may be induced with clomiphene citrate (Clomid), 50 mg orally daily for 5 days.

Pain due to a prolapsed adherent ovary may require uterine elevation. Ovariectomy is justified in cases of disabling and chronic or recurrent salpingitis.

2. Lutein cysts–There are 2 types of lutein cysts: granulosa lutein cysts, which are found within corpora lutea; and theca lutein cysts, which are only found in association with hydatidiform mole, choriocarcinoma, or treatment with clomiphene or hCG.

a. Granulosa lutein cysts–Corpus luteum cysts are functional, nonneoplastic ovarian enlargements caused by an unusual increase in secretion of fluid by the corpus luteum, which occurs after ovulation or during early pregnancy. They are 4–6 cm in diameter, raised, and brown and are filled with tawny serous fluid. A contracted blood clot is often found within the cavity.

A cystic corpus luteum must be distinguished from a corpus luteum cyst. The former is much smaller and is a normal variation of no clinical importance.

Corpus luteum cysts are usually readily palpable. They may cause local pain and tenderness and either amenorrhea or delayed menstruation, followed by brisk bleeding after resolution of the cyst. A cyst may lead to torsion of the ovary, causing severe pain; or it may rupture and bleed, in which case laparotomy is usually required to control hemorrhage into the peritoneal cavity. Unless these acute complications develop, symptomatic therapy is adequate. The cyst will disappear within 2 months in nonpregnant women and will gradually become smaller during the last trimester in pregnant women.

b. Theca lutein cysts–Theca lutein cysts range in size from minute to 4 cm in diameter. They are multiple and usually bilateral and are filled with clear straw-colored and occasionally bloody serous fluid.

Abdominal symptoms are often minimal. A sense of pelvic weight or ache may be described. Rupture of a cyst may result in intraperitoneal bleeding. Continued signs and symptoms of pregnancy, especially hyperemesis and breast paresthesias, are also reported.

Laboratory studies disclose persistently high plasma levels of hCG. Curettage should be done if there is any question of retained products of conception, a proliferative hydatidiform mole, or choriocarcinoma. Extrauterine pregnancy and contralateral cyst should be considered. The remote possibility of bilateral papillary cystadenoma should be included in the differential diagnosis.

Ovarian surgery is not required, because the cysts disappear spontaneously following elimination of hydatidiform mole, destruction of the choriocarcinoma, or discontinuation of hCG or clomiphene.

B. Inflammatory Cysts (Tubo-Ovarian Cysts): Distortion and adherence of the tube and ovary as the result of salpingitis or pelvic peritonitis cause a restricted, inflammatory adnexal mass up to 15 cm in diameter, with cyst formation.

Severe, persistent pelvic pain and tenderness are typical. Metrorrhagia or hypermenorrhea occurs concomitantly. If the pain is unilateral, acute appendicitis, intrapelvic bleeding, and endometriosis must be ruled out.

The white blood count and sedimentation rate are moderately elevated. Pregnancy tests are negative.

Antibiotics, analgesics, and local heat or cold will give relief. Surgery is not indicated if appendicitis and ectopic pregnancy can be excluded; however, if symptoms do not subside in 3–4 weeks, laparotomy is justified.

C. Endometrial Cysts (Endometriomas): Functional ectopic endometrium implants on the ovary and retains its ability to bleed periodically with the proper hormonal stimulus (endometriosis; see p 617). Alternate oozing and healing with each period results in formation of endometrial cysts. Patients with functioning endometriosis are in the premenopausal age group; tumors are more commonly seen during the perimenopausal years.

Endometrial cysts vary in size from microscopic ("powder burns") to 10–12 cm in diameter. Dense adhesions to neighboring viscera are common. The interior of the cyst is filled with thick, chocolate-colored old blood. The cyst wall contains active endometrial tissue, and local bleeding occurs from these foci at the time of the period. Hemosiderin, pseudoxanthoma cells, and chronic inflammatory elements with fibrosis are present.

Endometrioid adenocarcinoma of the ovary is histologically similar to endometrium. It may arise by metaplastic change from basic mesothelium without showing the histologic characteristics of classic endometriosis—hence, it is termed endometrioid. Cancer arising in identifiable areas of endometriosis is less common than endometrioid adenocarcinoma.

Symptoms of endometrial cysts include infertility, hypermenorrhea, dyspareunia, and secondary or acquired dysmenorrhea. Dysmenorrhea is generally pre- or comenstrual and is of an aching, crescendo, or curious "grinding" type, with the pain referred toward the sacrum and rectum. Laboratory tests are not diagnostic.

Not all "chocolate cysts" are endometrial in origin. Bleeding into any cystic cavity will later yield decomposed blood. The wall of a corpus luteum will show a yellowish lining zone. Papillary processes or thickened areas of actual cancer will be seen in cystadenomas.

For treatment of endometriosis, see p 621. In general, large ovarian endometriomas are treated by surgical resection of the cyst to leave as much functioning ovarian tissue as possible. Smaller points of endometriosis may disappear after prolonged hormone therapy, or they can be destroyed by fulguration. If cancer is present in endometriosis or if endometrioid adenocarcinoma is present, total ablation of the internal genital organs and affected pelvic tissues is indicated.

D. Inclusion Cysts: These small, often microscopic cysts just beneath the surface of the ovary occur in postinflammatory states or after the menopause. A minute amount of serous fluid fills the single loculus. The germinal epithelium becomes inverted or buried in one small area, perhaps within a fissure, to form one or more cysts.

No discomfort or disability results from these cysts, which are usually found by the pathologist. It is postulated that cystadenomas may originate from inclusion cysts as a result of unknown growth stimuli.

No treatment is required for inclusion cysts. Larger cystadenomas are easily recognized and should be resected.

E. Parovarian Cysts: Parovarian cysts lie between the tube and ovary, usually near the distal end of the broad ligament. Although they are commonly 3–4 cm in diameter, they may on rare occasions be 10 cm in diameter. They develop from the remnants of the mesonephric or paramesonephric system. The lining elements may be flattened as a result of pressure within the cystic cavity, but where they are intact, the classic cell types seen in the uterine tube can be found.

Parovarian cysts are only found in postpubertal women and, like most nonmalignant cysts, are asymptomatic unless they reach palpable size, produce pressure symptoms, or become infarcted by torsion.

FIBROMAS & SARCOMAS OF THE OVARY

Fibromas of the ovary are unilateral, firm, nonfunctional benign tumors of mesenchymal origin and are composed principally of fibrous connective tissue. They usually occur in postmenopausal women, and they represent about 5% of ovarian tumors.

Classification

A. Fibromas: Fibromas are smooth, round, and lobulated. Most are small; however, a few will weigh as much as 2 kg. Their weight may cause pedunculation of the gonad, leading to torsion and degeneration. Fibromas are poorly encapsulated and rarely adherent. Sectioning discloses dense grayish or white tissue. Calcific inclusions sometimes are found. Zones of degeneration with gelatinous or small cystic spaces are often seen within the soft portions. On microscopic examination, there is a monotonous pattern of fibrous connective tissue and smooth muscle elements in whorls and trabeculations of variable density.

B. Adenofibromas: This variation of fibroma appears rough, fissured, and coarsely lobulated and is covered by a single layer or pseudostratum of darkly staining cuboidal cells. Strands and clumps of cells suggestive of smooth muscle are occasionally interspersed between the fibrocytes.

C. Fibromyomas: Fibromyomas differ from fibromas only microscopically in the inclusion of smooth muscle.

D. Sarcomas: Sarcoma of the ovary, one of the rarest of gonadal tumors, also develops in fibromas. These cancers are usually of the spindle cell type, although chondrosarcomas, osteosarcomas, and myxosarcomas also have been reported. Many ovarian sarcomas are probably of teratogenous origin.

Clinical Findings

Fibromatous tumors are associated with Meigs' (Demons-Meigs) syndrome, which is characterized by a solid benign tumor of the ovary, with transudative hydrothorax and ascites. Ascites accompanies approximately 20% of fibromas, but Meigs' syndrome is far less common (about 130 authentic cases have been reported). Ascites (with or without hydrothorax) can occur with cardiac, renal, and hepatic disorders in the absence of a pelvic mass. Carcinoma, particularly of the tail of the pancreas, also may cause ascites.

The abdomen enlarges, and the patient complains of orthopnea, tachycardia, and a feeling of oppression in the chest. Torsion often occurs, causing agonizing pain in the affected lower quadrant and nausea and vomiting. Larger tumors cause a sense of pelvic heaviness. The tumor is usually palpable on pelvic examination, and shifting dullness of the abdomen and hydrothorax are apparent upon palpation and percussion. The tumor may not be felt until after abdominal paracentesis.

Peritoneal and thoracic fluid in Meigs' syndrome is a clear, pale yellow transudate. Epithelial cells are few, and leukocytes are rare. No malignant elements are present. Chest x-ray may demonstrate fluid in one or both sides of the thorax. Ultrasonography will reveal a tumor. Pneumoperitoneum after paracentesis may clearly delineate the fibroma on x-ray films.

Differential Diagnosis

Meigs' syndrome should be considered in every woman over 40 years of age in whom a relapsing, unexplained pleural or peritoneal transudate is discovered. The syndrome must be distinguished from primary pulmonary, cardiac, and abdominal disease causing hydrothorax and ascites.

Fibromas must be differentiated from granulosa-theca cell tumors.

Treatment & Prognosis

Laparoscopy or exploratory laparotomy should be performed. Upon removal of the fibroma, abdominal and chest fluid will usually disappear spontaneously within a week. Most patients recover following the removal of a fibromatous ovarian tumor. If sarcomatous change has occurred, the prognosis is grave.

CYSTADENOMAS & CYSTADENOCARCINOMAS
(Pseudomucinous & Serous Cystadenomas)

Cystadenomas are the most common ovarian cancers, representing about 70% of all ovarian tumors. They produce no hormone and are most common in women between the ages of 45 and 65. Serous cystadenomas and pseudomucinous cystadenomas occur with equal frequency.

Classification

A. Pseudomucinous Cystadenomas: These tumors grow more sluggishly and become larger than the serous type; some have been reported to weigh over 45.5 kg (100 lb). They may be derived from the ovarian surface epithelium, or they may be of teratogenous origin. They are usually multilocular; contain a thick, viscid, brownish liquid; are lined by tall columnar epithelial and goblet cells; and are sheathed by a tough membranous capsule. They may develop a well-defined pedicle. At surgery, about 5% of these tumors are found to be malignant.

Malignant primary pseudomucinous ovarian tumors may superficially resemble adenocarcinoma of intestinal origin.

B. Serous Cystadenomas: These tumors do not become very large; most weigh 4.5–9 kg (10–20 lb). Originally, they are unilocular, filled with a thin yellowish fluid, and lined by cuboidal or low columnar cells. Subsequently, they tend to develop multilocular spaces and papillary excrescences on both their inner and outer surfaces. Small sandlike, sharp, calcareous concretions (psammoma bodies) are often present within the tumor. Serous cystadenomas are believed to arise from invagination of the germinal epithelium of the surface of the ovary.

Serous cystadenomas, like the pseudomucinous type, are also contained in a parchmentlike capsule. While pseudomucinous cystadenomas may develop a pedicle, the serous type usually does not. Unless perforation, infection, or rupture ensues, the tough fibrous capsule is rarely adherent.

C. Cystadenocarcinomas: Malignant change in cystadenoma is characterized by (1) excessive proliferation and extensive stratification of cells; (2) an intricate pattern with increased glandular elements; (3) sparse stroma in proportion to epithelial cells; (4) anaplasia characterized by immature cells, variation in size and shape of cells and nuclei, numerous nucleoli, many undifferentiated cells, and numerous mitotic figures; and (5) invasion of the stroma or the capsule by glandular elements, with intralocular cyst formation.

Clinical Findings

Cystadenomas are endocrinologically silent tumors: they do not produce hormones. They are usually asymptomatic, and the patient is seen for evaluation of abdominal fullness or nonspecific abdominal discomfort. Symptoms are produced only when the tumor becomes large enough to cause increased abdominal girth and weight gain, pelvic heaviness, constipation, and urinary frequency.

Complications that may occur as a result of malignant change are due to extension or rupture. Intestinal obstruction may develop.

Abdominal examination generally discloses an insensitive, rounded pelvic-abdominal mass that may fill the entire true pelvis. The upper margin of the mass should be measured in centimeters above or below the umbilicus. A fluid wave should be sought by palpation of the abdomen. Although hydrothorax may also be noted, this cannot be classed as Meigs' syndrome, because malignant cells are often found in the tumor and in the abdominal fluid.

Laboratory findings are not diagnostic. The erythrocyte sedimentation rate may be elevated, and eosinophilia may be present.

Ultrasonography or abdominal x-rays reveal a rounded area of increased density. Psammoma bodies (small calcareous conglomerates) within the acini of the tumor can occasionally be seen on the films.

The differential diagnosis must include large dermoid cyst, semisolid tumor (especially dysgerminoma), secondary involvement by cancer from the gastrointestinal tract or breast, and thyroid and retroperitoneal tumors.

Treatment & Prognosis

Treatment is primarily surgical and depends upon the type of cystadenoma and whether it is thought to be malignant.

At least 50% of serous cystadenomas will become clinically malignant and will at least involve the opposite ovary. Only about 5% of pseudomucinous cystadenomas become definitely cancerous, with involvement of the opposite gonad and other structures.

Less than 40% of all patients with cystadenocarcinoma can be operated upon with the expectancy of 5-year arrest, because about 75% of such patients are found to have a far-advanced tumor, generally of the serous variety. Endometrioid carcinomas have a far better prognosis.

PRIMARY OVARIAN CANCER

Ovarian cancer, because of its insidious growth and relative inaccessibility, is rarely diagnosed early; most patients present with far-advanced tumors. Consequently, the 5-year survival rate and the age-adjusted mortality rate from ovarian cancer have not changed significantly during the past 40 years. Nonetheless, more aggressive surgical removal (debulking) of cancer, more extended radiation therapy, and improved chemotherapy have increased the mean survival time and enhanced the quality of life for many ovarian cancer victims.

Ovarian cancer is the most lethal common type of gynecologic cancer and the third most frequent type after cervical and endometrial cancer. Despite a decrease 20–30 years ago, the incidence of ovarian cancer has risen again in the USA. About 60% of ovarian cancers occur between ages 40 and 60, about 20% before age 40, and about 20% after age 60.

No causative factor has been identified. Nulliparity is the only significant risk factor for ovarian cancer.

Over 80% of ovarian carcinomas are of epithelial origin; most are of the serous cystadenocarcinoma type. Other less common cancers may be derived from special ovarian tumors (eg, dysgerminoma, teratoma).

Diagnostic Evaluation & Clinical Findings

A. Symptoms and Signs: These vary with the type of tumor, but patients frequently present with abdominal enlargement and complaints of abdominal or pelvic pressure or discomfort. A patient presenting with symptoms possibly due to ovarian cancer should receive a complete physical examination, with emphasis on abnormal findings in the breasts, abdomen, and pelvis; laboratory studies, including complete blood count, SMA 6 or 12, and urinalysis; endoscopic studies such as cystoscopy, proctoscopy, and laparoscopy, with inspection of the pelvis, omentum, liver, and diaphragm, together with biopsies of suspi-

Table 25—1. International Federation of Gynecology and Obstetrics (FIGO) classification of ovarian neoplasms (1976).

I. Histologic classification:
  A. Serous cystomas:
    1. Serous cystadenomas, benign.
    2. Serous cystadenomas with proliferation of epithelial cells and nuclear abnormalities but with no infiltrative destructive growth (low potential for malignant change).
    3. Serous cystadenocarcinomas.
  B. Mucinous cystomas:
    1. Mucinous cystadenomas, benign.
    2. Mucinous cystadenomas with proliferation of epithelial cells and nuclear abnormalities but with no infiltrative destructive growth (low potential for malignant change).
    3. Mucinous cystadenocarcinomas.
  C. Endometrioid tumors, similar to adenocarcinoma of the endometrium:
    1. Endometrioid cysts, benign.
    2. Endometrioid tumors with proliferation of epithelial cells and nuclear abnormalities but with no infiltrative destructive growth (low potential for malignant change).
    3. Endometrioid cystadenocarcinomas.
  D. Mesonephric tumors:
    1. Mesonephric tumors, benign.
    2. Mesonephric tumors with proliferation of epithelial cells and nuclear abnormalities but with no infiltrative destructive growth (low potential for malignant change).
    3. Mesonephric cystadenocarcinomas.
  E. Unclassified carcinomas: Tumors that cannot be placed in groups A, B, C, and D.

II. Staging: (Based on findings at clinical examination and surgical exploration.)
  Stage I   Growth limited to the ovaries.
  Stage IA   Growth limited to one ovary; no ascites.
  Stage IB   Growth limited to both ovaries; no ascites.
  Stage IC   Growth limited to one or both ovaries; ascites present with malignant cells in fluid.
  Stage II   Growth involving one or both ovaries with pelvic extension.
  Stage IIA   Extension or metastases to the uterus or tubes only.
  Stage IIB   Extension to other pelvic tissues.
  Stage III   Growth involving one or both ovaries with widespread intraperitoneal metastases to the abdomen (omentum; small intestine and its mesentery).
  Stage IV   Growth involving one or both ovaries with distant metastases outside the peritoneal cavity.
  Special category: Unexplored cases thought to be ovarian carcinoma (surgery or therapy not yet performed).

cious areas; and ultrasound scan of the abdomen and pelvis. X-ray studies should usually include a chest film, intravenous urogram, upper gastrointestinal series, small bowel follow-through, barium enema, and pelvic lymphangiography. Paracentesis may be indicated. Preoperative bowel preparation should be done in anticipation of bowel injury or the need for resection. Laparotomy may be limited to recovery of peritoneal washings or may be extended to include resection of primary ovarian tumor and sampling of pelvic and periaortic lymph nodes.

Either laparoscopy with biopsy or laparotomy is necessary for diagnosis and staging. Histologic classification and staging are summarized in Table 25–1.

B. Laboratory Findings: Papanicolaou smears rarely reveal ovarian cancer. If neoplastic elements are identified, the ovarian tumor is generally far-advanced.

C. X-Ray Findings: A pelvic mass may be found, though it will not be clear whether this is a primary ovarian cancer or cancer that has metastasized from a distant focus. Upper and lower gastrointestinal x-ray series are useful to confirm or rule out primary gastric or colonic malignancy and to identify functional compromise by the cancer.

D. Other Findings: Ultrasonography may identify a mass and may be helpful in paracentesis, eg, it may aid the operator to avoid the tumor or vital organs. Paracentesis or cul-de-sac aspiration is not recommended as a routine procedure, because of the possibility of spread of tumor. In patients with advanced or inoperable disease, paracentesis may permit a tentative diagnosis as a basis for palliative therapy.

Prevention

All women should have an annual physical examination. Early detection of ovarian cancer will reduce the rates of progressive disease and death.

Treatment

Cancer of the ovary eventually sheds malignant cells into the peritoneal cavity and then spreads to the inferior surface of the diaphragm and, via the lymphatics, to the retroperitoneal nodes, including those in the periaortic area. For this reason, ovarian cancer must be considered cancer of the peritoneal cavity. In all but early cases, patients with ovarian cancer probably will require combined therapy—ie, surgery plus chemotherapy or irradiation, or all 3.

A. Surgical Treatment: Operation is necessary for diagnosis as well as for therapy but must not be attempted without proper evaluation. Occasionally, in advanced cancer, definitive surgery may be deferred until the tumor burden has been reduced by chemotherapy or irradiation.

Primary cystic tumors should be removed intact. Total abdominal hysterectomy, bilateral salpingo-oophorectomy, and omentectomy should be done, if possible. Careful inspection of the entire abdominal cavity, including the liver, inferior aspect of the diaphragm, and the abdominal viscera, with biopsy of suspicious areas, is essential for staging and proper therapy. A careful search by the pathologist for evidence of spread of cancer is mandatory.

If all of the cancer cannot be removed, residual tumor must be debulked. The success of adjuvant therapy is directly proportionate to the amount and site of tumor left after surgery.

Occasionally, a "second look" operation may be warranted for removal of residual tumor following chemotherapy.

B. Radiation Therapy: Treatment must be individualized. Postoperative external pelvic irradiation is useful when macroscopic foci are likely or when gross cancer must remain after operation. Radioactive gold or iodine dispersed in a colloid may be used postoperatively to destroy microscopic foci over the peritoneal surfaces. Total abdominal irradiation, often by strip or serial approach, may be beneficial when cancer involves small, scattered malignant foci in both the lower and upper abdomen. Lymph node irradiation or diaphragmatic field irradiation is occasionally employed in specific cases.

C. Chemotherapy: Anticancer drugs are an important adjuvant to therapy because ovarian cancers are often advanced at diagnosis, numerous vital areas are affected, and many patients may not be able to withstand radical surgery or intensive irradiation. The newer anticancer drugs often are strikingly efficacious.

Ovarian cancer may be treated with a wide spectrum of anticancer agents:

1. Alkylating agents include melphalan, chlorambucil, and cyclophosphamide. Melphalan is favored by many. No one alkylating drug is superior to another, but some are less toxic. The objective response range of these drugs is 35–65%.

2. Combinations of drugs, eg, doxorubicin and cisplatin, are now recommended for initial treatment of patients with extensive cancer or for cancer unresponsive to single-drug therapy.

Unusual tumors, eg, secondary ovarian cancers of bowel origin, may respond best to fluorouracil alone or in combination with other anticancer drugs.

Complications of Therapy

Intestinal and ureteral injuries are potential problems with surgery. Irradiation and chemotherapy cause bone marrow suppression. Chemotherapeutic drugs are seriously toxic for many patients.

Prognosis

The stage of ovarian cancer is the most important factor influencing

Table 25—2. Five-year survival rates in patients with primary ovarian cancer.

Stage*	Surgery Alone	Surgery and Irradiation	Surgery and Chemotherapy
Stage I	67%	60%	94%
Stage II	24%	39%	75% (est)
Stage III	1%	9%	7%

*Stage is based on FIGO classification (see Table 25—1).

the success of therapy, although the type and grade of the tumor and the method of treatment must also be considered.

Table 25—2 shows 5-year survival rates based on the stage of ovarian cancer and modality of treatment.

In studies performed in 1971 and 1976, the 5-year survival rates for ovarian cancer patients were found to vary according to the extent of tumor in stage I disease and according to the amount of gross tumor removed in stage II and III disease. The survival rates for stage I cancer were as follows: intracystic tumor, 90%; extracystic excrescences, 68%; ruptured cyst, 56%; and adherent cyst, 51%. For stage II disease, the rates were 50% with complete removal and 15% with incomplete removal; for stage III, 28% with complete removal and 8% with incomplete removal.

SECONDARY OVARIAN CANCER

In 10% of cases of fatal cancer in women, the ovary is found to be secondarily involved; metastasis or extension of cancer is usually from the uterus or the other ovary, but in one-third of cases, metastasis is from stomach cancer. The gastrointestinal tract, breast, thyroid, kidney, or adrenals may also be primary foci.

Pathology

The Krukenberg tumor is an interesting carcinoma metastatic to the ovaries. It usually originates in the stomach, intestine, or gallbladder or, on very rare occasions, in the breast and thyroid. Grossly, it is moderately large, smooth, buff-colored, firm, solid, lobulated, often kidney-shaped, nonadherent, and bilateral. A heavy but easily stripped capsule covers the parenchyma, which is composed of firm and softer, often minutely cystic, tissue. Two microscopic features are diagnostic: (1) coarse, abundant, occasionally edematous stroma and (2) islands of moderately large epithelial cells with mucin-laden or vacuolated cytoplasm and eccentrically placed, small hyperchromatic nuclei. Such cells resemble signet rings. If the tumor does not display these classic details, it should not be termed a Krukenberg tumor but simply a secondary ovarian cancer.

The only justification for continuing to categorize certain metastatic ovarian tumors as Krukenberg tumors is the characteristic gross and histologic picture that may be associated with such tumors.

Other cancers metastatic to the ovary may be similar in morphology, but not in function, to their primary tumor.

Clinical Findings

There are no specific signs or symptoms. These tumors are generally insidious until the process is extensive. Hormones are not usually produced by most secondary ovarian cancers, including the Krukenberg tumor. The tumor is often outlined first in the abdomen by external or pelvic examination. Amenorrhea, dyspepsia, postprandial epigastric discomfort, slight weight loss, and mild anemia may then be noted. Ascites is rarely present.

Secondary ovarian cancer must be distinguished from primary ovarian cancer. Secondary involvement of the contralateral ovary is common in primary ovarian cancer. Only an occasional colon cancer involves both ovaries.

Treatment

Palliation is all that can be offered. Removal of the tumor mass will in many cases relieve local abdominal symptoms. Radiation therapy and radical gynecologic or other definitive surgery are futile because the cancer is widely disseminated by the time it reaches the ovary. Chemotherapeutic drug combinations may retard tumor growth. The drug regimen must be individualized.

For control of neoplastic effusions, quinacrine hydrochloride (Atabrine) ranks with radioisotopes and alkylating agents. The drug has inflammatory rather than cancericidal properties and causes surface fibrosis and adhesions that reduce fluid production. Quinacrine must be administered intraperitoneally. It is effective in limiting carcinomatous effusions originating in the ovaries, gastrointestinal system, breast, and lymphoid tissue. Fever, regional pain, nausea, and ileus are transient, dose-related side-effects. Discomfort is relieved by analgesics. Bowel stasis usually is self-limited.

For intracavitary therapy, initial trial dosage of quinacrine should not exceed 200 mg for peritoneal and 100 mg for pleural effusions. Partial evacuation of the fluid before treatment is recommended. Each 100 mg of drug should be diluted in 5 mL of effusion fluid or sterile water. The average dose of quinacrine for control of ascites of malignant origin is 400–800 mg daily for 3–5 consecutive days. For pleural effusions due to cancer, the usual dose is 200–400 mg daily for 4–5 days. A maintenance dose of quinacrine (0.2–1 g) depends upon the site and the extent of cancer and the patient's tolerance of the drug.

LIPOID CELL TUMORS OF THE OVARY

This category includes a number of rare unilateral, yellowish, glassy, semisolid, relatively small tumors that usually cause masculinization and occur most commonly in women over 50 years of age: luteomas, luteinomas, luteoblastomas, functional hypernephroid tumors, gynandroblastomas, masculinovoblastomas, corticoadrenal tumors, hormonally active adrenal carcinomas, and virilizing hilus cell tumors of the ovary.

There are at least 3 theories about the possible origin of these tumors. They may arise as (1) adrenal rest tumors of the ovary; (2) abnormally luteinized, atypical granulosa cell tumors or arrhenoblastomas; or (3) pseudo-Leydig cell tumors, perhaps of hilus cell origin.

Pathology

These poorly encapsulated tumors are rarely adherent unless they are malignant. About 20% are malignant. Areas of degeneration and internal hemorrhage are common. Clusters and sheets of at least 2 cell types are seen microscopically: (1) moderately large polyhedral cells with small basophilic nuclei and a generous eosinophilic cytoplasm containing lipoid inclusions, similar to cells in the reticular zone of the adrenal cortex; and (2) large, rounded cells with moderately to deeply staining basophilic nuclei containing prominent nucleoli and a clear cytoplasm. (This latter type is reminiscent of Leydig cells of the testis.) A light supporting framework of connective tissue is usually present.

Clinical Findings

Amenorrhea or oligomenorrhea and virilization often occur. Hypertension, polycythemia, and diabetes mellitus have occasionally been described. Because many of these tumors are small and nonpalpable, an adnexal enlargement may not be found.

17-Hydroxycorticosteroid or 17-ketosteroid excretion is elevated. The pregnanetriol level may be high.

Distant metastasis is a late complication of malignant tumors.

These tumors must be differentiated from other ovarian tumors (especially arrhenoblastoma), primary adrenal cortical tumors, and adrenal cortical hyperplasia.

Treatment & Prognosis

The adnexa on the affected side must be removed. These tumors often occur in young women, and conservation of the uterus and one tube and ovary may be important. The opposite ovary should be investigated thoroughly and biopsied for evidence of tumor or dysgenesis. If the tumor is due to metastases from the adrenal gland or a mesoblastic tumor, more radical surgery will be required. Results of palliation by irradiation have been disappointing.

Refeminization occurs after complete excision of a virilizing lipoid cell tumor. The deepened voice and coarse hair are not reversible changes, however.

MESONEPHROID TUMORS
(CLEAR CELL CARCINOMAS) OF THE OVARY

Mesonephroid tumors are a small group of ovarian tumors previously called mesonephromas (Schiller) because of scattered pseudoglomerular cell groupings suggestive of the mesonephros (the primordial kidney). Mesonephroid tumors are derived from the ovarian germinal epithelium, a mesothelial derivative. These tumors may occur in young women, but most patients are over age 40. At least 30% of mesonephroid tumors are malignant, and many are very aggressive.

Pathology

The tumor is grayish-brown, smooth, free, semisoft or cystic, and fairly well encapsulated. It is occasionally adherent. Friable tissue and thin serous fluid fill the loculi and tissue spaces, and there are areas of cystic degeneration and even hemorrhagic extravasation. Most tumors are 10–20 cm in diameter when first discovered.

There are 2 histologic types of mesonephroid tumors: a semisolid clear cell carcinoma and a more adenomatous papillary type with groups of prominent protruding "hobnail" epithelial cells studding the acinous spaces.

Clinical Findings

These tumors do not produce hormones but cause symptoms because of their size or location. Most are unilateral and tend to spread locally. They must be differentiated from cystadenomas, metastatic clear cell carcinomas of renal origin, and other poorly differentiated tumors.

The periodic acid–Schiff stain colors mesonephroid tumors and pseudomucinous cystadenoma cells red; serous cystadenoma elements do not take the stain.

Treatment & Prognosis

Excision of the adnexa is required. If malignant spread is found, bilateral salpingo-oophorectomy and panhysterectomy are indicated.

Radiation therapy is only palliative because these tumors are only slightly radiosensitive. Chemotherapy is of limited value.

The prognosis must be guarded. Patients with stage III or IV tumors rarely survive.

ARRHENOBLASTOMA

Arrhenoblastoma is a rare ovarian tumor (about 200 cases have been reported) that occurs most frequently during the reproductive years and is assumed to rise from sexually ambivalent cells present in the ovary of the 6- to 7-week embryo or to be of teratoid origin. The tumor is unilateral and may be minute or may fill the entire pelvis. These tumors rarely attain large size. Most are about 7 cm in greatest dimension, and occasionally they are discovered only on microscopic study. About 20% are malignant, but metastases usually occur late.

Pathology

Grossly, most arrhenoblastomas are grayish to yellow-brown, firm, and poorly encapsulated. They may become soft because of internal hemorrhage, degeneration, and cyst formation secondary to necrosis. The prominent large cells with abundant eosinophilic cytoplasm (Leydig type cells) are dispersed throughout the tumor and separated by tubular structures of varying degrees of organization (Sertolilike elements). Reinke's crystalloids may be seen as cytoplasmic inclusions in the Leydig type cells, as in hilar cell tumors.

Clinical Findings

Arrhenoblastomas are usually hormonally active, producing androgenic substances that cause defeminization and then virilization, which is manifested by varying degrees of amenorrhea, acne, hirsutism, recession of the hairline at the forehead, slight alopecia, loss of feminine contours, breast and genital atrophy (but clitoral hypertrophy), and deepening of the voice. Nonfunctional arrhenoblastomas (eg, Pick's adenoma) cause the signs and symptoms of a solid ovarian tumor.

Blood tests may reveal polycythemia. Levels of urinary 17-ketosteroids are slightly to moderately increased; etiocholanolone may represent 75% of the 17-ketosteroid fraction. The dehydroepiandrosterone level is strikingly high. Estrogen, hydroxysteroid, and FSH levels are normal or minimally reduced.

Arrhenoblastoma must be distinguished from adrenocortical disorders, which are a much more frequent cause of masculinization. Adrenocortical disorders usually produce less virilization and a much more pronounced elevation in the level of urinary 17-ketosteroids.

Treatment & Prognosis

Arrhenoblastoma should be removed surgically. Other pelvic reproductive organs should also be removed unless the patient desires children and the tumor is clinically and histologically benign, in which case unilateral oophorectomy and salpingectomy generally are sufficient. Estrogen therapy does not reverse the effects of androgenic hormones. Superfluous hair should be removed and acne treated. Hormonal evaluation should be repeated after several months to determine whether the tumor has recurred.

After the removal of an arrhenoblastoma, feminization recurs within several months in otherwise normal premenopausal women who have adequate function in the remaining ovary. Coarse hair, deep voice, and clitoral hypertrophy may persist. Pregnancy may be permitted after 1 year if the tumor has not recurred.

GRANULOSA CELL TUMOR
(Folliculoma)

Granulosa cell tumors, the most common functional ovarian tumors of stromal derivation, represent 3–4% of all ovarian tumors. These solid tumors vary in size from microscopic to 9 kg (20 lb) and often produce estrogens. A rare tumor may be virilizing, however. Granulosa cell tumors are most often seen in women 50–70 years of age. About 10% are bilateral. Granulosa and theca cells are invariably found together in these tumors. About 15–20% are malignant.

Pathology

The tumors are rounded or ovoid and somewhat lobulated. They are composed principally of granulosa cells arranged in pseudofollicles or rosettes that resemble primordial follicles. On section, the cell contents are soft and vascular with a poor supporting framework. In the more solid portions, the tumor is almost invariably yellowish-brown in color. Some division or trabeculation is occasionally seen. These tumors have a fragile, thin capsule; in large tumors, the capsule is easily damaged during examination or at surgery.

Granulosa cells are comparable to cells lining the antrum of the developing follicle. They are small, with scant cytoplasm and dark, granular, or vesicular nuclei that take a deep basophilic stain. Granulosa cells tend to occur in rather closely packed clusters. Circular or star-shaped groups of granulosa cells around a few degenerating central cells or small vacuolated areas (Call-Exner bodies, actually spaces) presumably represent attempted duplication of a graafian follicle. The difference, of course, is that there is no ovum in the center but only a few nondescript, degenerated connective tissue elements.

When the tumor is quite anaplastic, large areas of packed granulosa cells have no pattern, but here and there the folliclelike groupings distinguish the tumor. There may be considerable pleomorphism. There are no histologic criteria for grading malignant growth in granulosa cell tumors.

The stroma consists in large measure of elongated connective tissue cells that develop long, dendritic reticular fibrils. Less well differentiated cells are commonly insinuated between the connective tissue cells. Certain of the less differentiated cells appear to have epithelioid characteristics, and many are actually theca cells. Each such cell is found to be surrounded by a proliferation of reticulum fibrils, as shown by silver stains. In contrast, aggregations of well-differentiated granulosa cells form clusters that are surrounded as a group by whorls of reticular fibers.

In general, the higher the grade of differentiation or maturity of the granulosa cells, the greater the likelihood of hormone production, as is evidenced by luteinization.

Clinical Findings

The effect of the production of estrogen depends upon the age of the individual and her functional status. In children, this causes early development of pubic hair, hypertrophy of the breasts, and enlargement of the labia, cervix, and uterus (ie, pseudoprecocious puberty; these girls do not ovulate). Advanced bone age and early epiphyseal closure (dwarfism) will occur if hormonal stimulation is continued for a long time. Pelvic examination in such cases generally discloses an adnexal mass. In the reproductive years, menometrorrhagia is usually the only finding. In pregnant women, the principal problems are rupture of the tumor and hemorrhage. In postmenopausal women, refeminization occurs and uterine bleeding resumes. Generally speaking, however, this is not true menstruation but abnormal bleeding of an irregular type, and the flow is often more profuse and prolonged than with normal menses.

Granulosa cell tumors may cause pain due to torsion or pulsion of the mass. Abdominal distention usually occurs only with very large tumors or, in the case of malignant tumors, with regional spread or ascites. The rare occurrence of androgenicity in this group of otherwise feminizing tumors is not adequately explained.

The smallest granulosa cell tumors may not be palpable on pelvic examination; tumors that are palpable may be almost any size. They are generally mobile, rarely adherent, and often soft or semicystic. In slender women, firmer areas of tumor may be felt. Ascites and Meigs' syndrome may occur. Hemorrhagic ascites and fixation of the tumor suggest malignant changes. Metastases of the tumor to the opposite ovary, endometrium, and vagina are frequent, but distant spread is uncommon and almost never extensive.

Laboratory findings consist of elevated urinary estrogen levels and a high degree of cornification apparent in the vaginal cytologic smear.

The differential diagnosis includes multiple follicle cysts of the ovary; other functional ovarian tumors, such as theca cell tumors with cystic degeneration; ovarian adrenal rest or lipoid cell tumor of the ovary; and other causes of postmenopausal bleeding or abnormal menstruation. The probability of a granulosa cell tumor being present is about 1:500 in patients with postmenopausal bleeding; if postmenopausal bleeding is associated with an ovarian tumor, the chances are 1:5.

Treatment & Prognosis

Treatment consists of surgical removal of the tumor. In patients in the reproductive or prepubertal years, benign tumors are removed by ovariectomy; in postmenopausal women, total hysterectomy and bilateral salpingo-oophorectomy are indicated. If the patient is young or if it is uncertain whether cancer is present, it may be best to remove the tumor and await the pathologist's complete report. More radical surgery may be performed later if it is found that cancer is definitely present or has spread.

Radiation therapy may be of value, but adequate surgery is still the best therapeutic measure.

The histologic findings are not reliable for prognostic purposes, nor can cancer be judged by the degree of endocrine activity. The clinical course and stage of the tumor are the most helpful prognostic guides. Late recurrences (in one case, 33 years after surgery) have been recorded.

THECA CELL TUMOR
(Thecoma)

Theca cell tumors are uncommon, functional, usually feminizing, ovarian tumors derived from ovarian stromal anlagen. They occur most frequently in young girls and postmenopausal women and vary in size from minute nodules to masses 30 cm in diameter. The tumor is always unilateral and benign.

Granulosa cells and theca cells are almost always found together. The ratio of incidence of theca cell to granulosa cell tumors is often 1:8. A few thecal elements will be found even in a well-differentiated granulosa cell tumor. The tumor may be designated as a "granulosa-theca cell" or a "theca-granulosa cell" depending upon the predominant cell variety.

Pathology

Theca cell tumors are rounded, smooth, yellowish, and rarely adherent. A definite capsule is lacking. On section, the tumor is densely fibrous with much stromal connective tissue; vascularization is often deficient. Although the pattern of whorls (especially in older thecomas) may resemble that of a fibroma, the 2 can be differentiated on the basis of lipid staining; intracellular lipids are found in thecomas.

Stained sections of the tumor will show connective tissue elements with interspersed islands and strands of theca cells. Silver stains will reveal reticular fibrils. Sudan type stains reveal the presence of intracellular or extracellular lipids. Intracellular lipid material is doubly refractile with polarization and indicates luteinization; extracellular lipids indicate degeneration. Numerous luteinized theca and granulosa cells indicate that the tumor may have recently produced considerable steroid sex hormone. Distinctly pleomorphic nuclei with numerous mitoses and cells showing a tendency to invade are indicative of malignant changes.

Clinical Findings

Clinical and laboratory findings are identical with those of granulosa cell tumors (see above). As is true of granulosa cell tumors also, theca cell tumors may virilize rather than feminize in rare instances.

Theca cell tumors must be differentiated from other causes of abnormal uterine bleeding, including idiopathic precocious puberty, granulosa cell tumors, and uterine tumors. Meigs' syndrome (ascites and hydrothorax) may result, just as with ovarian fibroma. Partially degenerated theca-granulosa cell tumors are often mistaken for fibromas of the ovary. A definite diagnosis may require numerous sections and special stains.

Treatment & Prognosis

Unilateral oophorectomy will usually cure a patient with a benign theca cell tumor. Malignant tumors require total hysterectomy and bilateral salpingo-oophorectomy.

Experience with radiation therapy for treatment of the very rare cancers of the theca cell type is inadequate for evaluation.

Because of the low incidence of cancer ($<$ 1%) in theca cell tumors, the prognosis is excellent after surgery.

DYSGERMINOMA

Dysgerminoma is a nonfunctioning, potentially malignant ovarian germ cell tumor, the female counterpart of the male seminoma. (About 4% of all primary malignant ovarian tumors are dysgerminomas, and approximately one-third of dysgerminomas are clinically cancerous.) Dysgerminoma is bilateral in one-third of cases and occurs most commonly in females 10–30 years of age. Although usually small when found (4–7 cm in diameter), dysgerminomas may grow rapidly to fill the entire pelvis.

Pathology

The tumor is grayish-brown, smooth, rounded, thinly encapsulated, nonadherent, semisolid, and "rubbery." On section, the surface is edematous in appearance and soft, almost brainlike, in consistency. There are no septa—only a tenuous connective tissue framework.

Microscopically, 2 cell types are always seen: (1) unusually large, rounded cells with vesicular, coarsely granular cytoplasm and (2) many scattered small lymphocytes. The elements are loosely arranged with no typical pattern. The lymphocytes invariably infiltrate the tumor. Hemorrhagic extravasation and cystic degeneration are common. Anaplasia and pleomorphism may be found, but grading is impossible.

Clinical Findings

Symptoms are usually due to abdominal enlargement caused by rapid tumor growth and ascites. Acute pain may result if the thin capsule ruptures. Weakly false-positive pregnancy tests have been reported in some cases. Cancer must be suspected when a tumor grows rapidly, is firmly adherent or bilateral, or is accompanied by ascites.

Other nonfunctioning ovarian tumors (eg, teratoma, cystadenoma) must be considered in the differential diagnosis.

Treatment & Prognosis

Ovariectomy is required. If the dysgerminoma is unilateral and encapsulated, the salvage rate with simple unilateral adnexectomy approximates 85–90%. Because the tumors arise in young individuals, it is best to be conservative in such instances. Obviously, when the tumor has spread beyond the confines of the gonad, occurs in an older patient, or is bilateral, more extensive surgery will be necessary.

Dysgerminomas are very radiosensitive but not always curable by irradiation. Chemotherapy may be used to control recurrent cases.

The prognosis is generally guarded. The outlook is particularly serious in young patients and is very poor when extension or metastasis occurs.

BRENNER TUMOR OF THE OVARY

Brenner tumors are yellowish-brown, solid, nonadherent, fibroepitheliomatous mesenchymal tumors that usually affect postmenopausal women. They are almost always unilateral and very rarely secrete small amounts of gonadotropin. Brenner tumors represent about 1% of primary ovarian tumors, about 500 having been described in the medical literature. They may arise from teratomas but are occasionally found in the wall of a pseudomucinous cystadenoma. Rests are possible sites of origin also. Malignant change is very rare.

Pathology

This nonencapsulated tumor is composed of epithelioid cells surrounded by trabeculations of very dense connective tissue. The epithelioid cells have a clear cytoplasm and accept a pale basophilic stain. They are similar to transitional cells of the urinary tract. The dark nuclei have a longitudinal groove, which makes them resemble coffee beans. The epithelioid cells and the fluid within the tissue spaces stain positively for mucopolysaccharides in the same way as pseudomucinous cystadenoma cells. The basophilic connective tissue is unusually dense. Occasional areas of eosinophilic hyalinization are seen. Small degenerative cysts develop, but large, necrotic, or hemorrhagic zones are rarely observed. Degeneration destroys the epithelioid cells in occasional Brenner tumors; such a tumor might be described as a "fibroma with holes."

Clinical Findings

Unilateral pelvic discomfort and a sense of fullness and heaviness in the lower abdomen are described. Torsion results in severe pain. Ascites or Meigs' syndrome occasionally coexists with the larger Brenner tumors, which grow to about 30 cm in diameter. Most tumors, however, are less than 2–3 cm in diameter, are asymptomatic, and are discovered incidentally at surgery for other reasons.

On gross observation, Brenner tumors are occasionally mistaken for nonfunctional granulosa or theca cell tumors because of their color. Fibromas must also be considered; they also are firm but are usually pearl-gray, not yellow.

Treatment

Treatment consists of surgical removal, preserving the uninvolved portion of the ovary. If a pseudomucinous component is also present, oophorectomy is recommended.

TERATOID TUMORS OF THE OVARY
(Dermoid Cysts, Teratomas)

Teratoid tumors occur primarily in women 18–30 years of age. They are the most common ovarian tumors during this time of life.

Dermoid cysts account for 10% and semisolid teratomas for 0.1% of all ovarian tumors. About 15% are bilateral.

Classification

Teratoid tumors may represent an extension of haploid cell union or imperfect parthenogenesis. They are composed of one, 2, or 3 germinal layers that may grow into any possible combination of imperfectly formed organs or structures. If one type of tissue predominates, the appearance will be that of a single-tissue tumor; such is the case in struma ovarii, the thyroid tumor of the ovary.

Dermoid cysts, the most common type of teratoid tumor, contain ectodermal (and often mesodermal) tissue in the form of macerated skin, hair, bone, and teeth; the cyst is filled with a heavy, greasy sebaceous material and other structures as mentioned. A long pedicle is often present. Dermoid cysts may be minute; most weigh less than 0.5 kg (1 lb). Microscopically, dermoid cysts are lined by stratified squamous epithelium typical of epidermis. Sudoriparous and sebaceous glands and hair follicles are numerous.

Embryoma is the term applied to a semisolid teratoma containing poorly developed organs. Vestiges of many organs may be identified in teratoid cysts, depending upon their organization and development.

Epidermoid carcinoma occurs uncommonly in dermoid cysts. Sarcomatous change occurs much more rarely but is occasionally found in teratoid tumors during infancy and childhood.

Clinical Findings

Since the contents of dermoid cysts are light in weight, they "float" upward in the abdomen, elongating the ovarian pedicle. The symptoms are usually related to this freely shifting lower abdominal tumor. Constipation, reduced bladder capacity, and a sense of pelvic pressure occur in patients with teratoid tumors over 10 cm in diameter. Sudden, excruciating, continuous unilateral pelvic pain develops with torsion. Gangrene or trauma may rupture a teratoma, and severe chemical peritonitis often results. Ascites is rare with benign teratomas.

During pregnancy, a teratoma may become wedged in the true pelvis and obstruct the birth canal.

About 5% of struma ovarii produce T_4, which causes signs and symptoms of hyperthyroidism.

Urinalysis and blood studies will not identify most teratoid tumors. However, in the case of choriocarcinoma (a rare malignant teratoma), hCG is produced by the tumor and can be detected in the urine. A positive pregnancy test may be reported.

[131]I uptake studies of a woman with an adnexal tumor and hypermetabolism but no goiter may disclose radioactivity in the pelvis (struma ovarii) and not over the thyroid.

X-ray films occasionally disclose bone and teeth in dermoid cysts and a contrast in density between the cyst and nearby structures.

The differential diagnosis must include other adnexal tumors and pedunculated myomas. Most teratomas are found anterior and superior to the uterus (Küstner's sign).

Treatment & Prognosis

Even large dermoid cysts that have not twisted or ruptured often can be resected to preserve functional ovarian tissue. A twisted cyst must not be untwisted, since untwisting may discharge emboli; an oophorocystectomy should be performed instead. The opposite ovary should be incised or aspirated (with a large-bore needle) to determine if the tumor is bilateral. The incidence of malignant change is less than 0.5%.

The pregnant woman with a teratoma blocking the pelvic inlet should be placed in the knee-chest position so that vaginal manipulation can be attempted to displace the tumor out of the pelvis. If the tumor cannot be displaced, it should be removed immediately. Care should be taken not to spill the tumor contents into the pelvic cavity. Teratomas should never be aspirated through the cul-de-sac for diagnostic or therapeutic purposes, because leakage into the abdomen causes serious complications (chemical peritonitis, adhesion formation, and obstruction).

The immature malignant teratoma usually occurs in a young individual, and unilateral ovariectomy is the best therapy if the tumor is localized to one ovary. Obviously, if more widespread disease exists, every effort should be made to remove as much of the tumor as possible. When the lesion is localized to one ovary, removal of the opposite gonad and uterus has not been found to improve the salvage rate, but adjunctive chemotherapy may be beneficial, particularly if trophoblast is present. Older studies suggest that choriocarcinoma arising in a teratoma cannot be successfully treated by this means, but later reports are more encouraging. A combination of 3 chemotherapeutic agents may be best, because the prognosis with surgery alone is extremely poor.

POLYCYSTIC OVARY DISEASE
(Stein-Leventhal Syndrome)

Stein-Leventhal syndrome is an uncommon disorder characterized by bilaterally enlarged polycystic ovaries, secondary amenorrhea or oligomenorrhea, and infertility. About 50% of patients are hirsute, and approximately 10% are obese. The syndrome usually affects women between the ages of 15 and 30 years. About 2–3% of cases of infertility in women—those secondary to failure of ovulation—are due to polycystic ovary disease. The disorder is presumably of endocrine origin and may be familial.

The slightly enlarged, sclerocystic ovaries with smooth, pearl-white, shiny surfaces but without surface scarring or indentations have been called "oyster ovaries." Many small, fluid-filled follicle cysts lie beneath the thickened cortex. The ovarian stroma is often edematous but rarely luteinized. Hyperplasia and luteinization of the theca interna generally are observed, however.

Clinical Findings

A presumptive diagnosis of polycystic ovary disease often can be made from the history and initial physical examination. A normal puberty and early adolescence with reasonably regular menses are followed by progressively longer episodes of amenorrhea. The enlarged ovaries are identifiable on pelvic examination in about 50% of patients.

Urinary 17-ketosteroid levels are minimally elevated, but estrogen levels are normal. Some patients have increased 17α-hydroxyprogesterone output; others excrete considerable amounts of dehydroepiandrosterone. Adrenocorticosteroid hormone levels are normal. Occasionally, hyperprolactinemia may be found. Basal body temperature records and endometrial biopsies confirm anovulation.

Anovulation is related to abnormal production of androgens and estrogens. The normal ovary produces androgens and, if slightly but persistently stimulated by LH and FSH, will produce excessive amounts of androgens. In polycystic ovary disease, a relative excess of estrogens and abnormality in Δ^4 or Δ^5 steroid hormone metabolism may be the basic problem, resulting in persistent production and secretion of weak androgens. Conversion of androgens to testosterone (resulting in slightly elevated levels of testosterone) could explain why many patients with polycystic ovary disease are hirsute and fail to ovulate.

Women with polycystic ovary disease usually have low levels of FSH but normal or moderately elevated levels of LH. The androgens, together with converted estrogens, probably are sufficient to decrease FSH production. It is possible that the polycystic ovaries in these patients could result from the constant priming produced by low FSH levels and normal or slightly increased LH levels. This would explain the numerous partially stimulated follicles, theca luteinization, and moderate stromal maturation typical of polycystic ovary disease.

Laparoscopy, culdoscopy, culdotomy, pelvic pneumography, or laparotomy will reveal the ovarian abnormality.

Adrenocortical hyperplasia or tumor is ruled out if signs of defeminization and masculinization are absent and adrenal function is normal. The diagnosis of virilizing ovarian tumor is unlikely if the ovarian enlargement is bilateral and there are no voice changes or clitoral hypertrophy. If hyperprolactinemia occurs, pituitary microadenoma may be present and must be ruled out.

Treatment & Prognosis

Give hydrocortisone, 50 mg orally twice daily for 2–3 months. Clomiphene citrate (Clomid), 50 mg orally daily for 1–2 months, may be helpful. If ovulatory cycles are not resumed, wedge resection of one-third to one-half of each ovary should be considered. Most patients will respond, and infertility is often overcome. Hirsutism and obesity are not affected by corticosteroids or surgery and must be treated individually.

Endometrial cancer occurs more frequently in patients with polycystic ovary disease, perhaps because of unopposed estrogen stimulation.

OVARIAN CORTICAL STROMAL HYPERPLASIA

Focal or diffuse proliferation of partially luteinized stromal cells in the ovarian cortex is observed occasionally in menopausal and, particularly, postmenopausal women. The cause is not known, although its association with slightly increased estrogen production, endometrial hyperplasia, or cancer of the endometrium or breast is strikingly high. Whether hyperfunction of the ovary is primary or secondary is still debated.

Minimal enlargement and rounding of surface contours of the ovaries coincide with the accumulation of plump, ovoid, variably luteinized stromal cells in the cortex. No cysts develop. Multinodular, partially confluent stromal hyperplasia is the most common pattern. Small cortical granulomas composed of peripheral stromal cells and central epithelioid elements, chronic inflammatory cells, and lipid-containing debris are seen in histologic preparations.

Cortical stromal hyperplasia may be suspected when slight, persistently increased estrogen production continues after the menopause (in the absence of estrogen medication). Postmenopausal uterine bleeding may occur. Hyperestrogenism is best diagnosed on the basis of the vaginal cytologic smear.

The patient should be reexamined at frequent intervals. Laparotomy and resection of the ovaries are not justified on a presumptive diagnosis. If genital or breast cancer can be ruled out, spontaneous regression of the ovarian stromal hyperplasia is likely after age 60–70.

ARGENTAFFIN (CARCINOID) TUMORS

Argentaffin (carcinoid) tumors are not rare. Most originate in the appendix, but ovarian argentaffinoma may occur. The presence of an ovarian mass and vasomotor symptoms and a positive result in the urinary 5-hydroxyindoleacetic acid test suggest the diagnosis. Surgical removal is usually curative.

OOPHORITIS

Isolated infection of the ovary is very rare. However, oophoritis may accompany puerperal infection, mumps, tuberculosis, mycosis, severe regional infections (eg, appendicitis and tubal sepsis), and nematode infestations. Women in the reproductive years are most often affected.

Infective organisms may reach the ovary via the lymphatics (following D&C, attempted induced abortion, puerperal sepsis, salpingography); via the uterine tubes (gonorrhea, schistosomiasis); via the bloodstream (mumps, distant abscesses, wound infections, pulmonary tuberculosis); or via the peritoneal fluid and contiguous intra-abdominal infections (pelvic tuberculosis and actinomycosis). The microorganisms most often responsible for oophoritis are streptococci (usually hemolytic or anaerobic types), colon bacilli, staphylococci, gonococci, and tubercle bacilli (in that order).

The ovary is generally resistant to infection. Nevertheless, the point of rupture of the follicle or the forming corpus luteum itself may provide an entrance for bacteria. Little tendency toward healing is noted once deep cortical or medullary infection is established.

The symptoms of the suppurative form of oophoritis are similar to those of pyogenic salpingitis. Pain, fever, and menstrual abnormalities appear in the advanced stage of nonsuppurative oophoritis, together with ovarian (and other) adherent pelvic masses. Intestinal obstruction or fistula may develop.

Diagnosis and treatment are similar to those of acute salpingitis (see p 624).

When early oophoritis yields to medical management, the prognosis is good for fertility and normal ovarian function.

Urologic, Bowel, & Anorectal Problems in Obstetrics & Gynecology | 26

Urinary incontinence is one of the most common problems seen by the gynecologist. A patient with involuntary loss of urine may have one or more of the following types of urinary incontinence: (1) Stress incontinence is involuntary loss of urine only with increased intra-abdominal pressure, eg, with cough or lifting. (2) Urge incontinence is involuntary loss of small amounts of urine, preceded by a sudden and uncontrollable sensation of having to urinate. This is usually due to the presence of an irritable focus in or near the bladder, which initiates involuntary bladder contractions. (3) Neurogenic incontinence is unavoidable periodic loss of urine due to an uninhibited, hypotonic, or hypertonic neurogenic bladder. (4) Continuous incontinence is constant loss of urine from ureteral, vesical, or urethral fistulous openings or (very rarely) from an extrasphincteric ectopic ureter or exstrophy of the bladder.

Normal Bladder & Urethra Function

An understanding of normal bladder and urethra function is essential for the diagnosis of urinary incontinence.

The bladder and urethra resemble a long-neck flask when filled. The 2 parts should be considered to be a single entity because they must function together to allow the patient to retain a reasonable volume of urine, to initiate voiding without delay or discomfort when the natural urge occurs, and to terminate urination promptly.

A. Muscle Function: The nonstriated muscles of the bladder wall extend down the whole length of the urethra. This smooth (involuntary) muscle does not encircle the urethra, but it functions as a sphincter, normally closing the urethrovesical junction with the aid of strong elastic tissue. Strands of striated muscle on each side of the urethra arc laterally at about midurethra and join with fibrous tissue just above the urogenital diaphragm. This is the detrusor musculature, which functions as a voluntary or external urethral sphincter. The detrusor muscles must function properly for normal retention and voiding of urine.

B. Nerve Function: The bladder muscles have certain activities that are independent of the central nervous system. Notably, the smooth muscle of the lower urinary tract can exert persistent tension and adjust to the new pressure (compliance) as the bladder distends. Urethrovesical closure is also largely autonomous at low to moderate pressures, but changes in sensation are constantly mediated by the central nervous system.

Sympathetic nerves to the bladder and urethra originate in spinal cord segments T10–12 and travel to the pelvis via the second lumbar segment (L2). The hypogastric nerves contain most of the sympathetic nerve fibers. The sympathetic nervous system has α- and β-adrenergic components. Both the bladder and urethra receive α and β fibers. Beta fibers terminate principally in the detrusor muscle, whereas the urethra receives only minimal β-adrenergic innervation; the converse is true for the α fibers. Stimulation via the α fibers results in contraction of the bladder neck and urethra and relaxation of the detrusor muscle.

Parasympathetic nerves originating in the spinal cord segments S2–4 travel to the lower urinary tract via the pelvic nerve. Parasympathetic impulses cause contraction of the fundus of the bladder and the detrusor muscle and inhibit urethral smooth muscle activity.

The detrusor musculature is innervated by 4 reflex loops. Loops I and II, which involve cortical and cerebellar neural pathways, are necessary for voluntary control and complete emptying of the bladder. Central nervous system injury, tumor, or degenerative disorders (eg, Parkinson's disease) may interrupt loop I. Spinal lesions (eg, multiple sclerosis, diabetic atherosclerosis) may be responsible for failures of loop II. Relaxation of the bladder neck (internal sphincter) is effected via loop III, which involves sacral pathways. Detrusor dyssynergia may follow disorders involving this tract. Loop IV, also at the sacral level, mediates central and peripheral control of the striated muscles involved in voiding. Intermittent prolonged voiding and residual urine may accompany loop IV neuropathy.

C. Voiding: The first desire to void is perceived when the bladder contains about 150 mL of fluid. At this point (and even much later), normal women can voluntarily prevent voiding, even when there is a sudden increase in intra-abdominal pressure, as occurs with coughing. With more filling, the intravesical pressure remains fairly constant until the volume reaches 350–400 mL (a pressure of about 150 cm of water), at which point the individual feels the need to void. When bladder capacity (about 450 mL) is reached, the intravesical pressure exceeds the intraurethral pressure and triggers involuntary voiding.

To initiate urination, the periurethral striated muscles must relax, either reflexly or voluntarily. Then, as the bladder contracts, it descends posteriorly. This obliterates the posterior urethrovesical angle; concomitantly, the detrusor musculature contracts. This results in funneling of the bladder neck and apparent shortening of the urethra. Urethral tension is thus reduced, and a bolus of urine is propelled through and out of the urethra to initiate voiding. When voiding stops, these changes are reversed.

Some women aid voiding by consciously increasing intra-abdominal pressure. This augments normal urethral pressure to facilitate the passage of urine.

Diagnosis of Incontinence

The following measures are useful in the diagnosis of any type of urinary incontinence. The 4 specific types of urinary incontinence and their diagnosis, prevention, treatment, and prognosis are discussed below.

A. History and Physical Examination: A careful clinical history and physical examination usually will indicate the provisional diagnosis and the need for specific testing before treatment. The following information should be elicited: nature and extent of the problem (eg, the amount of urine lost in episodes of incontinence, the need to wear a pad, and the extent of inconvenience and social problems the incontinence causes); presence of neurologic problems or major illnesses (eg, diabetes mellitus); and history of pelvic or vaginal surgery or trauma. Reduced vesical or urethral support caused by obstetric trauma or restriction of the urethrovesical junction associated with scar tissue may cause or contribute to incontinence.

B. Laboratory Findings: Gross and microscopic urinalysis must be done initially in all incontinent patients. The polyuria of diabetes mellitus may be responsible for the symptoms of neurogenic incontinence. Urinary tract inflammation may cause urge incontinence. If increased numbers of white blood cells or bacteria are noted, urine specimens for culture should be taken before and after appropriate antibiotic therapy and before other studies are initiated. If there is convincing evidence of bladder or urethral disease, endoscopy should then be carried out.

C. Cystourethroscopic Findings: Cystourethroscopy is particularly valuable in the diagnosis of urge incontinence. A small-diameter cystoscope is ideal for visualization of the urethra and bladder. Erythema or granularity of the posterior urethra and trigone suggests chronic inflammation. Urologic abnormalities (eg, bladder trabeculation indicative of outflow obstruction) may be identified by cystourethroscopy, and stones or foreign bodies can often be detected and removed transurethrally. Fistulas and urethral diverticula should be sought.

D. Urodynamic Findings: Cystometry, intrarectal and intra-abdominal pressure studies, urethral closure pressure profile, uroflometry, and electromyography may be helpful in the diagnosis of urinary incontinence. The reader is referred to urologic texts for details of performing and evaluating these tests.

E. X-Ray Findings: Urodynamic studies are usually more informative than radiologic voiding studies. Nevertheless, cystourethrograms have demonstrated anatomic abnormalities in women with stress incontinence (see below).

1. STRESS INCONTINENCE

Stress incontinence is the most common type of incontinence in parous women. Because it is most frequently caused by childbirth injury (ie, loss of support of the bladder neck), this type of incontinence is rare in nulliparas. However, some obese nulliparas may lose urine with sudden increased intra-abdominal pressure. Postmenopausal women may have pelvic floor relaxation and incontinence secondary to marked estrogen deficiency. Scar tissue from surgery involving the bladder neck may cause or contribute to stress incontinence. Occasional patients, particularly elderly women, may have chronic urinary retention due to neuropathy; they void only with Valsalva's maneuver, and straining may cause loss of urine.

Clinical Findings

A. Symptoms and Signs: Loss of urine occurs only with increased intra-abdominal pressure (eg, with sneezing, running, straining). Except in severe cases, loss of urine usually occurs only when the patient is standing. A patient may state that she can prevent leakage of urine if she sits down quickly when she fears it may occur.

The physical examination should include identification of abdominal or pelvic masses, urethrocele, cystocele, rectocele, or uterine prolapse and measurement of residual urine. (Although cystocele or urethrocele may be present, they are not the cause of incontinence.)

B. Special Diagnostic Findings: The following tests may aid in the diagnosis of urinary stress incontinence:

1. Urethra measurement–The length of the urethra should be determined with the patient standing. (The length may be normal, ie, 3.8–4 cm, when the patient is supine.) The urethra of patients with stress incontinence is about 2–2.5 cm long. Urethral shortening is usually caused by inadequate musculofascial support to the bladder.

2. Stress test–Observe the urethral meatus when the patient is standing and has a full bladder. Stress incontinence is likely only if a spurt of urine occurs with each short cough. If leakage is delayed or considerable loss occurs, the diagnosis of uninhibited bladder should be considered.

3. Bonney test–Bonney found that elevating the bladder neck with 2 fingers placed in the vagina usually will prevent urine loss from a full bladder in patients with stress incontinence. In Read's modification of the test, a rubber-clad curved clamp is used to elevate the bladder neck. Compression of the urethra during either of these maneuvers will cause a false-positive result.

4. "Q-tip" test of Stamey–The patient is placed in the supine position, a lubricated Q-tip is inserted into the urethra to the urethrovesical junction, and the angle between the stick and the horizontal is estimated. In nulliparous women at rest, the angle will be 10–15 degrees above the horizontal. In patients with stress incontinence, the angle will often be 50–60 degrees above the horizontal because of lack of support to the vesical neck. The Q-tip test will be positive in most—but not all—patients with stress incontinence and in some patients without stress incontinence. In any event, a positive test indicates considerable descent of the vesical neck and urethra—important details when surgery is required.

C. Cystoscopic and Urodynamic Findings: Women with stress incontinence may require cystoscopy to identify urethral or bladder disorders. With pure stress incontinence, voiding will occur during cystometry at pressures of about 80 cm of water or less. Urodynamic studies may be required to diagnose or rule out associated neurogenic bladder dysfunction.

D. X-Ray Findings: X-ray cystourethrography is now an elective procedure, employed only occasionally. Lateral views are taken with the patient erect. The normal angle or inclination of the urethra to the perpendicular, ie, the anterior urethrovesical (UV) angle, is approximately 30 degrees; the normal posterior UV angle is 90–100 degrees. In the absence of childbirth injury or surgical compromise, these angles are not changed in women with true urge, neurogenic, or continuous incontinence. In most women with stress incontinence, the anterior UV angle is not greatly altered but the posterior UV angle is so severely reduced that the urethra and bladder trigone may even be aligned, especially with bearing down. In addition, funneling at the urethrovesical junction may be abnormal. This condition is often termed type I stress incontinence (Fig 26–1).

If obstetric injury strips the bladder and urethra from their normal supports posterior and inferior to the symphysis, the bladder will then rotate to sag backward and downward, irrespective of cystocele. Concomitantly, the urethra will sag to form a urethrocele. The anterior UV angle may exceed 90 degrees, and the posterior UV angle is usually considerably decreased. This condition is termed type II stress incontinence (Fig 26–1). In patients with type I or II stress incontinence, actual loss of urine with coughing can always be demonstrated.

Prevention

Methods for prevention of stress incontinence include ante- and postpartal exercises (Kegel) to strengthen the pelvic floor and sphincteric

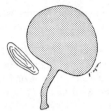

Normal support. (Continent.)

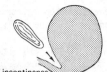

Type II stress incontinence.
(Loss of posterior urethrovesical angle, downward and
backward rotational descent
of urethra and bladder neck.)

Note: This is not a cystocele but
may simulate one. Often called
urethrocele, but this is a poor de-
scriptive term.

Type I stress incontinence.
(Loss of posterior urethrovesical angle, slight or no displacement of normal urethral axis,
minimal findings on pelvic
examination.)

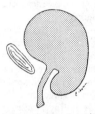

Cystocele. (Continent.)

Figure 26–1. Anatomic configuration of the bladder in normal (continent) women and women with stress incontinence. Drawn from cystourethrograms. (Reproduced, with permission, from Green TH Jr: *Gynecology: Essentials of Clinical Practice,* 3rd ed. Little, Brown, 1977.)

musculature; prevention of obstetric trauma, especially difficult forceps or breech deliveries; weight reduction in obese women; and use of estrogen supplements (if not contraindicated) in postmenopausal women who have a moderate degree of pelvic floor relaxation. The maintenance or surgical redevelopment of good UV angles, especially the posterior angle, is of major importance in the prevention or cure of stress incontinence.

Treatment

In less severe cases, especially in patients who desire more children, α-adrenergic drugs (eg, ephedrine, 25–50 mg orally 2–3 times daily) should be tried.

The success of almost all surgical operations for urinary stress incontinence depends upon whether the urethrovesical junction can be elevated in relation to the posterior bladder. This is usually accomplished more easily from above than from below. Thus, type I stress incontinence generally can be cured by transvaginal surgery (Kelly operation) or a suprapubic operation (Marshall-Marchetti-Krantz or comparable procedure). An anterior and posterior repair usually should also be performed if a large cystocele and rectocele are present. Sling operations may be effective, but they are more hazardous and are less commonly employed. Tupe II stress incontinence is best corrected by transabdominal cystourethropexy.

Prognosis

About 50% of cooperative, nonobese patients can achieve moderate to good continence with Kegel exercises. The overall cure rate with the first (vaginal) operation is about 80%, and approximately half of the remainder can be cured by a second (transabdominal) operation. The success rate is about 90% when the abdominal-vaginal approach is used.

Patients with extreme or complicated abnormalities are not cured easily. Women who have undergone 2 or more corrective operations have a very poor prognosis, owing to denervation of the bladder and the presence of scar tissue.

2. URGE INCONTINENCE

Urge incontinence is usually due to the presence of an irritable focus in or near the bladder, which initiates involuntary bladder contractions and results in loss of small amounts of urine. The causes include urinary tract infection, interstitial or radiation cystitis, atrophic (senile) urethritis and vaginitis, bladder tumor, calculus, and foreign body (see Renal Diseases in Chapter 13). Neuropathic unstable bladder, excessive use of drugs, and side-effects of drugs are less common causes of urgency incontinence.

Clinical Findings

Patients suddenly feel compelled to void but cannot hold back. Although under these circumstances they lose small amounts of urine, they are not wet after straining nor are they always wet. Patients with urge incontinence usually have frequency and urgency and may even have enuresis.

Prevention

Early, effective treatment of urinary tract, cervical, or vaginal infection often prevents urinary urge incontinence. Excessive use of drugs and ingestion of too much caffeine should be avoided.

Treatment

The cure of urge incontinence requires correction of the underlying cause (see Chapter 13). Cystourethritis may be treated by use of appropriate antibiotics and, possibly, by urethral stripping, repeated dilatation of the urethra under local anesthesia, or endoscopic topical therapy. In patients with chronic urethritis and urge incontinence, anticholinergic drugs such as nortriptyline or oxybutynin may be worthwhile adjunctive therapy. Estrogen supplements will be beneficial for many post-menopausal incontinent women. Interstitial cystitis may improve with bladder instillations of dimethyl sulfoxide (DMSO) or periodic over-distention of the bladder under light general anesthesia. Patients with radiation cystitis may benefit from anticholinergic medications such as propantheline or bladder sedative medications such as flavoxate hydrochloride.

Prognosis

With correct diagnosis and treatment, the prognosis for urge incontinence is excellent. Urinary tract infection and urge incontinence may recur, however.

3. NEUROGENIC INCONTINENCE

In neurogenic incontinence, periodic loss of urine is due to uninhibited, hypertonic, or hypotonic bladder.

Clinical Findings

Two clinical types of upper motor neuron uninhibited bladder are recognized. In type I, patients lose a slight amount of urine 10–20 seconds after the rise of intra-abdominal pressure and detrusor contraction. In these patients, a neurogenic bladder should be suspected even if no other neuropathy is identifiable. In type II, the patient has a hypertonic bladder with small capacity, and bladder irritability is related to bladder filling. In these individuals, a marked early rise of intravesical pressure is followed by abrupt early bladder contraction and loss of urine.

Neurogenic deficit of the lower motor neuron type usually results in hypotonic bladder. Despite their large bladder capacity, these patients are incontinent due to overflow urine loss.

Extensive urodynamic testing is required in patients with probable neurogenic incontinence.

Prevention

Neurogenic incontinence can be prevented by proper therapy of disorders capable of causing bladder dysfunction, eg, Parkinson's disease and diabetes mellitus.

Treatment

Use of anticholinergic drugs, eg, phenylpropanolamine, is beneficial in many cases, especially in women with slight neurogenic incontinence.

Many antihypertensive drugs (eg, methyldopa) are α-blockers. Therefore, women taking these drugs often become incontinent but can control urination when the antihypertensive drug is discontinued.

Patients with overflow retention are best managed by periodic self-catheterization after careful cleansing of the catheter and the urethral meatus. Supportive long-term therapy with low dose antibiotics such as nitrofurantoin (Macrodantin), 100 mg orally at bedtime, is warranted. Urine cultures will be required to monitor bacteriuria.

Surgery will not help patients with neurogenic bladder problems.

Prognosis

Well-selected drug therapy may be of considerable benefit, but cure is unlikely.

4. CONTINUOUS INCONTINENCE

Continuous urine leakage after pelvic or vaginal surgery or following difficult vaginal delivery or other trauma may be due to a lower urinary tract fistula. Fistulas may follow irradiation, particularly radium therapy for cancer of the vagina or cervix. Other fistulas may be associated with granulomas, schistosomiasis, or prolonged pressure by a vaginal pessary.

Clinical Findings

A fistulous opening and urine leakage often may be seen on vaginal examination. Cystourethroscopy or x-ray urography should reveal the fistula. Very small fistulas, especially where a "ball-valve" closure occurs, may be difficult to identify.

The following tests are useful to differentiate a ureterovaginal from a vesicovaginal fistula:

(1) Distend the bladder with a solution containing 5 mL of indigo carmine and 200 mL of water. In the absence of ureteral reflux (rare), a fistula will be revealed by the presence of blue fluid in the vagina. When reflux is present, add 50 mL of an aqueous x-ray contrast medium to the indigo carmine solution, fill the bladder, and take an anteroposterior film of the pelvis to demonstrate backflow as well as extravasation.

(2) Insert a vaginal pack or snug menstrual tampon that has been moistened with an aqueous solution of sodium carbonate or bicarbonate. Inject the bladder with 200 mL of water containing 10 mL of methylene blue. Remove the catheter, avoiding any spill that might discolor the

pack, and inject 1 mL (6 mg) of phenolsulfonphthalein (PSP) intravenously. Withdraw the vaginal pack in about 30 minutes. If the pack is
stained blue, the presumptive diagnosis is vesicovaginal fistula; if the
pack is red, the defect is probably a ureterovaginal fistula; if the pack is
multicolored, a ureterovesicovaginal fistula may be present.

Prevention

The incidence of urinary fistulas of obstetric origin can be reduced
by avoiding long labor or difficult instrumental delivery. Well-planned,
careful pelvic surgery, with suitable drainage and effective treatment of
postoperative sepsis, will limit postsurgical formation of fistulas. Proper
individualization of intravaginal or intracervical radiation therapy for
cancer should prevent fistulas.

Treatment

In the absence of serious infection, small postoperative fistulas may
close in 3–4 months. Others must be closed surgically. Accessory
ureters draining into the vagina must be ligated proximally or removed.

Prognosis

Surgery usually will correct urinary fistulas (see p 677) or continuous incontinence due to congenital anomalies.

URETHRAL CARUNCLE

A small, reddened, sensitive, fleshy excrescence at the urethral
meatus is called a caruncle. Most caruncles represent eversion (ectropion) of the urethra or infections at the urinary meatus (or both), but
vascular anomalies or benign or malignant tumors may also cause
caruncle formation. The vast majority of caruncles are benign; persistent
and progressive lesions may be cancerous. Caruncles may occur at any
age, but postmenopausal women are most commonly affected.

Caruncles are categorized according to type as follows (combined
types also occur): (1) Papillary caruncles are flame-shaped and delicate,
have a rich vascular supply, and are covered with stratified transitional or
squamous cells. Gross infection may or may not be present. (2) Granulomatous caruncles with a wide base are inflammatory processes, usually due to bacterial infection and less commonly due to lymphogranuloma venereum or syphilis. (3) Vascular caruncles usually
have an angiomatous pattern and are frequently infected.

Clinical Findings

A. Symptoms and Signs: A caruncle appears as a small, vividly
red, sessile or flattened mass protruding from the urethral meatus. It may

bleed, exude, or cause pain, depending upon its cause, size, and integrity. Dysuria, frequency, and urgency are uncommon.

B. Laboratory Findings: Specimens for cytologic examination and bacterial smear and cultures should be obtained. If cancer is suspected, biopsy should be performed.

Prevention

Estrogen therapy for postmenopausal women and avoidance of local irritation will probably prevent caruncle formation.

Treatment

Infections, including sexually transmitted diseases, must be treated with appropriate antibiotics. Estrogens (diethylstilbestrol vaginal suppositories, 0.5 mg every other night for 3 weeks) are given before specific therapy in postmenopausal patients who have not been receiving steroid sex hormone therapy.

If the caruncle is not infected or malignant, light fulguration under local anesthesia, cryosurgery, or excision may be done, taking care not to produce a stricture. Repeated cryosurgery is preferable to extensive fulguration initially and may be repeated if the caruncle recurs. Topical antiinfective therapy (eg, nitrofurazone) is indicated before and after cauterization or excision. If malignant change occurs, adequate resection or radiation therapy is required.

If stenosis develops, the urethral meatus must be dilated.

Prognosis

The prognosis is excellent in benign cases but guarded when malignant change has occurred.

URETHRAL DIVERTICULUM

Urethral diverticulum is a sacculation caused by (1) congenital cystic dilatation of paraurethral (wolffian) remnants; (2) infection of the paraurethral gland, with rupture or trauma to the urethra; or (3) urinary, obstetric, or gynecologic injury. Most patients are 40–50 years old and multiparous.

The mid or distal third of the urethra is the usual site. With congenital malformation, the cystic structure, usually 1–4 cm in diameter, may be a single or multiloculated cavity. One or more minute ostia connect the diverticulum with the urethra. Symptoms are due to sacculation and local inflammation. They may be acute or chronic and constant or intermittent, but chronic infection with periodic acute exacerbations is the most common clinical picture. Calculi are present in the diverticulum in 10–20% of patients.

Clinical Findings

A. Symptoms and Signs:

1. Urinary distress–The complaints (eg, urgency, frequency, and nocturia) are similar to those of cystitis, and there is often a feeling of inability to empty the bladder completely.

2. Dribbling after urination–The postvoiding leakage may be urine or purulent or bloody fluid and is the result of evacuation of the diverticulum.

3. Discharge–A urinous or bloody purulent discharge at the meatus following stripping of the urethra represents diverticulum contents.

4. Vaginal pain–Pain is usually more severe before and after the menses. Dyspareunia, urethral tenderness, and pelvic discomfort are caused by inflammation or distention of the diverticulum.

5. Vaginal fullness–There may be indefinite anterior vaginal fullness that is periodically painful. Soft masses may be found on digital examination after passage of a catheter or by cystoscopy.

6. Malaise, chills, fever–These indicate acute infection.

B. X-Ray Findings:
Radiopaque contrast fluid studies generally will outline the diverticulum.

C. Special Examinations:
Insertion of a small urethral sound may demonstrate a slight stricture of the urethra and the diverticulum just beyond. Air cystoscopy or panendoscopy with a large-caliber instrument to dilate the ostium will reveal the diverticular opening in most cases, although the opening may be small and obscured by mucosal folds or granulation tissue.

Complications

Urethrovaginal fistula may follow unsuccessful diverticulectomy or spontaneous rupture (often during labor), erosion by stone, incisional drainage, or fulguration of the cystic abnormality. Transitional cell carcinoma or adenocarcinoma may develop in urethral diverticula. Stricture of the urethra may be a consequence of extensive or complicated surgery.

Differential Diagnosis

Urethritis, sexually transmitted or nonspecific, is a diffuse process; urethral abscess is a phase of diverticulum development. Urethrocele is not a swelling or herniation but a disengagement of the urethra from the symphysis. Gartner's duct cysts and inclusion cysts do not communicate with the urethra. Tumors near or involving the urethra may be primary or secondary and are firm, semifixed, and nontender.

Treatment

Broad-spectrum antibiotic therapy and warm vaginal douches generally will resolve the acute inflammatory phase in about 5 days, but chronic infection almost always persists.

Transvaginal diverticulectomy usually is necessary for permanent relief in patients with all but very small or persistently asymptomatic (large ostium) sacculations. An indwelling urethral catheter should be left in place for 10 days.

URINARY TRACT INJURIES FOLLOWING OBSTETRIC & GYNECOLOGIC SURGERY

Iatrogenic fistulas may occur in any part of the urinary tract and result from direct or indirect injury. Occlusions usually involve the ureter and occur as a result of angulation or obstruction by a suture, scarring after injury or infection, or as a complication of the treatment of pelvic cancer. The incidence of urinary tract injury in large medical centers in the USA is about 0.8% following major gynecologic surgery and 0.08% following obstetric surgery.

Postpartum fistulas of the bladder and urethra are generally caused by continued pressure of the presenting part or by instrumentation. There is usually a history of prolonged labor or operative delivery. Many fistulas are the result of technical surgical errors (poor exposure, operative ineptitude, or distortion of anatomy); ischemia due to failure to preserve the blood supply; hematoma formation (incomplete hemostasis, failure to institute drainage when indicated); and infection (neglected hematoma or contaminated urinary extravasation). Deep sutures, mass ligatures, and overdistention of the bladder also cause bladder injuries and fistula formation.

The ureter is often involved in fistula formation or stenosis, but the kidney is rarely damaged directly during gynecologic surgery. Many types of fistulas (singly or in combination) may be diagnosed after operation or delivery: ureterovaginal, ureterovesical, ureteroperitoneal, ureteroenteric, vesicovaginal, vesicouterine, vesicocervical, and urethrovaginal. Some fistulas are minute; others represent loss of a major segment of the urinary tract. Strictures are confined to narrow structures, eg, the ureter and urethra. Partial or complete closure of one or both ureters is not uncommon, but stricture of the female urethra rarely occurs postoperatively.

Clinical Findings

A. Symptoms and Signs: The symptoms depend upon the site of the injury (unilateral or bilateral), the degree of damage (partial or complete), and the direction of urine drainage (external, intraperitoneal, or retroperitoneal).

Unilateral ureteral injury usually causes flank pain, tenderness, and fever but does not alter the urinary volume. It may indicate constriction of the ureter, fistula, or infection. Escape of urine from the abdominal or vaginal incision indicates ureteral or bladder fistulas (or both). Ileus often follows urinary obstruction, extravasation, and infection. Urinary infection, especially with partial obstruction of the ureter, results in chills, fever, renal pain, and costovertebral and loin tenderness. In the absence of preexisting bacteriuria, complete obstruction of one ureter usually is asymptomatic. If urine leaks into the peritoneal cavity, there will be signs of free peritoneal fluid and peritoneal irritation. Progressive degeneration and necrosis of a damaged area in the urinary system or temporary pocketing of extravasated urine may account for delayed leakage (up to 3–4 weeks postoperatively).

Uremia ordinarily does not follow unilateral ureteral injury. Signs of perirenal or psoas inflammation follow retroperitoneal extravasation of urine. Anuria and uremia follow complete bilateral ureteral occlusion. Dehydration, shock, lower nephron nephrosis, and congestive heart failure should be ruled out.

B. Laboratory Findings: The phenolsulfonphthalein (PSP) test is performed to determine the degree of renal tubular function. About 30 minutes before the test is started, the patient should drink 400 mL of water. Thirty minutes later, 1 mL (6 mg) of dye is injected intravenously. Urine specimens are collected 30 and 60 minutes after injection of the dye, and water is added to dilute the urine specimen to 1000 mL. A sample of the diluted mixture and a standard are compared in a colorimeter. Normally, 60–70% of the dye is excreted in 2 hours; excretion of less than 50% is an indication of renal insufficiency. Passage of the dye verifies the patency of at least one ureter in cases of postoperative oliguria provided adequate hydration and a normal blood pressure have been maintained.

C. X-Ray Findings:

1. Ureteral obstruction, fistula, or extravasation–

a. Excretory urography–Even the freshly occluded kidney will not excrete the contrast agent. Although the urogram is an excellent screening test, the presence of excessive intestinal gas reduces the clarity of the roentgenogram.

b. Retrograde urography–A ureteral catheter may be blocked by an occlusion. (A radiopaque catheter should be used so that the level of the obstruction can be observed on the film.) Injection of a contrast medium into a Braasch-bulb catheter may reveal a fistula above the bulb fixed in the most distal portion of the ureter.

c. Plain film–An anteroposterior film of the abdomen may suggest retroperitoneal extravasation of urine or psoas abscess by revealing a mass, obliteration of the psoas muscle contours, or displacement of intestinal gas shadows.

2. Bladder fistula and extravasation–An anteroposterior scout film of the pelvis should be obtained. The bladder should be filled with 50 mL of radiopaque medium (eg, iodopyracet or acetrizoate) in 200 mL of water, and a second film should be taken. The bladder must then be drained and a third film obtained at once. Slight extravasation not visible in the second film may be clearly seen in the third.

D. Special Examinations:

1. Passage of a urethral catheter should reveal an obstruction.

2. Urethroscopy often will expose an obstruction, perforating suture, or fistula.

3. Although cystoscopy will disclose large vesical fistulas, direct visualization may be disappointing in the identification of small fistulas.

4. Retrograde studies of the urinary tract may be used to rule out ureteral injury. If ureteral catheters pass readily to both renal pelves and clear urine is recovered, ureteral injury is excluded, except perhaps in cases of a crushing injury or a small perforation. If one of these complications seems likely, the catheter should be secured in the ureter for splinting and drainage for the 10–14 days necessary for healing.

Complications

Peritonitis is the most serious complication and may result in death. Anuria or oliguria may be associated with fatal uremia. Other complications are psoas or perirenal abscess, thrombophlebitis, and urinary incontinence. Urinary tract infection may follow obstruction, as may hydroureter, hydronephrosis, nephrolithiasis, and ureterolithiasis.

Differential Diagnosis

Some fistulas follow irradiation, particularly radium therapy, for cancer of the cervix. Some may be associated with treatment of granulomas, prolonged pressure by a pessary, or the presence of tuberculosis, lymphogranuloma venereum, or schistosomiasis. Clear, yellowish, odorless drainage from the abdominal wound may represent ascites or exudative peritoneal fluid, an antecedent of wound dehiscence. Thin, brownish discharge from an abdominal or vaginal suture line may be serum from a seroma or hematoma. In ureteral obstruction, oliguria or anuria may be due to shock, dehydration, or lower nephron nephrosis; abdominal distention may indicate dynamic ileus caused by intestinal obstruction or adynamic ileus due to peritonitis; fever may be due to an infected wound, peritonitis, or thrombophlebitis; and kidney pain and costovertebral or flank tenderness may be due to nephrolithiasis, ureterolithiasis, or pyelonephritis.

Prevention

Adequate preliminary studies of the urinary tract and full knowledge of the anatomy and pathologic processes involved are essential before surgery. The ureters should be catheterized and identified initially in all difficult cases, and the wire stylet should be left in a ureteral catheter for identification, ie, to prevent the ureter from being cut or clamped by mistake.

All structures must be identified before clamping, incision, and ligation; and care must be taken to prevent undue traction and needless denudation of the ureter and the base of the bladder. Only fine absorbable sutures should be used in or around the urinary tract. Multiple ligatures should not be used for hemorrhage; instead, pressure should be applied and a single bleeding point secured. The course of the ureters must be traced at the completion of each abdominal operation if surgery was near the ureter.

Antibiotics should be administered for treatment of infection. The surgeon should personally remove ureteral catheters after surgery if it is decided not to leave them in place. A "hang" may indicate ureteral constriction.

Treatment

A. Emergency Measures: Shock, blood loss, and dehydration are treated as indicated and the bladder catheterized. If oliguria or anuria is present, a PSP test should be performed. Specific gravity of the urine should be checked and the patient weighed.

B. Surgical Measures:

1. Bilateral ureteral obstruction–If both ureters are obstructed and the patient is a poor surgical risk, nephrostomy or unilateral tube ureterostomy is preferred. The largest child's urethral catheter that will enter the ureter should be used. The other kidney should not be left obstructed for more than a few days. As soon as the patient becomes a satisfactory operative risk, the second blocked kidney should be relieved by nephrostomy or tube ureterostomy. Deligation alone is not satisfactory unless this can be performed easily. If deligation is done, a splinting catheter should be inserted through a longitudinal incision several centimeters above the point of obstruction, passed to the kidney and bladder, brought out through the urethra, and fixed to a Foley retention catheter for 10–14 days, at which time both may be removed. The retroperitoneal area must be drained through a separate lower quadrant or flank stab wound.

A gallbladder T tube can be used in lieu of a catheter as follows: (1) The cross-arm of the T is notched at the vertical segment. (2) The ureter is incised longitudinally several centimeters above the defect. (3) The tube is inserted so that its lower arm splints the point of injury. (4) The upper arm of the tube is fixed in the proximal ureter and the long arm carried out retroperitoneally through a stab wound in the flank. (5) A drain is placed in the retroperitoneal space underlying the T tube and allowed to remain until drainage ceases (about 1 week after the removal of the tube).

2. Vesicoperitoneal fistula–Laparotomy should be performed as soon as the diagnosis is established. The edges are freshened and the fistula closed without tension in 2 layers: one continuous or both interrupted, using 000 chromic catgut. The mucosa should be avoided in suturing. The bladder must be drained by cystostomy or with a Foley retention catheter, and pelvic suction drainage should be employed for about 7 days.

3. Vesicovaginal fistula–Local infection should be treated by removing old sutures and concretions and by giving systemic antibiotics. Repair is indicated as outlined for vesicoperitoneal fistula. In general, attempts at closure should be delayed until 4 months or more after injury. If there are no other contraindications, one may take a calculated risk in selected cases and perform earlier repair after preparation with prednisone, 10 mg 4 times daily, and large doses of broad-spectrum antibiotics for 7 days. All but large, inaccessible, immobile vesicovaginal fistulas (85–90% of the total) should be closed transvaginally.

4. Ureterovesicovaginal fistula–The fistula should be closed abdominally. The procedure is to freshen the edges, excise scar tissue, free restrictions, and close without tension. Relatively few fine, absorbable, interrupted mattress sutures should be employed, avoiding the mucosa. Monofilament sutures should never be buried, and purse-string sutures should not be used.

Reimplantation of the severely damaged or severed ureter into the bladder (ureteroneocystostomy) is preferable to ureteroureterostomy on the same side. Ureteroneocystostomy should be attempted only when the proximal ureter is long enough to permit anastomosis without tension. The bladder should be drained by cystostomy or with a Foley retention catheter, and suction drainage should be used for about 7 days.

Ligation of the damaged ureter and sacrifice of the kidney on that side are almost always contraindicated. A renal abscess may develop, necessitating a much more serious operation (nephrectomy) than restoration of the continuity of the urinary system. Moreover, the opposite kidney may be deficient, or it may fail.

Prognosis

Most ureteral repairs are successful if carefully performed and if urinary and extraperitoneal drainage is ensured.

Very small vesicovaginal fistulas often close spontaneously if the bladder can be kept collapsed and infection prevented.

Urethral fistulas are notoriously resistant to spontaneous closure if a urethral catheter is used. Many heal well, however, when simply repaired and when a cystostomy is used instead of a urethral catheter.

BOWEL PROBLEMS

INTESTINAL INJURIES FOLLOWING
OBSTETRIC & GYNECOLOGIC SURGERY

Surgical accidents such as laceration, incision, crushing, or perforation of the intestine may be discovered at operation or soon thereafter. Such injury is usually associated with adhesions, distortion, unusual displacement of the abdominal contents, poor exposure, lack of surgical knowledge, or haste. Most operative damage occurs with pelvic tumor, chronic inflammation, or endometriosis or after previous surgery. About 5% of gynecologic operations involve primary or secondary bowel surgery exclusive of appendectomy.

Clinical Findings
Postoperative bleeding and infection follow extensive, initially unrecognized intestinal trauma. Even if a defect is closed at surgery, it may bleed or leak later. Peritonitis, pelvic abscess, possible fecal fistula, evisceration, septic embolization, and death are the sequelae.

Fever, severe anorexia, nausea and vomiting, abdominal pain, distention, tenderness, and guarding develop a few days after an operation with complications. A vague abdominal mass may be outlined. Spreading sepsis, purulent or fecal drainage from the incision, or dehiscence often follows 7–10 days after surgery. Laboratory tests indicate an acute infectious process; anemia may be evident. X-ray studies are rarely diagnostic. Moreover, the introduction of a contrast medium may enlarge the intestinal defect.

Differential Diagnosis
The differential diagnosis includes incisional, urinary, or respiratory tract infection and intestinal obstruction.

Prevention
The bowel should be inspected at surgery, bleeding controlled, and defects repaired. The suture line must be transverse, never longitudinal, or circular constriction will result. Interrupted intestinal nonabsorbable sutures are preferred. In wounds of the serosa and the muscularis, a single row of sutures will suffice. One or 2 mattress sutures will generally close puncture wounds satisfactorily.

When the mucosa of the bowel has been opened, contamination of the peritoneal cavity should be assumed and spill limited by suction, laparotomy packs, and elevation of the edges of the defect. Two layers of sutures should be employed: the first in the muscularis and the second in the superficial muscularis and serosa. Abdominal lavage with normal saline solution should be accomplished. A Penrose type drain is inserted through a stab incision to the site of repair. Antibiotic therapy, eg, penicillin and kanamycin, should be given in large doses if contamination is obvious.

When widespread bowel damage or invasion by tumor is noted, segmental resection, "aseptic anastomosis," and drainage should be considered, if feasible. Repair of the bowel, proximal tube enterostomy, peritoneal drainage, and later definitive surgery may be necessary for poor-risk patients.

Treatment

Initiation of gastric suction, reestablishment of fluid and electrolyte balance by parenteral means, and replacement of blood loss may be indicated. Enemas are contraindicated. Analgesics should be provided until bowel function is reestablished (in about 10 days).

If intestinal obstruction or dehiscence develops, the problem must be corrected by reoperation. A "pointing" pelvic abscess should be drained transvaginally or extraperitoneally. Critical sepsis is much more likely from injury to the large bowel than from injury to the small bowel.

Prognosis

When spreading peritonitis or large pelvic abscess develops, the prognosis becomes grave.

ANORECTAL PROBLEMS

Common lesions of the anal canal are shown in Fig 26–2.

PRURITUS ANI

Pruritus ani, a distressing symptom of an underlying local or general disorder, is often misdiagnosed or overtreated. It occurs because the sensitive, often moist pudendal skin is commonly exposed to irritating fecal material retained in anal recesses. Dermatitis may then develop. Women of any age may be affected, but it is most common among unhygienic middle-aged persons. Causes may be multiple. The major causes, in approximate order of frequency, are as follows:

A. Mechanical Problems: Faulty anal hygiene, tight nonabsorbent clothing, or scratching.

B. Local Proctologic, Gynecologic, or Urologic Disease: Hemorrhoids, fissure in ano, fistula, leukorrhea, or fecal or urinary incontinence.

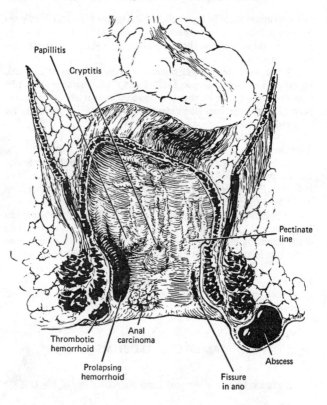

Figure 26–2. Common lesions of the anal canal. (Reproduced, with permission, from Wilson JL: *Handbook of Surgery*, 5th ed. Lange, 1973.)

C. Psychoneurosis and Habit: Continued inappropriate awareness of an unpleasant sensation, often following correction of a local condition (itch-scratch-itch sequence).

D. Infections: Proctitis or dermatitis due to bacteria, fungi, yeasts, trichomonads, or intestinal parasites (particularly *Enterobius vermicularis* and *Ascaris lumbricoides*).

E. Allergy or Sensitivity Reactions: Atopic eczema or contact dermatitis.

F. Systemic Diseases: Diabetes mellitus, jaundice, or Hodgkin's disease.

Clinical Findings

Pruritus is poorly localized. The lesion may be isolated, but the itching is usually circumanal, often spreading over the perineum or pudendum. It may extend to or from the vaginal introitus. The perianal skin may be erythematous, excoriated, dry, moist, or bleeding; secondary chronic changes are maceration, scaling, fissuring, or lichenification. A similar dermatologic condition (eg, fungal intertrigo, eczema) may also be present elsewhere. The itching sensation may be slight to almost unbearable.

Pruritus is invariably more acute at night or during periods of inactivity; it is heightened by warmth and scratching. Introspection also tends to aggravate the condition.

Treatment

If possible, treat the problem (eg, trichomoniasis) definitively. If the cause remains obscure, treat symptomatically. Complicated forms of treatment such as irradiation, surgery, or tattooing should not be used except in very persistent cases. Acute pruritus is much easier to relieve than chronic pruritus, which becomes complicated by secondary changes.

A. Specific Measures:

1. Tepid sitz baths or cool compresses of Burow's solution are soothing in acute cases.

2. If an allergic reaction is suspected, oral antihistamines (eg, diphenhydramine) may be helpful.

3. Sedatives induce sleep and reduce the sensation of itching, but bromides and barbiturates used extensively may themselves cause pruritus.

4. Hydrocortisone (1%) in lotion or nonoily cream is especially beneficial in idiopathic and allergic pruritus.

5. Treat local candidal infections with miconazole, 2% in a water-miscible base, applied twice daily. Tinea (fungal) infections usually yield to compound undecylenic acid ointment applied twice daily.

6. Topical anesthetics should be avoided because sensitization and increased itching may result.

B. General Measures:

1. The patient should keep the area clean. Bland, unscented, nonmedicated soaps or mild detergents such as hexachlorophene (pHisoHex) may be used. She should use moistened toilet tissue or cloth after each bowel movement and carefully blot (not wipe) the area dry to minimize irritation.

2. Regular bowel habits are important. Soften hard stools with hydrophilic agents such as psyllium hydrophilic mucilloid (Metamucil) and dioctyl sodium sulfosuccinate (Colace). Diarrhea must be controlled, because watery stools increase anal soiling and sensitivity.

Mineral oil in any form is contraindicated because the oil seals in irritants and prevents surface drying.

3. Shake lotions (eg, noncarbolated calamine) or dusting powders (eg, plain talc or cornstarch) are useful drying and protective agents.

PROCTALGIA FUGAX

Proctalgia fugax, so-called rectal spasm or rectal neuralgia, is a sudden cramping rectal pain of short duration. It is uncommon but often affects tense and introspective individuals. Its cause is not known, but partial intussusception of redundant rectal mucosa is suspected.

Clinical Findings

Cramping rectal pain begins without warning, ranges in intensity from marked to agonizing, and tends to recur after a few days or even after months. The discomfort starts low in the rectum and moves higher (perhaps combined with the urge to defecate). Pain is associated with sweating, agitation, and even collapse. It subsides gradually, leaving the patient weak and shaken.

Differential Diagnosis

Rectal examination readily differentiates proctalgia fugax from thrombosed hemorrhoids, fissure in ano, and abscess. The pain of factitial proctitis, which may follow intravaginal radium therapy or local treatment of acute rectal disease, is constant and is accompanied by rectal bleeding and ulceration. Sigmoidorectal obstruction causes extreme, unrelenting, progressive pain and is not likely to recur. Painful disorders of the sacroiliac joint, which may cause diagnostic confusion, are initiated and aggravated by movement. Cauda equina lesions may cause pelvic pain but are associated with paresthesia, hypesthesia, or weakness of the pelvic floor and sphincter muscles.

Treatment

Ample sedation and filling of the rectum with 200–300 mL of air or warm fluid may give dramatic relief. Investigation and correction of medical or social problems may prevent future attacks. Recurrent attacks should be treated by submucosal injections of a solution containing 4% phenol, 50% glycerine, and water. Injections of 1 mL each at 4 points—1 cm apart—just below the rectosigmoid junction may be curative.

ANAL CONDYLOMAS
(See Condylomata Acuminata, p 536.)

HEMORRHOIDS

Hemorrhoids (piles) are anorectal varicosities caused by lax pelvic veins and venous stasis. The condition is characterized by acute pain, protrusion, and tenderness due to thrombosis. Most women have hemorrhoids, which often develop during pregnancy or delivery. Causes include weakness of pelvic veins (aging), increased venous pressure (portal hypertension), reduced vascular drainage of the pelvic organs (pregnancy, constipation), or rectal disease (cryptitis). Hereditary factors predispose to hemorrhoids.

Inadequate perivascular support and the absence of vein valves permit reversed venous flow in the hemorrhoidal plexus. Repeated trauma to the terminal rectum and anus (eg, large or hard stool) is followed by mucosal fissures and ruptured blood vessels. Thrombosis, rupture, or infection often results.

Clinical Findings

Protrusion, pain, and bleeding are symptoms of hemorrhoids.

Internal hemorrhoids lie above the anorectal or mucocutaneous dentate) line and are derived from the superior and middle hemorrhoidal veins. They are usually located in the right anterior and both posterior quadrants of the rectum, are covered by thin rectal mucosa, and are innervated by autonomic nerves. External hemorrhoids develop below the mucocutaneous line and may appear in any quadrant. They are covered by skin, are supplied by the inferior hemorrhoidal vein, and are innervated by cutaneous nerves. An external hemorrhoid that has thrombosed becomes a small, coagulated perianal hematoma. Combined external and internal hemorrhoids are uncommon, but they may be serious if they involve at least one-third of the anorectal margin.

Differential Diagnosis

One must never assume that hemorrhoids are the cause of bleeding from the bowel until careful and complete physical, proctologic, and laboratory studies have failed to reveal tumor, cancer, or other local or systemic disease.

Prevention

Prevention includes good bowel habits, avoidance of straining at stool, and prompt treatment of diarrhea and anorectal disorders.

Treatment

A. Nonsurgical Measures:

1. Asymptomatic hemorrhoids–No treatment is required. Stool softeners and dietary advice regarding laxative foods and ample fluids should be given.

2. Hemorrhoids with mild or infrequent symptoms–Prescribe warm sitz baths, astringent ointments or suppositories (eg, Anusol), and oral analgesics. Avoid using sensitizing local anesthetics or antibiotics. Advise the patient to use moist cotton or cloth instead of toilet paper and take measures to correct faulty bowel function.

3. Hemorrhoids with moderate symptoms–Large or prolapsed hemorrhoids often cause moderate symptoms. Treat as for mild symptoms, and inject one hemorrhoid a week with 1 mL of 5% quinine and urea solution or 5% sodium morrhuate solution. Use a 22-gauge needle for injections.

4. Hemorrhoids with severe symptoms–Large or strangulated hemorrhoids often cause severe symptoms. Treat initially as for mild symptoms, and plan for early hemorrhoidectomy unless thrombosis has occurred. Acutely painful, thrombosed external hemorrhoids should be incised under local anesthesia and the clot removed. For the first 24 hours after clot formation, treat as for mild symptoms; later, consider hemorrhoidectomy.

5. Symptomatic hemorrhoids during pregnancy–Treat as for mild symptoms if possible. Hemorrhoidectomy should be deferred until after the puerperium.

B. Surgical Measures: Open type radial hemorrhoidectomy (ligation and excision) is the preferred surgical method. A cleansing enema should be administered before hemorrhoidectomy. No packs or drains should be used after surgery. Cover the incision with moist gel sponge. The patient should take daily sitz baths, mild laxatives, and parenteral analgesics. Antibiotics may be given if needed. Perform gentle digital rectal dilatation 5–7 days postoperatively, and repeat 2–3 times every 5–7 days to prevent bridging and formation of fistulas.

Complications of hemorrhoidectomy include postoperative bleeding, perianal hematoma, infection, fecal impaction, delayed healing (with granulation tissue), rectal stenosis, and recurrence of hemorrhoids.

Prognosis

Hemorrhoids are never precancerous, but cancer may coexist. Hemorrhoids are unlikely to be permanently cured by injection therapy, but complications are uncommon. Hemorrhoidectomy is curative.

CRYPTITIS & PAPILLITIS

Inflammation of the anal crypts and papillae causes brief pain and burning upon defecation. Digital and anoscopic examinations reveal hypertrophic papillae and infected, often indurated crypts.

Stool softeners such as psyllium hydrophilic mucilloid (Metamucil), several times daily by mouth, and analgesic suppositories (eg, Anusol), once or twice daily, help greatly. A single application of 5% phenol in oil into the crypts aids resolution of the inflammation. Surgical excision of involved crypts and papillae should be considered if these measures fail.

FISSURE IN ANO

Anorectal mucosal lacerations occur frequently as a result of sudden or marked distention during a difficult bowel movement. Acute fissures, although temporarily painful and perhaps associated with scant bleeding, generally heal rapidly. Chronic fissures may be persistent; either they fail to heal, or they heal and break down. They cause severe pain during and after defecation, and blood may be present in the stool or after evacuation. Recurrent fissures may be associated with the eventual development of a sentinel pile, hypertrophic papillae, and anal spasm (especially painful on rectal examination).

Treatment of acute fissures is the same as that for hemorrhoids with mild symptoms. A single application of a mild styptic such as 1% silver nitrate solution may be beneficial.

For chronic or recurrent fissures, prescribe sitz baths, analgesic suppositories, and stool softeners. Surgical excision of the sentinel pile or papilla and the fissure, preferably without suture closure, may be required. Postoperative care is similar to that after hemorrhoidectomy.

FISTULA IN ANO

Anal fistula (Fig 26–3) is a chronically suppurating rectoperineal tract caused by pyogenic, amebic, or tuberculous infections or by obstetric trauma. A complete fistula has an internal (rectal) opening and one or more external (perianal) openings. An incomplete or blind fistula has an internal opening only. A blind fistulous opening above the anorectal line is called an internal fistula; below the anorectal line, it is called an external fistula.

Over 90% of anal fistulas develop from an anal crypt, usually preceded by anal abscess. Anal fistulas are prevented from healing by persistent drainage of fecal material into or through the tract and by the activity of the sphincter and other pelvic floor muscles.

Clinical Findings
Pain is reported when the fistula closes temporarily and an abscess develops; drainage brings relief. Periodic soiling by fecal discharge is a common complaint. If the internal opening of a complete fistula is above the sphincter, involuntary passage of flatus may occur.

Devious sinus tracts may cause difficulty in identification of the

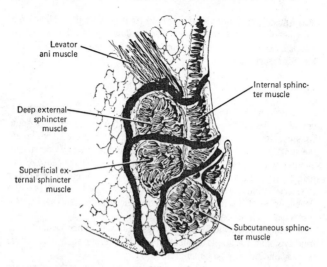

Figure 26–3. Cross section of muscles of anal wall showing usual paths of anal fistulas. (Reproduced, with permission, from Wilson JL: *Handbook of Surgery,* 5th ed. Lange, 1973.)

internal opening. Injection of one part hydrogen peroxide and 2 parts methylene blue into the external openings releases oxygen by contact with the discharges. The blue dye is carried through the tract; on anoscopic examination, the colored solution can be seen to bubble from the opening. For x-ray studies, injection of iodized oil (Lipiodol) may outline the fistulous tract.

Intestinal parasites should be identified by means of scrapings.

Prevention

Prompt and adequate treatment of proctitis usually will prevent fistula in ano.

Treatment

Chemotherapy should be used if parasites are present. Incision of the entire fistula with excision of all portions of the tract is the only curative treatment. Do not close with sutures; healing should occur by granulation. If the fistula is not totally exposed and removed, recurrence is likely.

ANAL ABSCESS

The acute stage of an anal fistula should be considered an anal abscess unless there is evidence to the contrary. The abscess should be adequately drained as soon as localization occurs. Localization may be expedited by hot sitz baths and large doses of broad-spectrum antibiotics. The internal orifice of the fistula rarely can be identified, owing to the presence of pain and swelling; this approach to drainage should therefore be avoided. Unfortunately, incision of the abscess may result in a persistent fistula.

BENIGN ANORECTAL STRICTURE

Anorectal stricture, contracture, or stenosis is a common problem of women and may cause pain, small or ribbonlike stools, and difficulty in achieving or completing a bowel movement. There are 3 forms: congenital, traumatic, and inflammatory.

Congenital Stricture

Congenital anorectal stricture occurs in newborns as a result of failure of disintegration of the anal plate in early fetal life.

Progressive and gentle dilatation of the terminal bowel to the diameter of the little finger usually is successful in resolving the problem.

Traumatic Stricture

Traumatic anorectal stricture is acquired as a complication of surgery (eg, hemorrhoidectomy, fistulectomy) or injury that denudes the epithelium of the anal canal. It predisposes to fissure, proctitis, and fistula. Stricture can generally be prevented by avoidance of infection and cautious postoperative digital dilatation of the anus.

In chronic cases, passage of graduated anal dilators by the patient is recommended. Correction by surgery is necessary in extreme cases.

Inflammatory Stricture

Inflammatory anorectal stricture may result from chronic infection after rectal surgery, from lymphogranuloma venereum, or from granuloma inguinale. Lymphogranuloma venereum causes early acute proctitis secondary to lymphatic spread of the organism, usually from the vagina or perineum. Perirectal mixed infection, sinus tract formation, and the growth of scar tissue cause the stricture. Granuloma inguinale may cause anorectal infection, fistulas, and stricture. Cellular viral inclusions (Donovan bodies) in a biopsy specimen indicate the presence of this sexually transmitted disorder.

Therapy with tetracyclines in the initial phase of lymphogranuloma venereum or granuloma inguinale is curative. Dilatation is helpful, but surgery to widen the stricture may be unsuccessful. Colostomy or abdominoperineal resection may be required.

About 5% of patients with chronic proctitis and stricture due to sexually transmitted disease develop squamous cell carcinoma of the anus or rectum.

ANAL INCONTINENCE

Anal incontinence follows obstetric lacerations, anorectal operations (especially fistulectomy), and neurologic disorders involving spinal nerves S2-4. When incontinence is the result of trauma or a complication of surgery, operative correction is indicated after the inflammation has subsided and initial healing is complete. Most serious lacerations due to childbirth injury should not be repaired until about 6 months after delivery.

ANAL CANCER

Anal cancer—almost always squamous cell type—represents only 1-2% of all cancers of the colon, rectum, and anus. (Carcinoma of the colon or rectum is discussed on p 350.) The cause is not known, but chronic granulomatous anal lesions are suspected.

In older women, anal cancer appears as a slightly raised, firm, ulcerative, and slightly tender area. Anal cancer is frequently confused with chronic fissure in ano or bleeding hemorrhoids and treated palliatively. It may be difficult to cure if it extends upward into the sphincter and around the anus and metastasizes to the inguinal glands.

Biopsy of suspect or frankly tumorous anal lesions should be done under local anesthesia. Ample excision of very small anal cancers is feasible. However, most lesions are large when they are first diagnosed accurately and require abdominoperineal resection and radical groin resection. Radiation treatment, even for palliation, is unsatisfactory.

The 5-year survival rate is currently only about 50%.

•   •   •

PROCTOSCOPY

All patients with symptoms of colorectal disease should be tested for occult blood in the stool (eg, Hemocult test) and should receive careful rectal and proctoscopic examinations for 2 reasons: (1) approximately 70% of all lesions of the lower gastrointestinal tract can be seen through an ordinary 25-cm proctoscope; and (2) about half of all large bowel cancers are in the anus, rectum, and lower sigmoid colon; moreover, at least half of these can be felt digitally.

The great majority of patients with cancer or other serious abnormalities associated with rectal pain or blood in the stool are over 40 years of age. Unfortunately, unless special precautions are taken, x-ray films of the lower bowel are unsatisfactory for tumor detection because of the configuration of the intestine and retained fecal material.

Positions for Proctoscopic Examination

The 3 positions for examination of the bowel are the knee-chest position, the left lateral (Sims) position, and the tipped-down lithotomy position on a proctoscopy table. The left lateral position is recommended because visualization is good; the patient stays in position even when experiencing pain; the position is feasible in the office, hospital, or home; and an expensive proctoscopy table is not required. This position is also less disturbing for the patient.

Procedure

(1) Administer tap-water enemas until the fluid is clear of fecal material.

(2) Place the patient in position.

(3) Examine the anus and rectum with the left index finger to identify such abnormalities as tumor or stenosis, which might indicate the need for a smaller proctoscope than is customarily used. If a painful anal lesion is present, topical anesthesia (eg, 1% dibucaine [Nupercaine] ointment) may be required.

(4) Insert the proctoscope into the anus with the right hand while holding the obturator firmly with the right thumb.

(5) Change hands, and remove the obturator with the right hand.

(6) Advance the proctoscope slowly with the left hand, maintaining careful visualization at all times. Use the right hand to steady the instrument and to adjust the light, swab, etc. (*Caution:* Do not advance the proctoscope blindly or forcefully; perforation may occur.) If a "blind pouch" or "blind alley" develops—actually a bowel segment blocking the field of the proctoscope—withdraw the instrument 2–6 cm to determine the site of the fold or valve. A slight deflection of the proctoscope in the opposite direction usually allows insertion beyond the fold. More than slight inflation of the bowel should be avoided; it may cause injury and pain.

Note: The 10-cm level, just beyond the first valve, is slightly above the floor of the nonherniated cul-de-sac.

(7) Record the location, characteristics, and extent of such single or

multiple abnormalities as erythema, ulceration and thickness of anal skin, hemorrhoids, anal stricture, fissures, drainage, bruises, scars, sphincter muscle defects, tumors, tenderness, and edema.

(8) Palpate the presacral space, levator ani muscles, cervix, rectovaginal septum, and ischiorectal space. Note narrowing or rigidity of the rectal walls and inflammatory or neoplastic masses.

(9) Remove tissue for biopsy from the margins of areas in which cancer is suspected; remove single, small sessile growths for evaluation by a pathologist.

(10) Refer the patient to a specialist for definitive treatment of unusual, large, or inflamed abnormalities.

Abnormalities of Menstruation; Anorexia Nervosa | 27

CLINICAL DISORDERS RELATED TO THE MENSTRUAL CYCLE

PREMENSTRUAL SYNDROME
(Premenstrual Tension)

The premenstrual syndrome is a recurrent variable cluster of troublesome symptoms and signs that develop during the 7–14 days before the onset of the menses and subside when menstruation occurs. The premenstrual syndrome affects about one-third of all premenopausal women, primarily those 30–40 years of age. In about 10% of these, the syndrome may be significantly debilitating. Although not every woman experiences all the symptoms or signs at one time, many complain of decreased energy, tension, irritability, depression, headache, mastalgia, and swelling of the abdomen, fingers, and ankles. Occasional patients may describe an increased craving for sweets or a decreased tolerance for alcohol before the menses.

The pathophysiology of premenstrual syndrome is still uncertain. It may be multifactorial. The many theories regarding its cause include the following:

A. Psychogenic Variability: Clearly, many affected women may be unreasonable and irascible and have difficulty with interpersonal relationships. These problems may be more the effect of premenstrual syndrome than its cause.

B. Fluid Retention: The fluid retention theory suggests that estrogen induces increased hepatic synthesis of angiotensinogen. This results in increased aldosterone production, which induces sodium retention and potassium depletion; concurrent release of norepinephrine causes irritability. However, even with spironolactone (an aldosterone blocking agent) or other diuretics, headache, mastalgia, and edema often persist.

C. Reactive Hypoglycemia: This hypothesis is based on the premise that a high level of progesterone after ovulation increases insulin secretion. The resulting hypoglycemia may follow even average glucose intake and may cause fatigue and a craving for sweets. However, even a carefully altered diet alone may not relieve premenstrual syndrome.

D. Estrogen Excess and Relative Progesterone Deficiency: This theory holds that premenstrual syndrome is due to an imbalance of estrogen and progesterone and can be relieved by the premenstrual administration of natural progesterone (not progestins, eg, medroxyprogesterone). However, this is by no means a certainty.

E. Alterations in Brain Stem Neurotransmitters: Decreased dopamine and serotonin levels in the central nervous system that result in elevated levels of prolactin have also been implicated in severe premenstrual syndrome. Moreover, dopamine has a direct natriuretic effect on the kidney, and serotonin may cause irritability. However, most patients with hyperprolactinemia do not have symptoms similar to those of premenstrual syndrome. Pyridoxine, which is involved in the synthesis of dopamine, seems to benefit some patients. Similarly, oral contraceptives may reduce or eliminate premenstrual syndrome. Bromocriptine mesylate reduces fluid retention and often improves mood in patients with premenstrual syndrome.

Treatment

Obviously, more careful investigation and better controlled therapeutic studies of this heterogeneous syndrome will be necessary before truly rational treatment is available. Current treatment recommendations (largely empiric) for the prevention and treatment of premenstrual syndrome include the following:

(1) Give the patient information about premenstrual syndrome and reassure her.

(2) Limit sodium, carbohydrates, and alcohol to reduce water retention and hypoglycemia. Increase exercise to reduce fluid retention and to augment the sense of well-being.

(3) Give pyridoxine, 500–800 mg orally daily for the 2 weeks before a period.

(4) Give spironolactone, 50 mg orally twice daily for 7–10 days before and through the menses. Avoid concurrent use of other diuretics and potassium supplements, and check electrolyte levels.

(5) Administer natural progesterone, 200–400 mg in rectal or vaginal suppositories, daily for 1 week before the menses. These suppositories must be made up from natural progesterone powder by a pharmacist.

(6) Prescribe oral contraceptive therapy if appropriate and acceptable.

PRIMARY DYSMENORRHEA
(Essential or Functional Dysmenorrhea)

Primary dysmenorrhea, in contrast to secondary dysmenorrhea (due to organic causes), is comenstrual pain for which no organic basis is evident. It accounts for about 80% of cases of painful menses. Dysmenorrhea and general menstrual discomfort often are described together as "menorrhalgia."

Dysmenorrhea rarely begins at menarche but has its onset 1 or more years later. It may be relieved after vaginal delivery of an infant or may continue through much of the woman's reproductive life and then fade, usually during the fourth decade of life.

Ovulatory, regular periods are associated with dysmenorrhea; anovulatory, irregular menses are not. Anovulation is usual during the early and late reproductive years.

Cramps—colicky pain radiating from behind the symphysis downward to the thighs and vulva—may precede the period. Usually, however, the distress is comenstrual for 1–2 days, followed by gradual relief. Premenstrual tension, nausea and vomiting, or diarrhea often accompanies the pain.

The fact that pain can be relieved by conversion of ovulatory to anovulatory cycles by means of hormone therapy suggests a basic organ dysfunction. Hypertonicity of the uterus and uterine dyskinesia have been reported in association with dysmenorrhea. These signs and nausea and diarrhea have been described as prostaglandin effects. Pain of this type may be analogous to angina pectoris.

Diffuse congestion of the pelvic viscera may be noted, but findings on gynecologic examination are usually essentially normal. Tension, anxiety, and fatigue may aggravate the pain.

Clinical Findings

Engorgement of the vagina and cervix, slight patulousness of the os, and bogginess of the uterus frequently occur before and during bleeding. Uterine, parametrial, and adnexal tenderness often are described as well, but none of these are diagnostic.

Significantly elevated prostaglandin ($PGF_{2\alpha}$) has been detected in the endometrium and menstrual fluid of women with primary dysmenorrhea. Abnormal prostaglandin levels can be reduced and relief of pain achieved with prostaglandin synthetase inhibitors or antiprostaglandin drugs. Anovulatory drugs do not constitute specific therapy for dysmenorrhea, but they are also effective.

Differential Diagnosis

A trial of estrogen or estrogen-progestogen therapy may be helpful in diagnosis. Anovulatory periods usually are painless in the absence of cervical obstruction or other genital disorders. Suppression of ovulation usually prevents dysmenorrhea during that month. The patient should keep a basal body temperature chart to document an ovulation.

Menstrual cramps that develop more than 8–10 years after the menarche are usually due to organic causes and may include generalized abdominal pain or particularly well localized right- or left-sided pelvic pain. Typical patterns of pain also suggest secondary dysmenorrhea, which often precedes the bleeding, continues during the flow, and may persist even after bleeding has stopped.

Treatment

A. Immediate Measures: Analgesics such as aspirin, 0.6 g, with codeine, 0.03 g, are warranted occasionally until the diagnosis of primary dysmenorrhea is established. Continued use of narcotics should be strictly avoided for fear of addiction.

B. General Measures: The patient should be encouraged to be normally active during menstruation. Sports and calisthenics are helpful.

C. Specific Measures:

1. Medical–The current treatment for primary dysmenorrhea involves nonsteroidal anti-inflammatory drugs to reduce uterine contractility and discomfort, either directly or by inhibition of prostaglandin production. Contraindications to use of these drugs include aspirin allergy and possible early pregnancy.

Effective drugs and their dosages are ibuprofen (Motrin), 400 mg orally 3 times a day, and naproxen (Naprosyn), 250 mg orally 2 or 3 times a day. Results may be better when the medication is begun 1–2 days before the onset of a menstrual period.

Undesirable side-effects, eg, nausea and vomiting, headache, or vertigo, are uncommon with the doses given. A curious but desirable side-effect of nonsteroidal anti-inflammatory drugs taken for dysmenorrhea is the unexplained reduction in blood loss during menstruation.

2. Surgical–A paracervical block may be performed in an attempt to evaluate the potential effectiveness of a Doyle paracervical neurectomy or a Cotte type presacral neurectomy in the patient unresponsive to other methods of treatment. Hysterectomy is never indicated in the treatment of primary dysmenorrhea.

Prognosis

In women with satisfactory psychobiologic integration, the prognosis is good.

THE ABNORMAL MENSTRUAL CYCLE

ABNORMAL UTERINE BLEEDING

Any bleeding from the uterus that differs significantly from that of the usual menstrual cycle is abnormal. Menstrual disturbances include uterine bleeding in excess of the normal amount, prolonged beyond 7 days' duration at the expected time of the menses (hypermenorrhea, menorrhagia), or more often than at 24-day intervals (polymenorrhea). Nonmenstrual disturbances include flow at times other than the menstrual period (metrorrhagia).

Abnormal uterine bleeding is a matter of concern to almost all women at some time from the menarche to the menopause. The bleeding is always annoying, often debilitating, and occasionally critical. Accurate diagnosis and prompt treatment are necessary to the well-being of the patient.

Abnormal uterine bleeding may be due to local or systemic disorders or psychogenic causes. It often is presumed to be caused by an enlarged, irregular uterus or an adnexal tumor, but additional studies or curettage frequently disclose an entirely different but serious abnormality as the cause. The amount and periodicity of blood loss are important measures of menstrual function. Regular menstrual periods of average flow, often with cramps, are generally ovulatory; abnormal uterine bleeding should not be ascribed to ovulation or anovulation without knowing the patient's history and performing a physical examination and laboratory studies.

Hypermenorrhea (menorrhagia) may be caused by carcinoma or sarcoma, myoma, endometrial polyposis, irregular shedding of the endometrium, functional hypertrophy of the uterus, blood dyscrasias, or psychic problems. Polymenorrhea may be due to a short cycle (proliferative phase less than 10 days or secretory phase less than 14 days) or to premature interruption of the cycle, often owing to physical or emotional stress. Metrorrhagia may be due to hormonal imbalance or miscellaneous benign or malignant pelvic abnormalities. Hormonal causes include endometrial hyperplasia (unopposed stimulation by estrogen), ovulation bleeding with fleeting midcycle abdominal pain (''mittelschmerz''), excessive estrogen administration, anovulatory bleeding, and hypo- or hyperthyroidism. Pelvic disorders that cause metrorrhagia include disturbed pregnancy (abortion, hydatidiform mole, choriocarcinoma); cervical and endometrial polyposis; submucous myoma; cancer of the cervix, uterus, or uterine tubes; and endometritis (postabortal or due to tuberculosis or cervical stenosis).

Dysfunctional uterine bleeding is abnormal bleeding for which no organic cause can be readily identified. The bleeding is likely to be irregular and painless and may be profuse or scanty. Ovulation does not occur. Every effort must be made to discover the cause.

There are 3 major types of dysfunctional uterine bleeding: (1) Estrogen breakthrough bleeding is intermittent spotting that often occurs in patients with prolonged low levels of endogenous estrogen or small doses of exogenous estrogen. Other patients may have amenorrhea followed by irregular, occasionally profuse or prolonged bleeding that is associated with high levels (or doses) of estrogen. (2) Estrogen withdrawal bleeding occurs with a sharp reduction of endogenous estrogen (eg, bilateral ovariectomy in a premenopausal woman) or with interruption of exogenous estrogen therapy (eg, termination of regular estrogen medication in a postmenopausal patient). (3) Progesterone breakthrough bleeding occurs after the excision of a corpus luteum. Termination of progestogen therapy after endometrial "priming" with estrogen up to the proliferative phase will also result in endometrial bleeding.

The differential diagnosis of dysfunctional uterine bleeding includes polycystic ovaries and pituitary, hypothalamic, thyroid, or adrenal diseases.

Clinical Findings

A. Symptoms and Signs: The symptoms are best revealed by the history, which must include the type, amount, and duration of flow; character of related pain; last menstrual period (LMP); and previous menstrual period (PMP). The patient's general health, previous illnesses, surgery, and accidents should be described. Congenital maldevelopment and metabolic abnormalities and bleeding tendencies in relatives are important. The menstrual record should be reviewed: menarche; usual interval between menses; average duration; amount of flow; discomfort before, during, and after menstruation; and previous leukorrhea, pruritus, or intermenstrual bleeding. All medications taken, including those for control of abnormal uterine bleeding, must be identified: estrogens may increase bleeding, and androgens may suppress the flow.

Significant signs include abdominal fullness due to enlarged organs, tumors, or fluid; tenderness and guarding of the abdominal wall due to inflammation, pulsion, traction, torsion, or obstruction; dullness due to an inflammatory or neoplastic process; shifting dullness due to ascites; herniation, often due to tumor or fluid; adenopathy due to infection or cancer; and swelling, tenderness, or discharge from Skene's or Bartholin's glands due to infection or tumor.

Rectovaginal examination may reveal tenderness, induration, nodulation, mass formation, and the presence of peritoneal fluid. A separate rectal examination may confirm, modify, or rule out previous impressions.

B. Laboratory Findings: Vaginal smears for cytologic and bacteriologic study should be obtained before digital examination. Smears may be taken during active bleeding. Specimens are fixed in alcohol-ether and cleared of red cells by use of 1% hydrochloric acid. The epithelial detritus that remains may reveal tumor cells or trophoblastic squamae from a uterine abortion.

Application of Schiller's or Lugol's iodine solution to the vaginal canal and cervix will identify abnormal zones. Scrapings or biopsies of ulcerated or hyperplastic areas should be obtained.

Other tests should include a hematocrit, urinalysis, and a serologic test for syphilis. Systemic diseases, some of which are revealed as bleeding diatheses, may be detected by measurements of bleeding time, clotting time, and clot retraction time and leukocyte and platelet counts and by use of the tourniquet test for capillary resistance (Table 27–1). The presence of infection or leukemia, which may also cause bleeding, may be detected by a white blood cell count plus a differential count and sedimentation rate determination. Leukorrheal discharges should be investigated and thyroid function appraised.

C. X-Ray Findings: A flat film of the abdomen, hysterosalpingography, cystography, and pneumoperitoneum and barium enema studies of the abdomen may reveal tumors, fluid levels, and distortions. These x-rays should be ordered only when abnormalities are suspected.

D. Special Examinations: Examination, biopsy, and surgical curettage in the anesthetized patient will usually be necessary to establish the diagnosis, eg, occult cancer, polyps, or submucous fibroids. Cancer of the cervix or endometrium may be revealed by colposcopy, directed or cone biopsies of the cervix, and differential curettage of the cervix and uterus.

Complications

Continued or excessive blood loss leads to anemia; and this, in turn, is often followed by local as well as systemic infection. Tumors cause bleeding, discharge, pain, and infertility. Cancer developing in the cervix, uterus, and tubes may be fatal when there is delay in diagnosis and treatment.

Prevention

Periodic medical and gynecologic evaluation and early treatment of disorders capable of causing uterine hemorrhage will prevent many cases of abnormal uterine bleeding.

Treatment

A. Emergency Measures: Patients with acute blood loss should be placed in the slight Trendelenburg position, and sedation, intravenous fluids, and blood transfusions should be given. Hemostasis can be achieved by surgical D&C, which is both diagnostic and therapeutic.

Table 27–1. Differential diagnosis of some hematologic causes of abnormal uterine bleeding.

Characteristics*	Idiopathic Thrombocytopenic Purpura	Vascular Hemophilia	Thrombasthenia (Glanzmann's)	Prothrombin Complex Deficiency	Fibrinogen Deficiency
Clinical findings					
Petechiae	+++	+	++	Ecchymoses.	Ecchymoses.
Hematoma, large	–	–	–	–	–
Hemarthrosis	–	±	–	–	–
Postsurgical bleeding	+	+++	+	++	++++
Onset in childhood	–	+	+	±	±
Hereditary association	–	+	+	–	–
Laboratory findings					
Bleeding time	Incr	Incr	N or incr	N	N
Clotting time	N	N	N	N or incr	No clot.
Clot retraction time	Incr	N	Incr	N	No clot.
Prothrombin time	N	N	N	Incr	Incr
Partial thromboplastin time (PTT)	Only platelets abnormal.	Abnormal.	Incr. Only platelets abnormal.	N	N
Platelet count	Decr	N	Platelets abnormal.	N	N
Capillary fragility (tourniquet test)	Incr	N or incr	N or incr	N	N

*Frequency expressed on a scale of – to ++++. N = normal; Incr = increased; Decr = decreased.

Excessive uterine bleeding due to almost any cause may be checked temporarily (1–2 days) by use of hormonal preparations. The choice of medication must be determined by the condition of the endometrium, the severity of bleeding, and the availability of drugs. Use of steroid sex hormones will check bleeding by suppressing pituitary production of gonadotropins and reducing endometrial vascular dilatation and permeability. Large doses will strikingly modify the morphology of the endometrium in 2–3 days.

B. Medical Measures: Premenopausal patients with abnormal uterine bleeding include those with early abortion, salpingitis, or pelvic tumors, to mention only a few possible causes. Definitive therapy depends upon the cause of the bleeding.

1. Estrogen-progestogen medications–Most patients with dysfunctional bleeding can be treated successfully with estrogen-progestogen medication and without regular surgical procedures such as D&C. The objective is to reestablish the normal mechanism of control of endometrial bleeding. Control usually can be established by giving oral estrogen-progestogen combination contraceptive tablets in high doses. Side-effects such as nausea may occur but are tolerable. Any commercially available oral contraceptive (eg, Ortho-Novum 1/50) can be used, and the plan of therapy, irrespective of the individual dosage of each tablet, is 1 tablet orally 4 times daily for 5–7 days. In most cases, bleeding will slacken markedly or even cease within 24 hours; nonetheless, the full course of therapy should be administered. Meanwhile, iron replacement therapy and other supportive measures can be instituted.

The week of therapy provides an opportunity for strengthening the structural stromal support in the endometrium, which includes progestogen-induced pseudodecidual changes. Treatment will also result in a less fragile endometrial vasculature in which irregular breakdown of the delicate endometrium (hyperplastic endometrium) no longer occurs, so that bleeding is checked and healing can go forward. Even so, excessive tissue often remains to be sloughed or normalized by estrogen-progestogen withdrawal at the end of the treatment period. Therefore, the patient must be warned that a heavy, perhaps painful period may follow termination of the medication.

To ensure control of the several menstrual periods following, a low-dosage oral contraceptive (eg, Modicon or Brevicon), 1 tablet orally daily, should be begun on the fifth day of the period and continued for 3 weeks, followed by 1 week off medication, for a total of 3 months. Maturation and limitation of endometrial growth should allow regular periods without cramps or excessive flow. Patients who wish to use this method to prevent pregnancy should continue taking this or a similar medication for a longer time.

Women who are not sexually active, who are using a barrier method of contraception, or who do not wish to continue oral contraceptives may develop abnormal bleeding again after the 3-month period of combination hormone therapy. In these patients—provided that they have adequate endogenous estrogen—administration of medroxyprogesterone acetate (Provera), 10 mg orally daily for the last week of each cycle, should ensure regular, limited bleeding; thick proliferative or hyperplastic endometrium will not develop or persist. If ovulation occurs, average periods may make progestogen therapy unnecessary.

If uterine bleeding is not controlled promptly by endocrine therapy as described above, the provisional diagnosis was inaccurate. Other diagnostic procedures (eg, D&C) or therapeutic measures (eg, salpingectomy for ectopic pregnancy) should be instituted without delay.

Certain patients should not be given estrogen-progestogen medication immediately for direct control of dysfunctional uterine bleeding:

a. Women over 35 years of age should have an initial endometrial or suction biopsy before hormone therapy in order to rule out endometrial carcinoma.

b. Patients who have had continued excessive bleeding or prolonged intermittent spotting often have low estrogen levels in plasma or 24-hour urine samples. Thus, the residual endometrium may be extremely thin and inadequate for a good estrogen-progestogen effect. Therefore, D&C would only intensify the bleeding problem by denuding the endometrium. In such cases, initial administration of conjugated estrogens (Premarin), 25 mg intravenously every 4 hours for 3–4 doses, will check the bleeding and prepare the endometrium for the high-dosage estrogen-progestogen regimen, which can be started the following day.

c. Patients who have received intramuscular depot medroxyprogesterone (Depo-Provera) for contraception and patients who have been taking a high-progestogen, low-estrogen oral contraceptive (eg, Ovral) for a long time may have progestogen breakthrough bleeding. In such cases, a few glands with stroma similar to pseudodecidua and with scattered, fairly straight arterioles typify the endometrium. Preparatory therapy should consist of conjugated estrogens (Premarin or equivalent), 1.25 mg orally daily for 5 days, before and concurrently with the estrogen-progestogen tablets for the first cycle of therapy. This will thicken the inactive, thin endometrium; control the bleeding; and allow regulation over the next few months.

2. Use of thyroid hormone–Hypermenorrhea and metrorrhagia often are noted in clinical hypothyroidism. Oligomenorrhea or amenorrhea may be due to hyperthyroidism. Thyroid hormone will improve menstrual function if a deficiency in thyroid hormone production is the only problem, but it should not be used for all patients with abnormal menstrual periods. Euthyroid individuals may be harmed by this medication. Endogenous T_4 production is suppressed during and for several weeks after treatment with thyroid hormone.

3. Corticosteroids–Patients with Stein-Leventhal syndrome may be treated with prednisone, 5 mg/d (or equivalent dose of other cortico-steroid) orally for 2–3 months. Corticosteroids are not indicated for patients with excessive or intermenstrual bleeding.

C. Surgical Measures: Surgical curettage may reveal polyps, submucous myomas, and abnormal endometrium. Intractable abnormal uterine bleeding, particularly after age 40, may require hysterectomy, but ovaries that appear to be normal need not be removed.

D. Other Measures: Radiation therapy should be reserved for poor-risk (often perimenopausal) patients. To eliminate the possibility of cancer, cervical cytologic smears must be taken and an endometrial biopsy performed first. Radiation should be limited to the amount required for biologic sterilization, which varies directly with ovarian functional capacity and age. In women under age 35, approximately 1250 R to the ovaries will be required; in those over age 35, 800 R will usually suffice.

Prognosis

The medical management outlined above for menorrhagia and metrorrhagia will be effective in at least 85% of patients.

In the absence of cancer, large tumors, or salpingitis, about 50% of patients with hypermenorrhea and almost 60% of patients with metror-rhagia will resume normal menstrual periods after curettage alone. Results are not likely to be so favorable in teenage patients. The addition of thyroid hormone or progesterone to the treatment regimen, when indicated, will increase recoveries by an additional 10–15%. Abnormal uterine bleeding due to uncorrectable blood dyscrasias often recurs with a hematologic crisis.

POSTMENOPAUSAL VAGINAL BLEEDING

Postmenopausal vaginal bleeding is bleeding from the reproductive tract 6 months or more after cessation of menstrual function. The type, amount, and duration of bleeding are unrelated to the cause. Bleeding may be due to local pelvic disorders, systemic diseases, or malignant lesions anywhere in the reproductive tract.

Pelvic cancer is the most serious cause of postmenopausal vaginal bleeding. Cancer of the cervix or endometrium accounts for 35–50% of cases. Other causes, in approximate order of frequency, include exces-sive or prolonged estrogen administration, atrophic vaginitis, physical injury, cervical or endometrial polyposis, hypertensive cardiovascular disease, submucous myomas, trophic ulcers of the cervix associated with prolapse of the uterus, blood dyscrasias, and endogenous estrogen produced by feminizing ovarian tumors.

Postmenopausal women, like premenopausal women, may bleed

from any type of endometrium. Endometrium from postmenopausal women can be divided into 3 basic types: (1) functioning (implying hormone stimulation), (2) nonfunctioning (inactive, atrophic), and (3) malignant (cancerous). Many endometrial specimens obtained from postmenopausal patients will be actively proliferative. The most exaggerated variety is cystic glandular hyperplasia, with unequal glandular development, stromal edema, and increased vascularity. The relative number of benign mitotic figures in the endometrium is a good index of estrogen stimulation.

Adenomatous or atypical hyperplasia of the endometrium is diagnosed occasionally. It is characterized by disparity in the size and shape of the glands, invaginations and pseudostratification of the glandular epithelium, and slight to moderate activity of the stroma. No positive evidence of malignant change is present in this type of specimen, and whether the pattern represents a neoplastic trend, a "premalignancy," or overactivity is still being debated. Nevertheless, atypical hyperplasia and actual adenocarcinoma are often discovered together. Whether this is coincidental or indicates progression to cancer is not known.

Bleeding from a proliferative or hyperplastic endometrium is probably breakthrough bleeding. There is ample proof of endocrine activity (vaginal cytology, endometrial histology, and blood and urinary sex steroid assay) in postmenopausal women. The ovaries probably continue to produce estrogen for 10–15 years after cessation of the menses. In addition, even small granulosa or theca cell tumors may produce considerable estrogen during the climacteric. The adrenal cortex also produces estrogenic steroids. Exogenous or endogenous estrogens may account for postmenopausal endometrial activity and subsequent bleeding.

Other causes of bleeding from any type of endometrium include infection, vascular fragility, and varices or congenital vascular anomalies.

Inactive endometrium is atrophic or senile. Some dilatation of the glands occurs, but a dormant epithelium and a sparse, shrunken stroma is the rule. Bleeding from an atrophic endometrium is often due to senile thinning of the functionalis layers that virtually exposes capillary loops, which may rupture during episodes of increased intravascular pressure, especially with hypertensive cardiovascular disease.

A benign polyp bleeds from its surface or pedicle as the result of mechanical trauma, circulatory disturbances, infection, or a combination of these causes. Bleeding from submucous myomas results from torsion and infection.

Adenocarcinoma may be focal or extensive. Except in early "in situ" cancers, the midzonal and basilar layers are usually involved in adenocarcinoma. Anaplasia and pleomorphism will be present. Carcinomatous invasion of vascular channels and sterile as well as bacterial necrosis may account for bleeding in cancer patients. Carcinogenesis by therapeutic doses of steroids is possible; certainly, estrogen may create a favorable environment for the development of cancer induced by other (unknown) agents. There is no evidence that either parity or nulliparity predisposes to postmenopausal vaginal bleeding.

Clinical Findings

A. Symptoms and Signs: Postmenopausal vaginal bleeding may be painless or painful. Discomfort depends upon the patency of the cervix, the amount and rapidity of blood loss, the presence of infection, or torsion of a tumor. Bleeding varies from a bright ooze or brownish discharge to frank hemorrhage. Patients may report a single episode of spotting or profuse bleeding for days to months.

B. Laboratory Findings: Vaginal cytologic examination may disclose the presence of exfoliated cancer cells, infectious organisms (eg, trichomonads, *Candida,* bacteria) diagnostic of specific forms of vaginitis, or free basal cells and leukocytes (but no cornified epithelial cells). The latter indicates probable vaginal atrophy or infection. Plasma estrogen or FSH values are rarely significant in diagnosis.

C. Special Examinations: Passage of a sound through the cervix into the uterus will demonstrate cervical stenosis and hematocolpos, will cause an intracervical or endometrial cancer to bleed, or may outline a cervical or uterine tumor. Aspiration biopsy or suction curettage often provides adequate endometrial tissue to diagnose cancer, endometrial hyperplasia, or endometritis.

Complications

Although it is not known whether atypical endometrial hyperplasia can or will progress to adenocarcinoma, atypical hyperplasia that persists or recurs after thorough curettage may presage cancer. An undiagnosed pelvic carcinoma or inadequately treated malignant tumor may be fatal. Unsuccessful therapy of a genital or urinary tract infection may lead to abscess formation or septicemia. A neglected functional granulosa cell tumor of the ovary may grow and develop malignant characteristics.

Differential Diagnosis

Bleeding may originate from a disease process in the lower genital tract. Bleeding from the urethra (caruncle, carcinoma of the urethra or bladder) or the anus (hemorrhoids, fissure in ano, cancer) may be erroneously reported as vaginal hemorrhage.

When a postmenopausal patient is receiving unspecified medication for ''nervousness,'' flushes, or arthritis, the possibility of exogenous estrogen therapy must be considered and the drug identified. Estrogens prescribed in uninterrupted dosage may cause breakthrough bleeding.

A functional ovarian tumor or carcinoma of the uterine tube may cause bleeding but may not be palpable.

Prevention

Periodic (6–12 months) vaginal cytologic smears and gynecologic examinations should be scheduled and indiscriminate or excessive estrogen treatment avoided. Examination and surgical curettage in the anesthetized patient are important when repeated vaginal cytologic smears show class III or IV results (Table 22–2). Inadequate or improperly applied radiation therapy may palliate but not eliminate an occult cancer missed at previous surgery. D&C should be repeated.

Treatment

Treatment depends upon the cause of bleeding. Surgical D&C, together with polypectomy when indicated, are adequate operative treatment for almost two-thirds of patients with postmenopausal vaginal bleeding.

A. Emergency Measures: The patient should be hospitalized at once and all possible causes of bleeding investigated. D&C should be performed if bleeding is coming from above the external cervical os. The site of bleeding must be biopsied.

B. Specific and Surgical Measures:

1. All steroid sex hormone therapy must be discontinued until the cause of bleeding has been determined and the bleeding controlled for at least 3 months.

2. A complete gynecologic evaluation and urinary, gastrointestinal, and hematologic examinations are necessary to determine the cause of bleeding.

3. Vaginal cytologic studies and biopsies of vaginal or other possibly cancerous lesions also are necessary.

4. The cervix should be thinly coned and endometrial biopsies or a differential curettage performed if bleeding is from the upper genital tract. If cancer is not found but atypical endometrial hyperplasia is diagnosed, vaginal cytologic smears should be obtained each month and curettage repeated in 3 months, during which time the patient should not receive hormone therapy.

5. Laparotomy must be considered if an adnexal tumor is palpated in association with persistent endometrial hyperplasia (in the absence of estrogen therapy).

6. Cancer from any source requires definitive treatment.

7. Exploratory laparotomy and total hysterectomy and bilateral salpingo-oophorectomy may be indicated for recurrent postmenopausal bleeding after the second curettage (in the absence of estrogen therapy).

8. If atrophic vaginitis alone is determined to be the cause of the bleeding, cyclic estrogen therapy should be instituted.

C. Supportive Measures: Explanation, reassurance, and mild sedatives are important supportive measures for the anxious patient. Antibiotics, hematinics, or dietary supplements should be given for infection, anemia, and nutritional deficiency, respectively. Daily acetic acid vaginal douches should be prescribed for clinical vaginitis.

D. Treatment of Complications: If the uterus is perforated during curettage, bleeding into the peritoneal cavity, bladder, or rectum may occur, in which case a total abdominal hysterectomy may be required and other damage must be repaired. Infection should be treated with antibiotics.

Prognosis

D&C and estrogen therapy will generally correct postmenopausal vaginal bleeding in the absence of cancer or a feminizing ovarian tumor. The prognosis in women whose bleeding is due to cancer depends upon the extent of invasion and the success of anticancer therapy.

AMENORRHEA

Amenorrhea (failure to menstruate) is a symptom rather than a disease. Pregnancy is the most common cause. The regularity of the menses is a delicate index of physical and mental health and may be the first indication of a physiologic disorder. When menstrual periods have not begun by mid adolescence, an abnormality must be assumed to exist.

Amenorrhea is physiologic before puberty, during pregnancy and the puerperium, and after the menopause. The average age at menopause is 51; only about 5% of women cease to menstruate normally before age 40. Menstruation is the end point in a complex intraglandular coordination. Disorders involving one area of function will often be reflected in other areas, with resultant amenorrhea.

Exercise-associated amenorrhea is common in long-distance runners and other women involved in intense physical training. These women have more preexisting menstrual irregularities, less body fat, and greater weight loss from running than women athletes who menstruate regularly. Athletes with regular menstrual cycles often have fewer premenstrual symptoms and shorter, lighter periods than is usual. When women with exercise-associated amenorrhea reduce their physical activity and gain weight, menstruation resumes. It is not known whether women who have had prolonged exercise-associated amenorrhea have fertility problems after menses are reestablished. Exercise-associated amenorrhea is probably not a variant of hypothalamic (psychogenic) amenorrhea; women athletes usually have no serious emotional problems, and they have higher LH and lower FSH and TSH levels than do patients with psychogenic amenorrhea.

Amenorrhea has traditionally been classified as primary (if the woman has never had a period) or secondary (if uterine bleeding has occurred on one or more occasions). Except for the suspicion that the former might be more serious, the distinction is not helpful in either diagnosis or treatment. A more practical definition based on the age of the patient is as follows:

(1) Amenorrhea is present in an adolescent (a) if by age 14 there are no menses and no secondary sex characteristics or (b) if by age 16 there are no menses despite the presence of secondary sex characteristics.

(2) Amenorrhea is present in a mature woman (a) if there have been no menses for 3 months or longer without the use of oral contraceptives or (b) if there have been no menses for 6 months or longer after stopping oral contraceptive use.

Pregnancy must always be excluded as a cause of amenorrhea. Anomalies such as congenital absence of the vagina, Turner's syndrome, and testicular feminization must be identified.

Methodical investigation of a case of suspected amenorrhea consists of assessment of function at 4 anatomic-physiologic levels.

Level I: Uterus, Cervix, & Vagina

The uterus should have a functional endometrium, a cervix, and a patent outflow tract. To determine whether a patent outflow tract is present, proceed as follows:

(1) Examine the patient to confirm the presence of a uterus and an unobstructed vagina and cervix.

(2) Administer a progesterone preparation, eg, progesterone in oil, 250 mg intramuscularly, or medroxyprogesterone acetate, 10 mg orally, for 5 days. Bleeding—even spotting—constitutes a positive withdrawal response, which indicates the presence of a reactive endometrium primed by endogenous estrogen and lack of obstruction in the cervix or vagina. Moreover, the presence of estrogen confirms secretory function of the ovary and the pituitary, but central nervous system integration may still be uncertain. Of course, such a patient is anovulatory.

(3) Determine the serum prolactin level (normal = 0–20 ng/mL). If the level is less than 20 ng/mL or if galactorrhea is noted, pituitary polytomography must be performed to identify possible microadenoma despite a bleeding response.

Disorders at level I are uncommon causes of amenorrhea. Obliterative uterine synechiae (Asherman's syndrome) may occur following excessive curettage after abortion or delivery or may be due to tuberculous endometritis. Anomalies such as an abnormally small and functionless uterus, obstructions to outflow (as in congenital vaginal obstructions or imperforate hymen), or testicular feminization (absent uterus) will prevent induced bleeding. These problems can be diagnosed on the basis of a good history and pelvic examination.

If progestogen administration does not induce bleeding, either the endometrium has not been primed by adequate endogenous estrogen or the outflow tract is blocked. The latter can be ruled out by giving conjugated estrogens, 2.5 mg/d orally for 3 weeks, and adding medroxyprogesterone acetate, 10 mg/d orally for the last 5 days of the course. Withdrawal bleeding several days after stopping the drugs establishes the presence of a satisfactorily receptive uterus and a patent outflow tract.

Level II: Ovaries

If bleeding can be induced by progesterone or estrogen-progesterone administration, the next step is to determine whether the ovaries are capable of secreting adequate estrogen and progesterone (after ovulation). Estrogen production requires an adequate number of normal follicles and sufficient FSH and LH (pituitary gonadotropins) to stimulate these follicles. Serum FSH and LH levels should be determined by radioimmunoassay. However, if exogenous estrogen has been given, it is important to delay hormone determination for at least 2 weeks to restore homeostasis.

The normal values for FSH and LH vary in different laboratories. However, an abnormally low FSH level indicates hypogonadotropism, which may extend to pituitary failure; an abnormally high value indicates ovarian failure. An abnormally low LH level indicates hypogonadotropism; high levels do not necessarily establish ovarian failure, because LH peaks are occasionally noted if ovarian follicles are adequate. Obviously, several hormone determinations should be done to ensure accuracy. If the FSH level is consistently abnormally low, the diagnosis of ovarian failure is conclusively established, and other procedures (laparoscopy, gynecography) are unwarranted.

Early ovarian failure may represent gonadal dysgenesis or agenesis (Turner's syndrome), mosaicism, or the rare resistant ovary syndrome.

Level III: Anterior Pituitary Gland

If problems at levels I and II can be ruled out, anterior pituitary function must be assessed. Amenorrhea may be due to the presence of a small, slowly growing pituitary tumor—in some cases, it may take years before the tumor is detectable by traditional roentgenography. Suspicion of a pituitary tumor may be aroused by the development of acromegaly, Cushing's syndrome, or galactorrhea. Nevertheless, amenorrhea may be the sole symptom of a hormonally "silent" tumor of the anterior pituitary.

Improved diagnostic x-ray techniques such as polytomography or CT scan (with 1-mm increments) may now identify microadenomas as small as 5–10 mm in diameter. There is a positive correlation between the size of the sella turcica and the presence of a pituitary tumor. If there is a true sellar bulge, the tumor will usually be at least 10 mm in diameter. The frequency with which these small tumors occur is not definitely known, but an autopsy incidence of 10–20% (in both sexes), with a peak in the sixth decade of life, has been reported.

About 25–30% of women with secondary amenorrhea will have one or more pituitary microadenomas; and approximately 50% of patients in whom galactorrhea accompanies amenorrhea will have one or more pituitary tumors.

The serum prolactin level is a useful screening test. About 75% of women with a pituitary tumor (in the absence of acromegaly or Cushing's syndrome) have high serum prolactin levels, as do about 20% of amenorrheic women (ie, those with anorexia nervosa or chromosomal abnormalities). Microadenomas may also be found in women with amenorrhea and normal or only slightly elevated prolactin levels. Galactorrhea occurs in about 30% of women with significantly elevated serum prolactin levels. It may be that women with amenorrhea and prolactinemia but no galactorrhea produce too little estrogen for the prolactin to cause breast secretion.

Patients with abnormal findings on polytomography or high serum prolactin levels (> 30 μg/mL) should be admitted to hospital for endocrinologic, ophthalmologic, and neurosurgical consultation. Baseline hormone studies of TSH, FSH, LH, prolactin (repeat), and morning and evening cortisol levels may be most revealing. Pneumoencephalography with tomography (to identify possible suprasellar tumor extension, "empty sella syndrome," or sellar aneurysm) is most important, especially if the serum prolactin level is less than 50 μg/mL.

In general, if an anterior pituitary tumor is identified—particularly in an amenorrheic woman with a prolactin level greater than 50 μg/mL and impaired function—transsphenoidal microsurgery for removal of the tumor is indicated.

If results of polytomography are normal and the serum prolactin level is also normal—or even if the latter is significantly elevated—the patient may harbor a tumor too small to be identified. Treatment with bromocriptine and reassessment in the hospital after 1 year may be justified in such cases. If fertility is an important consideration, induction of ovulation should be attempted. Pregnancy may or may not stimulate the growth of pituitary microadenomas, but the pregnancy is almost never compromised. Polytomography should be repeated in late pregnancy or if unusual central nervous system or ocular symptoms develop. It should again be repeated several months after delivery.

Level IV: Central Nervous System & Hypothalamic Factors

If pituitary abnormalities can be ruled out, amenorrhea is probably caused by a problem within level IV. Actually, hypothalamic disorders are the most common cause of hypogonadotropic amenorrhea. Stress and travel are frequently responsible for secondary amenorrhea. Reassurance, situational adjustments, and informal psychotherapy may be effective, but hormone replacement therapy is often necessary even when pregnancy is not desired. Because patients with hypothalamic amenorrhea can become pregnant if normal function unexpectedly returns, nonhormonal or oral contraceptives are useful; if oral contraceptives are chosen, 50–75 μg of estrogen will usually be required, since lower amounts in combination pills may not permit withdrawal bleeding. Even so, low-dose pills should be tried in order to minimize undesirable side-effects such as fluid retention and headache.

The patient should be reassured that if she wishes to become pregnant, ovulation usually can be induced with either clomiphene citrate or menotropins (hMG). However, these medications are not helpful in the basic therapy of hypothalamic amenorrhea, because they will not restore normal function even when given periodically.

Amenorrhea occurs in about 2% of patients who stop taking oral contraceptives (post-pill amenorrhea). In most such cases, it persists for less than 6 months and is followed by resumption of periods and no serious reduction in fertility. For this reason, reassurance and patience may be all that is required. Amenorrhea lasting longer than 6 months requires investigation as outlined above.

Neurologic symptoms develop in about 10% of amenorrheic women with pituitary microadenomas who achieve pregnancy by induced ovulation or bromocriptine suppression of hyperprolactinemia. With this significant risk, careful follow-up during pregnancy by a neurologist or ophthalmologist should be arranged. Symptoms that suggest tumor enlargement include unusual headaches, visual aberrations, bitemporal visual field changes, and abnormalities involving cranial nerves III, IV, and VI. In rare instances, blindness may result.

Central nervous system disorders usually resolve with removal of the tumor. In the absence of obstetric contraindications, vaginal delivery is recommended for patients who have only mildly symptomatic pituitary adenomas or those who have had transsphenoidal microsurgery during pregnancy.

Prognosis

Success in reestablishing menstruation in the nonpregnant woman is inversely proportionate to the duration of amenorrhea and the seriousness of the underlying disorder.

HIRSUTISM

Marked normal variations in the amount of body hair occur on a racial, familial, or genetic nonendocrine basis. Hirsutism is one of the

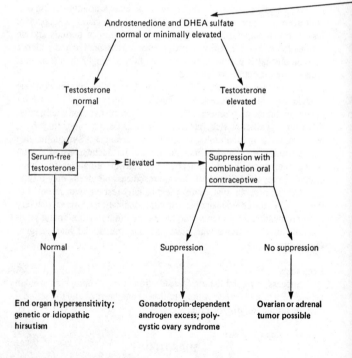

Figure 27–1. Laboratory investigation of hirsutism. (Reproduced, with permission, from Goldfien A, Monroe SE: Chapter 14 in *Basic & Clinical Endocrinology*. Greenspan FS, Forsham PH [editors]. Lange, 1983.)

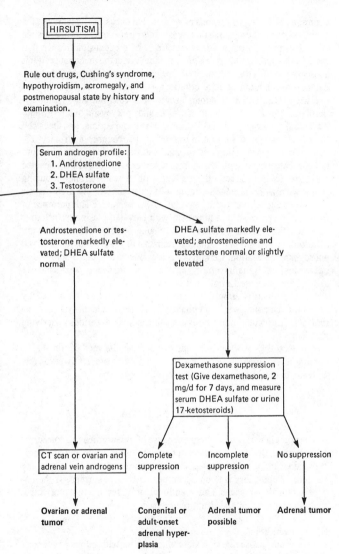

Figure 27–1 (cont'd). Laboratory investigation of hirsutism. (Reproduced, with permission, from Goldfien A, Monroe SE: Chapter 14 in *Basic & Clinical Endocrinology.* Greenspan FS, Forsham PH [editors]. Lange, 1983.)

common presenting complaints of women, but occasionally it may be the first sign of a serious neoplastic disease. It is rarely completely reversible even if a tumor is removed. Hirsutism is of greater significance if it occurs other than at puberty, with pregnancy, or at the menopause; if it is associated with other features of virilization such as voice changes, balding, or enlargement of the clitoris; and if the onset is sudden. Always investigate the patient's adrenal status and rule out tumor and hyperplasia (Fig 27–1). Ovarian causes include polycystic ovaries (Stein-Leventhal syndrome), hilar cell tumors, arrhenoblastoma, and theca cell luteinization. As a minimum screening procedure, a urinary 17-ketosteroid determination and plasma testosterone level should be obtained. The patient with an adrenal disorder will often have elevated 17-ketosteroids, whereas the patient with a testosterone-producing tumor such as an arrhenoblastoma will have abnormally high plasma testosterone level but usually normal 17-ketosteroids. The presence of obesity, amenorrhea, and hirsutism with elevated plasma testosterone and high tonic levels of LH is highly suggestive of polycystic ovary syndrome. It is important to make certain that the patient has not received androgenic medication. Certain drugs (eg, phenytoin, diazoxide) and an occasional malignant tumor (eg, arrhenoblastoma) will cause a generalized increase in body hair.

If hirsutism is simply a cosmetic problem, it can be treated by bleaching, shaving, wax or depilatory epilation, or electrolysis or thermolysis. The patient should be assured that there is no serious underlying problem.

If hirsutism is drug-induced, discontinue the medication that is causing it. Hirsutism may regress but will not be completely reversible with treatment of more serious underlying problems.

ANOREXIA NERVOSA

Anorexia nervosa is a frequent cause of amenorrhea in adolescents and young adults. Great dissatisfaction with body image and an abnormal preoccupation with losing weight become obsessions with these patients. Weight loss is soon accompanied by amenorrhea. If the patient's nutritional status and emotional attitudes are not corrected, anabolic deprivation and death may ensue.

Clinical Findings

Bulimia, nausea, and anxiety when eating with others are characteristic symptoms. With weight loss, carbohydrate and protein metabolic abnormalities develop. Malnutrition causes liver dysfunction. Vitamin deficiencies occur. Sleep disturbances develop along with decreased central nervous system production of catecholamines and somatomedins. Growth hormone secretion is accelerated, but height is unaffected because epiphyseal closure has already occurred. FSH and LH titers fall to prepubertal levels. As a result, estrogen production is drastically reduced, and conversion of other estrogens to estriol is decreased. Concomitantly, 2-hydroxyestradiol, a nonactive estrogen that competitively inhibits the normal inactivation of catecholamines, is produced.

Prevention

Prevention requires adequate childhood social adjustment, good relationships with the parents, and inculcation of appropriate psychosexual attitudes.

Treatment & Prognosis

The treatment of anorexia nervosa is controversial, and the reader is referred to other texts for discussions of psychotherapy and nutritional management. With improvement, a reversal of the abnormal metabolic and endocrine changes will occur. As median weight is approached, menstruation usually resumes. However, amenorrhea, oligomenorrhea, or anovulatory cycles may persist despite reasonable nutritional improvement. Long-term follow-up and repeat treatment, if necessary, are most important. Pregnancy should be avoided until the patient's adjustment is sustained.

The prognosis depends upon the age of the individual at the time of diagnosis, the duration of amenorrhea, associated serious psychiatric problems, and the severity of weight loss. About half of patients with anorexia nervosa will achieve a satisfactory emotional state with proper therapy. An occasional patient will experience a schizophrenic break. Two to 6% of patients with anorexia nervosa will die as a consequence of the disorder.

28 | The Menopause & Climacteric

Physiologic menopause, or "change of life," is the gradual decline and eventual cessation of menstruation. It is an endocrine deficiency state that marks the termination of reproductive function in women. Natural or physiologic menopause due to eventual ovarian failure occurs between ages of 46 and 52 years, the mean age in the USA being 51 years. This represents an increase of at least 5 years of reproductive life in the past century. Where health and nutritional standards are poor, the menopause may occur 5–10 years earlier. The time of onset and termination of manifestations of natural menopause are unpredictable.

Artificial menopause may occur at any age after the menarche as the result of pituitary or ovarian destruction or surgical ablation or devastating ovarian disease (eg, tuberculosis).

The climacteric is the period following menopause, normally after middle age, when marked involution or deterioration (aging) due to sex hormone hypofunction or dysfunction occurs. Actually, the climacteric is evidence that physiologic decline is in progress.

Some authors use the terms menopause and climacteric synonymously. Others believe that the menopause is that period during the climacteric when ovarian function diminishes gradually and menstruation ceases. Later, the body undergoes marked involution. Although noticeable changes begin at about age 35 (eg, stiffness of joints, skin wrinkles), these findings are only coincidentally related to menstrual function and certainly are not to be considered menopausal. Hence, it is this author's belief that the terms "menopause" and "climacteric" should be distinguished as defined above.

Although it is true that diminished ovarian function causes physical symptoms, cessation of menstruation does not itself impair physical capacity. Nevertheless, the menopause is emotionally disturbing and may cause psychosomatic complications. Fewer than 15% of women require therapy during the menopause, but many eventually seek medical treatment for disorders pertaining to the climacteric.

PHYSIOLOGIC MENOPAUSE

As a result of gonadal failure, the normal reciprocal relationship between the production of ovarian estrogens and progesterone and secretion of FSH and LH changes prior to the menopause. Occasional anovulation begins at about age 35 and is common after age 40; therefore, no ovarian progesterone is produced. The declining plasma estrogen level releases the "brake" on the hypophysis; FSH then rises from the usual normal level of 4–30 mIU to more than 100 mIU after the menopause. Similarly, the level of LH rises to at least 100 mIU postmenopausally.

Estrogen depletion is the most significant factor in the production of menopausal symptoms. Menopausal flushes are associated with surges in circulating LH and small increases in FSH but not with elevations in circulating neurohormones or prolactin.

Major changes occur in the levels of virtually all hormones after the menopause as follows:

(1) The estradiol level decreases by almost one-third and that of estrone by about one-fifth. Estriol depletion is comparable. Most of the estrogen produced postmenopausally comes from the adrenal cortex. However, the continued gradual decline in estrogen production until about age 65 finally leads to marked estrogen deficiency.

(2) Small amounts of progesterone are secreted (by the adrenal cortex alone) after the menopause.

(3) Androstenedione production is reduced by about one-third, and dehydroepiandrosterone and dehydroepiandrosterone sulfate levels together are reduced by about three-fourths. Reasonable levels of these androgens are maintained by the adrenal gland. Moreover, after about age 50, conversion of the androgens to estrogens, mainly by fat, muscle and the liver, increases considerably.

Testosterone secretion is reduced by about one-third. After menopause, testosterone production is principally by the ovary rather than the adrenal gland. The relative increase of testosterone over estrogen may explain the slight virilization that may occur in older women.

(4) Gonadotropin levels increase. That of FSH increases markedly, reciprocating the fall in estrogen; that of LH increases moderately.

(5) The thyroid and parathyroid hormone levels may be slightly reduced after the menopause.

There is only a rough correlation between the alteration of normal plasma or urinary estrogen and FSH or LH levels and the degree of discomfort reported by the patient. However, estrogen deprivation is undoubtedly the primary cause of such disorders as atrophic vaginitis and cystitis. Vasomotor symptoms generally are more severe in women with preexisting vasomotor instability. They are due to a decline in estrogen or an increase in circulating FSH (or both).

Women who are emotionally unstable before the menopause are prone to suffer more during this time than well-adjusted individuals.

Clinical Findings

The diagnosis of menopause cannot be made solely on the basis of menstrual aberration, "nervousness," and vasomotor symptoms; ovarian deficiency must be established by inspection and laboratory tests.

A. Menopausal Symptoms and Signs: This discussion will include also those complaints commonly but inappropriately attributed to hormonal changes during this period of life.

1. Alteration in menstrual flow–Irregular and occasionally profuse menstrual periods are common after age 40; they can usually be related to anovulatory cycles. Biopsy and curettage will rule out cancer and benign tumors.

2. Cessation of menses–Menstrual periods usually become irregular, with wider intervals, scanty flow, and episodes of amenorrhea (oligomenorrhea). Symptoms are apt to be more severe if the periods cease abruptly than if oligomenorrhea precedes cessation of menses.

3. Vasomotor flushes and flashes–These are the most distressing complaints concomitant with or following the menopause. The patient describes a sensation of heat felt first in the epigastrium or over the chest, spreading suddenly over the entire body and accompanied by a facial flush or blush. These unpleasant sensations may occur rarely or many times an hour. Associated tachycardia and subsequent perspiration are frequent. Vasomotor disturbances occur at short intervals and are most disturbing at night and during periods of fatigue, illness, or emotional tension.

With appropriate therapy, flushes can be eliminated or reduced to an occasional mild sensation of warmth. Even with no treatment, they usually cease after 1–2 years. However, in some women these symptoms persist until age 65–68. If the patient records the number of hot flushes experienced during a day, the degree of disability or success of therapy can be appraised.

4. Atrophic vulvar and vaginal changes–Contracture of the introitus and thinning of the vulvovaginal tissues occur about 6 months after the menses cease. Irritation, vaginal dryness, and dyspareunia will promptly improve following appropriate estrogen therapy.

5. Local manifestations of depressed ovarian function–These include gynatresia, pallor and thinning of the mucosa, atrophy of the rugae, loss of elasticity of the vagina, involution of the cervix, diminution of vaginal mucus, and reduced size of the uterus and ovaries.

6. Other problems–Other problems commonly reported at the menopause or during the climacteric are independent of pituitary or ovarian hormonal alterations; these include emotional instability, headaches, dyspnea, vertigo, and digestive disorders. Medical disorders capable of causing such symptoms must be diagnosed and treated or excluded. Certainly, estrogen therapy will not relieve these complaints.

B. Postmenopausal Symptoms and Signs: Estrogen lack is responsible for disorders that may not occur until a year or more after menstruation ceases.

1. Atrophic (senile) vaginitis–Diminished estrogen levels cause target organs to show variable atrophic changes: shrinkage of the labia and narrowing of the introitus (kraurosis), loss of rugae, blanching of the mucosa, and fissure formation and dryness of the vaginal canal.

2. Atrophic (senile) cystitis–The bladder and urethral mucosa are also responsive to estrogen; atrophy may occur in the lower urinary tract during the climacteric. Cystourethritis, more troublesome in the perimenopausal period, causes frequency, nocturia, and urgency— sometimes to the point of urge incontinence. Bacterial infections must also be considered.

3. Osteoporosis–Demineralization of the skeleton, particularly the vertebrae and long bones, occurs 3–5 years after cessation of menses. Decline in production of steroid sex hormones causes some rarefaction of bone, with the result that pathologic fractures may occur following trivial accidents, coughing, or sudden rising to an erect posture. The lumbar vertebrae are most susceptible; fracture of the rarefied head or neck of the femur is also common. Inactivity and inadequate intake of protein, calcium, and vitamin D are contributing factors.

The clinical symptoms of osteoporosis are back pain and disability upon movement. Backache (in the absence of fractures) may be due to contracture of the periarticular structures; compression of the cartilaginous intervertebral disks contributes to pain. Arthritic changes may occur concomitantly.

In advanced osteoporosis, x-ray studies reveal decreased density of bone due to demineralization of trabeculae, particularly in the vertebrae. The cortex may appear dense by comparison. Pathologic fractures of the vertebral bodies (due to compression) are identifiable radiologically.

The diagnosis of osteoporosis is supported by the Sulkowitch test for hypercalciuria.

The differential diagnosis must include radiculitis and osteoarthritis. Decalcification of bone also occurs in Cushing's syndrome, hyperthyroidism, hyperparathyroidism, multiple myeloma, metastatic carcinoma, and osteoporosis of disuse.

4. Arteriosclerosis and coronary heart disease–Although estrogen supplementation seems to delay or minimize the acceleration of atherosclerosis that occurs after early ovariectomy, estrogen replacement in postmenopausal women has not been shown to limit or reduce the incidence of coronary or cerebral thrombosis. Estrogen therapy may actually increase the likelihood of thromboembolic disease in older women.

5. Skin and hair changes–The aging process after the menopause causes progressive wrinkling and thinning of the skin, loss of skin pigmentation, and hyperkeratosis. Slight generalized alopecia may be noted.

6. Mental and emotional deterioration–These cannot properly be attributed to the climacteric.

C. Laboratory Findings Indicative of Ovarian Deficiency:

1. Vaginal cytology–Scanty mucus, fewer than 5% cornified cells, numerous basal cells and leukocytes (in the absence of specific infection).

2. Plasma FSH and LH levels over 100 mIU.

3. Endometrial biopsy reveals atrophic endometrium.

Differential Diagnosis

Amenorrhea and depressed gonadal function may result from severe metabolic and psychic disorders such as adenohypophyseal or adrenocortical insufficiency, anorexia nervosa, and myxedema. The incidence is low, but such patients are seriously ill and may present many medical problems.

Prevention of Senile Atrophic Changes

The increasing longevity of women (women in the USA lived an average of 47 years in 1900, 74 years in 1968, and 75 years in 1976) has placed greater importance on the need for continued prophylactic support and treatment of problems in the postmenopausal years. The aging changes that characterize this period of life in women include the following: (1) Progressive attenuation of the genitalia and pelvic floor structures. (2) Osteoporosis (normal calcification but little bone). (3) Slowly developing kyphosis ("dowager's hump") due to muscle weakness, poor posture, and an attitude of "peering" due to failing vision. (4) Increased atherosclerosis and increased incidence of ischemic heart disease. (5) Keratodermia climactericum, seborrheic keratosis, and neurodermatitis.

Early and adequate steroid sex hormone therapy will usually reduce the extent of mucosal, muscular, fascial, osseous, and, frequently, vascular degenerative changes, but such therapy can only rarely prevent or reverse them. Postmenopausal women receiving sex hormone therapy should have periodic examinations of the breasts and genital organs, because hormone administration may accelerate the growth of premalignant lesions or dormant cancers in these anatomic areas.

Treatment

Amelioration of discomfort and prevention of future disability must be achieved with a minimum of medication. Therapy should be governed by symptomatic responses, not by results of laboratory tests alone.

A. General Measures:

1. Education–Explain the menopause and climacteric and allay unrealistic apprehensions. Reassure the patient that her enjoyment of life will continue as before.

2. Sedation–Mild vasomotor symptoms can be controlled with phenobarbital, 15 mg 2–4 times daily. More severe discomfort is relieved by sedatives combined with antispasmodics. If barbiturates are contraindicated, prescribe flurazepam, 30 mg, or equivalent, at bedtime for sleep. Tranquilizers will control anxiety, eg, perphenazine, 2–4 mg 3–4 times daily. Avoid giving dangerous amounts of tranquilizers and sedatives to depressed patients.

B. Specific Measures: Estrogens, progestogens, and androgens afford relief of menopausal symptoms due to hormonal imbalance, and all have protein anabolic effects. The estrogens alone reduce vaginal irritation, contracture, and dryness. The androgens increase libido and do not cause mastalgia and uterine bleeding. Progestogens given in doses appropriate for menopausal complaints have no side-effects.

1. Estrogens–Most menopausal women have only mild symptoms and therefore do not need hormone supplements. Others may require estrogens for 4–6 months or longer while they adjust to lower levels of estrogen production. Estrogens should be prescribed first unless contraindicated. To avoid overstimulation, particularly of the endometrium, administer orally for the shortest time necessary the smallest cyclic dose that gives relief, eg, 3 weeks of pills followed by 1 week without pills or accompanied by a progestogen for 10 days (days 15–25), as discussed below. Monitor for the possible development of carcinoma of the endometrium. Mastopathy and endometrial hyperplasia may thus be avoided.

An unusually sensitive endometrium may be induced to bleed after even minute doses of estrogen. If so, an endometrial biopsy should be obtained. If no malignant trend is revealed, interrupt therapy for 2 months to see if bleeding continues. Investigate other local causes of bleeding.

Although long-term estrogen therapy may be beneficial for the treatment of osteoporosis, for example, there is no proof that taking estrogens for years after the menopause maintains a soft and supple skin and 'keeps the woman feeling "young."

Because a postmenopausal woman has low levels of estrogen without treatment, adequate hormone levels should be restored and maintained by endocrine therapy if the woman is symptomatic (unless contraindicated). Both natural estrogens and nonsteroidal estrogens in appropriate doses will relieve the symptoms. Natural conjugated estrogens (Premarin) may be given in a dosage of 0.3–0.625 mg orally every day for 3 weeks per month if undesirable side-effects do not develop. (A dose of 0.625 mg of natural conjugated estrogens is comparable to diethylstilbestrol, 0.25 mg, or ethinyl estradiol, 0.025 mg.)

Overdosage may be harmful. Parenteral estrogen is indicated only when the patient is in great distress and must have immediate relief or when oral administration is not feasible. In such cases, prescribe depot estrogen such as estradiol valerate (Delestrogen), 1 mL (10 mg) in lieu of the first 7 days of oral estrogen. A preliminary examination of the breasts and pelvis for tumors is required. Uterine bleeding is more likely to occur after depot estrogen because of the large initial dose and occasional rapid assimilation.

Recent reports suggest that there is an increased risk of endometrial cancer if estrogens are used in the postmenopausal period for over 1 year. A postmenopausal woman not taking estrogens has about 1 chance in 1000 each year of developing endometrial cancer, but the risk is 5–10 times greater for a woman taking estrogens. Hence, it is important to prescribe estrogens only when they are really needed. The risk of cancer seems to increase with the duration of estrogen therapy and the dosage. Therefore, the lowest dose of estrogen that will control the symptoms should be prescribed, and for only as long as it is required. If estrogens are prescribed for several years or more, reevaluation of need and endometrial sampling every 6 months are recommended. On the other hand, after hysterectomy, the danger of carcinogenesis is no longer a threat, because no good evidence is available to implicate the usual menopausal estrogen therapy in causing cancer of the breast, cervix, liver, or other organs.

Theoretically, progestogen, eg, medroxyprogesterone acetate (Provera), 5–10 mg administered orally daily for 10 days (days 15–25) together with 3 weeks of daily estrogen therapy, should reduce the threat of endometrial carcinoma by "medical curettage" or even periodic normalization. A similar approach is the administration of progestogen at 6-month intervals. Whether this protects against endometrial cancer, however, is moot. Moreover, slight periodic withdrawal bleeding, which occurs in 5–10% of patients on this regimen, is generally unacceptable to postmenopausal women. Hence, low-dosage estrogen for the shortest required time, with endometrial sampling every 9–12 months, is the most popular current plan of therapy.

Women who have had cholestatic jaundice of pregnancy should not take estrogens at the menopause because icterus or pruritus may recur. Patients on prolonged estrogen therapy are more likely to develop cholecystitis-cholelithiasis than those not taking estrogen. Women who take oral contraceptives may be at greater risk of thromboembolism than those who do not, but the use of estrogens during the menopause is not known to cause such problems. Nonetheless, if there is a history of thrombophlebitis, heart attack, stroke, or evidence of abnormal clotting, estrogens should be used with great caution, if at all.

2. Progestogens–Some progestogens, eg, norethindrone, are partially converted by intermediate metabolism to estrogen. Nonetheless, medroxyprogesterone or medroxyprogesterone acetate contributes no estrogen. The 2 are effective in controlling vasomotor reactions when given in ample doses.

Progestins are also useful when estrogens are contraindicated (eg, endometrial cancer). Medroxyprogesterone acetate (Provera), 5–10 mg orally daily, will suppress vasomotor reactions in most cases.

3. Androgens–Androgens may be beneficial if estrogens cause mastalgia or uterine bleeding; if uterine fibroids, pelvic endometriosis, or cachexia is present; or if an increase in libido is considered desirable. Prescribe cautiously, because masculinization may occur. Methyltestosterone (buccal), 10 mg, approximates the efficacy of diethylstilbestrol, 0.5 mg, in the immediate postmenopausal years; however, individual variation in response cannot be predicted.

4. Combined therapy–Combined estrogen-androgen therapy controls symptoms and minimizes the undesirable effects of both hormones. Commercial preparations containing half the usual individual dose of each are no longer available in the USA.

5. Local sex steroids–Local sex steroid therapy should be given for vulvovaginal or urinary disorders secondary to ovarian deficiency. Regional application of small doses of sex steroids will relieve pelvic symptoms without the undesirable effects of larger oral or parenteral doses, although measurable absorption occurs. Local estrogens are available as diethylstilbestrol in suppositories, 0.1 and 0.5 mg; dienestrol in suppositories, 0.7 mg; dienestrol creams, 0.01%; and conjugated estrogen creams, 0.625 mg/g. The physician should consult the manufacturer's insert for details of dosage and administration.

Satisfactory symptomatic and metabolic adjustments may be difficult to achieve, and sex steroid hormone therapy may have to be continued indefinitely—regardless of hormone contribution by the adrenal cortex.

C. Treatment of Osteoporosis:

1. General measures–Provide analgesics, eg, codeine, 30 mg, or aspirin, 0.6 g, every 4 hours as necessary, and braces or back supports for pain and fractures. Do not keep the patient in bed for protracted periods; further demineralization may ensue. A high-protein, high-vitamin diet is required. Additional small amounts of calcium may be beneficial.

2. Sex steroid therapy–Backache due to osteoporosis in the climacteric is ameliorated in 2–3 weeks after beginning moderately large doses of estrogen or androgen. A high-protein diet and calcium and vitamin D supplementation are helpful. Fractures naturally prolong discomfort. Although marked improvement usually follows therapy, x-ray films will not demonstrate increased bone density until much later. Prolonged treatment is required. Interruption of treatment is often followed by recurrence of pain, and further skeletal damage is likely.

Prognosis

The prognosis for an uncomplicated, only mildly disturbing meno-pause and climacteric is excellent for the well-adjusted, informed woman. Neurotic patients or those who are intolerant of therapy (or for whom medication is contraindicated) may have to endure considerable distress before they "settle down" to a relatively more agreeable old age.

ARTIFICIAL MENOPAUSE

Oophorectomy, intense radiation therapy to the pelvic viscera, or hypophysectomy causes prompt onset of the menopause. The signs and symptoms of the climacteric develop prematurely (1–2 months after surgery or radiotherapy). Endocrine therapy must be instituted to prevent metabolic disorders such as osteoporosis and coronary heart disease. The treatment of artificial menopause and its sequelae is similar to that given for natural cessation of ovarian function. However, hormone administra-tion is contraindicated if endometriosis or carcinoma of the breast were the reasons for the ovarian excision, irradiation, or hypophysectomy.

The benefits of continued ovarian function far outweigh the alleged advantages of routine removal of the ovaries after age of 40 for surgical convenience or to avoid ovarian carcinoma.

INFERTILITY

Infertility is defined as failure to conceive after 1 year of regular coitus without contraception.

No longer are infertility patients mostly young people; they are now more apt to be older couples who have used oral or other contraceptives and are anxious to have a family.

Infertility is a disorder of couples, and both partners must be evaluated. The man is responsible in about 30% of cases, the woman in approximately 40% of cases, and both in the remainder. Treatment may correct infertility but not sterility, which is the absolute inability to reproduce.

Infertility in Women

Ovulation and conception may occur at any time from menarche to menopause. Conception is most likely during the period of reasonably regular ovulation, which begins after adolescence and usually ends about 5–8 years before menopause. Normal pregnancy and delivery of a viable infant depend upon the following sequence of events: (1) A fertile ovum is extruded from the ovary. (2) The ovum finds its way into the uterine tube within a few hours. (3) Insemination occurs, and the spermatozoa migrate to the tube. (4) The ovum is fertilized in the mid portion of the tube. (5) The fertilized, segmenting ovum implants and develops in a favorable site in the endometrium. (6) Maturation proceeds until delivery.

Infertility in women may be due to the following causes:

A. Metabolic: Vitamin deficiency, protein deficiency, or severe iron deficiency anemia may cause infertility. Metabolic disorders, eg, diabetes mellitus, may also cause infertility.

B. Endocrine:

1. Pituitary–Ovulation and pregnancy depend upon the normal production of thyrotropin, corticotropin, and the gonadotropins (FSH and LH). Secondary ovarian failure occurs when pituitary function is significantly altered. Hypopituitarism may be due to circulatory collapse resulting from hemorrhage and pituitary necrosis (Sheehan's syndrome), cysts or tumors, or starvation. Pituitary cachexia (Simmonds' disease) is quite rare. Hyperpituitarism is most often due to benign adenoma.

2. Thyroid–Hypothyroidism results in anovulation, infertility, and abortion. Severe hyperthyroidism causes infertility.

3. Adrenal–Adrenocortical overactivity (Cushing's syndrome) results in decreased ovulation. Adrenal failure (Addison's disease) causes gonadal atrophy. Hypo- or hyperfunction of the adrenal medulla does not affect fertility.

C. Vaginal: Congenital vaginal anomalies (absence of vagina, gynatresia, imperforate or cribriform hymen, stenosis, septate vagina) prevent intromission and insemination. Vaginitis due to infection causes leukorrhea, which may kill the sperms. Sperm immobilization (SI) or sperm agglutination (SA) antibodies may develop in vaginal or cervical fluid and cause infertility.

D. Cervical:

1. Developmental abnormalities ("pinhole" or double cervix) may prevent sperm migration.

2. Cervical tumors (polyps, myomas) may partially occlude the passage of sperms or cause a discharge inimical to sperms.

3. Cervicitis produces acid, viscid, sometimes purulent secretions noxious to sperms. Chlamydial, T mycoplasma *(Ureaplasma urealyticum),* enterococci, trichomonad, and mixed infections are the most common.

4. Cervical incompetence is a common cause of second-trimester abortion.

E. Uterine:

1. Congenital uterine anomalies (hypoplasia, bicornuate or septate uterus) rarely impede implantation, but they prevent normal maturation to viability by reducing the capacity of the uterus.

2. Uterine tumors (polyps, myomas) thin the endometrium, cause bleeding and discharge, alter the blood supply, and distort the uterus or limit its capacity.

3. Endometrial disorders, eg, polyps, endometritis, or refractoriness to hormonal stimuli, prevent nidation or maintenance of pregnancy.

F. Tubal: Total or partial occlusion of the tubal lumen usually is due to infection. Congenital atresia or false passages are unusual.

G. Ovarian:

1. Congenital abnormalities (eg, ovarian dysgenesis) are associated with primary ovarian failure.

2. Infections involving the ovaries cause infertility by preventing follicle maturation and ovulation. Thickening of the tunica ovarii caused by prolonged infection prevents release of the ova.

3. Ovarian tumors may disrupt function or destroy the ovary.

4. Endometriosis disorganizes and scars the ovary, impairing all ovarian functions.

H. Psychic: Anxiety, fear, overconcern, severe psychoneurosis (eg, anorexia nervosa), or psychosis (eg, schizophrenia) often causes amenorrhea or anovulation.

I. Coital: Douches, lubricants, or antiseptics may dilute, inactivate, or destroy sperms.

Infertility in Men

Male reproductive ability begins at about age 16. After approximately age 45, fertility decreases, although men over age 80 have fathered children.

Infertility in men may be due to the following causes:

A. Coital: Incomplete vaginal penetration is caused by chordee, epispadias, hypospadias, or extreme obesity.

B. Sperm Abnormalities: The normal values of spermatic fluid are as follows:

> Volume: 3.4 mL (mean)
> pH: 7.4
> Viscosity: Moderately liquefied after 30 minutes.
> Motility (at 26.5 °C [75 °F]): More than 70% motile at ejaculation; 60% at 2 hours; 25–40% at 6 hours; a few still active after 24 hours.
> Count: 50–120 million/mL
> Morphology: Fewer than 30% abnormal spermatozoal heads.

Fresh ejaculate is a whitish, semigelatinous fluid with small opalescent flecks that contain most of the sperms. The first portion of the ejaculate contains the largest number of sperms per volume and the fewest abnormal forms. After 30 minutes, the specimen should become homogeneous, translucent, and liquefied. The presence of blood or pigment is abnormal.

Sperms survive longest in alkaline cervical secretions and are destroyed quickly if they remain in the acid vaginal fluid. The optimal pH for maintenance of sperms is 8.5–9.0. Motility is arrested at pH 6.0 and does not return after sperms have been exposed to a pH below 4.0.

Sperms travel at a rate of about 1 cm/h by their own propulsion. They maintain proper direction by their tendency to swim along polymerized cervical mucous strands, against fluid currents and toward the alkaline, glycogenic medium of the upper female genital tract. They enter the cervix, traverse the uterus, and are propelled toward the ovum by the ciliary activity of the tubal epithelium, which beats in the direction of the fimbria.

Fertility is assumed to be high when the sperm count approaches 185 million/mL and low when the count of active sperms is less than 50 million/mL. No definite minimum can be given, but conception rarely occurs when the sperm count is below 35 million/mL.

Endocrine studies may be important in diagnosis of the cause of sperm problems.

1. Azoospermia–

a. Low serum testosterone levels, elevated LH and FSH levels–These men have primary testicular failure involving Leydig and germinal cells.

b. Normal serum testosterone and LH levels, elevated FSH level–Primary germinal tubular failure with sparing of Leydig cells is likely.

c. Low serum testosterone, LH, and FSH levels–These patients have hypogonadotropic hypogonadism, either congenital or acquired.

d. Normal serum testosterone, LH and FSH levels–Failure of ejaculation is the probable cause of azoospermia. Either retrograde ejaculation or obstruction of the ejaculatory system is likely.

2. Oligospermia–

a. Low serum testosterone level, elevated LH and FSH levels–These men have primary gonadal insufficiency.

b. Normal serum testosterone and LH levels, elevated FSH level–Secondary gonadal insufficiency, probably from acquired damage to germinal elements, is present.

c. Low serum testosterone levels and low or normal LH and FSH levels–A central nervous system neuroendocrine disorder is likely. These patients may have partial deficiencies of gonadotropin secretion secondary to hypothalamic or pituitary disease. An elevated serum prolactin level suggests a pituitary tumor.

d. Normal serum testosterone, LH, and FSH levels–Varicocele is present or the diagnosis is uncertain. Check for varicocele or other lower genital abnormality.

e. High to normal or slightly elevated serum testosterone and LH levels but low normal to low FSH level–This unusual category includes men with partial androgen resistance that results in a secondary increase in serum LH.

3. Abnormal sperms–Necrospermia and abnormal sperm morphology or motility may be found.

C. Testicular:

1. Developmental defects–Agenesis of the testes is extraordinarily rare; small testes are present in Klinefelter's syndrome. Absence of the testes from the scrotum is usually due to cryptorchidism, but migratory or ectopic testes must be considered. In 2% of postpuberal boys, both testes are cryptorchid, and these individuals are usually sterile at maturity. Unilateral cryptorchidism does not affect fertility, but varicocele may.

2. Endocrine–Hypopituitarism, Cushing's disease, and anterior pituitary tumors cause infertility. Hypothyroidism is associated with infertility, but the reason is not known. Atrophy of the testes occurs in

Addison's disease. In Klinefelter's syndrome, infertility is due to failure of development of the seminiferous tubules. Cushing's syndrome suppresses spermatogenesis. Anemia and poorly controlled diabetes mellitus result in infertility for unexplained reasons.

3. Immunologic–Abnormal spermatogenesis (eg, oligospermia, aspermia) or incomplete spermatogenesis may result from immunologic alteration of germinal cells following genital injury or vasectomy.

4. Infections–Fertility is reduced during and shortly after high fever. Mumps in prepuberal boys only rarely involves the testes; after puberty, mumps is complicated by orchitis in 20% of cases. If orchitis is bilateral, sterility usually results. Chronic debilitating infections (eg, malaria, tuberculosis, brucellosis) cause temporary infertility.

5. Physical injury–Irradiation, direct trauma to the testes, and reduced circulation following complicated herniorrhaphy or varicocele repair reduce or destroy testicular function.

D. Penis and Urethra: Congenital malformations or scarring may interfere with erection and intromission. Urethral stricture may prevent ejaculation.

E. Prostate and Seminal Vesicles: These organs produce the liquid vehicle for the sperms; only 5% of the ejaculate is semen. Prostatic fluid contains fibrinogen and fibrinolysin, which cause the ejaculate to coagulate initially and subsequently to liquefy. Infections of the prostate and seminal vesicles are detected by digital rectal examination and microscopic examination of the fluid expressed.

F. Epididymides and Vasa Deferentia: These structures conduct sperms from the testes to the seminal vesicles and provide nutritional or maturational factors for the sperms. Most mechanical obstructions (congenital, inflammatory, or traumatic) occur here. Varicocele and hydrocele may increase scrotal temperature and thus impair spermatozoal maturation.

Impairment of seminal fluid formation or variations in its constitution may be due to immunologic factors. The acrosome of the spermatid and the spermatozoon contains a polysaccharide-polypeptide antigen that activates the immune system. Anti-seminal fluid antibodies in men react only with adnexal gland cells and seminal sperm; testicular cells are spared.

Diagnostic Survey

Infertility can be treated successfully only if an accurate diagnosis can be established. This requires an energetic and systematic approach by the physician and the cooperation of both partners. Over a period of at least 3 months, with 4 office visits for the wife and 2–3 for the husband, both partners usually can be evaluated and the cause of infertility determined (Table 29–1). Obscure or multiple causes of infertility may require more time and special techniques of investigation.

Table 29–1. Suggested 4-visit routine for evaluation of infertility.

	Wife	Husband
First visit	Joint discussion of problem of infertility.	
	Medical history. Explanation. Taking and recording of basal body temperature.	Medical history. Explanation of semen collection and analysis.
Second visit (2–4 weeks later) at mid-cycle	Physical examination. Routine and indicated laboratory tests. Preliminary evaluation of basal body temperature chart.	Physical examination. Routine and indicated laboratory tests, including thyroid hormone determinations. Discuss results of semen analysis.
Third visit (3 weeks later)	Hysterosalpingography (best done in early proliferative phase). Evaluation of basal body temperature chart.	Repeat semen analysis if first was deficient. Sperm agglutination and immobilization tests.
Fourth visit (5 weeks later)	Spinnbarkeit and fern test. Sims-Huhner test.	Testosterone, LH, and FSH determinations if second semen analysis was abnormal.
Later (tests and procedures as indicated)	Sex chromatin analysis. Endometrial biopsy. Laparoscopy. Laparotomy to correct problems (eg, endometriosis).	Testicular biopsy if indicated. Cystoscopy. Definitive genitourinary surgery.

A. First Visit: (Wife and husband.) In a joint interview, the physician explains the problem of infertility and its causes to the husband and wife. Separate private consultations are then conducted, allowing appraisal of marital adjustments without embarrassment or criticism. A routine history should be taken. Pertinent details (eg, sexually transmitted disease or prior pregnancies) must be obtained. The husband should be asked if he has had mumps; both partners should be asked about chronic infections, anemia, and medical therapy for these. Past surgical procedures should be discussed. The gynecologic history should include information about the menstrual pattern and any menstrual abnormalities (eg, pain, metrorrhagia, and leukorrhea) as well as the number of pregnancies, abortions, deliveries, lactation, and complications. Occupational stresses and hazards of both partners, prior marriages and fertility, pregnancies, and previous tests for infertility, including tests and therapy, must be elicited. The present history should include marital adjustment, difficulties in the marriage, use of contraceptives and the types used, douches, libido, sex techniques, orgasm, frequency and success of coitus, and correlation of intercourse with ovulation.

The husband is instructed to bring a complete ejaculate for spermatozoal analysis at the next visit and to abstain from sex for at least 4 days before the semen is obtained. Semen may be collected by either coitus interruptus or masturbation into a clean, dry, wide-mouthed bottle (preferred) or a vaginal (Doyle) spoon. Condoms should not be used, because residual rubber solvents and sulfur, which are noxious to sperms, cannot be eliminated. The corked bottle should be transported to the laboratory in a paper bag held away from the body in order to prevent stimulation and dissipation of the sperms by warmth and reduced oxygen tension. The bottle should not be allowed to become chilled, since cold slows and may damage the sperms.

Semen should be examined within 1–2 hours after collection. The experienced physician should examine the specimen personally.

B. Second Visit: (Wife and husband; 2–4 weeks after first visit.) The physician should explain abnormal findings briefly but avoid identifying one or the other partner as being responsible for infertility, because blame is invariably followed by guilt feelings and resentment. Both husband and wife are often found to have problems that contribute to infertility.

The woman should have a complete physical and pelvic examination. The man's general physical examination is performed next, with emphasis on the genital and rectal examination. The results of the sperm analysis should be explained to the couple without undue optimism or pessimism. Laboratory studies for both husband and wife include urinalysis, complete blood count and hematocrit determination, serologic test for syphilis, and thyroid function tests. The physician must explain that the optimal time for conception is at ovulation. The most accurate way to determine the time of ovulation is by the serum LH "surge" (peak) at midcycle.

C. Third Visit: (Wife: 1 month after second visit. The husband is not required to return for a third visit if his physical examination and initial semen analysis are normal.)

Hysterosalpingography (Fig 29–1) is preferred for determination of uterotubal patency because the site and degree of occlusion usually are clearly identified by this method.

If the first semen analysis was abnormal, a second should be done together with sperm agglutination and immobilization tests.

D. Fourth Visit: (Wife; 1 month after third visit.) The woman returns within 6 hours after coitus just prior to ovulation. The cervical mucus should be thin, clear, and alkaline. Spinnbarkeit (see p 39) should be 4 cm or more in length. A small drop of cervical mucus should be obtained, using a Knight or Kerner forceps, for the fern test and the Sims-Huhner test. The fern test should show clear arborizations: frondlike crystal patterns in the dried mucus. In the Sims-Huhner test, cervical mucus is examined microscopically for active sperms. The presence of 10–15 active sperms per high-power field constitutes a satisfactory test. If no motile sperms are found but active sperms were present in the semen analysis, the Sims-Huhner test should be repeated.

If the second semen analysis shows azoospermia or oligospermia,

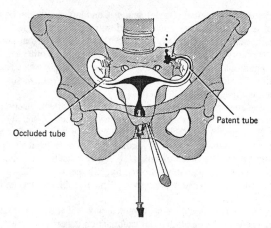

Figure 29–1. Hysterosalpingography.

the man's serum testosterone, LH, and FSH levels should be determined
to aid in diagnosis (see p 711).

    E. Later Tests: (As indicated.) A vaginal smear and an endome-
trial biopsy (see Fig 29–2) may be required to determine if ovulation is
occurring. To avoid a pregnancy, which usually implants high in the
uterus anteriorly or posteriorly, samples are best taken from the side wall
in the fundus. Laparoscopy may be required if tubal adhesions or
endometriosis is suspected. Laparotomy will be necessary for salpingostomy, lysis of dense adhesions, and elimination of ovarian abnormalities.

    The following tests should be performed in infertile women with
prolonged amenorrhea: (1) Serum prolactin determination, because the
prolactin level is often elevated with pituitary tumors, especially when
galactorrhea is present; (2) urinary gonadotropin determination for appraisal of anterior pituitary function; (3) urinary 17-ketosteroid and
17-hydroxycorticosteroid determination if adrenal or ovarian hyperfunction is likely; and (4) buccal smear and chromosomal studies in women
with primary amenorrhea.

    In men, the need for special studies, eg, prolactin determination, is
determined by the results of other hormone determinations. Testicular
biopsy is indicated if azoospermia or oligospermia is present. Cystoscopy and catheterization of ejaculatory duct orifices, using a fluid x-ray
contrast medium, may be required to demonstrate duct stenosis. Vasog-
raphy by direct injection of the vas near its origin may demonstrate an
occlusion. If no spermatozoa are recovered upon needle aspiration of the

upper pole of the epididymis (globus major), inflammatory closure of the tract is suggested.

F. Antisperm Antibodies: Occasional instances of unexplained infertility may be caused by immune processes: (1) circulatory or tissue antibodies against spermatozoa in women, (2) autoimmunization antibodies against spermatozoa in men, or (3) both.

Approximately 15% of women have antisperm antibodies, presumably developed in response to vaginal deposition (inoculation) of sperms. Such serum IgG or IgM antibodies may also be present in cervical mucus and may impair sperm migration by immobilizing or agglutinating sperms. Therefore, in the absence of demonstrated causes of infertility, tests for sperm immobilization and agglutination should be done, although the true significance and reliability of these tests are still debated. However, if the tests are positive, the use of condoms for at least 6 months should reduce antisperm antibody production in most women. About 75% of women with sperm agglutination antibodies will become pregnant, but less than 33% of patients with sperm immobilizing antibodies will become pregnant despite a reduction in antibody titer.

Autoantibodies in men may interfere with normal spermatogenesis or alter sperms so that pregnancy does not occur.

In autoimmune spermatogenesis, development of the sperms is altered within the seminiferous tubules; the seminiferous tubules themselves are not affected. Infection, trauma, or surgical occlusion of the ductus deferens may induce oligospermia or azoospermia. In these cases, there are increased titers of immobilizing or agglutinating sperm antibodies in the blood and seminal fluid. This may be the reason for the low sperm count and reduced pregnancy rate in some cases of successful vas reanastomosis.

Testosterone therapy for men with autoimmune serum and seminal vesicle antisperm antibodies has been a logical but limited method of treatment. With high doses of testosterone, temporary azoospermia is eventually produced; theoretically, this should eliminate the source of antigen. Certainly, antigen titers are reduced, and in most cases the semen quality improves when spermatogenesis is allowed to resume. However, only an occasional pregnancy results.

Treatment

Treatment in all cases depends upon correction of the underlying disorder or disorders suspected of causing infertility.

A. Infertility in Women:

1. General measures–Infertility due to nutritional deficiencies is frequently corrected by an adequate, well-balanced diet and nutritional supplements. Psychotherapy may be of value in women who are fearful of pregnancy and those in whom infertility is related to deep-seated psychiatric problems.

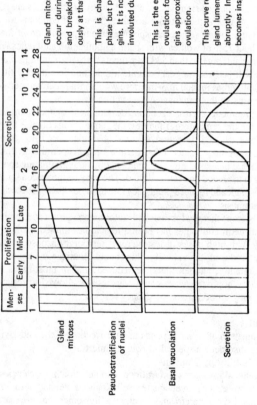

Gland mitoses indicate proliferation. They occur during menstruation because repair and breakdown are progressing simultaneously at that time.

This is characteristic of the proliferative phase but persists until active secretion begins. It is not resumed until the glands have involuted during menstruation.

This is the earliest morphologic evidence of ovulation found in the endometrium. It begins approximately 36–48 hours following ovulation.

This curve represents visible secretion in the gland lumen; active secretion falls off more abruptly. In the later stages, the secretion becomes inspissated.

Figure 29–2. Dating the endometrium. (Approximate relationship of useful morphologic factors.) (Modified slightly after JPA Latour and reproduced, with permission, from Noyes, Hertig, and Rock: Dating the endometrial biopsy. *Fertil Steril* 1950;1:3.)

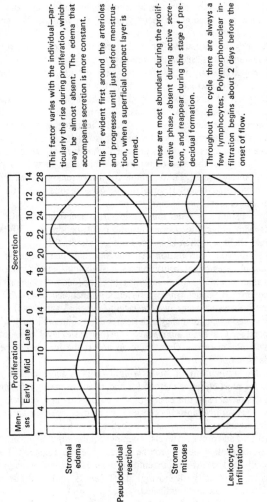

This factor varies with the individual—particularly the rise during proliferation, which may be almost absent. The edema that accompanies secretion is more constant.

This is evident first around the arterioles and progresses until just before menstruation, when a superficial compact layer is formed.

These are most abundant during the proliferative phase, absent during active secretion, and reappear during the stage of predecidual formation.

Throughout the cycle there are always a few lymphocytes. Polymorphonuclear infiltration begins about 2 days before the onset of flow.

Figure 29–2 (cont'd). Dating the endometrium. (Approximate relationship of useful morphologic factors.)

2. Medical measures–Fertility may be restored by proper treatment in many patients with endocrine imbalance, particularly hypo- or hyperthyroidism. Treatment of cervicitis is of value in the return of fertility. If sperm immobilization or sperm agglutination antibodies are present, use of a condom for about 6 months may result in their spontaneous dissipation.

3. Surgical measures–Surgical correction of congenital or acquired abnormalities (including tumors) of the lower genital tract or uterus may frequently renew fertility. Surgical excision of ovarian tumors or ovarian foci of endometriosis frequently restores fertility. Surgical relief of tubal obstruction due to salpingitis will reestablish fertility in about 30% of favorable cases. New microsurgical techniques have improved the success rate considerably. In instances of cornual or fimbrial block, the prognosis after surgery is much better.

Ovarian wedge resection is indicated when medical measures are not effective or in the case of progressive hirsutism in women with polycystic ovary disease. The technique consists of removing a wedge of ovary (cortex and medulla) equal to 40–50% of one ovary on the antimesenteric side. Ensure hemostasis.

The operation is often only temporarily beneficial; 60–80% of patients with polycystic ovaries resume menstruation, and 30–60% conceive. Hirsutism often is arrested but not eliminated.

4. Induction of ovulation–An attempt should be made to induce ovulation in cases of infertility due to anovulation that has persisted longer than 6 months (this includes brief secondary amenorrhea, oligomenorrhea), galactorrhea, recurrent dysfunctional uterine bleeding, and polycystic ovary disease (Stein-Leventhal syndrome). It is recommended when pregnancy is desired and not contraindicated; when the general medical evaluation is favorable (normal T_3 level, gonadotropin levels not markedly elevated, etc); and if the husband's sperm analysis is normal.

a. Normalization of body weight–This is the simplest and perhaps the most effective method for under- and overweight patients, but many women resist this easiest of all measures to improve fertility.

b. TSH suppression–In occasional women, compensated primary hypothyroidism causes anovulation. Such women have normal T_4 but elevated TSH and prolactin levels. Therapy requires suppression of TSH with replacement by levothyroxine. Usually levothyroxine, 0.1 mg orally daily, will be sufficient to reinitiate ovulation. Thyroid therapy for euthyroid patients with normal TSH levels and without hyperprolactinemia is contraindicated.

c. Bromocriptine–The dopamine agonist bromocriptine, 1.25–2.5 mg orally 2–3 times daily, may be given to women with hyperprolactinemia. If the patient misses a period, discontinue the medication and obtain a pregnancy test.

d. Clomiphene citrate (Clomid)–Clomiphene, 50–250 mg orally daily, may be given for 5 days beginning on the fifth day of the cycle to induce ovulation. Recent studies indicate that daily dosages of 50–100 mg of clomiphene are more effective because they produce a more normal rise in serum FSH levels. Higher doses seem to be self-defeating because they are associated with unfavorable cervical mucus and even luteal phase defects. If ovulation still does not occur, repeating the course of clomiphene and adding hCG, 10,000 units intramuscularly on the 15th day of the cycle, followed by 2000–5000 units intramuscularly on the 17th and 19th days may result in ovulation.

e. Menotropins (hMG, Pergonal)–Each ampule of Pergonal contains 75 IU of LH and 75 IU of FSH. hMG is used exclusively to induce ovulation in cases of hypogonadotropic hypogonadism or luteal phase defects or when clomiphene and hCG fail to induce ovulation.

In amenorrheic patients, induce menstrual bleeding with progesterone, 100 mg intramuscularly. On the fifth or sixth day following the onset of bleeding, give Pergonal, 1–2 ampules intramuscularly daily for 2 days. Later doses will depend upon the serum estrogen levels and the status of the ovaries.

An optimal serum estrogen concentration is 800–1000 pg/mL. (Higher amounts risk multiple ovulation.) Over the next 1–2 days, palpation and ultrasonography should identify a follicle about to ovulate. When such a follicle is found, give hCG, 10,000 units intramuscularly, to trigger ovulation. Pregnancy may result if the patient has intercourse that day and 24–48 hours later. The cost of the drug and laboratory tests may be about \$400–500 per month, and there is no guarantee of pregnancy. Often, 4–6 months of Pergonal therapy will be required to achieve pregnancy.

Ovulation is likely to occur after induction in women with polycystic ovary disease and those who are amenorrheic after having used oral contraceptive agents. In other types of patients, the results are unpredictable. The incidence of multiple pregnancy is one in 16; abortion occurs in 20–25% of pregnancies. Induction of ovulation is short-term therapy; its long-range effectiveness is poor.

f. Corticosteroids (glucocorticoids)–In patients with hyperadrenocorticism (hyperplasia) and polycystic ovary disease, corticosteroids act by reducing production of ACTH, which results in suppression of androgen production; this makes the ovary more receptive to gonadotropin stimulation, and ovulation results. This treatment must be used cautiously in patients with chronic infections, peptic ulcer, hypertension, diabetes mellitus, or mental depression.

Give prednisone (minimal sodium retention) or equivalent, 7.5–15 mg orally in 3–4 divided doses daily. Treatment must be continued indefinitely for women with adrenal hyperplasia; for others, a therapeutic trial of 6–8 months is indicated

About 30% of patients with polycystic ovary disease will ovulate as a result of corticosteroid therapy. Discontinue treatment if ovulation does not occur after 6 months. Polycystic ovary disease patients are generally improved for months after cessation of therapy.

Complications of induction of ovulation include multiple pregnancy, mild to moderate ovarian enlargement associated with abdominal pain, and ascites in 20% of patients. Spontaneous regression occurs in 2–3 weeks. Gross ovarian enlargement with pain, ascites, and hydrothorax or hematoperitoneum indicates hyperstimulation of the ovaries and requires hospitalization. Repeated vaginal examination is unwarranted because large cysts may be ruptured. Paracentesis should be avoided. Emergency surgery may be necessary to control bleeding.

5. In vitro fertilization ("test-tube pregnancy")–The first successful term delivery of an infant conceived by in vitro fertilization occurred in England in 1978. Many other normal "laboratory-conceived" newborns have been delivered since then.

Many women whose uterine tubes are obstructed or have been removed are now potential candidates for similar treatment. However, it is likely that use of this complex procedure to cure infertility must remain very limited for the near future, although many medical centers have or are developing programs for in vitro fertilization.

The following steps are involved in in vitro fertilization: (1) Ovulation is induced by gonadotropin therapy. (2) Mature follicles are identified by laparoscopy, and ova are removed by needle aspiration. (3) Ova are transferred to tissue culture media, and the sperms are added. (4) After fertilization, a second tissue culture transfer allows division to approximately a 12-cell blastocyst (3–6 days). (5) During this interval, progesterone therapy is given to the mother to induce formation of late secretory type endometrium in the uterus. The blastocyst is then transferred to the uterus, where it nidates, and embryonic development proceeds as in normal conception.

The Roman Catholic Church is strongly opposed to in vitro fertilization.

B. Infertility in Men: No form of treatment has been successful for azoospermia due to primary testicular failure or primary germinal tubular failure or for oligospermia due to secondary gonadal insufficiency. Necrospermia and abnormal sperm morphology or motility in the absence of infection usually defy treatment. Other causes of infertility in men can be treated as follows:

1. Surgical measures–Surgical correction of congenital or acquired abnormalities of the penis and urethra may permit successful vaginal penetration and normal insemination. Testicular hypofunction secondary to hypothyroidism or diabetes mellitus is often corrected by appropriate treatment. Surgical correction of varicocele or hydrocele may restore fertility. Mumps orchitis requires prompt testicular decompression by surgical excision of the tunica albuginea to preserve fertility. Microsurgery may correct failure of ejaculation.

2. Medical measures–Testicular hypofunction secondary to endocrine or metabolic dysfunction is often corrected by appropriate treatment. Azoospermia due to congenital or acquired hypogonadism may be corrected by hCG and hMG replacement. Treatment of oligospermia due to central nervous system neuroendocrine disease will depend on central nervous system findings. Treatment of oligospermia due to varicocele or to unknown causes with testosterone rebound therapy, clomiphene, or hCG and hMG has been disappointing.

3. Artificial insemination–In instances where the husband has poor sperm quantity, quality, or motility, eg, oligospermia due to primary gonadal insufficiency or that due to unknown causes when varicocele is not present, the spermatozoa-laden first portion of split ejaculates may be collected for artificial insemination (AIH [artificial insemination, homologous]). A number of split ejaculates may be frozen and later pooled for insemination. Rapid freezing and thawing do not cause genetic damage, and pooling increases the sperm count. However, AIH is usually unsuccessful, probably because poor motility or low count reflects only part of the sperm deficiency.

In contrast, the success of donor artificial insemination (AID) is about 70%. Numerous inseminations may be necessary to ensure proper timing at ovulation, which is usually determined by the basal body temperature record. With AID, about 50% of pregnancies occur within 2 months and almost 90% within 6 months.

Many emotional, ethical, and legal questions arise concerning AID. Both husband and wife must be strongly in favor of the procedure. They must know that there is no guarantee of pregnancy and that the frequency of fetal anomalies ($< 5\%$) and obstetric complications (5–10%) is the same whether insemination is achieved by coitus or by AID.

The physician must maintain the anonymity of the donor and must attest to the donor's genetic background, health, and fertility. The Rh factors of the donor and the woman should be compatible.

Instillation of semen into the uterine cavity should be avoided because of severe cramping (prostaglandin effect) and possible infection. Most of the specimen should be instilled into the cervical canal, with the remainder deposited in a cervical cap or a cleanly washed contraceptive diaphragm to be worn by the patient for about 1 hour.

Prognosis

The prognosis for conception and normal pregnancy is good if minor (even multiple) disorders can be identified and treated properly; poor if the causes of infertility are severe or poorly treatable.

No treatment is effective for infertility due to marked uterine hypoplasia. Congenital deficiency or absence of the ovaries is a hopeless sterility problem. Perioophoritis defies medical and surgical treatment. Agenesis or dysgenesis of the testes resists all treatment. Infertility due to marked or resistant prostatitis, seminal vesiculitis, or obstructions in the sperm conduit system rarely is correctable.

If treatment is not successful within 1 year, the physician should obtain consultation. If improvement is unlikely, adoption may be recommended.

CONTRACEPTION
(Birth Control)

The voluntary and temporary prevention of pregnancy may be indicated or desired for socioeconomic, medical, genetic, or personal reasons.

The following types of contraceptives are in current use:

(1) Biologic: Abstinence, including natural family planning and the "rhythm method"; coitus interruptus; hormonal suppression of ovulation; and tubal or ductal sterilization.

(2) Mechanical: Condoms and sheaths; cervical or intrauterine occlusion, eg, pessaries, diaphragms, intrauterine devices.

(3) Chemical: Spermicidal jellies, gels, creams, and suppositories.

(4) Mechanical and chemical: Foam, powder and sponge, douches, suppositories, diaphragm and cream or jelly.

(5) Immunologic methods are still investigational.

A woman seeking contraceptive advice should be examined and carefully instructed about the types, advantages, disadvantages, and use of appropriate methods of contraception and alternatives. Ideally, she should be given simple written or printed instructions to follow. A woman who is married or has a long-term relationship may wish to discuss contraception with her partner, since both should be satisfied with the choice of contraceptive.

The physical examination should detect all abnormalities, especially those that require treatment and those that might contraindicate certain contraceptive devices or methods.

Complete Abstinence

If faithfully practiced, this is completely effective as a birth control method. However, it is unphysiologic and generally is unacceptable and impractical for most couples.

Natural Family Planning; "Fertility Awareness"

Proponents of so-called natural family planning or "fertility awareness," a system that uses the basal body temperature chart, ovulation, or sympto-thermal methods, claim that a 98% effectiveness rate was achieved for each method in a limited series in a 1980 report from the US Department of Health, Education, and Welfare. However, the "use effectiveness" in this group permitted 6–10 unexpected pregnancies per 100 woman years of use with the basal body temperature method; 10–25 with the ovulation method; and 10–15 with the sympto-thermal method. This corresponds to an 80–90% overall effectiveness in pregnancy prevention.

Although these methods may be highly effective when used conscientiously after proper training, actual use compliance has been disappointing, especially in uneducated or poorly motivated individuals, eg, adolescents. Although these methods are promising, large-scale controlled studies on their reliability must be completed before their practicality can be regarded as established.

"Rhythm Method"

Ovulation occurs approximately 14 days before the onset of the next menstrual period regardless of the length of time between periods; when the cycle is regular, the time of ovulation (the "unsafe" period) can be anticipated.

The ovum and the sperms are probably fertile for about 24 hours. Coitus on the day of ovulation is most likely to result in pregnancy. If one allows 2 days of abstinence before ovulation to make certain that viable sperms will not be in the tube when the ovum descends, and 2 days afterward to make certain that a fertile ovum will not be in the tube when sperms are deposited, the "unsafe" period may be considered to extend from the 12th through the 16th days of a 28-day cycle. The "safe" periods are the 1st–11th and the 17th–28th days. However, ovulation may occur at virtually any time before the 14th day and is delayed in long cycles. Because these calculations are of no value in women recently delivered and when the cycle is irregular, the "calendar" method of determining the time of ovulation is usually unreliable.

The time of ovulation can be determined more certainly by the use of the basal body temperature record (Fig 29–3). The vaginal or rectal temperature must be taken immediately upon awakening, before any activity whatever. A drop in temperature occurs 24–36 hours after ovulation; the temperature rises about 0.4 °C (0.7 °F) 1–2 days after ovulation and remains at this plateau throughout the remainder of the cycle. The third day after the rise marks the end of the fertile period. This method requires a great deal of effort and interest on the part of the patient to be sure a true basal temperature chart is being recorded.

Oral Contraception; "The Pill"

"The pill" is a popular term for more than 20 different oral contraceptives commercially available in the USA. The products are of

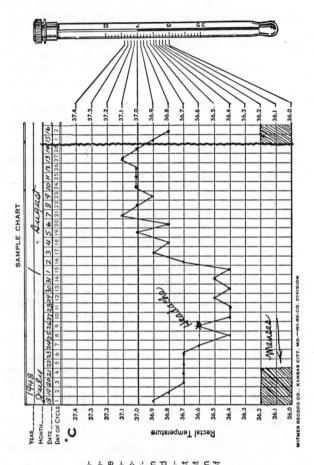

Figure 29-3. Basal body temperature recording. The temperature (vaginal or rectal) must be taken immediately upon awakening every morning, before any activity whatsoever. The thermometer is allowed to remain in place for at least 5 minutes and the recording is made immediately. This procedure must be continued over a period of at least 3 cycles in order to obtain an accurate chart. (Courtesy of Witmer Record Co.)

different hormone combinations and dosage and represent many variable but comparable medications (Table 29–2).

A. Types: There are 5 basic types:

1. Ethinyl estradiol alone ("morning after" pills), 25 mg orally twice daily for 5 days, preferably beginning within 24 hours but not later than 72 hours of coitus, prevents ovulation or speeds transport of the ovum through the uterine tube and prevents fertilization or nidation. Medroxyprogesterone acetate, 100 mg intramuscularly, is also effective as "morning after" contraception.

2. The combination pill (Ortho-Novum, Ovcon, etc) contains estrogen plus a progestogen. The dosage is 1 tablet daily for 20 or 21 days beginning on the fifth day of the cycle. With the combination pill, LH release is blocked so that ovulation does not occur; tubal motility is altered and fertilization is impeded; endometrial maturation is modified so that implantation is unlikely; and cervical mucus is thickened and sperm migration blocked.

3. The "sequential pill"* (eg, Oracon, Ortho-Novum SQ) contains estrogen only for 15 days and then estrogen plus progestogen for 5 days. The pills are resumed on the fifth day of the next cycle. The sequential compounds owe their contraceptive properties mainly to estrogen, which blocks LHRH, the hypothalamic releasing factor for FSH and LH, and thus inhibits ovulation. Certain tubal, endometrial, and cervical alterations add some minor protection.

Despite precise dosage, ovulation (and pregnancy) may occur rarely. The sequential pills are not quite as effective as the combination products. Maximal protection against pregnancy is not reached until the second cycle of treatment.

4. In biphasic estrogen-progestogen tablets (eg, Ortho-Novum 10/11), all 21 tablets contain 35 μg of the estrogen ethinyl estradiol; the first 10 tablets also contain 0.5 mg of progestogen, but the last 11 contain 1 mg of progestogen. This biphasic design more nearly approximates the normal cycle while minimizing undesirable side-effects, eg, breakthrough bleeding, amenorrhea, nausea, headache, etc. Protection against pregnancy is equivalent to that with other compounds containing similar amounts of estrogen.

5. Progestogen alone ("mini-pill"), eg, norethindrone, 0.35 mg daily without a break, makes the cervical mucus impervious to sperm or alters the endometrium slightly, making implantation unlikely. The advantages of this method are that (1) because no estrogen is given, the side-effects attributable to the estrogen component of conventional oral

---

*Sequential agents have been withdrawn in the USA because of the associated occurrence of endometrial carcinoma in some patients. They are still available in many other countries, and although they are not recommended, they are mentioned here for completeness.

Table 29–2. Oral contraceptives available in the USA in 1983.

	Progestogen Content (mg)						Estrogen Content (mg)	
	Norethindrone	Norethindrone Acetate	Norethynodrel	Ethynodiol Diacetate	Norgestrel	Levonorgestrel	Ethinyl Estradiol	Mestranol
Combination tablets								
Brevicon	0.5						0.035	
Modicon	0.5						0.035	
Ortho-Novum 1/35	1						0.035	
Ortho-Novum 10/11	0.5/1						0.035	
Norinyl 1 + 35	1						0.035	
Ovcon-35	0.4						0.035	
Ovcon-50	1						0.05	
Loestrin 21 1/20 (Fe)		1					0.02	
Loestrin 1.5/30 (Fe)		1.5					0.03	
Norlestrin 1/50 (Fe)		1					0.05	
Norlestrin 2.5/50 (Fe)		2.5					0.05	
Demulen 1/35				1			0.035	
Demulen				1			0.05	
Lo/Ovral					0.3		0.03	
Ovral					0.5		0.05	
Nordette						0.15	0.03	
Norinyl 1 + 35	1							0.035
Norinyl 1 + 50	1							0.05
Ortho-Novum 1/50	1							0.05
Ortho-Novum 10/11	0.5/1						0.35	
Norinyl 1 + 80	1							0.08
Ortho-Novum 1/80	1							0.08
Ortho-Novum 2	2							0.1
Norinyl 2	2							0.1
Enovid E			2.5					0.1
Enovid 5			5					0.075
Ovulen				1				0.1
Daily progestogen tablets								
Micronor	0.35							
Nor-QD	0.35							
Ovrette					0.075			

contraceptives are eliminated; (2) because ovulation occurs in a high percentage of the cycles, anovulatory bleeding abnormalities are largely eliminated; and (3) no special sequence of pill-taking is necessary because the mini-pill is taken every day.

B. Beneficial Effects:

1. Prevention of pregnancy–When properly used, oral contraceptives are almost 100% effective in preventing pregnancy. There is no increase in the rate of spontaneous abortion or fetal abnormalities in former users of oral contraceptives, and no long-term reduction in pregnancy potential has been demonstrated.

2. Relief of menstrual problems–The incidence of iron deficiency anemia is reduced by about 65% in oral contraceptive users because excessive blood loss, particularly from menometrorrhagia, is checked by anovulatory drugs. Combination oral contraceptives usually limit premenstrual tension and eliminate midcycle pain or dysmenorrhea. Acne, particularly the premenstrual type, often is benefitted by the estrogens in oral contraceptives.

3. Prevention of salpingitis–The incidence of salpingitis in women who take oral contraceptives is approximately 50% that of other women. Hence, pelvic inflammatory disease and infertility are greatly reduced.

4. Reduced risk of cancer–Oral contraceptive users are about 25% as likely to develop benign breast disease or ovarian cysts as other women and also have a lesser risk of developing ovarian cancer.

5. Reduced risk of arthritis–Users of oral contraceptives are about 50% as likely to suffer from rheumatoid arthritis as nonusers.

C. Adverse Effects: Although oral contraceptives suppress the pituitary gonadotropins by negative feedback, such medication stimulates production of other tropic factors such as MSH and prolactin; thus, increased skin pigmentation (melasma or chloasma) and even breast secretion may occur. These undesirable side-effects are reversed when the contraceptive is discontinued. TSH and corticotropin levels are not increased, although increased binding of TSH and cortisol occurs during estrogen-progestogen therapy, as it does during pregnancy.

Women synthesize and tolerate different amounts of estrogen and progestogen. In women who ovulate normally, homeostatic mechanisms act as checks; therefore, symptoms of hormone imbalance do not occur except during hormone excess (premenstrually and during pregnancy) or depletion (puerperium or menopause). Natural controls do not operate with oral contraceptives, so that over- and understimulation by steroid sex hormones may occur. If the oral contraceptives approximate the patient's normal hormone production and tolerance, there will be no unpleasant side-effects, but if the amount of hormone given is more or less than normal for the patient, troublesome complaints may occur.

The side-effects of the oral contraceptives are actually direct effects due to estrogen or progestogen "sensitivity." The undesirable effects may be classified as common (usually only annoying) or uncommon (often serious). Even some women who know they have moderate problems with oral contraceptives may insist upon using them.

Several common but minor side-effects are attributable to one or the other (or both) of the steroidal components of the pills. Estrogen excess may cause gastrointestinal upset (nausea), fluid retention (edema, acute weight gain, headache, breast congestion), and stimulation of estrogen-sensitive tissues (cervical mucorrhea, chloasma). Many of these complaints are also common during pregnancy. Estrogen deficiency does not occur in women who take oral contraceptives. Progestogen excess may cause increased appetite, progressive (anabolic) weight gain, tiredness, depression, decrease of libido, and (occasionally) increased blood pressure.

The following uncommon complications of oral contraceptive use, some of which also occur during pregnancy, are far more dangerous—even life-threatening—in susceptible patients:

1. Dermatologic–Melasma (chloasma) may be a cosmetic problem, especially for brunettes in areas where the sun is bright.

2. Cardiovascular–Cardiovascular complications are the most life-threatening side-effects of oral contraceptives. Evidence to date suggests that the late development of cardiovascular disease is related to the dosage, duration of use, and overuse of oral contraceptives even after the drug has been discontinued.

a. Myocardial infarction–Oral contraceptive users who smoke or are hypertensive have a greatly increased incidence of coronary occlusion, with a higher mortality rate than nonusers, nonsmokers, or normotensive controls. The risk is further increased if the woman is over age 35, is obese, or has diabetes mellitus or hypertension. It is estimated that if only nonsmokers used oral contraceptives, at least 50% of the deaths associated with this method of birth control could be avoided.

b. Venous thromboembolism–Oral contraceptive users have a slightly higher mortality rate from venous thromboembolism than nonusers, and this is related to the estrogen dosage. Therefore, the smaller the estrogen dose, the safer the drug.

c. Hypertension–The progestogen component of oral contraceptives is probably responsible for hypertension in occasional patients. If diagnosed early, the hypertension is reversible upon discontinuation of the drug.

d. "Transient vascular attacks"–These rare occurrences presumably represent localized cerebral vascular insufficiency and may cause severe headache, seizures, stroke, diplopia, or hemianopia. Whether oral contraceptives are a primary cause or a trigger factor is uncertain.

3. Metabolic–

a. Carbohydrate metabolism–Oral contraceptive ingestion may alter plasma insulin levels and glucose tolerance. This is probably a progestogen effect. Nonetheless, there is no evidence that oral contraceptives increase the occurrence of clinical diabetes mellitus. However, it may be more difficult to manage diabetes in women who take oral contraceptives than in those who use barrier or natural contraception.

b. Weight gain–Anabolic effects and fluid retention may be problems. Corneal edema may occasionally make contact lens correction abnormal.

c. Vitamins–Although blood analyses have indicated minor changes in vitamin absorption or utilization with use of oral contraceptives, the variations are subclinical; thus, vitamin supplements are not necessary.

d. Liver disorders–There is an increased risk of development of very rare benign hepatoma. These tumors may rupture to cause even lethal hemorrhage. Cholestatic jaundice is an unusual complication of oral contraceptive users. It is more likely to occur in women who had this problem during pregnancy.

4. Tumors–

Oral contraceptives appear to prevent endometrial carcinoma, but it is not clear whether malignant melanoma is more frequent in women who take these drugs.

Galactorrhea may occasionally occur after oral contraception is discontinued. However, numerous studies have failed to disclose a causal relationship between the use of oral contraceptives and prolactinomas or other pituitary tumors.

D. Contraindications: Do not prescribe oral contraceptives for any young woman whose bone growth is still not completed and who has not reached physical maturity. Based upon the seriousness of the effects listed above and the patient's past history, the following contraindications to oral contraceptive therapy have few exceptions:

1. Strong family history of stroke.
2. Severe migraine or convulsive disorder.
3. Cerebral arterial insufficiency.
4. Borderline cardiac decompensation.
5. Recent hepatitis or hepatic insufficiency.
6. Severe diabetes mellitus.
7. Severe renal disease.
8. Genital or breast cancer.
9. Thromboembolic disease, sickle cell disease, heavy smoker over age 35, familial hyperlipidemia.

E. Pharmacologic Properties and Drug Interactions: So-called breakthrough ovulation may occur in oral contraceptive users who are also taking antibiotics (eg, ampicillin, tetracyclines, amoxicillin, rifampin) or anticoagulants (eg, phenytoin, barbiturates). In such cases, ovulation may result from multiple causes, including acceleration of sex hormone metabolism or increased capacity of sex hormones to bind globulin. The latter results in reduction of free circulating steroids and increases the likelihood of an LH surge and ovulation. When antibiotics or anticoagulants are to be used in combination with oral contraceptives, a supplementary method of contraception, eg, use of condoms, should be suggested.

Oral contraceptives potentiate the effects of oral anticoagulants, although this is usually not clinically significant. Slight adjustments in the dosage of anticoagulant will maintain prothrombin activity within the therapeutic range. Nonetheless, oral contraceptives and anticoagulants should only rarely be prescribed together because hormonal contraceptives should not be used by women at risk of thromboembolism.

Estrogen or progestogen dominance can be estimated for each oral contraceptive product. Most are progestogen dominant.

F. Selection of Product for Particular Patients: Selection of patients for oral contraception and identification of the proper oral contraceptive for each patient should be based upon knowledge of the composition of various pills and estimation of the woman's natural hormonal status and menstrual pattern. The FDA recommends that products containing more than 50 μg of estrogen not be used by women over age 35 because of the increased risk of coronary occlusion and myocardial infarction. Hence, another method of contraception, including sterilization, should be considered by women over age 35.

Knowledge of the effects of estrogen and progestogen and the patient's past and present hormonal status will help in choosing an oral contraceptive or a later substitution. The physician should inquire about the type of periods, fluid retention, acne, nausea during pregnancy, etc.

The length of the period will determine the potency of the progestogen needed. When the flow is heavy and long, the patient will need a potent progestogen or a larger dose combination (Norlestrin, 2.5 mg, or Norinyl, 2 mg), or both. Patients with a short flow do best on a weaker progestogen.

The protection afforded by oral contraceptives is best when they are taken at the same time every day, and the best time is upon arising. Oral contraceptives are a poor choice for patients who are careless or those with chronic gastrointestinal disorders. Some patients may find the "mini-pill" easiest to use because it is taken daily without interruption.

G. Effectiveness: The antiovulatory drugs are the most effective contraceptive agents available (Table 29–3).

H. Complications of Oral Contraceptive Therapy: A decision about the use of oral contraceptives or other forms of contraception must not be a unilateral choice by the physician but one arrived at with the patient and based upon an assessment of the risks, benefits, and alternatives of the various forms of contraception.

Table 29–3. Efficacy of various methods of contraception.*

Method	Pregnancy Rate Per 100 Woman-Years	1-Year Continuation Rate
Tubal closure	0.04–0.08	99%
Vasectomy	0.15	99%
Oral pills		60–82%
Combined type	0.03–0.1	60–82%
Sequential type	0.2–0.56	60–82%
Intrauterine devices (in situ)	0.8–5.8	50–92%
Lippes Loop D	1.8–2.7	77–80%
Double coil	0.4–2.8	70–88%
Copper 7 (Gravigard)	2.7	65%
Condom	7–28	
Diaphragm with jelly	4–35	
Coitus interruptus	10–38	
Postcoital douche	21–41	
Spermatocides	5–20	
Aerosol foam	?–29	
Foam tablets	12–43	
Suppositories	4–42	
Jelly or cream	4–38	
Breast feeding	24–26	
Rhythm	2.4–38	

*Reproduced, with permission, from Tatum HJ: Chapter 23 in *Current Obstetric & Gynecologic Diagnosis & Treatment*, 4th ed. Benson RC (editor). Lange, 1982.

An apparent association exists between the use of estrogen-progestogen oral contraceptives and the occurrence of thromboembolic phenomena, including pulmonary embolism, cerebral thrombosis, and coronary thrombosis. The risk of thromboembolic phenomena is increased in smokers and women over age 35 and also increases with the estrogen dosage; thus, smokers and women over age 35 should consider other methods of contraception, and if oral contraceptives are prescribed, the lowest effective estrogen dose should be offered. It has been suggested that blood lipid determinations should be made before and occasionally during oral contraceptive therapy for women at increased risk.

The incidence of hepatic focal nodular hyperplasia, hepatic adenomas, or hamartomas of the liver seems to be increased among users of oral contraceptives. Products containing mestranol or norethindrone seem to be most likely to cause these rare hepatic tumors, but almost all contraceptive steroids have been implicated. Genetic differences in the intermediate metabolism of synthetic steroids with a long half-life may be responsible for susceptibility to hepatic tumors, or the tumors may be dose-related. Early diagnosis of hepatic tumors is difficult because symptoms are not present early. Pre- and posttherapy hepatic enzyme studies may indicate hepatic dysfunction. Periodic palpation of the liver, especially in patients who develop pain, is important because most women with hepatic tumors develop intralesional bleeding and intraperitoneal hemorrhage that can often be avoided.

Although the incidence of thromboembolism and hepatic adenomas appears to be higher in women who have used oral contraceptives over an extended period of time, their death rate, estimated at 3 per 100,000, must be compared with the risk to maternal life in pregnancy and delivery (excluding deaths from illegal abortion), which in the USA and the UK is about 25 per 100,000.

Injectable Contraceptive Hormones

Steroid sex hormones may be injected intramuscularly to provide a depot that, depending on the drug, dosage, and formulation, may provide contraception for 1 or more months or even a year. A pure progestogen may be used, or the injection may consist of a combination of a progestogen with an estrogen. Most of these regimens prevent ovulation by suppression of FSH and LH.

Although not approved for use in the USA, medroxyprogesterone acetate, 150 mg intramuscularly every 3 months, is very effective as a contraceptive, and this method is used widely abroad. Irregular scanty periods or slight spotting are the rule during treatment. The reestablishment of menses may be delayed, but ovulatory cycles usually return after 6 months.

Condom or Animal Membrane Sheath

These devices give good to excellent protection. Failures are mainly due to mechanical faults or procedural errors, eg, applying the condom after initial intromission. Sheaths have the additional advantage of protecting against sexually transmitted disease but the disadvantage of impairing sensation and gratification.

Vaginal Diaphragm

The diaphragm is almost as reliable as the condom or cap, but the patient must be taught how to insert it, and it must be inserted in advance of coitus. The diaphragm should be left in place for 6–12 hours after intercourse. Vaginal or pelvic relaxation may interfere with accurate fitting or wearing. The patient should be refitted for a diaphragm after vaginal delivery or after a weight gain or loss of 7.5 kg (15 lb).

Intrauterine Device (IUD), Intrauterine Contraceptive Devices (IUCD) (See Figs 29–4, 29–5, and 29–6.)

The intrauterine device (IUD) or intrauterine contraceptive device (IUCD) is a plastic or metal form inserted through the cervix into the endometrial cavity to prevent pregnancy. Those most widely used in the

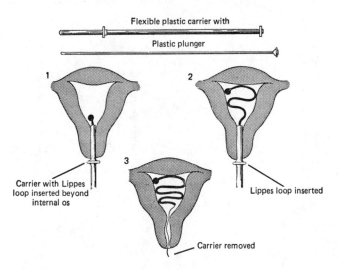

Figure 29–4. Insertion of the Lippes loop (a plastic device with configuration recall).

USA are shaped like an open loop (Lippes loop), a double coil (Saf-T-Coil), the letter T (Tatum-T), or the numeral 7 (Cu-7). The application of a few turns of fine copper wire about the tail of T or 7-shaped IUDs reduces the failure rate (ie, the incidence of pregnancy) by more than half. It is postulated that metallic copper or zinc may alter the enzyme systems required for fertilization or implantation. The approximate efficacy of IUDs are listed in Table 29–3. Millions of IUDs have been inserted in the USA alone, and a continuation rate of about 80% is recorded at the end of the first year of use when the device is retained.

The mode of action of the IUD is still debated. Single or multiple factors may be responsible: (1) Implantation of the blastocyst may be prevented by endometrial alteration (slight endometritis) or slow progestogen release (Progesterone T). (2) Cytotoxic substances (eg, copper) may prevent embryonic development. (3) Very early abortion may occur, but this seems unlikely.

Women who cannot afford contraceptive supplies, those who are ignorant or unreliable, those who fear or have had problems using oral contraceptives, and those who strongly request it may be suitable candidates for an IUD.

Absolute contraindications to an IUD are pregnancy, subacute or acute pelvic inflammatory disease, congenital uterine anomalies, gonorrhea, severe cervicitis, abnormal uterine bleeding, marked cervi-

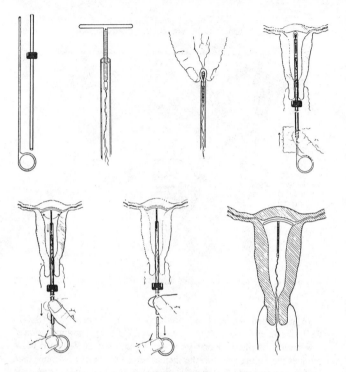

Figure 29–5. Insertion of the Tatum-Zipper Copper T. (Reproduced, with permission, from Tatum HJ: Chapter 23 in *Current Obstetric & Gynecologic Diagnosis & Treatment,* 4th ed. Benson RC [editor]. Lange, 1982.)

cal stenosis, and coagulopathy or other blood disorders, and conditions in which infection may be disastrous (eg, women taking immunosuppressive drugs). Relative contraindications include a history of ectopic pregnancy and menstrual disorders.

Preparation for insertion of an IUD requires a careful pelvic examination to rule out pregnancy or cervical, uterine, or tubal disease and to determine the shape and position of the uterus. Sterile technique must be employed. A tenaculum is applied to the cervix; traction is exerted to straighten the cervico-uterine angle; and the uterus is sounded to avoid misdirection of the IUD. The device is then inserted so that it will be in the transverse plane of the uterus.

Insertion is easier and fewer unpleasant side-effects occur when the patient is a multipara. However, smaller sizes and certain devices, eg,

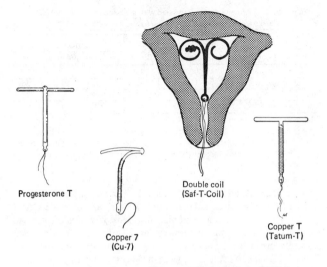

Progesterone T

Copper 7
(Cu-7)

Double coil
(Saf-T-Coil)

Copper T
(Tatum-T)

Figure 29–6. Some intrauterine contraceptive devices (IUCDs).

size A Lippes loop, often can be inserted successfully in nulligravidas. Insertion is easiest during the puerperium or the last few days of the menses. The straightened device is passed through a plastic cyclinder and resumes its shape in situ. A monofilament strand attached to its tail or body should protrude through the cervix for verification of its presence and to facilitate removal.

Perforation of the uterus (IUD translocation), usually during insertion, occurs in about 1:2500 cases with the loop. Perforation is less common with a ring or T form. Intraperitoneal bleeding is an early complication of open loop IUDs (eg, the now outmoded Birnberg bow); intestinal obstruction may be a late complication, especially with closed loop devices. If a copper-clad IUD is discovered in the peritoneal cavity, it must be removed promptly. All others discovered in this location probably should also be removed whether or not symptoms are present.

Pelvic inflammatory disease can be a serious problem. Slightly over 2% of patients develop salpingitis during the first year after insertion of an IUD. Many such cases are exacerbations of an old infection. Pelvic inflammatory disease can usually be treated successfully with broad-spectrum antibiotics even when the device is allowed to remain in place, but removal of the IUD prior to therapy probably is the better policy.

About 3% of women who received an IUD become pregnant even though the device is still in the uterus; others become pregnant after

Table 29–4. Births and deaths associated with pregnancy exposure in 100,000 fertile women during 1 year (induced abortions excluded).*†

Method of Contraception	Pregnancies	Births	Deaths		
			Pregnancy	Method	Total
None	60,000	50,000	12	0	12
Condom and/or diaphragm	13,000	10,833	2.5	0	2.5
Pills	100	83	0	3	3
Intrauterine devices	2,190	1,825	0.4	0.3	0.7

*Reproduced, with permission, from Tatum HJ: Chapter 23 in *Current Obstetric & Gynecologic Diagnosis & Treatment*, 4th ed. Benson RC (editor). Lange, 1982.
†Data from Jain AK: Safety and effectiveness of intrauterine devices. *Contraception* 1975;11:243; and Tietz C: Mortality with contraception and induced abortions. *Stud Fam Plan* 1969;45:6.

undetected expulsion of the IUD. About 20% of pregnancies occurring with an IUD still in place end in abortion. At least 30% of patients fitted with an IUD report cramps and bleeding. Most instances of pain and spotting occur during the first few cycles, and the incidence decreases markedly thereafter. Nonetheless, these symptoms account for about 60% of IUDs removed, most of them in the first 6 months. Lippes loop removals average about 20% for medical and 10% for personal reasons during the first 5 years.

Most patients with IUDs have increased vaginal secretion, and many report heavier periods. Endocervicitis may also occur and may not heal while the tail or cord of the device extrudes through the cervix. Cytologic and other studies are necessary to rule out trichomonal and other infections and carcinoma. If actinomycetes are reported, the IUD should be removed and the infection treated. If no cause for leukorrhea except the IUD is found, management depends upon whether the patient is determined to retain the device.

The rate of expulsion is about 30% in puerperal women and almost 10% for nonpuerperal women at the end of the first year. Few women persistently expel an IUD if one size or shape is substituted for another. If expulsion was asymptomatic and spontaneous, it is best to reinsert the next larger size. If the IUD is removed because of pain or bleeding, the next smaller size or another design should be substituted.

In a review of IUD safety, Jain (Table 29–4) compared the relationship between births and deaths associated with pregnancy exposure during 1 year of use. This comparison suggests that the IUD has the best safety record, followed by pills and combined use of a condom and diaphragm. No other methods can be recommended that are safer and more effective.

Vaginal Jellies, Gels, Creams, Suppositories

These chemical substances, often containing spermatocidal drugs such as phenylmercuric nitrate in a low surface-tension cream base, are easily applied to the upper vaginal canal, but they are not as effective as the best of the mechanical and biologic methods, eg, IUDs or oral contraceptives. Their expense, undesirable lubricating effects, and possible irritating quality are disadvantages. Gels and creams interfere with gratification because they are often considered "slick" or "greasy."

Foam
This is a combined mechanical and chemical method. Aerosol foam, eg, Delfen or Emko, is available for use within the vagina. It is inserted by means of an applicator, and no sponge is needed. It is slightly less effective than the diaphragm. This simple, effective method may be unaesthetic to some women, and the foam may be irritating.

Douche
Douching with vinegar solution or a proprietary acid douche after coitus is not an effective method of contraception because sperms cannot be either adequately washed out of the cervix and vagina or destroyed by the medication. Sperms are actually aspirated into the cervix immediately after ejaculation, and the semen is often beyond the reach even of potent germicides under dangerously high pressure.

Diaphragm & Vaginal Cream or Jelly
This logical combination of 2 good methods of contraception is utilized widely with good results.

Abortion
See p 439.

Coitus Interruptus
This method of contraception is rarely acceptable, and its effectiveness is low because of the small but active sperm content of the preejaculate secretion.

Prolongation of Lactation
Women are less fertile while breast feeding than after the infant has been weaned. Deliberate continuation of breast feeding beyond the point of necessity for the child has long been a widespread contraceptive method in emerging countries. The delay in recurrence of ovulation after delivery is due in part to hypophyseal or hypothalamic stimuli from the nursing, and there is a corresponding amenorrhea. However, the duration of the suppression of ovulation is quite variable. At 6 weeks postpartum, about 5% of lactating women will ovulate; at 12 weeks postpartum, approximately 25% will ovulate; and at 6 months after delivery, about 65% will ovulate. These women may become pregnant.

30 | Psychosomatic & Other Gynecologic Problems

PSYCHOGENIC (ATYPICAL) PELVIC PAIN

Psychogenic (functional) pelvic pain, pain for which no organic cause can be found, is usually chronic or recurrent and is caused by unresolved emotional conflicts. It may be due to the unperceived presence of disturbing subliminal impulses or the precognition of sensations without conscious awareness. Women 25–45 years of age are most susceptible. The reported incidence in gynecologic patients in the USA varies from 5 to 25%, depending upon the interests and skills of the reporting physician.

Psychogenic pelvic pain is genuine. The pain is a manifestation of unease or unhappiness and serves as a warning of a potentially serious chronic emotional disorder. It represents an abnormal need for solicitude or gratification in the masochistic woman; resentment in the frustrated woman; anxiety in the hypochondriacal woman; guilt in the strict, introspective woman; and a psychic defense mechanism in the borderline schizophrenic woman. The type and degree of pain and the circumstances in which it appears or intensifies vary in accordance with age, temperament, and the culture in which the woman lives.

Pain unattributable to physical causes may result from exaggeration of normal physiologic impulses by ignorance, fear, or tension or from a lowered perceptual threshold to disturbing stimuli. The mind associates the pain with past or present environmental factors, and repeated episodes augment and solidify the association, producing sensory conditioning. The patient's complaints may be fixed on one anatomic area or organ system.

Patients with psychogenic pelvic pain are often hysterical personality types. All degrees of intelligence are represented. The principal emotional and personality characteristics of these women are as follows: They are egotistic, self-indulgent, and vain; demanding and dependent; emotionally immature and shallow; prone to dramatize, exaggerate, and seek attention; excitable; deficient in emotional control, inconsistent in emotional reaction; and coquettish and sexually provocative but sexually fearful and often relatively unresponsive. Most have unhappy family histories. Their parents and husbands are frequently described as shown in Table 30–1.

Table 30–1. Typical personality characteristics in mother, father, and husband of women with psychogenic pelvic pain.

Mother (Often)	Father (Often)	Husband (Often)
Domineering, critical.	Inadequate, repeatedly unemployed.	A passive, friendly "nice guy."
Unaffectionate, cruel.	Alcoholic, epileptic, brutal.	Hard-working, dependable.
Old-fashioned, prudish.	Too serious, unaffectionate toward daughter.	Less than normally demanding of coitus.
A religious fanatic.	A faithless woman-chaser.	Subject to premature ejaculation.
Complaining, chronically ill, tense.	Frequently like mother.	Uncomplaining, stoical, long-suffering.

There is often a history of long-standing conflict between the patient and her mother, whom the patient perceives as unloving and unsupportive. The patient's resentment and guilt are repressed, and the result is a masochistic personality with hysterical tendencies. The patient has never been able to confront her mother; her father is frequently unacceptable and therefore is rejected. Women with such a background are led to believe that sex is "dirty" and best avoided.

The girl often marries young to escape the situation at home, and her marriage is usually loveless, even though she may marry a kindly man unlike her father (but not a dominant, virile man). She is unable to achieve satisfaction with adult life and its responsibilities, and her attitudes toward sex are dominated by dread of coitus and aversion to pregnancy.

Clinical Findings

A. Symptoms and Signs: Complaints are almost invariably multiple. In addition to pelvic pain, which is often in the right lower quadrant and worse before and during menses, most patients also report dyspareunia, lack of orgasm, dysmenorrhea, abnormal menses, urinary and bowel dysfunction, headache and backache, "nervousness," agitation, or depression. The signs are usually those of so-called pelvic congestion: persistent vaginal and pelvic hyperemia, excessive cervical mucus in the absence of infection, and generalized pelvic tenderness and sensitivity to even gentle palpation of the pelvic viscera. There may be numerous abdominal scars, indicating repeated surgery.

The patient insists she is in great pain, but in at least 25% of cases no physical abnormality can be found; in the remainder, insignificant physical variations or minimal lesions may be present. The other extreme of the spectrum of pain is illustrated by the patient who reports only slight distress despite gross demonstrable organic disease; this may be a psychologically diminished reaction to somatic pain.

Table 30–2. Differentiation of organic and psychogenic pain.

	Organic	Psychogenic
Type	Sharp, cramping, intermittent.	Dull, continuous.
Time of onset	Any time. May awaken patient.	Usually begins well after waking, when social obligations are pressing.
Radiation	Follows definite neural pathways.	Bizarre patterns or does not radiate.
Localization	Localizes with typical point tenderness.	Variable, shifting, generalized.
Progress	Soon becomes either better or worse.	Remains the same for weeks, months, or years.
Provocative tests	Often reproduced or augmented by tests or manipulation, not by mood.	Not triggered or accentuated by examination but by interpersonal relationships.

B. Special Examinations:

1. Psychologic testing–Tests (Cornell Medical Inventory, Taylor Anxiety Score, Saslow Anxiety Quotient, etc) may reveal definite abnormal traits. If the anxiety score is low, however, the pain is probably organic.

2. Psychiatric evaluation–Clues to psychoneurosis may include heavy makeup, etc), agitation, and rapid breathing ("acting-out" of the problem). A woman who wears dark glasses indoors may be sensitive to minor annoyances. Personification of organs or blaming certain viscera may be revealing. ("My right ovary is diseased." "My uterus has given me trouble all my life.") Psychosis may be suggested by crude, illogical, or incongruous remarks or behavior.

Complications

Surgery does not relieve the pain and underlying emotional distress but may intensify the psychic disorder and lead to medical and surgical complications. If the uterus or ovaries are removed, the symptoms may be transferred to the gastrointestinal or urinary tract. Psychoneurosis may progress to psychosis. A despondent patient may commit suicide.

Differential Diagnosis

Psychogenic disease can be differentiated from organic disease by ruling out the latter or by recognition of psychoneurosis or psychosis while investigating organic pathology. Because most patients with psychogenic pelvic pain present many characteristic features that make a direct diagnosis possible without extensive studies, direct diagnosis is preferred.

It is curious that popular lay concepts may be prominent in the physician's mind as causes of pelvic pain but rarely occur to the patient as such. "Chronic appendicitis," adhesions, a "painful ovary," or "tipped uterus" are often suspected by physicians as possible causes of pain. Appendicitis is invariably acute, and pelvic adhesions themselves rarely cause pain. Ovarian cysts without adherence or torsion are almost never painful, and an adherent ovary is sensitive only in the second phase of the menstrual cycle or during intercourse. Uterine retroposition may cause specific, periodic pain (dyspareunia, dysmenorrhea) but not the many complaints mentioned by the patient.

Chronic salpingitis or urinary tract infection, spastic and other types of colitis, and endometriosis must be ruled out, perhaps by laparoscopy.

A comparison of organic and psychogenic pelvic pain may be helpful in diagnosis (Table 30–2).

Prevention

Sex education, marriage counseling, and early recognition and treatment of emotional illness are the best preventive measures for this psychic disorder.

Treatment

Ideally, the patient should be admitted to the hospital for examination, observation, and treatment. She should be reassured and given simple symptomatic therapy. A complete history and thorough physical examination are necessary. The physician must be sympathetic, unhurried, and a good listener.

Once the diagnosis is established, the disorder must be explained to the patient and her husband in direct, convincing terms. The patient should be given an acceptable "escape," with explanations such as "Our nerves often play tricks on us," "Emotions tie us in knots," or "The mind governs the body." The physician must gain the patient's cooperation in a basic, perhaps lengthy reorientation and reeducation program.

Occasional warm douches, external heat (or cold), diathermy, massage, and similar physical measures may be helpful.

Simple analgesics are useful. Do not give sedatives, amphetamines, or narcotics because these patients tend to be prone to addiction. Be particularly wary of prescribing sedatives, because their use may lead to suicidal depression. Tranquilizers are contraindicated because the patient must adjust to her circumstances and solve her problems without therapeutic crutches.

Do not perform operative procedures except on definite surgical indications. Psychotherapy or referral to a psychiatrist may be required.

When the patient is discharged to office care, it is wise to schedule frequent visits to maintain contact and ensure the continuity of therapy. Be prepared to spend a great deal of time talking to the patient. Every effort must be made to assist her to adjust socially.

Prognosis

Because these patients often refuse psychotherapy, withdraw from a treatment program after it is under way, and change physicians frequently, their medical future is bleak. In general, they are unwilling to abandon invalidism as a way of life.

Reassurance and symptomatic therapy result in temporary improvement in about three-fourths of cases. Psychiatric treatment may result in lasting improvement in many patients.

GYNECOLOGIC BACKACHE

The initial investigation of all complaints of back pain is the same regardless of cause. A comprehensive history of the backache is most important to the diagnosis. Answers to the following questions should be helpful:

(1) When did the backache begin? (2) Has there been similar backache before? If so, what studies and treatment were ordered, and what was the result? (3) What initiated the current pain (eg, lifting, intercourse, other activity)? (4) Was the onset sudden or gradual? (5) What aggravates the pain (eg, coughing, menses, etc)? (6) What relieves it? (7) Is there also pain in the legs or bladder or other complaints?

Backache of gynecologic origin is generally due to a well-defined, significant pelvic disorder. It is rare before puberty and uncommon after the menopause but frequent during reproductive life. Multiparas are more often afflicted than nulliparas. Less than 25% of gynecologic patients who complain of backache will be found to have genital disease but no orthopedic or other causes of discomfort; 15% will have no gynecologic problem; most will have an orthopedic disorder; and a few will have urologic or neurologic disease.

Gynecologic backache may be due to any of the following causes: traction or pulsion on the pelvic peritoneum or the supportive structures of the reproductive organs or pelvic floor (tumors, ascites, uterine prolapse); inflammation of the pelvic contents due to bacteria (eg, peritonitis or salpingitis) or chemicals (eg, lipids used in salpingography or fluid from a ruptured dermoid cyst); invasion of pelvic tissues or bone by tumor or endometriosis; genital tract obstruction (cervical stenosis); torsion or constriction of the pelvic viscera (ovary enmeshed in adhesions, twisted ovarian cyst); congestion of internal genitalia (turgescence of the retroposed uterus, backache during menstruation); or psychic tension (anxiety, apprehension, psychogenic pain).

Most cases of gynecologic backache represent referred pain, but cancer metastatic to the spine or spinal nerves causes direct pain due to irritation of the afferent nerves from the organ involved or abnormal nerve impulses from the site of the disorder to the back via the sympathetic nervous system. The distribution of back pain depends upon the site, type, and extent of the problem.

Tumors produce pressure, vascular engorgement, and nerve involvement. Pelvic tumors may cause pain depending upon their size and type. Small tumors rarely cause backache. Moderately large tumors, such as ovarian cysts 8–12 cm in diameter, or even the uterus itself in advanced pregnancy may cause backache due to traction on the pelvic ligaments. Very large tumors often do not cause back pain, because they tend to be immobile and may even rest upon the bones of the pelvis.

Clinical Findings

A. Symptoms and Signs:

The patient's back should be assessed for abnormal curvatures while she is standing and sitting. Palpate for tense muscles or pain trigger points. Note any limitation of motion on flexion, extension, or lateral bending.

Observe the patient's walk for limp or other abnormalities. Weakness of the plantar or dorsiflexion muscles will be apparent when she walks on her heels and then on her toes.

Straight leg raising with the patient supine may elicit the pain or cause it to radiate down the leg. The latter suggests an intervertebral disc herniation. Determine muscle strength and possible atrophy.

Check knee and ankle reflexes and skin sensation of the lower back, upper legs, and pudendum.

The gynecologic examination is not normally painful. Note any unusual appearance of the cervix or vagina, and determine the size, position, consistency, contour, mobility, and descent of the uterus. Pain on movement of the cervix or uterus is abnormal. Hypersensitivity, restriction, enlargement, or nodulation of the adnexa or thickening in the cul-de-sac is abnormal and may be related to backache.

Gynecologic backache is almost invariably associated with other major signs and symptoms of pelvic disease. Fairly constant lumbosacral or sacral backache often occurs with salpingitis, pelvic abscess, or twisted ovarian cyst. Discomfort is usually more pronounced on the involved side. Back pain due to endometriosis of the cul-de-sac is referred to the coccygeal region or rectum. Backache due to ovarian, renal, and ureteral lesions commonly radiates toward the inguinal region; and that due to orthopedic and neurologic disease often radiates down into the buttocks or along the distribution of the sciatic nerve. Faulty posture, bony deformity, muscle spasm, or spinal cord or other back injury may cause or contribute to back pain. In cases of herniated intervertebral disk, hypesthesia, reduced reflex responses, and regional lumbar tenderness are apparent on neurologic evaluation.

Uterine bleeding, vaginal discharge, pelvic tumors, prolapsed uterus or ovaries, marked retroposition of the fundus, and similar findings may be observed.

B. Laboratory Findings: Leukocytosis and an elevated sedimentation rate may indicate infection. The vaginal cytologic smear may reveal neoplastic changes. Bacteriuria, pyuria, or hematuria in a catheterized or clean-catch specimen suggests urinary tract disease as a possible cause of backache.

C. X-Ray Findings: Anteroposterior and lateral films of the spine often show a postural, degenerative, neoplastic, or other orthopedic cause of backache. Myelograms may be required to demonstrate a herniated intervertebral disk.

D. Orthopedic Tests: Bone or joint disease may be indicated by orthopedic tests.

Prevention

Many cases of gynecologic backache can be prevented by avoidance of obstetric trauma, immediate repair of cervical and other obstetric lacerations, prompt and adequate treatment of cervicitis and pelvic infections, and periodic examination so that tumors, hernias, and similar lesions can be detected and treated early.

Treatment

A. Specific Measures: The underlying problem should be treated definitively. Relief of backache will ensue in most instances.

B. Supportive Measures: The patient should be placed at bed rest in the most comfortable position on a firm mattress. Apply heat to the back as necessary for pain. Warm water douches twice daily may be beneficial.

Aspirin with or without codeine may be given every 4 hours as required. Phenothiazines such as prochlorperazine (Compazine), 5–10 mg 3 times daily, may be given to induce relaxation.

C. Local Measures: Cervicitis may respond to topical therapy (see p 556).

D. Surgical Measures: Tumors, malpositions of the uterus, pelvic hernias, herniated intervertebral disk, etc, may require surgery.

Prognosis

Although persistent low backache may be a manifestation of serious disease, about 80% of women with this complaint have only a minor, usually curable, musculoskeletal problem. However, multiple causes of backache cloud the prognosis. If the backache is of gynecologic origin, successful treatment of the pelvic problem will almost always eliminate the backache.

COCCYGODYNIA

Persistent pain in the region of the coccyx is a fairly common presenting complaint among women 30–50 years of age of any parity. The causes and treatments are as follows:

A. Pelvic Disorders: Endometriosis, such neoplasms as glomus tumor, and sepsis (ie, retrorectal abscess) should be sought and treated definitively.

B. Sacrococcygeal Arthritis, Injury, or Congenital Anomalies: Physical therapy is often helpful. Improved sitting posture and use of a straight-backed chair with a firm seat are beneficial. Revision of the sacrum or coccygectomy may be required for gross deformity or pain that cannot be relieved medically.

C. Lumbosacral Joint Dysfunction: Abnormal posture and mechanical irritation of the dura mater may cause pain referred to the coccyx. The pain may be felt during sitting but not during standing or manipulation of the coccyx. Exercises to flex the pelvis often bring relief.

D. Attention Fixation: Inconsistency of symptoms and exaggerated attitudes and responses are characteristic. A fall, a "fractured coccyx" during childbirth, or a similar imprecise occurrence may initiate the problem. The coccyx remains sensitive, often in spite of ankylosis without deformity. Strong reassurance, suggestion, and physical therapy may be helpful. Analgesics should be prescribed. Injection of 1% lidocaine and hydrocortisone may be tried. Coccygectomy should be avoided. Patients with little or no insight are rarely cured.

E. Undetermined Cause: The onset is gradual, and there is no history of trauma or other specific cause. The coccygeus muscles are extremely tense and tender on both sides, but pressure on the coccyx does not cause discomfort. In many cases, the pain is self-limited and gradually disappears. Brief transrectal "stripping" or massage of the tender muscles every day for 3–4 days and administration of analgesics generally brings relief.

DYSPAREUNIA

Dyspareunia (painful coitus) may be functional (psychogenic) or organic or due to a combination of organic and emotional causes. Functional dyspareunia occurs most frequently and is more difficult to treat. Either type may occur early (primary) or late (secondary) in the sexually active period of life. The site of discomfort may be external (at the introitus) or internal (deep within the vagina or beyond), and some women describe both types of pain.

Functional dyspareunia may be caused by psychosexual problems, especially fear of genital damage, sexually transmitted disease, or pregnancy. Vaginismus, an involuntary spasm of the muscles around the introitus and levators when the thighs are adducted, is an indication of extreme anxiety. It may be due to psychologic factors (eg, marital disharmony, personal emotional problems) or occur in anticipation of or response to pain. Pain may also be feigned to avoid intercourse or to "punish" the sexual partner, who may be poorly informed regarding sex techniques, inept, selfish, or unsympathetic. Marital disharmony, coitus interruptus, or failure of orgasm may lead to emotionally induced vaginismus and dyspareunia.

External organic dyspareunia may be due to an occlusive or rigid hymen, vaginal contracture due to any cause, or inflammatory disorders of the vulva, vagina, urethra, or anus. Traumatic or infectious processes are often seen in younger patients and atrophic vulvovaginitis in postmenopausal women.

Organic causes of internal dyspareunia include hourglass contracture of the vagina, septate vagina, severe cervicitis, marked fundal retroposition, uterine prolapse or neoplasm, tubo-ovarian disease, pelvic endometriosis, and severe disorders of the lower urinary tract or colon.

Functional and organic problems are often related, and their relative importance as components of dyspareunia varies. For example, in women who are tense or newly sexually active, a rigid hymen may be a less important cause of dyspareunia than emotionally induced tautness of the introital and pelvic musculature; in contrast, dyspareunia due to senile vaginal atrophy may disturb the patient more physically than emotionally.

Clinical Findings

A. Symptoms and Signs: The physician should accept the patient's statement that coitus is painful and then differentiate between functional primary external dyspareunia and the less common types.

Pelvic examination often reveals marked contraction of the perineal and levator musculature with adduction of the muscles of the thighs, even when the patient is "relaxed," and such specific signs as: genital hypoplasia, virtually complete or rigid hymen, septate vagina, urethral or subvesical tenderness, postpartal or postoperative scarring or contracture of the vagina, vulvovaginitis, kraurosis vulvae, prolapse of the cervix and uterus, uterine retroposition or tumor, tubo-ovarian inflammation or tumor, pelvic endometriosis, or rectal or vesical abnormalities.

The physician should inquire about fear of pregnancy and the success of the woman's relationship with her partner.

B. Special Examinations: Psychiatric evaluation is indicated if complex psychosexual problems seem to be present. Specialized techniques of physical examination, eg, cystoscopy, may be required.

Complications

If not corrected, dyspareunia frequently leads to infidelity or divorce. Psychoneuroses in both the wife and husband often develop or become intensified. The woman also may experience menstrual difficulties and bladder and bowel dysfunction. The man may develop premature ejaculation, impotence, or other sexual problems if his partner's difficulties (or their joint problems) are not resolved.

Prevention

Preventive measures consist of sex education of children at home, in the schools, and by religious organizations. Personal or premarital counseling, courses in "preparation for marriage," scientific films emphasizing pelvic anatomy and genital function, and premarital examination by a physician are helpful.

Treatment

A. Specific Measures: Functional dyspareunia can only be treated by counseling and psychotherapy. Both partners should be interviewed. Information on contraception is often helpful. The importance of foreplay before sexual intercourse must be emphasized. An appropriate water-soluble vaginal lubricant may be useful. Adequate estrogen treatment is often required for postmenopausal women. The treatment of organic dyspareunia varies and depends upon the basic underlying cause.

B. General Measures: Mild sedation, eg, the benzodiazepines, phenobarbital, or prochlorperazine, is of value for the relief of extreme emotional tension.

C. Local Measures: For functional dyspareunia, hymenal-vaginal dilatations by the patient with a conical (Kelly) dilator or test tubes of graduated sizes may give confidence. Such dilatation or daily dilatation with fingers over a period of 2–4 weeks may also stretch a tight hymen to adequate size to allow coitus without pain. Anesthetic ointment applied to the introitus gives some relief but is of no permanent value. Organic dyspareunia due to vaginal dryness may be treated with a water-soluble lubricant. Estrogen therapy is indicated for senile vulvovaginitis.

D. Surgical Measures: Hymenotomy (Fig 30–1), hymenectomy, perineotomy, and similar procedures should be performed only on clear indications. Significant obstructive lesions should be corrected. Treat chronic symptomatic cervicitis by cauterization or shallow conization.

Prognosis

Few patients with functional dyspareunia are quickly and easily cured, even with psychotherapy. Organic dyspareunia subsides promptly after elinination of the cause.

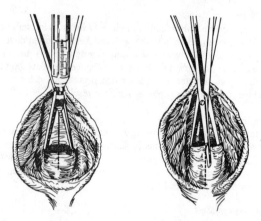

Figure 30–1. Hymenotomy under local anesthesia.

FRIGIDITY

Frigidity is a symptom. It is defined as the absence of a pleasurable reaction to coitus. The spectrum ranges from (at worst) revulsion, vaginismus, and severe dyspareunia; through indifference and lack of pleasure; to vaginal hypesthesia and sexual pleasure without orgasm. Relative frigidity is common, but absolute frigidity is rare. In so-called facultative frigidity, the patient is responsive to one partner but not to another. Nymphomania is a type of frigidity characterized by a constant quest for sexual gratification, always without success.

About 60–70% of married women experience orgasm "usually or always"; about 25% "some of the time"; and 5–10% "rarely or never." Women may be happy with their partners and feel sexually gratified without frequent orgasm.

Etiology

A. Psychologic Problems: Problems may be deep-seated disorders, eg, infantile fixations, hostility toward men, homosexuality, residua of rape or incest; or less serious and perhaps transitory, eg, faulty coital technique, fear of pregnancy, the partner's premature ejaculation.

B. Environmental and Social Difficulties: Barriers to full sexual expression and orgasm in the woman are generally considered to have a psychologic basis in social and cultural conditioning during childhood. However, with increasing education and sexual freedom, women are discovering their own sexual responses through childhood masturbation, earlier heterosexual activity, and other investigations. Early constraints may be less operative than they were, but many women, because of inhibitions, may never have learned what is erotically stimulating. Environmental factors include lack of privacy, fatigue, or general unhappiness.

C. Physical Disorders: A frigidity "reaction" may result from pain due to anatomic abnormality or inadequate vaginal lubrication.

Clinical Findings

Out of reluctance to admit lack of sexual gratification, women may seek medical advice by describing other symptoms (often dyspareunia).

Lack of ability to achieve orgasm may lead to chronic or prolonged pelvic congestion.

Treatment

There is no treatment for frigidity as such; treatment must be directed at resolution of underlying causes and related problems.

In many instances, frigidity is a more intricate problem than the rather superficial causes often recorded would indicate. The background of the patient's sexual difficulty must be explored cautiously but carefully. Simple discussion may often be useful in correcting misconceptions and allaying fears, and the physician can sometimes give advice about sex practices that will be of value to both partners.

The male contribution in frigidity is large. The man may be inept, crude, inconsiderate, or perhaps personally inhibited in love-making. He may be generally uncommunicative or unsupportive.

Review of the problem and correction of obvious medical and interpersonal difficulties may be all that is necessary. Suggesting "social engineering" to ensure the couple's privacy or adequate rest for the woman may be helpful. Deep-seated conflicts may require psychotherapy or perhaps behavior therapy (systematic desensitization), or marriage counseling may be needed.

Androgens and aphrodisiac drugs are worthless in the treatment of frigidity and may be harmful.

The prognosis in severe long-standing frigidity is extremely poor.

PREMARITAL COUNSELING

Counseling before marriage can be a worthwhile and satisfying aspect of preventive medicine. Premarital counseling offers a unique opportunity for the physician to deal with any fears or misconceptions the couple may have about sexual matters and explain certain physical and emotional problems that may interfere with sexual fulfillment in marriage.

Couples who request premarital counseling may be seeking information and reassurance that they are "doing the right thing," because they are anxious to ensure a good and enduring marriage and may have doubts about whether they are suited to marriage. The physician must help them to identify these concerns and make a suitable decision. This does not include advising about whether or not to marry except in rare situations in which a critical or intolerable problem is present that would doom the marriage or make the couple unsuitable as parents.

The couple should be given an opportunity to talk about what they expect from marriage and any anxieties they may have about any aspect of it. The counselor should use the occasion to offer information and guidance about the responsibilities, needs, goals, values, and difficulties of marriage.

The following areas should be explored:

(1) Courtship: How did the couple meet, and what made them decide to get married?

(2) Personal background: Racial, ethnic, social, educational, cultural, family, and religious.

(3) Family attitudes: Will each accept the other's parents as in-laws? Will there be possible domination by one family? Is the couple financially dependent on one family, and will this persist?

(4) Planning: Are both individuals realistic and responsible in preparing for the wedding and for future projects, eg, buying a house? Is there an attitude of consideration, compromise, communication, and cooperation to work toward mutual goals?

(5) Psychologic and personality factors: Does each individual approve of and accept the other's physical and behavioral characteristics (life-style), including habits, dress, grooming, and manners?

(6) Sexual compatibility and plans for a family: Is there a clear understanding and agreement on sex roles? Are there possible problems regarding sexual fulfillment and parenting? Are children desired by only one partner, both, or neither?

Counseling should include both discussion and a physical examination. Each of the following is important, although they are not necessarily listed in order of importance:

(1) Pelvic examination: If the findings are normal, the patient should be told this. If not, plans should be made for correction of problems.

(2) Anatomy and physiology: Include a basic discussion of male and female reproductive biology with illustrations.

(3) Coitus: Explain coital physiology.

(4) Contraception: Present an overview of contraception that is detailed enough to allow a choice of method. The advantages, disadvantages, problems, and alternatives should be considered. Provide a prescription if necessary.

(5) Virginity: A virgin may wish to have her hymen dilated or incised. Self-dilatation with fingers or graduated test tubes or dilators is effective if time will permit; otherwise, hymenotomy may be performed under anesthesia.

(6) Questions: Provide an opportunity for the couple to ask questions, eg, the "normal" frequency of coitus (whatever is satisfactory to both parties is normal).

(7) Follow-up discussion.

Both parties should be involved in the discussion and decision-making. If indicated, a visit with and examination of the man alone should be arranged to discuss differential anatomy, physiology with special reference to sex differences, and preference regarding the method of contraception.

A return visit 2 months after marriage is suggested. The 2-month interval is recommended because at 4 weeks, if trouble has developed, the partners cannot admit even to themselves that there is a problem; at 6 weeks, each knows there is a problem but cannot admit it to the other; and at 8 weeks, they know they have a problem, are quite certain whose it is, and are willing to discuss it. The physician usually can help to correct it.

MARRIAGE COUNSELING IN THE MANAGEMENT OF SEXUAL PROBLEMS

Sexual problems in marriage are a major cause not only of annulment, divorce, and abandonment but also of protracted emotional distress for both partners and the children.

Much marital discord in developed countries, at least, is related to relaxed social attitudes; equalization of the status of the sexes; differences in ethnic, religious, and socioeconomic backgrounds; and money problems. Conflicts may be manifested by sexual difficulties for one or both partners to the marriage; and sexual problems, in turn, may aggravate other stresses the couple may be undergoing. Marital disharmony often develops because one or both partners have unrealistic marriage attitudes and expectations.

There can be no successful marriage without sexual fulfillment, and this puts a great burden on what often seems to be a fairly tricky mechanism. Female sexuality is complex and a satisfactory self-image is mandatory for good sexual performance. A woman who is poorly adjusted, tense, frustrated, or unhappy is not likely to be able to maintain a satisfactory sexual relationship.

The differences between male and female sexuality have been emphasized by many sexologists and will not be outlined in detail here.

Healthy men have a 48- to 72-hour libidinal cycle, are easily aroused by visual stimuli, and are more apt than women to be able to find sexual gratification with casual partners. In normal women, sexual desire, the spontaneous initiation of sexual activity, and orgasmic response depend to some degree upon adequate steroid sex hormone levels. Genital sensitivity and sexual responsiveness are usually heightened at the time of ovulation and just before and after menstruation, and response to tactile stimulation is greatest at this time. Sexual responsiveness in women is reduced in hypoestrogenic states.

Etiology

Sexual difficulties usually are symptoms of other problems. The following must be considered:

A. Stress: Tension, anxiety, and frustration may initiate or aggravate sexual problems. When one or both partners are under stress, the couple may become confused and not know whom to consult.

B. Physical Illness: Sexual incapacity may be due to neuropathic impotence. Premature ejaculation may be due to urinary tract infection. Gynatresia or pelvic endometriosis may be associated with failure of orgasm. Patients with such problems come for therapy voluntarily.

C. Psychologic Problems: These usually pertain to the more basic difficulties that have existed all during the marriage, eg, emotional immaturity, egocentricity, alcoholism, or use of dangerous drugs. Such patients often seek the physician's help upon insistence by the spouse.

D. Psychiatric Disorders: Loss of libido and potency may be an expression of serious depression or of psychosis or organic brain syndrome; a marked increase in sexual aggressiveness may suggest mania or schizophrenia. These patients represent a small percentage of the total, and in any case, they usually refuse to come to the physician or marriage counselor.

Prevention

Much can be done to prevent sexual maladjustment in marriage by early sex education and premarital counseling. Many physicians fear to discuss the subject and prevent their patients from raising the question of sex problems early, when they are most easily corrected. Both partners should be seen and counseled together when such problems arise. The physician should encourage the partners to trust each other and tell them that successful marriages require continual effort. The couple should discuss and try to solve their problems promptly and strive for common interests and realistic answers to their needs.

Treatment

Marital problems can often be managed successfully by the practicing physician who is knowledgeable, interested, and nonjudgmental.

The physician should try to reduce tensions between wife and husband and attempt to help them talk about and think through their difficulties and solve them at the conscious, intellectual level. Marriage counseling, whether in the physician's office or at a family service agency, differs from psychotherapy in that the counselor must be persuasive and occasionally directive. The major focus is on the marriage relationship rather than on personality deficiencies; personality reorganization is not sought in most counseling programs.

The couple should be encouraged to make time to be together by themselves, eg, they should get away from the family occasionally (many seem to think that leaving the children for a weekend is a crime). Encourage them to take short vacations alone in surroundings that are conducive to a satisfactory sexual experience. It is important to set the stage for success rather than failure. Instruct them in ways to achieve pleasure through various ways of making love.

Organic disorders should be identified and treated promptly. (**Note:** The presence of physical disease does not mean that emotional factors are not present also or can be ignored.) Causes of stress should be identified and eliminated if practical, and other problems should be explored. Encouragement must be offered.

Patients involved in a neurotic marital relationship may require a sympathetic and impartial referee. They may need a brief explanation that stresses the normal aspects of the interreactions and gives specific direction and firm assurance.

Arrange psychotherapy for difficult cases, eg, alcoholic, homosexual, or bisexual patients. Psychotic patients must also be referred to a psychiatrist unless the illness is chronic and socially manageable. Such individuals may benefit from reassurance, supportive measures, and tranquilizing drugs.

The physician should help the couple to formulate a plan of reconciliation and support their determination to pursue it. A basis should be provided for a logical approach to the solution of future problems.

Prognosis

Immature, severely neurotic, or drug-dependent patients probably cannot or do not want to get well. In most instances, however, marriage partners who are willing to strive for improvement in their relationship and seek a happier life for each have a very good chance of doing so. Unfortunately, a marital problem may sometimes be without practical solution because neither the individuals themselves nor available social institutions can afford to pay for the cost of counseling and rehabilitation.

Continued marriage is no longer a rigid social requirement. Divorce is common, and for many couples, the marriage contract includes this "escape clause" even though it may never be mentioned. Incompatible individuals may find it easier to live apart than together because the desire for personal satisfaction and fulfillment is more important for one or both partners than the drive to seek happiness in family life.

If the answer to the question, ''Do you love your husband (or wife)?'' is negative, the marriage cannot be saved. If the answer is affirmative and the couple is willing to make the effort and compromise to resolve their differences, the outlook for reconciliation is good.

MANAGEMENT OF THE TERMINAL CANCER PATIENT

Cancer is a fearsome diagnosis that evokes thoughts of pain, invalidism, mutilation, social exile, and death. The physician should be sensitive to these implications and must be prepared to extend both his personal and professional resources to help the patient live even while she is dying. Management must always be individualized. Patients with family and financial obligations usually should be told the diagnosis; others should be told as much as they wish to know about their diagnosis and prognosis despite family opinions to the contrary. The exceptions usually are elderly or pediatric gynecologic patients who are emotionally unstable or cannot reason. Unfortunately, severe illness and hospitalization may be interpreted by these patients as punishment for wrongdoing, and this false view must be corrected.

Hope must be kept high. Spontaneous regression of tumors does occur, and new methods of treatment constantly are being developed. Nevertheless, patients and their families must be kept from impoverishing themselves in a futile search for nonexistent cures. Much can be done for the patient's comfort and peace of mind. She should know that everything will be done to prevent suffering. Depression must not go unnoticed or untreated. The thought of suicide to avoid terminal agony or helplessness or to save the expense of prolonged hospitalization must occur to most patients who know they have cancer, but only a few patients actually attempt suicide.

The consolation of religion is the greatest source of strength and comfort for many patients in the face of suffering and impending death. The physician should be prepared to cooperate with the patient's religious adviser so that she will derive the greatest possible benefit from her spiritual beliefs. The management of terminal illness requires emphasis on daily experience. The patient should not be allowed to look back with regret or forward with fear. Insofar as possible, the drugs used should not impair the mental faculties, so that reading, visiting, and entertainment still can be enjoyed. When death is near, heroic measures to preserve life for brief periods are seldom justified. The patient should be permitted to die with dignity.

Hospice

The word hospice derives from a Latin word meaning a place of shelter and rest for travelers. This "good Samaritan" concept was revived in the 1960s when St. Christopher's Hospital in London initiated comprehensive medical and nursing care and unrestricted pain relief for dying patients—mostly cancer victims—when many institutions were refusing to provide terminal care. Currently, the term hospice connotes institutions committed to the relief of physical and emotional suffering of the terminally ill.

In the last decade, many hospice programs have been established in the USA and abroad. There are some variations, but the fundamental characteristics of a true "hospice" include the following essentials proposed by the American Cancer Society:

(1) The hospital program includes an autonomous, centrally administered program of home care and, when necessary, hospital admission of the dying based upon need rather than ability to pay. This comprises complete nursing care, including the complex needs of the dying patient.

(2) Control of symptoms–Relief of physical symptoms such as pain, nausea, and vomiting, insofar as possible, is achieved by medication administered as needed and not according to a routine. Useful oral analgesics include Brompton mixture (Brompton Hospital, England), a compound containing morphine and cocaine; and Schlesinger's solution, which contains morphine. These drugs are given upon request. The goal should be prevention of pain. Waiting for pain to reappear (as with an "as needed" order) only accentuates the problem of pain control. Anxious anticipation and memory of pain is lessened by successful pain prevention; thus, the amount of analgesic medication needed will frequently decrease.

Epidural administration of morphine or alcohol gives protracted relief of pain due to localized pelvic cancer. Percutaneous retrograde arterial infusion of nitrogen into the cancerous area may relieve pain for weeks. Unilateral selective cordotomy will permanently eliminate pain, but numbness will result.

Treatment of emotional symptoms is by psychologic reinforcement to help the patient and the family carry the burden of catastrophic illness and death. Ministerial guidance must be generously available so that the patient's spiritual needs can be met.

(3) Interdisciplinary care may be provided by one or more physicians to integrate and implement treatment by various means.

(4) Trained volunteers–Specially trained volunteer workers are available to provide transportation, recreation, and companionship.

(5) On-call services–Nursing and medical staff are available 24 hours a day, 7 days a week.

(6) Staff support and communication includes scheduled and impromptu evaluation of patients' problems and their management.

(7) Bereavement follow-up–Hospice services are available to the family during the period of grieving.

The building, its appointments, and especially the attitude of the staff must convey a spirit of welcome, understanding, and dedication to serving the terminally ill in a compassionate, holistic manner.

Although a formally established hospice may not exist in a particular community, most aspects of a hospice program can still be incorporated into the management of terminally ill cancer patients and will be of great benefit to them.

Appendix |

Metric System Prefixes
(Small Measurement)

In accordance with the decision of several scientific societies to employ a universal system of metric nomenclature, the following prefixes have become standard in many medical texts and journals.

k	kilo-	10^{-3}
c	centi-	10^{-2}
m	milli-	10^{-3}
μ	micro-	10^{-6}
n	nano- (formerly millimicro, mμ)	10^{-9}
p	pico- (formerly micromicro, μμ)	10^{-12}
f	femto-	10^{-15}
a	atto-	10^{-18}

Apothecary and Metric Equivalents of Common Measures

Household Measures	Apothecary	Metric
1 teaspoon	1 fl dr (f℈)	4 mL
1 tablespoon	½ fl oz (f℥)	15 mL
1 teacup	4 fl oz (f℥)	120 mL
1 glass (tumbler)	8 fl oz (f℥)	240 mL
1 cup	8 fl oz (f℥)	240 mL
1 pint	16 fl oz (f℥)	480 mL
1 quart	32 fl oz (f℥)	946 mL

Conversion of Celsius to Fahrenheit Temperatures

°C		°F	°C		°F	°C		°F
35	=	95	37.5	=	99.5	40	=	104
35.5	=	95.9	38	=	100.4	40.5	=	104.9
36	=	96.8	38.5	=	101.3	41	=	105.8
36.5	=	97.7	39	=	102.2	42	=	107.6
37	=	98.6	39.5	=	103.1	43	=	109.4

Conversion of Metric Weights (grams) to Approximate Avoirdupois Weights (pounds and ounces)

Metric g	Avoirdupois lb	oz	Metric g	Avoirdupois lb	oz	Metric g	Avoirdupois lb	oz
2000	4	7	3050	6	12	4050	8	15
2050	4	8	3100	6	13.5	4100	9	1
2100	4	10	3150	6	15	4150	9	3
2150	4	12	3200	7	1	4200	9	4
2200	4	14	3250	7	3	4250	9	6
2250	4	15.5	3300	7	4.5	4300	9	8
2300	5	1.5	3350	7	6	4350	9	10
2350	5	3	3400	7	8	4400	9	11
2400	5	5	3450	7	10	4450	9	13
2450	5	7.5	3500	7	11.5	4500	9	15
2500	5	8	3550	7	13.5	4550	10	
2550	5	10	3600	7	15	4600	10	2.5
2600	5	12	3650	8	1	4650	10	4
2650	5	14	3700	8	3	4700	10	6
2700	5	15.5	3750	8	4.5	4750	10	8
2750	6	1	3800	8	6	4800	10	10
2800	6	3	3850	8	8	4850	10	11
2850	6	5	3900	8	10	4900	10	13
2900	6	6.5	3950	8	11.5	4950	10	15
2950	6	8	4000	8	13	5000	11	
3000	6	10						

Feet and Inches to Centimeters
(1 cm = 0.39 in; 1 in = 2.54 cm)

ft	in	cm	ft	in	cm	ft	in	cm	ft	in	cm
0	6	15.2	2	7	78.7	3	10	116.8	5	1	154.9
1	0	30.5	2	8	81.2	3	11	119.3	5	2	157.5
1	6	45.7	2	9	83.8	4	0	121.9	5	3	160.0
1	7	48.3	2	10	86.3	4	1	124.4	5	4	162.6
1	8	50.8	2	11	88.8	4	2	127.0	5	5	165.1
1	9	53.3	3	0	91.4	4	3	129.5	5	6	167.6
1	10	55.9	3	1	93.9	4	4	132.0	5	7	170.2
1	11	58.4	3	2	96.4	4	5	134.6	5	8	172.7
2	0	61.0	3	3	99.0	4	6	137.1	5	9	175.3
2	1	63.5	3	4	101.6	4	7	139.6	5	10	177.8
2	2	66.0	3	5	104.1	4	8	142.2	5	11	180.3
2	3	68.6	3	6	106.6	4	9	144.7	6	0	182.9
2	4	71.1	3	7	109.2	4	10	147.3	6	1	185.4
2	5	73.6	3	8	111.7	4	11	149.8	6	2	188.0
2	6	76.1	3	9	114.2	5	0	152.4	6	3	190.5

Desirable Weights (in pounds) for Women Age 25 and Over*†

Height‡ Feet	Inches	Small Frame	Medium Frame	Large Frame
4	10	92– 98	96–107	104–119
4	11	94–101	98–110	106–122
5	0	96–104	101–113	109–125
5	1	99–107	104–116	112–128
5	2	102–110	107–119	115–131
5	3	105–113	110–122	118–134
5	4	108–116	113–126	121–138
5	5	111–119	116–130	125–142
5	6	114–123	120–135	129–146
5	7	118–127	124–139	133–150
5	8	121–131	128–143	137–154
5	9	126–135	132–147	141–158
5	10	130–140	136–151	145–163
5	11	134–144	140–155	149–168
6	0	138–148	144–159	153–173

*This table was derived primarily from data of the Build and Blood Pressure Study, 1959, Society of Actuaries.
†For women between 18 and 25, subtract 1 pound for each year under 25.
‡With shoes with 2-inch heels.

Average Height and Weight (in pounds) for Girls

Age	Height Feet	Inches	Weight Pounds
Birth	1	8	7.5
6 months	2	2	16
1 year	2	5	20
2 years	2	9	25
3 years	3	0	30
4 years	3	3	33
5 years	3	5	38
6 years	3	8	45
7 years	3	11	49
8 years	4	2	56
9 years	4	4	62
10 years	4	6	69
11 years	4	8	77
12 years	4	10	86
13 years	5	0	98
14 years	5	2	107

Drug selection, 1982–1983.[*]

Suspected or Proved Etiologic Agent	Drug(s) of First Choice	Alternative Drug(s)
Gram-negative cocci		
Gonococcus	Penicillin,[1] ampicillin, tetracycline[2]	Spectinomycin, cefoxitin
Meningococcus	Penicillin[1]	Chloramphenicol, sulfonamide
Gram-positive cocci		
Pneumococcus (*Streptococcus pneumoniae*)	Penicillin[1]	Erythromycin,[3] cephalosporin[4]
Streptococcus, hemolytic groups A, B, C, G	Penicillin[1]	Erythromycin,[3] cephalosporin[4]
Streptococcus viridans	Penicillin[1] plus aminoglycoside(?)[5]	Cephalosporin,[4] vancomycin
Staphylococcus, nonpenicillinase-producing	Penicillin[1]	Cephalosporin,[4] vancomycin
Staphylococcus, penicillinase-producing	Penicillinase-resistant penicillin[6]	Vancomycin, cephalosporin[4]
Streptococcus faecalis (enterococcus)	Ampicillin plus aminoglycoside[5]	Vancomycin
Gram-negative rods		
Acinetobacter (Mima-Herellea)	Aminoglycoside[5]	Minocycline
Bacteroides (except *B fragilis*)	Penicillin[1] or chloramphenicol	Clindamycin, cephalosporin[4]
Bacteroides fragilis	Clindamycin, cefoxitin	Metronidazole, chloramphenicol
Brucella	Tetracycline plus streptomycin	Streptomycin plus sulfonamide[7]
Enterobacter	Aminoglycoside[5]	Chloramphenicol
Escherichia *Escherichia coli* sepsis	Aminoglycoside[5]	New cephalosporin,[8] ampicillin
Escherichia coli urinary tract infection (first attack)	Sulfonamide[9] or TMP-SMX[10]	Ampicillin, cephalosporin[4]
Haemophilus (meningitis, respiratory infections)	Chloramphenicol	Ampicillin, TMP-SMX[10]

[*]Reproduced, with permission, from Jawetz E: Chapter 28 in *Current Medical Diagnosis & Treatment 1983.* Krupp MA, Chatton MJ (editors). Lange, 1983.

[1] Penicillin G is preferred for parenteral injection; penicillin V for oral administration. Only highly sensitive microorganisms should be treated with oral penicillin.

[2] All tetracyclines have similar activity against microorganisms and comparable therapeutic activity and toxicity. Dosage is determined by the rates of absorption and excretion of different preparations.

[3] Erythromycin estolate is the best-absorbed oral form but carries greatest risk of hepatitis. Also erythromycin stearate, erythromycin ethylsuccinate.

[4] Cefazolin, cephapirin, cephalothin, cefamandole, and cefoxitin are parenteral cephalosporins; cephalexin and cephradine the best oral forms.

Drug selection, 1982–1983 (cont'd).*

Suspected or Proved Etiologic Agent	Drug(s) of First Choice	Alternative Drug(s)
Gram-negative rods (cont'd)		
Klebsiella	New cephalosporin,[8] aminoglycoside[5]	Chloramphenicol
Legionella pneumophila (pneumonia)	Erythromycin[3]	Tetracycline[2]
Pasteurella (Yersinia) (plague, tularemia)	Streptomycin or tetracycline	Sulfonamide,[7] chloramphenicol
Proteus		
Proteus mirabilis	Penicillin or ampicillin	Aminoglycoside[5]
Proteus vulgaris and other species	Aminoglycoside[5]	Chloramphenicol
Pseudomonas		
Pseudomonas aeruginosa	Aminoglycoside plus carbenicillin	New cephalosporin,[8] polymyxin
Pseudomonas pseudomallei (melioidosis)	Tetracycline	Chloramphenicol
Pseudomonas mallei (glanders)	Streptomycin plus tetracycline	Chloramphenicol
Salmonella	Chloramphenicol or ampicillin	TMP-SMX[10]
Serratia, Providencia	Aminoglycoside[5]	TMP-SMX[10] plus polymyxin
Shigella	Ampicillin or chloramphenicol	Tetracycline, TMP-SMX[10]
Vibrio (cholera)	Tetracycline	TMP-SMX[10]
Gram-positive rods		
Actinomyces	Penicillin[1]	Tetracycline
Bacillus (eg, anthrax)	Penicillin[1]	Erythromycin
Clostridium (eg, gas gangrene, tetanus)	Penicillin[1]	Tetracycline, cephalosporin[4]
Corynebacterium	Erythromycin	Penicillin, cephalosporin[4]
Listeria	Ampicillin plus aminoglycoside[5]	Tetracycline
Acid-fast rods		
Mycobacterium tuberculosis	INH plus rifampin or ethambutol[11]	Other antituberculosis drugs

[5] Aminoglycoside: Gentamicin, tobramycin, amikacin, selected by local pattern of susceptibility.

[6] Parenteral nafcillin or oxacillin. Oral dicloxacillin, cloxacillin, or oxacillin.

[7] Trisulfapyrimidines and sulfisoxazole have the advantage of greater solubility in urine over sulfadiazine for oral administration; sodium sulfadiazine is suitable for intravenous injection in severely ill persons.

[8] New cephalosporins (1982): Cefotaxime, moxalactam, cefoperazone, etc.

[9] For previously untreated urinary tract infection, a highly soluble sulfonamide such as sulfisoxazole or trisulfapyrimidines is the first choice. TMP-SMX[10] is acceptable.

[10] TMP-SMX is a mixture of 1 part trimethoprim plus 5 parts sulfamethoxazole.

[11] Either or both.

Drug selection, 1982–1983 (cont'd).*

Suspected or Proved Etiologic Agent	Drug(s) of First Choice	Alternative Drug(s)
Acid-fast rods (cont'd)		
Mycobacterium leprae	Dapsone, rifampin, clofazimine	Amithiozone
Mycobacteria, atypical	Ethambutol plus rifampin	Rifampin plus INH
Nocardia	Sulfonamide[7]	Minocycline
Spirochetes		
Borrelia (relapsing fever)	Tetracycline	Penicillin
Leptospira	Penicillin[1]	Tetracycline
Treponema (syphilis, yaws)	Penicillin[1]	Erythromycin, tetracycline
Mycoplasma	Tetracycline	Erythromycin
Chlamydia trachomatis, Chlamydia psittaci	Tetracycline	Erythromycin
Rickettsiae	Tetracycline	Chloramphenicol

*Reproduced, with permission, from Jawetz E: Chapter 28 in *Current Medical Diagnosis & Treatment 1983*. Krupp MA, Chatton MJ (editors). Lange, 1983.

[1] Penicillin G is preferred for parenteral injection; penicillin V for oral administration. Only highly sensitive microorganisms should be treated with oral penicillin.

[7] Trisulfapyrimidines and sulfisoxazole have the advantage of greater solubility in urine over sulfadiazine for oral administration; sodium sulfadiazine is suitable for intravenous injection in severely ill persons.

Index